ANNALS OF
THE NEW YORK ACADEMY
OF SCIENCES

Volume 438

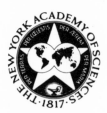

EDITORIAL STAFF
Executive Editor
BILL BOLAND
Managing Editor
JOYCE HITCHCOCK
Associate Editor
MARY KATHERINE BRENNAN

The New York Academy of Sciences
2 East 63rd Street
New York, New York 10021

THE NEW YORK ACADEMY OF SCIENCES
(Founded in 1817)
BOARD OF GOVERNORS, 1984

CRAIG D. BURRELL, *President*
KURT SALZINGER, *President-Elect*

Honorary Life Governors

SERGE A. KORFF

H. CHRISTINE REILLY

IRVING J. SELIKOFF

Vice Presidents

WILLIAM S. CAIN
FLORENCE L. DENMARK
PETER M. LEVY
(on leave in 1984)

HARRY LUSTIG
NORBERT J. ROBERTS
FLEUR L. STRAND

ALAN J. PATRICOF, *Secretary-Treasurer*

Elected Governors-At-Large

1982-84

WILLIAM T. GOLDEN
DENNIS KELLY

HERBERT SHEPPARD
DONALD B. STRAUS

1984-86

MURIEL FEIGELSON

Past Presidents (Governors)

JACQUELINE MESSITE

WALTER N. SCOTT

HEINZ R. PAGELS, *Executive Director*

MORRIS H. SHAMOS

ANNALS OF THE NEW YORK ACADEMY OF SCIENCES
Volume 438

HORMONE ACTION AND TESTICULAR FUNCTION

Edited by Kevin J. Catt and Maria L. Dufau

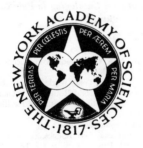

The New York Academy of Sciences
New York, New York
1984

Cover: Electron microscopy autoradiograph of a rat Leydig cell after incubation with $[^{125}I]hCG$. The hormone is mainly localized on cell surface receptor (shown on front cover in detail), particularly on microvilli with only minor internalization.

Library of Congress Cataloging in Publication Data

Main entry under title:

Hormone action and testicular function.

(Annals of the New York Academy of Sciences, ISSN 0077-8923 ; v. 438)
Proceedings of the 8th Testis Workshop sponsored by the National Institute of Child Health and Human Development, held at National Institute of Health, Oct. 14-17, 1983.
Includes bibliographies and index.
1. Testis—Congresses. 2. Hormones, Sex—Congresses. I. Catt, Kevin J. II. Dufau, Maria L. III. Testis Workshop (8th : 1983 : National Institute of Health) IV. National Institute of Child Health and Human Development (U.S.) V. Series. [DNLM: 1. Testicular Hormones—physiology—congresses. 2. Testis—physiology—congresses. Wl AN626YL v.438 / WJ 830 H8118 1983] Q11.N5 vol. 438 [QP255] 500 s [599'.0166] 85-2931
ISBN 0-89766-270-9
ISBN 0-89766-271-7 (pbk.)

BCP/PCP
Printed in the United States of America
ISBN 0-89766-270-9 (cloth)
ISBN 0-89766-271-7 (paper)
ISSN 0077-8923

ANNALS OF THE NEW YORK ACADEMY OF SCIENCES

Volume 438

December 30, 1984

HORMONE ACTION AND TESTICULAR FUNCTION[a]

Editors

KEVIN J. CATT AND MARIA L. DUFAU

CONTENTS

[a] The papers in this volume were presented at the Eighth Testis Workshop, which was sponsored by the National Institute of Child Health and Human Development and held in Bethesda, Maryland on October 14–17, 1983.

Introduction

KEVIN J. CATT and MARIA L. DUFAU

Endocrinology and Reproduction Research Branch
National Institute of Child Health and Human Development
National Institutes of Health
Bethesda, Maryland 20205

The proceedings of the conference on Hormone Action and Testicular Function, held at the National Institutes of Health in October 1983, provide ample evidence of the active progress that continues to be made in the field of male reproductive biology. The National Institute of Child Health and Human Development series of Testis Workshops, of which this was the eighth since their origin as a satellite symposium to the International Congress of Endocrinology in 1972, has become an established venue for local and international investigators to meet for discussion and debate about recent advances in reproduction research and for the presentation of new findings on the endocrine control and cell biology of the testis. Over the same period, the introduction of related series of meetings including the National Institute of Child Health and Human Development Workshops on the Ovary and the European Testis Workshops, has indicated the growth of basic and clinical research on reproduction and the expanding needs for international colloquia on the progress of research in reproductive science.

The Eighth Testis Workshop was opened by introductory lectures by notable investigators in the field of hormone action. For those attending the meeting, the introductory talks by Anthony Means on peptide hormone action, Donald Coffey on the nuclear matrix, and Bert O'Malley on steroid regulation of gene expression were a splendid overture to the program. Their contributions provided the background and set the standards for many of the findings presented in subsequent lectures. These guest lecturers were not requested to provide manuscripts, and the reader is directed to their recent reviews for information on advances in these fundamental aspects of hormone action.

In addition to the focus on hormone action in male reproductive tissues, topics including developmental and immunological aspects of testicular function, regulatory mechanisms of sperm motility, and the clinical management of hypogonadotropic hypogonadism were also covered by both lectures and posters. A session on techniques in reproduction research, which has come to be a valued aspect of the Workshop, was once again of major interest in presenting the applications of newly developed methods to problems of the male reproductive tract. The role of gonadal peptides in testicular function continued to be a source of lively debate, especially on the functional significance of GnRH receptors and actions in the testis of certain species. This field was expanded by the recognition of POMC-derived peptides in the Leydig cell and by the search for potential roles of gonadal peptides in communication between testicular compartments and in the control of testicular development. Given its complex and functionally integrated structure, the testis may represent a major site of paracrine and other local regulatory mechanisms that operate during maturation and in the adult gonad. Other new topics of interest were the role of the extracellular matrix in the development and function of reproductive tissues and the functions of reproductive tract proteins, including transferrin and alpha-lactalbumin.

In each of these areas, new information about the testis and accessory tissues provided further insight into reproductive function, yet at the same time revealed additional questions to be answered by increasingly refined methods of investigation at the molecular level. Two important features of the Testis Workshop series have been its topical nature and the excitement generated by the interactions between investigators with widely differing special interests within the one fundamental topic of male reproductive biology. It can be anticipated that future Workshops will provide increasingly detailed information about the processes involved in testicular function and its disorders, and that the interdisciplinary nature of reproduction research will ensure that our understanding of testicular regulation will continue to develop in an integrated and productive manner.

Control of Transferrin mRNA Synthesis in Sertoli Cells[a]

JODI HUGGENVIK, STEVEN R. SYLVESTER, and
MICHAEL D. GRISWOLD

Biochemistry/Biophysics Program
Washington State University
Pullman, Washington 99164-4460

The biochemical products of the Sertoli cells of the testis are presumed to be of primary importance in the maintenance, protection, support, and regulation of spermatogenesis.[1,2] Two important activities of the Sertoli cells are the formation of tight intercellular junctions and the secretion of the components of the tubular fluid. The tight junctions between adjacent Sertoli cells allow for the existence of a unique intratubular environment in which germinal cells undergo meiosis and development.

The Sertoli cells secrete glycoproteins that become components of the tubular fluid, interact directly with germinal cells, or have hormone-like activities in tissues other than the testis.[3] Some of the secreted proteins from rat Sertoli cell cultures have been identified and characterized, while others are known only as spots or bands on an electrophoretic gel or by their biological activities. The total spectrum of major Sertoli cell–secreted proteins has been analyzed in detail by two-dimensional gel electrophoresis and fluorography.[4]

We have identified one of the major proteins secreted by cultured rat Sertoli cells as testicular transferrin.[5] Antibodies to serum transferrin cross-reacted with testicular transferrin but the extent of structural similarity between the two proteins was unknown. We purified serum transferrin from rat serum and testicular transferrin from spent medium obtained from cultured Sertoli cells. The amino acid analysis and tryptic peptide map of serum and testicular transferrin were essentially identical. These results indicate that both transferrins could be the product of the same gene expressed in two different tissues.

The function ascribed to transferrin is that of an iron transport protein.[6] Testicular transferrin could provide a means of supplying spermatozoa with iron, as they are excluded from contact with serum transferrin by the blood-testis barrier. Since the tubular environment is also excluded from the immune system, testicular transferrin may provide a biological defense mechanism by sequestering any available iron.[7]

We utilized a radioimmunoassay (RIA) and micropuncture techniques to measure the amount of transferrin in rete testis fluid, seminiferous tubule fluid, and testicular lymph. Rete testis fluid and seminiferous tubule fluid were found to contain 47 μg/ml and 141 μg/ml, respectively.[8] Since these amounts are relatively small compared to that found in serum and testicular lymph (3.8 mg/ml), the function of testicular transferrin is probably not for defense.

[a] Supported by National Institutes of Health (grant HD 10808). M.D.G. is supported by Grant HD 00263.

1

In our current perception, the function of testicular transferrin in spermatogenesis involves the transport of iron to developing spermatids. Ferric ion is required by all living cells and because of the insolubility of Fe^{3+} it must be transported by carrier molecules. The testis has had to evolve mechanisms of transport that circumvent the tight junctional complexes of the Sertoli cells, which exclude the serum transferrin.

To learn more of the protein's function in the testis, immunoreactive transferrin was localized in testis paraffin sections by indirect immunofluorescence. FIGURE 1 shows that transferrin is associated with the acrosome and nuclear cap regions of developing spermatids. The interstitial tissue was also brightly fluorescent but this is probably due to serum transferrin.

In some of the immunofluorescence experiments, we incubated the testis sections first with transferrin, and then with the anti-transferrin and fluorescent second antibody. In these experiments, which presumably would be specific for cells that could bind the added transferrin, a large number of germinal cells were fluorescent. In particular, pachytene and meiotic spermatocytes were intensely fluorescent. We speculate that the fluorescence on these cells was due to the presence of unoccupied receptors.

From these studies we propose the following model for Fe^{3+} transport to developing germinal cells (FIGURE 2). The basic steps in the mechanism are:

(1) Serum diferric transferrin binds to receptors on the basal surface of the Sertoli cell.

(2) The transferrin-receptor complex is internalized by endocytotic mechanisms into vesicles.

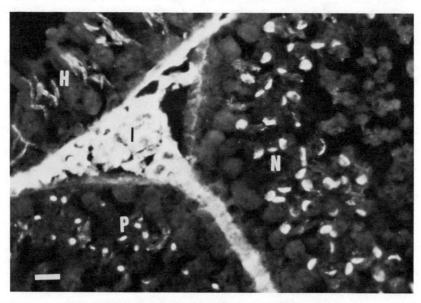

FIGURE 1. Fluorescence photomicrograph of paraffin section of rat testis stained with rabbit anti-rat transferrin. Tissues were treated with the antibody, biotinylated goat anti-rabbit IgG, and then FITC-avidin. The fluorescence is localized in the interstitium (I), on proacrosomes (P) and nuclear caps (N) of early spermatids, and on the heads (H) of late spermatids. Bouin's fixation; bar represents 10 μm.

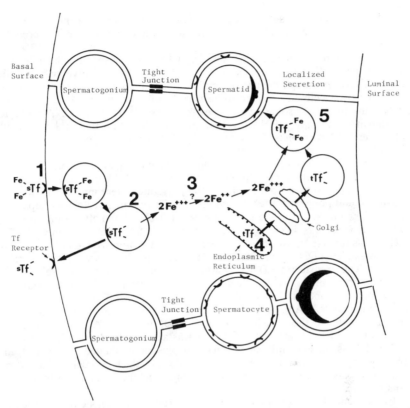

FIGURE 2. Proposed model of iron transport mechanism in the testis. Serum transferrin (sTf) binds to transferrin receptors at the basal surface of seminiferous tubules. The receptor ligand is internalized and iron is released to be taken up by newly synthesized testicular transferrin (tTf). The iron and testicular transferrin then bind to germinal transferrin receptors and become a part of developing germ cells.

(3) The vesicles are acidified and the iron is released to other carrier molecules or is free in solution as ferrous ion. The vesicle then fuses with the plasma membrane, the apotransferrin is released, and the receptor is available to bind more diferric transferrin. Steps 1 through 3 are based on the known mechanism of action of serum transferrin.[9] Sertoli cells appear to contain either no or very little ferritin, the storage form of iron (unpublished observations).

(4) Testicular apotransferrin is synthesized in the endoplasmic reticulum, transported to the Golgi, and secreted in vesicles. The iron in the form of Fe^{3+} or Fe^{2+} may interact with the testicular apotransferrin before, during, or after secretion. Testicular ceruloplasmin is another protein secreted by Sertoli cells, that may function as a ferroxidase to convert Fe^{2+} to Fe^{3+}.[10,11]

(5) Secretion may be into the lumen at low levels but more likely the Fe^{3+} is delivered directly to early spermatids.

The key elements in this model are the requirement for net unidirectional Fe^{3+} transport by the Sertoli cells, the existence of transferrin receptors on spermatocytes and spermatids, and the selective secretion of diferric testicular transferrin to early spermatid stages during defined stages of the spermatogenic cycle. This model is still speculative, in parts, and the available data could be interpreted in a different way.

The secretion of transferrin measured by RIA has been shown to be influenced by hormones.[12] These hormones may contribute to the selective secretion described above. Although the use of a radioimmunoassay to measure secretion by cultured Sertoli cells has proven to be very fruitful, we wished to extend these studies and to initiate some new studies requiring the use of a cDNA probe for transferrin to measure mRNA levels in Sertoli cells. With this probe we could determine if the hormones that stimulated transferrin secretion acted at the level of transcription or post-transcription.

We therefore constructed our own plasmid containing rat transferrin cDNA.[13] The plasmid was constructed by first isolating the mRNA from the transferrin-synthesizing polysomes from rat liver. The polysomes were incubated with anti-transferrin and polysome-antibody complex collected on a protein A–Sepharose column. The mRNA from these polysomes was isolated and after translation in a cell-free system was found to be approximately 80% transferrin mRNA. The mRNA was reverse transcribed, the second strand synthesized, and the resulting double-stranded cDNA was dC·dG-tailed into the Pst I site of the plasmid, pBR322. The transferrin cDNA bearing bacterial colonies were selected by differential screening in which each tetracycline-resistant colony was hybridized to radioactively labeled cDNAs prepared from total liver mRNA or from transferrin-enriched mRNA. Approximately 90 of 850 colonies were obtained that hybridized specifically to the transferrin-enriched cDNA probe. A plasmid that contained a large (1.5 kb) insertion of cDNA was selected for further hybridization studies. It was subsequently shown that this plasmid contained cDNA for transferrin by a hybridization release experiment in which the liver mRNA that hybridized to that plasmid was recovered and translated and the product was found to be transferrin.

Cytoplasmic RNA was isolated from cultured Sertoli cells essentially as described by White and Bancroft.[14] Cells were resuspended in ice-cold hypotonic buffer and lysed by the addition of Triton X-100 and deoxycholate, 1% and 0.5%, respectively. The nuclei were pelleted by centrifugation and later assayed for DNA content by a fluorescence-enhancement assay with bisbenzimidazole (Hoechst 33258) reagent.[15] The protein in the supernatant fraction was digested with proteinase K (50 μg/ml) for 20 min at 45°C in the presence of 1% SDS and then extracted with phenol : chloroform (1 : 1). The aqueous phase was precipitated with two volumes of ethanol. The RNA pellet was resuspended in 6% formaldehyde in 17×SSC [0.15 M NaCl/0.015 M sodium citrate (standard saline citrate)], heated five minutes at 70°C, cooled, and applied to nitrocellulose by suction. The nitrocellulose "dot blot" was baked for two hours at 80°C, prehybridized, and hybridized as described by Thomas.[16] Hybridization was for 18–24 hours at 42°C using a ^{32}P-labeled nick-translated cDNA probe ($\sim 1 \times 10^8$ cpm/μg). A nick-translation kit was obtained from Bethesda Research Laboratories and used according to the supplied instructions. The blots were washed and exposed to X-ray film. For quantitative analyses, the dot blots were cut out and the amount of ^{32}P-cDNA hybridized was determined in a liquid scintillation counter.

FIGURE 3 shows the results of the hybridization of ^{32}P-labeled transferrin cDNA to RNA isolated from FIRT (FSH, insulin, retinol, and testosterone)-treated and control Sertoli cell cultures. Cells that received no hormones show a steady decline of transferrin mRNA with time in culture, while FIRT-treated cells show an increase in transferrin mRNA production. The maximum transferrin mRNA accumulation in treated cells occurs on day 4 of culture and represents a 3.6-fold stimulation over control mRNA levels.

A second experiment was designed to measure the rate of transferrin mRNA accumulation over a shorter time interval. Cells were plated without hormones and then stimulated with hormones on day 2 of culture. FIGURE 4 shows the levels of transferrin mRNA at indicated hours after hormone treatment or after change

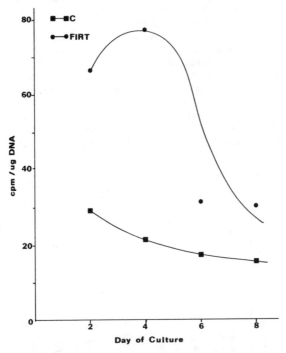

FIGURE 3. Influence of hormone and retinol supplements on transferrin mRNA in Sertoli cells cultured from 20-day-old rat testes. Cell culture was performed as previously described[4] and cells were plated in Falcon 60 mm dishes in 7 ml of Ham's F-12 medium. The hormones were (F) FSH, 25 ng/ml (NIH S-13); (I) insulin, 5.0 μg/ml; and (T) testosterone, 0.7 μM. Retinol (R) was 0.3 μM. Medium with or without hormones was replaced every two days. Duplicate RNA samples were applied to nitrocellulose and transferrin-specific mRNA was measured by hybridization to ^{32}P-labeled cDNA. The counts per minute were adjusted to μg DNA measured in the sample fraction.

of medium only. There is a steady increase in transferrin mRNA levels up to 24 hours with addition of FIRT, while control cultures show a slow decline in transferrin mRNA.

To examine further the influence of individual hormones on transferrin mRNA levels, we treated cultures with various agents and isolated mRNA on day 4 of culture. The results of these studies are shown in FIGURE 5. FSH- and testosterone-treated cultures show little stimulation of mRNA accumulation, while retinol imparts a 2.4-fold increase over control cultures. Insulin alone, insulin/retinol, and FIRT demonstrate similar stimulation capabilities. Previous studies in our laboratory have shown that FSH, insulin, retinol, or testosterone does not appreciably affect the accumulation of total RNA or mRNA.[17] However, only insulin produced a dramatic increase in $^{32}P_i$ incorporation into total RNA and mRNA. Thus the increase in specific activity may reflect a stimulation in synthesis of a very small population of mRNAs. Our results suggest that insulin is the major influencing factor in transferrin mRNA synthesis of the hormones we tested.

The amount of transferrin secreted by Sertoli cells under these conditions has also been measured by radioimmunoassay (FIGURE 5). It was found that the secretion of transferrin was regulated by the interaction of insulin with FSH, testosterone, and retinol. Each of these four agents would stimulate transferrin secretion if added singly to the cultures although the stimulation by testosterone was minimal. Maximum secretion of 164 ng transferrin/10^5 cells was obtained only in the presence of all four agents. The presence of insulin in the medium resulted in at least a twofold increase in transferrin secretion whether or not the cells were treated with FSH, testosterone, or retinol.

A comparison of transferrin mRNA levels to transferrin secretion suggests that FSH enhances some aspect of transferrin synthesis and/or secretion, while insulin appears to have a more dramatic effect on transferrin mRNA production.

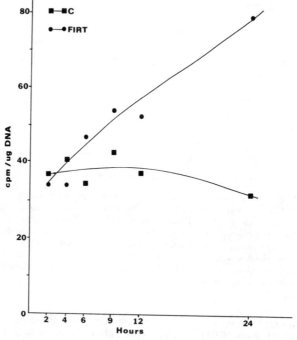

FIGURE 4. Stimulation of transferrin mRNA production by hormones and retinol in cultured Sertoli cells. Sertoli cells were plated initially in unsupplemented medium. On day 2 of culture the medium was replaced with or without supplementation of FIRT. Total RNA was isolated at the indicated interval after supplementation and Tf-specific mRNA measured as described in the text.

FIGURE 5. Influences of hormones and retinol on the relative amounts of mRNA in cultured Sertoli cells and on the amounts of secreted transferrin. Cells were plated in culture with the selected treatments and the medium (with treatment) was changed every two days. On day 4 of culture total mRNA was isolated from cells under each treatment and hybridized to ^{32}P-labeled cDNA as before (*solid bars*). In a separate experiment the medium was collected on day 6 and the amount of transferrin secreted during the preceding 48 hours was determined by radioimmunoassay (*striped bars*).

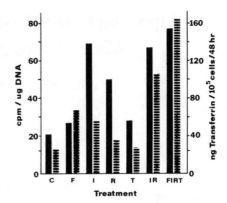

In summary, Sertoli cells synthesize and secrete transferrin. We propose that the function of transferrin in the testis is to transport Fe^{3+} to selected stages of developing germinal cells. The secretion of transferrin and the accumulation of transferrin-specific mRNA is regulated by hormones and retinol. Insulin alone or in combination with various treatments produced the most dramatic increase in transferrin mRNA accumulation.

ACKNOWLEDGMENTS

The authors gratefully acknowledge the expertise of Drs. G. Stanley McKnight and David C. Lee for their help in the construction of the plasmid containing the transferrin cDNA and the technical help of Alice F. Karl in cell culture. We wish to thank Holly Schumacher for her assistance in preparing this manuscript.

REFERENCES

1. FAWCETT, D. W. 1975. Handb. Physiol. **5:** 21–55.
2. FRITZ, I. B. 1973. Curr. Topics Cell Reg. **7:** 129–174.
3. WAITES, G. M. H. 1977. *In* The Testis. A. D. Johnson & R. Gomes, Eds. **4:** 91–117. Academic Press. New York.
4. KISSINGER, C., M. K. SKINNER & M. D. GRISWOLD. 1982. Biol. Reprod. **27:** 233–240.
5. SKINNER, M. K. & M. D. GRISWOLD. 1980. J. Biol. Chem. **255**(20): 211–221.
6. AISEN, P. & LISTOWSKY. 1980. Ann. Rev. Biochem. **49:** 357–393.
7. EMERY, T. 1980. Nature **287:** 776–777.
8. SYLVESTER, S. R. & M. D. GRISWOLD. 1984. Biol. Reprod. **31:** 195–203.
9. DAUTRY-VARSAT, A., A. CIECHANOVER & H. F. LODISH. 1983. Proc. Natl. Acad. Sci. USA **80:** 2258–2262.
10. SKINNER, M. K. & M. D. GRISWOLD. 1983. Biol. Reprod. **38:** 1225–1229.
11. FRIEDIN, E. & P. AISEN. 1980. Trends Biochem. Sci. **6:** 5.
12. SKINNER, M. K. & M. D. GRISWOLD. 1982. Biol. Reprod. **27:** 211–221.
13. HUGGENVIK, J., D. C. LEE, G. S. MCKNIGHT & M. D. GRISWOLD. 1984. (Manuscript in preparation.)
14. WHITE, B. A. & F. C. BANCROFT. 1982. J. Biol. Chem. **257**(15): 8569–8572.
15. DOWNS, T. R. & W. W. WILFINGER. 1983. Anal. Biochem. **131:** 538–547.
16. THOMAS, P. S. 1980. Proc. Natl. Acad. Sci. USA **77:** 5201–5205.
17. GRISWOLD, M. D. & J. MERRYWEATHER. 1982. Endocrinol. **111**(2): 661–667.

Alpha-lactalbumin–like Proteins in the Male Reproductive Tract[a]

STEPHEN W. BYERS and MARTIN DYM

Department of Anatomy
School of Medicine-School of Dentistry
Georgetown University
Washington, DC 20007

INDIRA K. HEWLETT and PRADMAN K. QASBA

Laboratory of Pathophysiology
National Cancer Institute
National Institutes of Health
Bethesda, Maryland 20205

INTRODUCTION

Alpha-lactalbumin, the modifier or B protein of the lactose synthetase complex, had until recently only been detected in the mammary gland. In this tissue alpha-lactalbumin participates in a unique mechanism for the control of an enzymatic reaction. The A protein of lactose synthetase is a ubiquitous galactosyl transferase (UDP-galactose: N-acetylglucosamine − B1 → 4 galactosyl transferase) that catalyzes the incorporation of galactose in a B1 → 4 linkage with N-acetylglucosamine during the synthesis of the oligosaccharide prosthetic groups of certain glycoproteins in many tissues (*reaction 1*).[1] In the lactating mammary gland however, alpha-lactalbumin is produced and forms a manganese-dependent complex with the transferase. This results in a change in the substrate specificity of the enzyme such that the free glucose now becomes the preferred acceptor and the milk sugar lactose is produced (*reaction 2*).[2]

$$\text{UDP-Gal} + \text{GlcNAc} \dashrightarrow \text{Gal-GlcNAc} + \text{UDP} \qquad (1)$$

$$\text{protein} \qquad \text{protein}$$

$$\text{UDP-Gal} + \text{Glc} \dashrightarrow \text{GalGlc} + \text{UDP} \qquad (2)$$

$$\text{lactose}$$

The mammary lactose synthetase system, particularly the role and characteristics of alpha-lactalbumin, has been extensively studied in many laboratories (see Hill and Brew[2] for review). Consequently, a great deal is known about the mechanism and hormonal control of alpha-lactalbumin production as well as the requirements for its association with the A protein of the complex.[2,3] Alpha-lactalbumin itself has been purified and both polyclonal and monoclonal antibodies[4–6] as well as complementary (c) DNA are available to study the expression and localization

[a] Supported by a Rockefeller Fellowship (S.W.B), a grant from the National Institutes of Health (No. HD 16260 to M.D.), and a grant from the Mellon Foundation (M.D.).

8

of this protein.[7,8] For many years it was thought that as lactose production only occurred in the mammary gland alpha-lactalbumin and lactose synthetase would also be restricted to this tissue. In 1981 however, Hamilton showed that alpha-lactalbumin–like activity could also be detected in epididymal fluid.[9] In this communication we report on the galactosyl transferase modifier characteristics, hybridization with cDNA probes, immunocytochemical localization, and possible role of alpha-lactalbumin–like proteins in the male reproductive tract.

GALACTOSYL TRANSFERASE MODIFIER ACTIVITY

Although it has been known for some time that galactosyl transferase, the A protein of lactose synthetase, occurs on sperm as well as in rete testis fluid,[10,11] the

TABLE 1. Amino Acid Composition of Rat Mammary Alpha-lactalbumin and Epididymal Alpha-lactalbumin–like Proteins[a]

Amino Acid	Amino Acid Composition (mol/100 mol recovered)				
Aspartic acid	11.9	11.8	11.2	9.9	8.8
Threonine	4.8	4.9	4.4	7.3	7.7
Serine	8.2	9.8	8.9	7.2	6.7
Glutamic acid	13.9	13.7	11.8	11.8	11.5
Proline	4.9	5.9	7.6	4.3	2.9
Glycine	5.5	5.8	10.5	7.4	7.7
Alanine	7.2	6.5	6.1	7.4	8.7
Valine	5.6	6.0	7.7	6.9	7.5
Methionine	1.4	1.9	1.3	2.4	2.2
Isoleucine	7.9	6.9	2.5	3.7	3.5
Leucine	7.4	5.8	8.7	9.4	9.8
Tryosine	2.9	2.2	3.1	4.0	4.4
Phenylalanine	4.4	4.1	3.0	4.2	4.2
Histidine	2.0	1.7	3.2	3.2	3.1
Lysine	8.0	7.0	6.5	7.6	7.9
Arginine	1.4	1.6	3.5	3.3	3.0
Protein	LA 1	LA 2	23K	18.5K	19K
	Mammary		Epididymal		

[a] Modified from Qasba and Chakrabarrty[5] and Jones *et al.*[13]

possible role of this has not been studied extensively. Hamilton[9] first showed that rat epididymal fluid also had some alpha-lactalbumin activity. It could make lactose with the appropriate substrates, i.e., glucose, UDP-Gal, and rete testis fluid galactosyl transferase. The activity was associated with proteins of similar molecular weights and amino acid composition to rat mammary alpha-lactalbumin (TABLE 1).[5,12,13]

Hamilton[9] and Jones and Brown[19] have already shown that epididymal alpha-lactalbumin activity differs from bovine mammary gland alpha-lactalbumin in that it transfers galactose from UDP-Gal to either glucose or myoinositol with equal efficiency. We have now compared the alpha-lactalbumin–like activity of epididymal extract with an extract of five-day lactating mammary gland and with pure rat mammary alpha-lactalbumin.[18] FIGURE 1 shows the galactosyl transferase and sugar dependence of lactose synthase activity in these preparations. All the alpha-

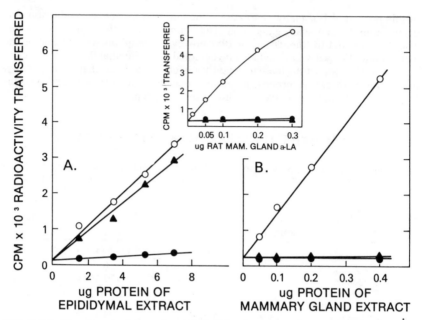

FIGURE 1. Transfer of galactose from UDP-(^{3}H)-galactose to glucose (O) and inositol (▲) by epididymal extract (A), five-day lactating mammary gland extract (B), and purified rat mammary alpha-lactalbumin (*insert*) in the presence of bovine milk galactosyl transferase. Values obtained without added sugar are represented by solid circles. (From Qasba *et al.*[18] With permission from *Biochemical and Biophysical Research Communications.*)

lactalbumin preparations will modify the activity of exogenous galactosyl transferase to allow transfer to galactose from UDP-Gal to glucose, but only the epididymal extract will allow transfer to inositol. Neither epididymal extract nor bovine milk galactosyl transferase alone catalyzes this reaction. The products of these reactions, lactose and galactinol, were further characterized by paper chromatography (results not shown). FIGURE 2 (B, C, and D) shows that alpha-lactalbumin–like activity can also be detected in extracts from mouse and rabbit epididymis and in human semen. Curiously, the preparations failed to transfer galactose to myoinositol. We have no explanation for these species differences although epididymal levels of inositol in these species are not as high as in the rat.[20]

HYBRIDIZATION WITH cDNA PROBES

The availability of cloned rat mammary gland alpha-lactalbumin complementary DNA (cDNA)[4] allowed us to determine homologous messenger (m) RNA sequences in the epididymis. We have recently shown that this cDNA probe will hybridize with epididymal RNA.[18] Homologous RNA sequences could be detected by dot-blot analysis in 5–10 μg of total epididymal RNA while electrophoresis of the RNA through agarose gels containing formaldehyde and subsequent analysis on Northern blots showed that the size of this RNA is very similar to mammary gland alpha-lactalbumin mRNA. Both these methods showed that the epididymal total RNA contained about 50 to 75 times less homologous alpha-lactalbumin RNA sequences than in five-day lactating rat mammary gland total RNA. However, as whole epididymides were used in the preparation of mRNA this value may underestimate the specific mRNA concentration in the proximal caput epididymis. Under similar conditions of hybridization, mRNA sequences homologous to other mammary specific cDNA clones, such as whey-phosphoprotein and casein clones, could not be detected in the epididymis.

LOCALIZATION AND IMMUNOLOGICAL SIMILARITIES

We have demonstrated that an antiserum specific for rat mammary alpha-lactalbumin does cross-react with something in the male reproductive tract.[14] Immunocytochemical experiments showed that specific staining in the epididymis is con-

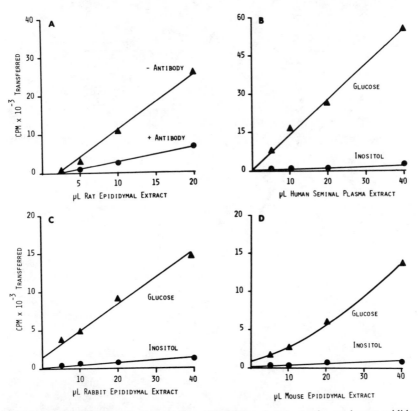

FIGURE 2. (A) Transfer of galactose from UDP-(^{3}H)-galactose to glucose by rat epididymal extract in the presence of bovine milk galactosyl transferase with normal rabbit serum (▲) or (●) anti-mammary alpha lactalbumin serum (1:20 final dilution). (B) Transfer of galactose from UDP-(^{3}H)-galactose to glucose (▲) or inositol (●) by human seminal plasma extract. (C) Rabbit epididymal extract. (D) Mouse epididymal extract. For details of the procedure see Qasba *et al.*[18]

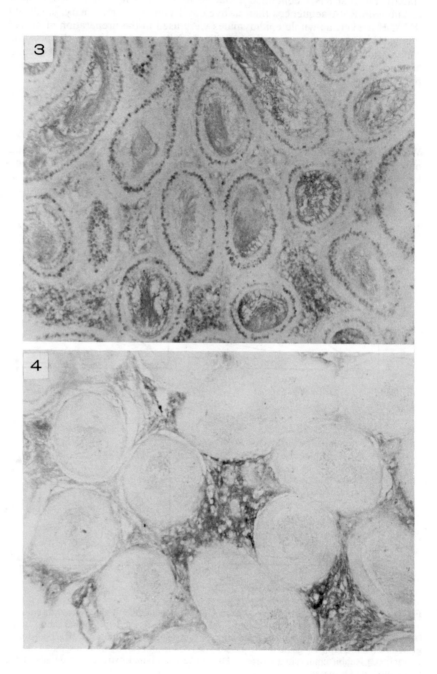

fined to the supranuclear cytoplasm of principal cells from the proximal caput epididymidis but is rarely found in cells from other parts of the duct (FIGURE 3).[14] At the electron microscope level it can be seen that this area is crowded with elements of the Golgi apparatus.[15] In the mammary epithelial cell it is well known that the lactose synthetase complex is localized on Golgi membranes,[16] and we interpret our results as showing that alpha-lactalbumin–like molecules are also present in the Golgi of the principal cell. Staining extended into the apical cytoplasm of these cells and was always associated with the luminal surface and with spermatozoa, which suggests that the immunoreactive material is secreted by principal cells and is taken up by maturing spermatozoa. Klinefelter and Hamilton[17] have now shown that tubules from the caput epididymis will secrete alpha-lactalbumin–like proteins *in vitro*. Alpha-lactalbumin–like immunoreactivity also occurs in post-meiotic germ cells in the testis and appears to be associated with the Golgi-acrosome region of these cells.[14] Alpha-lactalbumin immunoreactivity can be demonstrated in the epididymides of rats as young as 10 days of age while specific staining in mature rats disappears after castration.[14] Specific immunoreactivity can be abolished by preadsorbing the primary antiserum with pure mammary alpha-lactalbumin, milk, or epididymal fluid (FIGURE 4). In addition, this antiserum will inhibit the galactosyl transferase modifier activity of epididymal alpha-lactalbumin (FIGURE 2A), while normal rabbit serum has no effect on this reaction. It should be pointed out however that the antiserum is more potent in inhibiting mammary alpha-lactalbumin modifier activity than the epididymal activity. These results suggest therefore that we are detecting a molecule or molecules in the epididymis immunologically similar, but probably not identical, to rat mammary alpha-lactalbumin.

OTHER CHARACTERISTICS AND POSSIBLE FUNCTIONS

Although the immunological similarity and apparent homology of messenger RNAs suggest that rat epididymal and mammary alpha-lactalbumin are related molecules, we feel that there are enough differences between them to make it unlikely that they are identical. For instance, while both epididymal and mammary alpha-lactalbumins will modify the activity of galactosyl transferase in a way that permits the synthesis of lactose, only rat epididymal alpha-lactalbumin will promote the transfer of galactose to inositol. Jones and Brown[19] have shown that the three epididymal proteins with activity are considerably less potent than bovine mammary alpha-lactalbumin. We also find that the purified epididymal proteins are only 10–20% as active as purified rat mammary alpha-lactalbumin.

FIGURE 3. A light micrograph of a section through the proximal caput epididymidis showing specific immunocytochemical staining for alpha-lactalbumin using anti-mammary alpha-lactalbumin serum. Specific staining occurs in the supranuclear region of the principal epithelial cells and is associated with spermatozoa in the lumen. Magnification × 100. (From Byers *et al.*[4] With permission from *Biology of Reproduction*.)

FIGURE 4. An adjacent section of the proximal caput epididymidis showing the loss of specific epithelial staining after the primary antiserum is preadsorbed with pure mammary alpha-lactalbumin. Non-specific interstitial staining remains. Magnification × 100. (From Byers *et al.*[14] With permission from *Biology of Reproduction*.)

However, definitive identification of molecular differences between the two alpha-lactalbumin species awaits protein sequence analysis and sequence analysis of the cDNA clone corresponding to the epididymal alpha-lactalbumin gene. These studies are currently underway.

The function of alpha-lactalbumin, galactosyl transferase, and perhaps their combination as a lactose synthase complex in the male reproductive tract is not known. It is unlikely that lactose synthesis takes place as this sugar has not been detected there, and free glucose levels are very low.[9] It is possible, in the rat, that the epididymal alpha-lactalbumin–like proteins may interact with galactosyl transferase in transferring galactose to inositol, linked to membrane-bound glycoproteins. However, this galactose-inositol linkage has not been reported on any glycoproteins so far isolated from the epididymis and the disaccharide galactinol has not been detected there.

The demonstration that the initial binding of mouse sperm to the egg zona pellucida involves sperm surface galactosyl transferase[21] suggests that epididymal alpha-lactalbumin may have a role in this interaction. Indeed, exogenous mammary alpha-lactalbumin will prevent sperm-egg binding in vitro in a dose-dependent manner.[22] This work indicates that epididymal alpha-lactalbumin may act as a sort of decapacitation factor. Further evidence for a role of galactosyl transferase and alpha-lactalbumin–like proteins in capacitation and fertilization comes from work on the t-mutant mouse. Sperm from these animals have increased fertilizing ability at least partly because of a fourfold increase in the activity of sperm surface galactosyl transferase.[10] Interestingly, freshly isolated sperm from the cauda epididymis of these mice also show the hyperactivated, non-progressive, whiplash type of motility characteristic of capacitated sperm.[23] Olds-Clark[24] has now shown that progressive motility can be restored to a significant number of these sperm by the addition of mammary alpha-lactalbumin but not other proteins. It is not known at this time whether this effect of alpha-lactalbumin is due to its association with sperm surface galactosyl transferase or to a previously unrecognized function of this protein. In this regard it is interesting to note that alpha-lactalbumin has a number of other characteristics apparently unrelated to its role in lactose synthesis (TABLE 2). For example, neither the protein itself nor its modifier activity is affected by high temperature (80°C for 10 minutes). We find that alpha-lactalbumin activity in the epididymis is similarly unaffected by high temperatures. Mammary alpha-lactalbumin is also a calcium binding protein with two binding sites for calcium although there is some dispute as to their exact binding affinities.[25–28] However these calcium binding sites do not seem to be important in the interaction of alpha-lactalbumin with galactosyl transferase, in vitro at least.[27]

Many of the properties of mammary alpha-lactalbumin and the epididymal alpha-lactalbumin–like protein are similar to those of another enzyme modulator found in the reproductive tract and elsewhere, namely calmodulin[29] (TABLE 2). These proteins have similar molecular weights, are heat stable, and also have effects on sperm motility. Both proteins are hydrophobic under certain conditions. Calmodulin becomes hydrophobic upon binding calcium and can be separated from other proteins on the basis of its calcium-dependent binding to phenyl sepharose.[30] Mammary alpha-lactalbumin, in contrast, is hydrophobic in the absence of calcium and becomes less hydrophobic upon binding calcium,[31–35] its behavior on phenyl sepharose therefore being unlike calmodulin. Preliminary experiments indicate that the epididymal alpha-lactalbumin–like proteins behave like mammary alpha-lactalbumin rather than calmodulin on phenyl sepharose columns.

Perhaps one of the most intriguing characteristics of alpha-lactalbumin is its association with artificial lipid bilayers. Physical biochemists have in fact used the unusual properties of this protein in their studies of membrane fluidity and lipid transition temperatures.[31–35] Briefly, alpha-lactalbumin can be either a peripheral or an integral membrane protein depending on pH or on whether it is binding calcium or not. The effects of pH are thought to be due to protons displacing the bound calcium. When integrated into a lipid bilayer, alpha-lactalbumin effectively raises the transition temperature by 4°C. Thus, incorporation of this protein into a membrane can alter its fluidity without a change in temperature. Changes in sperm membrane fluidity and mobility of proteins within the membrane have been described during sperm maturation and capacitation.[36–38] It also appears that many membrane-bound enzymes, including certain glycosyl transferases, are sensitive to the gel-fluid state of neighboring membrane lipids.[39,40] In addition some

TABLE 2. Properties of Mammary Alpha-lactalbumin, Calmodulin, and Epididymal Alpha-lactalbumin–like Proteins

Properties	Mammary Alpha-lactalbumin	Calmodulin	Epididymal Alpha-lactalbumin– like Proteins
Modifies galactosyl transferase	+ (2,18)	?	+ (9,18,19)
Heat stable	+ (27)	+ (41)	+ (*)
Molecular weight	16K–23K (4)	16K–18K (29)	16K–23K (9,19)
Affects sperm motility	+ (24)	+ (29)	?
Binds Ca^{2+}	+ (28)	+ (29)	?
Detectable on spermatozoa		+ (29)	+ (19)
Regulates phospho- diesterase and Ca^{2+}- dependent ATPase	?	+ (29)	?
Prevents sperm-egg interactions	+ (22)	?	?
Hydrophobic interactions with other proteins or with membranes	+ (32,33)	+ (29,43)	+ (19,44)

Number in parentheses indicates selected references and * indicates this paper. Known properties are indicated by (+) and properties not yet tested by (?).

epididymal fluid proteins, particularly those with alpha-lactalbumin activity, do become integral components of the sperm membrane.[19,44] One of these binds far more effectively at acid pH although the effects of calcium on this binding have not yet been investigated.[41]

The existence of alpha-lactalbumin–like molecules in the male reproductive tract as well in the mammary gland raises a number of interesting questions about possible roles of this protein in mammalian reproduction. A function of alpha-lactalbumin in the mammary gland other than in lactose synthesis has already been proposed by Nakhasi and Qasba[42] who showed that alpha-lactalbumin appears in the mammary gland during early gestation, in the absence of any lactose production, then does not reappear until late gestation. Perhaps the calcium binding properties, hydrophobicity, and membrane interactions of alpha-lactalbumin or epididymal alpha-lactalbumin–like molecules as well as their galactosyl transferase modifier effects are important in the mammary gland and the male reproductive tract.

REFERENCES

1. SCHACTER, H, I. JABBAL, R. L. HUDGIN & L. PINTERIC. 1970. J. Biol. Chem. **245:** 1090–1100.
2. HILL, R. L. & K. BREW. 1975 Adv. Enzymol. Related Areas Mol. Biol. **43:** 441–490.
3. TOPPER, Y. T. & C. S. FREEMAN. 1980. Physiol. Rev. **60:** 1049–1106.
4. QASBA, P. K. & P. K. CHAKRABARRTY. 1978. J. Biol. Chem. **253:** 1167–1173.
5. RAY, D. B., I. A. HORST, R. W. JANSEN & J. KOWAL. 1981. Endocrinology **108:** 573–583.
6. KAETZEL, C. S., D. B. RAY & J. KOWAL. 1982. J. Cell Biol. **95:** 23014 (abstract).
7. DANDEKAR, A. M. & P. K. QASBA. 1981. Proc. Natl. Acad. Sci. USA **78:** 4853–4857.
8. HALL, L., R. K. CRAIG, M. R. EDBROOKE & P. N. CAMPBELL. 1982. Nucleic Acids Res. **10:** 3503–3515.
9. HAMILTON, D. W. 1981. Biol. Reprod. **25:** 385–392.
10. SHUR, B. D. & D. BENNETT. 1979. Dev. Biol. **71:** 243–259.
11. HAMILTON, D. W. 1980. Biol. Reprod. **23:** 377–385.
12. BROOKES, D. E. & S. J. HIGGINS. 1980. J. Reprod. Fert. **59:** 363–375.
13. JONES, R., C. R. BROWN, K. J. VON GLOS & M. G. PARKER. 1980. Biochem. J. **188:** 667–676.
14. BYERS, S. W., H. L. PAULSON, P. K. QASBA & M. DYM. 1984. Biol. Reprod. **30:** 171–178.
15. HAMILTON, D. W. 1975. In Handbook of Physiology. Section 7. Male Reproductive System. D. W. Hamilton & R. O. Greep, Eds. **5:** 259–30. American Physiology Society. Bethesda, MD.
16. KEENAN, T. W., D. J. MOORE & R. J. CHEETHAM. 1970. Nature **228:** 1105–1106.
17. KLINEFELTER, G. R. & D. W. HAMILTON. 1983. Proceedings of the Society for the Study of Reproduction. Abstract 205.
18. QASBA, P. K., I. K. HEWLETT & S. W. BYERS. 1983. Biochem. Biophys. Res. Commun. **177:** 306–312.
19. JONES, R. & C. R. BROWN. 1982. Biochem. J. **206:** 161–164.
20. HINTON, B. T., R. W. WHITE & B. P. SETCHELL. 1980. J. Reprod. Fert. **58:** 395–399.
21. SHUR, B. D. & N. G. HALL. 1982. J. Cell Biol. **95:** 567–573.
22. SHUR, B. D. & N. G. HALL. 1982. J. Cell Biol. **95:** 574–579.
23. OLDS-CLARK, P. 1983. J. Androl. **4:** 136–143.
24. OLDS-CLARK, P. 1984. Ann. N. Y. Acad. Sci. (This volume.)
25. HIRAOKA, Y., T. SEGAWA, K. KUWAJIMA, S. SUGAI & M. MURAI. 1980. Biochem. Biophys. Res. Commun. **95:** 1098–1104.
26. PERMYAKOV, E. A., V. V. YERMOLENKO, L. P. KALINCHENKO, L. A. MOROZOVA & E. A. BURSTEIN. 1981. Biochem. Biophys. Res. Commun. **100:** 191–197.
27. KRONMAN, M. J., S. K. SINHA & K. BREW. 1981. J. Biol. Chem. **258:** 8582–8587.
28. KRONMAN, M. J. & S. C. BRATCHER. 1983. J. Biol. Chem. **258:** 5707–5709.
29. MEANS, A. R., J. S. TASH & J. G. CHAFOULEAS. 1982. Physiol. Rev. **62:** 1–39.
30. GOPALAKRISHNA, R. & W. B. ANDERSON. 1982. Biochem. Biophys. Res. Commun. **104:** 830–836.
31. HANSSENS, I. & F. H. VAN CAUWELAERT. 1978. Biochem. Biophys. Res. Commun. **84:** 1088–1096.
32. HANSSENS, I., C. HOUTHUYS, W. HERREMAN & F. H. VAN CAUWELAERT. 1980. Biochim. Biophys. Acta **602:** 539–557.
33. HERREMAN, W., P. VAN TORNOUT, F. H. VAN CAUWELAERT & I. HANNSENS. 1981. Biochim. Biophys. Acta **640:** 419–429.
34. DANGREAU, H., M. JONAI, M. DE CUYPER & I. HANNSENS. 1982. Biochemistry **21:** 3594–3598.

35. VAN CAUWELAERT, R., I. HANNSENS & W. HERREMAN. 1983. Biochim. Biophys. Acta **727:** 273–284.
36. GOFER, G. P. & R. A. SCHEGEL. 1982. J. Cell Biol. **95:** 8011 (abs).
37. O'RAND, M. 1977. Dev. Biol. **55:** 260–270.
38. O'RAND, M. 1982. Ann. N.Y. Acad. Sci. **383:** 392–404.
39. BLANQUET, P. R. 1983. Biochem. J. **213:** 479–484.
40. HOCHMAN, Y. & D. ZAKIM. 1983. J. Biol. Chem. **258:** 11758–11762.
41. WONG, P. Y. D. & A. Y. F. TSANG. 1982. Biol. Reprod. **27:** 1239–1246.
42. NAKHASI, H. L. & P. K. QASBA. 1979. J. Biol. Chem. **254:** 6016–6025.
43. JOHNSON, J. D. & L. A. WITTENHAUER. 1983. Biochem. J. **211:** 473–479.
44. BROWN, C. R., K. I. VON GLOS & R. JONES. 1983. J. Cell Biol. **96:** 256–264.

The Sperm Adenylate Cyclase[a]

DOMINIQUE STENGEL and JACQUES HANOUNE

Unité de Recherches INSERM U-99
Hôpital Henri Mondor
94010 Créteil, France

INTRODUCTION

The role of cyclic AMP in spermatozoa physiology and mobility is now being recognized, albeit little is known about the intimate mechanisms by which cyclic AMP acts.[1-4]

Cyclic AMP is synthesized from ATP by the enzyme adenylate cyclase (EC 4.6.1.1.) and we shall only deal with this aspect of cyclic AMP metabolism in the present report. We will summarize recent data from our laboratory concerning the characterization of ram sperm adenylate cyclase, the proteolytic activation and solubilization of the enzyme, and recent progress made in its purification.

Characterization of Ram Sperm Adenylate Cyclase

In mammalian spermatozoa, adenylate cyclase is essentially a membrane-bound enzyme, with the exception of the immature forms where it is soluble, as described by Braun and Dods.[5] Unlike all the other adenylate cyclase systems, spermatozoa adenylate cyclase cannot be stimulated by hormones, guanine nucleotides, or cholera toxin.[6] Ram sperm adenylate cyclase is also not regulated by calcium, adenosine, and forskolin[7] (TABLE 1). Also, no stimulation has been observed by the addition of tubulin purified to homogeneity, whether at low or high MgATP concentration (TABLE 2).

Garbers and coworkers[8] have reported a Ca^{2+} activation of guinea pig spermatozoa adenylate cyclase that is dependent on bicarbonate concentration. In ram sperm, we also observed a marked stimulation of the cyclase activity by bicarbonate (FIGURE 1), but we were unable to observe any regulation by Ca^{2+}.

Ram sperm adenylate cyclase activity is optimal in the presence of a large excess of manganese (10 mM) or magnesium (40 mM) concentration over that of ATP. In these conditions, the apparent K_m values determined by Lineweaver-Burk plots for MnATP and MgATP are rather high, 1.6 and 16.1 mM, respectively, with V_{max} values between 2.0 and 1.3 nmol/mg protein/min. Thus the enzyme can utilize magnesium to reach almost the same final maximal velocity as with manganese, provided that adequate concentrations of magnesium and ATP are used.

[a] Supported by the Institut National de la Santé et de la Recherche Médicale and by the Délégation Générale de la Recherche Scientifique et Technique.

TABLE 1. Effect of Various Effectors on Ram Sperm Adenylate Cyclase Activity

	Adenylate Cyclase Activity (pmol/mg prot/min)
Basal	7.2
GTP 10 μM	7.0
Gpp(NH)p 10 μM	6.9
NaF 10 mM	6.2
Epinephrine 10 μM	8.0
PGE$_1$ 10 μM	7.1
hCG 10 μM	7.6
Forskolin 100 μM	7.0
Adenosine 10 μM	7.9
Ca^{2+} 10 μM	7.0

Mg-dependent adenylate cyclase activity was measured in the presence of 0.5 mM ATP and 5 mM MgCl$_2$ at 30°C

Proteolytic Activation and Solubilization of Adenylate Cyclase System

In most tissues tested (liver, fat cells, platelets, kidney, etc.) a mild proteolytic treatment of isolated membranes results in an activation of the adenylate cyclase system (for a recent review, see Hanoune et al.[9]). In sperm membranes, the effect of proteases is more complex as it leads to the solubilization of the enzyme.[10]

Proteolytic treatment was performed by incubation of sperm particles (1.8 mg of protein per ml) for 15 min at 30°C in the presence of increasing amounts of alpha-chymotrypsin. The reaction was stopped by the addition of soybean trypsin inhibitor (2 mg/ml final concentration) and further incubation at 30°C for 2 min. One-half of the membrane suspension was then centrifuged for one hour at 49,000 rpm. In the non-centrifuged membrane preparation, we observed (FIGURE 2A) a biphasic effect of alpha-chymotrypsin upon adenylate cyclase assayed in the presence of MnATP as the substrate: activation at low concentrations of the proteolytic enzyme and inhibition at high concentrations. The activation was half-maximal for 3 μg alpha-chymotrypsin per ml, in the presence of 1.8 mg of membrane

TABLE 2. Tubulin Effect on Ram Sperm Adenylate Cyclase Activity

Concentrations	Adenylate Cyclase Activity (pmol/mg prot/min)		
ATP (mM)	1	5	18
MgCl$_2$ (mM)	41	45	58
Basal	35	120	220
Tubulin 0.6 μM	36	118	230
Gpp(NH)p 10 μM	34	135	210
Tubulin + Gpp(NH)p	36	127	210

Tubulin, purified from brain, was a kind gift of Dr. D. Pantaloni (Gif sur Yvette, France).

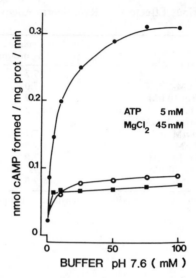

FIGURE 1. Buffer activation of sperm adenylate cyclase activities. Adenylate cyclase activity was measured in the presence of increasing amounts of $NaHCO_3$ (●), Tris-HCl (○), or Na-HEPES (■) at pH 7.6 in the presence of 5 mM ATP and 45 mM $MgCl_2$. Adenylate cyclase activity is expressed in nmol cyclic AMP formed per mg protein per min.

protein per ml; a maximal twofold activation was observed at 10 μg/ml of alpha-chymotrypsin. Activation of the adenylate cyclase was not observed when measured in the presence of magnesium as cosubstrate (FIGURE 2B), with which only inhibition at the highest concentrations of alpha-chymotrypsin was observed. These results are in agreement with our previous finding in the cyc⁻ S49 lymphoma cell line,[11] also devoid of a functionally active regulatory component (Ns) and where mild proteolysis increased the catalytic activity only when assayed in the presence of MnATP.

Proteolytic treatment also resulted in solubilization of ram sperm adenylate cyclase in a manner independent of the activation process. Thus, after high-speed centrifugation of the membranes treated with 10–15 μg/ml of alpha-chymotrypsin, up to 100 percent of the initial adenylate cyclase activity appeared in the supernatant fraction (FIGURE 2A), corresponding also to 60 percent of the measurable activity after proteolytic activation, when the enzyme was assayed in the presence of 21 mM $MnCl_2$ and 1 mM ATP, and up to 50 percent when the enzyme was assayed in the presence of 45 mM $MgCl_2$ and 5 mM ATP (FIGURE 2B). In this experiment, optimal solubilization was obtained at 8 μg alpha-chymotrypsin per mg of sperm membrane protein. At higher concentrations of alpha-chymotrypsin, the adenylate cyclase activity in the supernatant, as well as that remaining in the pellet, was inhibited, probably due to proteolytic degradation of the catalytic site. Trypsin treatment also caused activation and solubilization of the adenylate cyclase from ram sperm membranes in an analogous manner. However, the concentration range of trypsin over which activation occurred was narrower than for alpha-chymotrypsin. Proteolytic activation and solubilization were also observed with the bull sperm adenylate cyclase. The physiological meaning of such a phenomenon, if any, is unclear. Since proteolytic enzymes are well known to be involved in the acrosomal reaction, such an effect upon adenylate cyclase at that stage cannot be ruled out.

Kinetics Parameters and Cation Dependency of the Solubilized Adenylate Cyclase

The requirement for magnesium and manganese after solubilization by proteolytic treatment was the same as for the membrane-bound enzyme. The apparent K_m values for MgATP (12.8 versus 16.1) obtained was not modified after proteolytic treatment but it was lower for MnATP (1.1 versus 1.6). The V_{max} values obtained after proteolytic treatment were 10 and 2.8 nmol cyclic AMP/mg protein/min for MnATP and MgATP, respectively. Thus, the proteolytic treat-

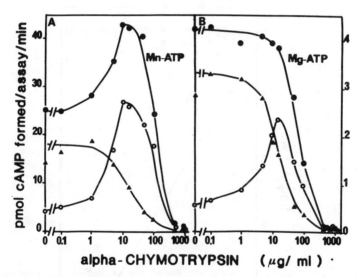

FIGURE 2. Effect of increasing concentrations of alpha-chymotrypsin upon activation and solubilization of adenylate cyclase from sperm membranes. Membranes (1.8 mg protein/ml) were preincubated in the presence of increasing concentrations of alpha-chymotrypsin for 15 min at 30°C. The reaction was stopped by the addition of 2 mg/ml of soybean trypsin inhibitor. Thereafter, aliquots of the membrane suspension were centrifuged for one hour at 165,000 × g(Spinco rotor Ti 50). Pellets were resuspended in the initial volume of buffer. The initial membrane solutions (●), the supernatants (○), and the pellets (▲) were assayed for adenylate cyclase activity in the presence of 1 mM ATP, 21 mM MnCl₂ (panel A) or in the presence of 5 mM ATP and 45 mM MgCl₂ (panel B) for 10 min at 30°C. Results are expressed in pmol of cyclic AMP formed/assay/min.

ment and the solubilization did not modify the apparent affinity of the enzyme for its substrates, and the apparent increase in the V_{max} of the enzyme reaction is mainly due to partial purification of the enzyme.

Thermodegradation

The enzyme from spermatozoa was solubilized under the conditions described in Stengel et al.[10] and was kept at 4°C, 20°C, 30°C, and 40°C for various periods of time, from 10 min up to 19 hours. The residual activity was then measured for 10 min at 30°C in the presence of 1 mM ATP and 21 mM $MnCl_2$. The chymotrypsin-solubilized adenylate cyclase was stable at 4°C and 20°C for at least one day. At 30°C, the adenylate cyclase lost 20% of its activity in four hours and 60% in 19 hours. At 40°C, the adenylate cyclase was degraded very rapidly. A semilogarithmic transformation of the data (FIGURE 3) allowed a more rigorous assessment of thermolability of the enzyme at the various temperatures studied, yielding half-life values of 15 min, 11 hours, and 25 hours at 40°C, 30°C, and 20°C, respectively.

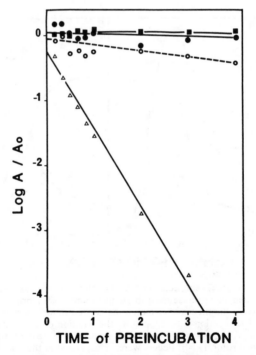

FIGURE 3. Thermodenaturation of adenylate cyclase solubilized by proteolytic treatment. The solubilized preparation was incubated at 4°C (■), 20°C (●), 30°C (○), and 40°C (△) for various periods of time. Adenylate cyclase was measured in the presence of MnATP for 10 min at 30°C. Residual adenylate cyclase is expressed in Log A/A_0

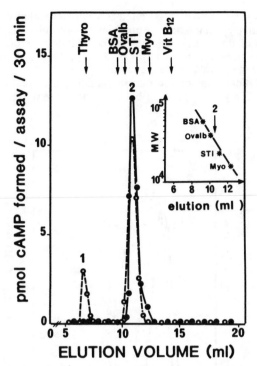

FIGURE 4. BioSil TSK 250 high performance liquid chromatography of adenylate cyclase activity. The proteolytically solubilized adenylate cyclase, prepared as described in Reference 10, and the cytosolic adenylate cyclase from ram testis, were used after filtration through a 0.2 μm Millipore filter. The amounts of protein injected into the BioSil TSK 250 column were 10 μg for the proteolytically solubilized cyclase (●———●)(this includes alpha-chymotrypsin and trypsin inhibitor) or 700 μg for the cytosolic cyclase (○————○). Aliquots (40 μl) of each elution fraction were assayed in duplicate for adenylate cyclase activity in the presence of 11 mM MnCl₂ and 1 mM ATP for 30 min at 30°C. Arrows refer to the position of marker proteins that were chromatographed under the same conditions. The inset refers to the calibration curve of the marker proteins.

Thus, it appears that the solubilized enzyme is rather stable at low temperature, which should facilitate its further purification.

Determination of the Hydrodynamic Parameters of the Solubilized Adenylate Cyclase

The solubilized preparation of adenylate cyclase was chromatographed at room temperature on a BioSil TSK 250 Biorad high performance gel permeation column, which had previously been equilibrated in 50 mM Tris-HCl pH 7.6 containing 100 mM NaCl. The elution profile of a typical run is shown in FIGURE 4.

The adenylate cyclase activity was eluted as a symmetrical peak between ovalbumin and soybean trypsin inhibitor. Approximate molecular weight was estimated by comparison of the elution volumes of the calibrating proteins. An apparent value of 38,000 corresponding to a Stokes radius of 2.8 ± 0.05 nm was calculated for the solubilized sperm adenylate cyclase.

The proteolytically solubilized ram sperm adenylate cyclase was centrifuged through a 3 to 12% sucrose gradient buffered with 50 mM Tris-HCl pH 7.6. The

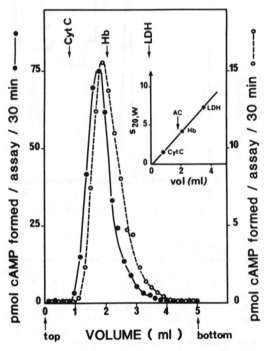

FIGURE 5. Sucrose density gradient centrifugation of the proteolytically solubilized adenylate cyclase. Gradients, 3–12% sucrose, were performed and run as described in Ref. 10. Aliquots (40 μl) of each fraction were assayed in duplicate for adenylate cyclase activity in the presence of MnATP, for 30 min at 30°C. Closed circles refer to the proteolytically solubilized cyclase and open circles to the cytosolic cyclase from ram testis. Arrows refer to the position of marker proteins that were run in parallel (Cyt C: cytochrome C, Hb: hemoglobin, LDH: lactate dehydrogenase). *Inset:* Calibration curve for the marker enzymes.

elution profile obtained are depicted in FIGURE 5. An apparent $S_{20,w}$ value of 3.85 was obtained.

From the apparent $S_{20,w}$ value and the apparent Stokes radius, one can calculate a molecular weight of 46,000 for this adenylate cyclase, assuming a partial specific volume of 0.735 ml/g (TABLE 3). This value (46,000) is similar to that obtained for cytosolic cyclase from ram,[10] rat,[12] or human testis.[13]

TABLE 3. Hydrodynamic Parameters of the Solubilized Ram Sperm Adenylate Cyclase

Stokes radius (nm) ± 0.05	2.8 ± 0.05
Apparent molecular weight	38,000
$S_{20,w}$ (S)	3.85 ± 0.10
Electrophoresis (Rf)	0.776 ± 0.02
Electrofocusing (pI)	6.0 ± 0.20
Calculated molecular weight	46,000

Purification of Ram Sperm Adenylate Cyclase

In order to further purify the ram sperm adenylate cyclase, semen was stored in liquid nitrogen before preparation of membrane particles. Sperm particles (about 6 mg proteins/ml) were incubated in the presence of 0.15 mg alpha-chymotrypsin/ml for 30 min at 30°C. The proteolytic action was stopped by the addition of 0.4 mg/ml of soybean trypsin inhibitor at 30°C for 5 min. Solubilized cyclase was obtained after one hour centrifugation in Ti 50 rotor (Spinco) at 49,000 rpm at 4°C.

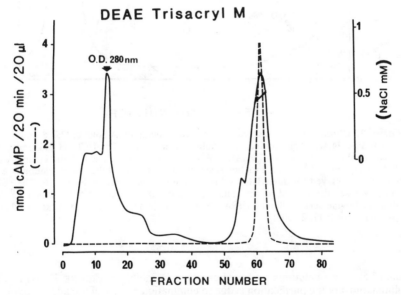

FIGURE 6. DEAE Trisacryl M chromatography of solubilized extract from ram sperm particules. DEAE Trysacryl M was equilibrated with 50 mM Tris-HCl, pH 7.6. Solubilized extract was applied at 4°C at a flow rate of 30 ml/hr and then the column was washed with the same buffer. From fraction 40, the column was eluted with a linear gradient of NaCl from 0 to 1 M. Fractions of 3 ml were collected, 20 µl aliquots of each fractions were assayed for adenylate cyclase activity in the presence of 1 mM ATP and 11 mM MnCl₂ for 20 min at 30°C. Adenylate cyclase activity is expressed in nmol cyclic AMP formed per 20 µl fraction per 20 min.

The solubilized enzyme was applied directly on a DEAE Trisacryl M (IBF) column (11 × 3 cm) preequilibrated in 50 mM Tris-HCl pH 7.6, at a flow rate of 30 ml/hr. The retained enzyme was eluted by increasing concentration of NaCl from 0 to 1 M. Adenylate cyclase activity coeluted at 0.5 mM NaCl, with soybean trypsin inhibitor (FIGURE 6). Fractions containing adenylate cyclase activity were pooled and applied on an Ultrogel AcA 34 column (90 × 2.7 cm) preequilibrated in 50 mM Tris-HCl pH 7.6 at a flow rate of 30 ml/hr. Fractions of 3 ml were collected and assayed for adenylate cyclase activity. Peak of the enzyme activity was

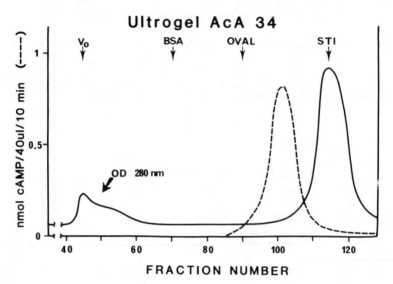

FIGURE 7. Ultrogel AcA 34 molecular size chromatography. A column (2.7 × 90 cm) of Ultrogel AcA 34 was equilibrated and calibrated in 50 mM Tris-HCl pH 7.6. Partially purified adenylate cyclase from DEAE Trisacryl column was applied to the column and eluted at a flow rate of 30 ml/hr. Fraction size was 3 ml. Aliquots of the eluted fractions were removed and assayed for adenylate cyclase activity as described in FIGURE 6. The void volume (V_o) was determined by the elution position of blue dextran. Arrows indicate the position of bovine serum albumin (BSA: 68,000), ovalbumin (Oval: 46,000), and soybean trypsin inhibitor (STI: 21,500).

eluted between ovalbumin and soybean trypsin inhibitor (FIGURE 7). With this column, most of the purification is due to elimination of 90% of the added soybean trypsin inhibitor. After concentration of the eluate on an Amicon membrane filter (PM 30) and equilibration in 25 mM imidazole-HCl at pH 7.2, the enzyme was applied on a column of chromatofocusing PBE 94 (Pharmacia), pH gradient was formed by polybuffer 74 diluted $^1/_{15}$ and preequilibrated at pH 3.8. Fractions of 3 ml were collected, quickly neutralized with Tris at pH 7.6, and assayed for adenylate cyclase activity. The cyclase peak was eluted at pH 4.6. The recovery of this

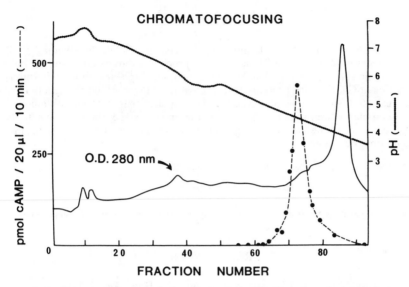

FIGURE 8. Chromatofocusing of adenylate cyclase. The peak from AcA 34 column was concentrated and applied to a chromatofocusing column (0.6 × 16.2 cm) equilibrated in imidazole-HCl buffer pH 7.2. A linear pH gradient from 7.2 to 3.8 was set up by passing 250 ml of eluent polybuffer (⅟₁₅) pH 3.8 through the column. A flow rate of 30 ml/hr was used and 2.5 ml fractions were collected. (——): protein profile at 280 nm; (●●●●●●●●): pH gradient; (●————●): adenylate cyclase activity.

column is low but it considerably increased the specific activity of the enzyme (FIGURE 8).

Finally, specific activity was calculated after a final Ultrogel AcA 54 column step that eliminated the polybuffer component. We thus obtained at this step an adenylate cyclase activity that is the highest obtained to date for mammalian enzyme (0.5 μmol cyclic AMP formed/mg protein/min). The catalytic subunit of the adenylate cyclase appeared essentially pure by SDS-gel electrophoresis. TABLE 4 summarizes the procedure.

TABLE 4. Purification of the Manganese-dependent Adenylate Cyclase of Ram Sperm after Solubilization by Proteolytic Treatment

	Total Protein (mg)	Total Activity (nmol/min)	Yield (%)	Specific Activity (nmol/mg/min)	Fold Purification (×)
Sperm	1470	150.0	100.0	0.10	1
Sperm Particules	570	205.0	136.0	0.36	3.6
Solubilized Fraction	400	200.0	134.0	0.51	5.1
DEAE Trisacryl M	88	261.0	174.0	2.90	29.0
ACA 34	10	88.0	58.0	9.00	90.0
Chromatofocusing	—	5.0	3.3	—	—
ACA 54	0.0012	0.6	0.4	538.00	5380.0

CONCLUSION

The procedure described here to purify cyclase has the following advantages: (1) no detergent and only classical biochemical procedures are needed and (2) only the catalytic subunit is purified, as the system does not appear to contain hormone receptors or GTP binding proteins. This is clear from the molecular weight that we obtained (46,000), a molecular weight much smaller than that one obtained in more complex systems such as liver.[14] At the present stage, the specific activity obtained is one of the highest for a mammalian enzyme and complete purification should now be at hand.

ACKNOWLEDGMENTS

We are grateful to V. Poli and C. Petit for their expert secretarial assistance.

REFERENCES

1. HOSKINS, D. D. & E. R. CASILLAS. 1975. Adv. Sex Horm. Res. **1:** 283–321.
2. LINDEMANN, C. B. 1978. Cell **13:** 9–18.
3. GARBERS, D. L. & G. S. KOPF. 1980. Adv. Cyclic Nucleotides Res. **13:** 251–306.
4. AMANN, R. P., S. R. HAY & R. H. HAMMERSTEDT. 1982. Biol. Reprod. **27:** 723–733.
5. BRAUN, T. & R. F. DODS. 1975. Proc. Natl. Acad. Sci. USA **72:** 1097–1101.
6. STENGEL, D. & J. HANOUNE. 1981. J. Biol. Chem. **256:** 5394–5398.
7. STENGEL, D., L. GUENET, M. DESMIER, P. INSEL & J. HANOUNE. 1982. Mol. Cell. Endocrinol. **28:** 681–690.
8. GARBERS, D. L., D. J. TUBB & R. V. HYNE. 1982. J. Biol. Chem. **257:** 8980–8984.
9. HANOUNE, J., D. STENGEL & M-L. LACOMBE. 1982. Mol. Cell. Endocrinol. **31:** 21–41.
10. STENGEL, D., L. GUENET & J. HANOUNE. 1982. J. Biol. Chem. **257:** 10818–10826.
11. STENGEL, D., P. M. LAD, T. B. NIELSEN, M. RODBELL & J. HANOUNE. 1980. FEBS Lett. **115:** 260–264.
12. GORDELADZE, J. O. & V. HANSSON. 1981. Mol. Cell. Endocrinol. **23:** 125–136.
13. GORDELADZE, J. O., D. ANDERSEN & V. HANSSON. 1981. J. Clin. Endocrinol. Metab. **53:** 465–471.
14. STENGEL, D. & J. HANOUNE. 1979. Eur. J. Biochem. **102:** 21–34.

Translation of Messenger RNA from Rat Epididymis and Identification of Poly(A)RNA Coding for Acidic Epididymal Glycoprotein[a]

R. J. BARTLETT,[b] O. A. LEA,[c] E. C. MURPHY,[d] and
F. S. FRENCH[e]

Department of Pediatrics
Laboratories for Reproductive Biology
School of Medicine
University of North Carolina
Chapel Hill, North Carolina 27514

INTRODUCTION

It has been established that mammalian spermatozoa undergo biochemical, morphological, and functional changes during passage through the epididymis and that these changes result in their ability to fertilize ova.[1-3] Changes in the properties of the sperm surface during epididymal transit have been well documented. These include alterations in antigenic properties,[4-7] in surface charge,[1,8] and in lectin binding.[9-12] It has been suggested that these changes result from alterations in the protein composition of the sperm plasma membrane caused by addition of new proteins and perhaps by modification of existing proteins. Indeed, striking differences in proteins extracted from cauda sperm as compared with caput sperm have been described.[11,13-16]

Epididymal sperm maturation is androgen dependent and requires protein synthesis.[3,12,17] Evidence from several mammalian species has indicated that proteins are secreted by the epididymis[10,18-26] and that some of these proteins bind to spermatozoa.[15,16,25] One such protein, referred to as forward motility protein from bovine epididymis, has been shown to bind to caput spermatozoa and act in concert with cyclic AMP to increase forward motility.[27] A secretory protein, with a molecular weight of 32,000, from rat epididymis referred to as acidic epididymal glycoprotein (AEG),[1] was previously purified in this laboratory.[25,28] Antibody raised against highly purified AEG was purified by affinity chromatography on a column of AEG-Sepharose. Immunoperoxidase staining showed AEG to be present in caput, corpus, and cauda epithelium.[25] Staining was present in principal cells of these regions but absent in similar epithelial cells of the major portion of

[a] Supported by United States Public Health Service, National Institutes of Health Grant HD 04466.

[b] Recipient of a postdoctoral fellowship grant from the University of North Carolina Cancer Research Center.

[c] Present address: Department of Pharmacology, University of Bergen, Bergen, Norway.

[d] Department of Tumor Virology, University of Texas System Cancer Center, M.D. Anderson Hospital and Tumor Institute, Houston, Texas 77030.

[e] Address correspondence to F.S.F.

initial segment. Sperm within the lumen of the initial segment showed no staining for AEG while sperm within the lumen of caput, corpus, and cauda were heavily stained. AEG is retained on the surface of caudal sperm after extensive washing and centrifugation through heavy sucrose.

AEG is secreted by epididymal epithelial cells grown in culture.[29] In epithelial cells cultured from immature (20–22 day old) and mature (20 month old) caput, AEG could be detected by immunoperoxidase staining in 80% of the cultured cells. Secretion of AEG into the culture medium, measured by radioimmunoassay, was maintained for several days.[29] More recent studies have shown AEG to be secreted by epithelial cells cultured from caput, corpus, and cauda.[30] *In vitro* synthesis and secretion of AEG by isolated tubules in these regions have also been demonstrated by immunoprecipitation of [^{35}S]methionine-labeled AEG.[31]

Jones and co-workers have purified rat epididymal secretory proteins from cauda luminal fluid collected via retrograde injection of saline through the vas deferens.[21] In addition to AEG (32,000 MW), two acidic proteins (19,000 and 18,500 MW) comigrated with [^{35}S]methionine-labeled proteins synthesized in incubations of minced caput. Two other proteins (23,000 and 80,000 MW) were unique to the initial segment.

As a preliminary to studies on the regulation of gene expression in rat epididymis, we prepared polyadenylated RNA (poly(A)RNA) from different segments of the epididymis and examined its translation products using a cell-free system. Messenger RNAs coding for AEG and other epididymal secretory proteins have been identified by immunoprecipitation and/or SDS-polyacrylamide gel electrophoresis. AEG messenger RNA was present in the caput plus corpus and cauda epididymis.

MATERIALS AND METHODS

Animals and Tissues

Epididymides used in the whole cell synthesis of proteins and in the isolation of total RNA were obtained from 250–450 g Sprague-Dawley rats (Zivic Miller).

Materials

Chemicals, except where otherwise noted, were from Fisher Scientific or Sigma. Radioactive amino acids were from New England Nuclear. Proteinase K was from P& L Biochemicals. Oligo(dT)-cellulose (T-3) was from Collaborative Research. JLS-V16 cell extract was prepared as described.[32] IgG-sorb (protein-A absorbent) was from the Enzyme Center. X-ray film, X-OMAT AR, was from Kodak.

EXPERIMENTAL PROCEDURES

Isolation of Poly(A)RNA

Sprague-Dawley rats weighing 300–350 g were decapitated using a guillotine. Epididymides were quickly separated into initial segment,[33] caput plus corpus, and cauda. They were frozen in liquid nitrogen and total RNA was extracted using guanidine-HCl.[34]

Poly(A)RNA was prepared using a modification of the oligo(dT)cellulose chromatography method of Aviv and Leder.[35] With this modification, the temperature of the oligo(dT) column was set at 30°C for the original binding of total RNA samples and was raised in steps of 10°C up to 50°C while washing the oligo(dT)-bound RNA with binding buffer (10 mM Tris, pH 7.4, 0.5% SDS, 0.5 M NaCl). After UV absorbance (A_{260}) had fallen to baseline level at each temperature increment, poly(A)RNA was eluted at 50°C with eluting buffer (10 mM Tris, pH 7.4, 0.05% SDS). Typically, 10–20 mg of total RNA were applied to a 0.5 g column of oligo(dT) cellulose and 200–1000 μg of poly(A)RNA were recovered. RNA was desalted on a 5 ml G–25 column, lyophilized to dryness, and suspended in distilled, deionized, filtered (0.2 μ filter) water at a concentration of 200 μg/ml.

Translation of Poly(A)RNA in the JLS-V16 System

In vitro translation of poly(A)RNA was carried out in a mouse embryo fibroblast extract as described. The extract and a high-salt wash of rabbit reticulocyte lysate[32,36] were incubated at 32°C for 2 hr with carrier-free labeled and 19 unlabeled amino acids and 0.5–1.5μg of poly(A)RNA. Trichloroacetic acid–precipitable radioactivity was measured as described.[37]

SDS-Polyacrylamide Gel Electrophoresis

Sample preparation and polyacrylamide gel electrophoresis in either 10% or 12% gels was performed as described previously.[38] Where indicated, some gels contained 4.0 M urea. Fluorography of gels was performed using Enhance (New England Nuclear) according to the manufacturer's instructions.

Immunoprecipitation of Labeled Protein

Immunoprecipitation of labeled proteins was with primary antibody adsorbed to fixed *S. aureus* protein A. To reduce non-specific binding, all immunoprecipitation mixtures were pre-adsorbed with IgG-sorb (10% suspension) prior to addition of primary antibody. Pre-adsorbed mixtures in 1.5 ml microfuge tubes were centrifuged in an Eppendorf microfuge and supernatants were transferred to 13 × 100 mm polystyrene tubes containing appropriate dilutions of antisera. Incubation with AEG antisera was at 2°C for up to 72 hr with continuous shaking. Antibody adsorption was with 50 μl of 10% IgG-sorb added to each sample followed by incubation at 23°C for 30 minutes with occasional shaking. Precipitation of adsorbed antigen-antibody complexes and preparation of samples for electrophoresis was performed as described previously.[36]

RESULTS

Regional differences in mRNA of rat epididymis were examined by cell-free translation of poly(A)RNA extracted from initial segment, caput plus corpus, and cauda. Labeled peptides translated from the poly(A)RNA preparations show dis-

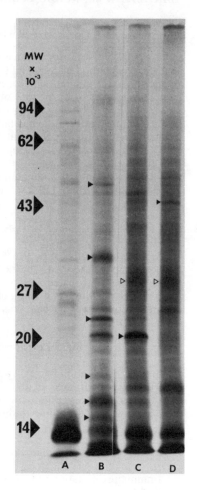

FIGURE 1. SDS-gel electrophoresis of [35S]cysteine-labeled proteins translated in the JLS-V16 system. Guanidine-HCl extracted, oligo(dT)-selected poly(A)RNA from initial segment (lane B), caput and corpus (lane C), cauda (lane D) was translated in the JLS-V16 cell extract system. Lane A is a control containing no added RNA. 1.0 μg of each RNA was added to a 25 μl reaction mixture containing 25 mM HEPES (pH 7.5), 90 mM KCl, 1 mM Mg(OAc)$_2$, 150 μM spermine, 8 mM 2-mercaptoethanol, 1 mM ATP, 150 μM GTP, 600 μM CTP, 10 mM creatine phosphate, 16 ng/ml creatine kinase, 400–800 μCi/ml of [35S]cysteine (<800 Ci/mmole), 100 μM each of unlabeled amino acids (minus cysteine), 5.25 μl of nuclease-treated cell extract, and 0.10 to 0.125 A$_{280}$ units of reticulocyte ribosome high salt wash–initiation factors. Protein synthesis proceeded at 32°C for 2 hr and acid-precipitable radioactivity was determined. 50,000 cpm each of the products were analyzed by SDS-polyacrylamide gel electrophoresis on 12% gels. Solid arrowheads indicate radioactive proteins that are unique to a particular region of epididymis. However, the 20,000 MW caput protein appears also in the initial segment as a lighter band and the 23,000 MW initial segment protein appears as a faint band in caput. This may have resulted from some overlap in the dissection of these regions. Open arrowheads indicate the location of acidic epididymal glycoprotein.

tinct regional patterns (FIGURE 1) indicating the presence of different populations of mRNA.

Cell-Free Translation of Epididymal Poly(A)RNA from Initial Segment

In initial segment mRNA (FIGURE 1, lane B), a radioactive band of 23,000 MW may correspond to a major initial segment protein synthesized in tissue minces and purified from epididymal fluid by Jones and co-workers.[21] Other prominent bands synthesized from initial segment mRNA corresponded to apparent molecular weights of 50,000, 35,000, 20,000, 17,500, 16,500, and 15,000.

Caput and Corpus

The 20,000 MW peptide that is more prominent in caput plus corpus (FIGURE 1, lane C) but absent from the cauda (Figure 1, lane D) corresponds to an androgen-dependent 20,000 MW protein synthesized in rabbit reticulocyte lysate from caput mRNA by D'Agostino *et al.*[39]

Cauda

Translations with [^{35}S]cysteine (FIGURE 1) revealed three radioactive bands of greater abundance in the cauda (lane D) than in caput plus corpus (lane C) or initial segment (lane B). Proteins of 47,000 and 25,000 MW were apparent both in [^{35}S]cysteine and [^{35}S]methionine (FIGURE 2) translations while a major band of approximately 16,000 MW was obvious only in translations with [^{35}S]cysteine.

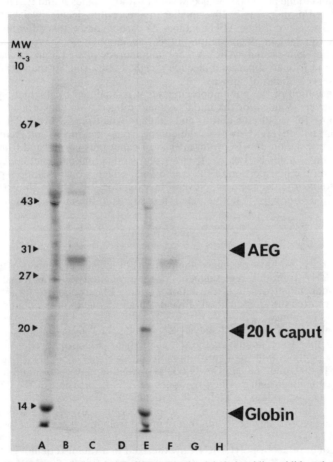

FIGURE 2. Immunoprecipitation of [^{35}S]methionine-labeled acidic epididymal glycoprotein. ^{35}S-labeled proteins were translated from epididymal poly(A)RNA as described in FIGURE 2. Lanes A–D are from cauda and lanes E–H from caput plus corpus. Labeled proteins in lanes A and E are without added antiserum; B and F are immunoprecipitated with AEG antiserum in 1 : 500 final dilution; C and G contain AEG as competitor, D and H contain rat transferrin antiserum in a final dilution 1 : 500. Arrowheads on the right indicate electrophoretic mobility of purified AEG, which is added to the sample as standard, and radiolabeled globin, which is translated from globin mRNA present in the JLS-V16 system.

Acidic Epididymal Glycoprotein

Aliquots containing 5×10^6 cpm of trichloroacetic acid–precipitable radioactivity were precipitated with AEG antisera as indicated in the METHODS section. In all cases, specificity of precipitation was determined by comparing the precipitates of homologous antisera, precipitates of homologous antisera competed with unlabeled purified AEG, and precipitates of heterologous antisera (anti-rat transferrin). Immunoprecipitates of translated proteins from caput plus corpus and from cauda epididymis were run on 10% SDS-PAGE in 4.0 M urea (FIGURE 2). Specific precipitation of AEG translation products from both caput and corpus (FIGURE 2, lane B) and cauda (FIGURE 2, lane F) translation corresponded to a minor band found at 29,000–30,000 MW in FIGURE 2, lanes A and E. The immunoprecipitated protein was 7–10% smaller in apparent molecular weight than purified AEG standard. Since AEG contains 7% carbohydrate, this difference is probably due to a lack of glycosylation in this translation system. Proteins translated from initial segment poly(A)RNA were immunoprecipitated in like manner and a minor band with an apparent molecular weight 7–10% smaller than purified AEG was observed (data not shown).

Quantitation of the immunoprecipitates was hindered by fluctuation in background levels. Values for the initial segment ranged from background to 0.09%, while those for caput plus corpus and cauda ranged from 0.29 to 1.4%, and 1.1% to 3.5%, respectively. However, the comparisons seen in FIGURE 2 clearly indicate the translation of AEG from mRNA of caput plus corpus and from cauda.

Previous studies by Lea et al.[25] have shown that immunoreactive AEG is not detected in the first portion of the epididymis, which would include a portion of the anatomical initial segment. Several investigators[21,31,40] have shown that synthesis of AEG in vitro is not detected in tissue from the initial segment.

DISCUSSION

In this study, we have examined the patterns of labeled proteins produced when poly(A)RNA from different segments of the rat epididymis was translated in an mRNA-dependent cell-free translation system. Electrophoresis of labeled proteins permitted the identification of bands either unique to or in common with the segments examined.

Initial segment–enriched poly(A)RNA coded for no less than six abundant peptides that were unique to the initial segment. Electrophoretic mobilities of these six peptides indicated apparent molecular weights of 50,000, 35,000, 23,000, 17,500, 16,500, and 15,000. The 23,000 MW peptide may correspond to a unique initial segment protein purified by Jones et al.[21] Expression of the 23,000 MW protein was dependent on factors in testicular fluid.[21]

The pattern of translation of caput plus corpus poly(A)RNA was especially interesting when contrasted with that obtained from initial segment. In the caput, a major 20,000 MW translation product corresponded with an abundant translation product of caput poly(A)RNA synthesized in a rabbit reticulocyte lysate by D'Agostino et al.[39] They further demonstrated that this 20,000 MW protein was processed in minced caput tissue and secreted as glycoproteins of 19,000 and 18,500 MW, which were caput specific and androgen dependent. These correspond to proteins B and C of Cameo and Blaquier,[18,40] and of proteins II and III of Jones et al.[21] Hamilton[41] has shown that α-lactalbumin activity isolated from rat epididymis migrates as 18,000–19,000 MW bands on SDS gels. He has suggested that rete testis fluid galactosyltransferase is secreted by Sertoli cells while the regulator protein α-lactalbumin, is synthesized and secreted by the epididymis.

In cauda epididymis the 47,000 MW protein may correspond to a basic (pI 7.2) caudal protein of similar molecular weight identified by Jones *et al.*[21] and found to be highly androgen dependent.

Several of the major proteins synthesized in this cell-free system are similar in size to major proteins secreted *in vitro* by tubules isolated from diffferent regions of the epididymis.[31] One difference, however, is the relative abundance of AEG. In contrast to our cell-free translations of total poly(A)RNA in which AEG is a relatively minor product, AEG is a relatively major protein secreted *in vitro* by tubular segments from corpus and cauda.[31]

A protein that appears similar to AEG had been partially purified by Garberi *et al.*[20] Their protein D resembles AEG with respect to its isoelectric point, gel filtration radius, and ability to bind to sperm. Brooks and Higgins[40,42] have separated proteins D and E and have suggested that protein D and AEG are identical. Incubation of minced epididymal segments with [35S]methionine indicated that protein D is synthesized from caput to cauda but not in initial segment. A glycoprotein extracted from epididymal sperm by Fournier-Delpech *et al.*[10] may also prove to be identical to AEG. Jones and co-workers[15] using the galactose-oxidase sodium boro[3H]hydride method, labeled membrane-associated proteins on sperm extracted by micropuncture from different regions of the epididymis. They found that the major glycoprotein on testicular sperm is 110,000 MW. As sperm pass through the caput and corpus, labeling of this protein disappears and is replaced by a 32,000 MW protein thought to be AEG. Recent studies by DePhilip *et al.*[31] have shown that AEG synthesis and secretion is higher in principal cells cultured from corpus than from the caput. Thus, AEG is secreted in large amounts and is inserted into or adsorbed onto the sperm plasma membrane in the region where sperm maturation is taking place. Because of the positive correlation between the amount of AEG bound and the fertilizing capacity of sperm as they reach the distal corpus, AEG may play a role in fertilization, perhaps in cellular recognition or in the acrosome reaction.

The marked differences in the translation products of epididymal segments imply an exquisite and finely tuned control of the genes for these products.

SUMMARY

Different proteins are secreted by the various regions of rat epididymis. We have examined the messenger RNA dependence of this varied gene expression by cell-free translation of poly(A)RNA extracts from initial segment, caput plus corpus, and cauda. Labeled translation products were analyzed by polyacrylamide gel electrophoresis under denaturing conditions. Poly(A)RNA from initial segment coded for several unique bands of labeled protein, including a 23,000 MW protein that may correspond to an initial segment protein reported previously to be regulated by testicular fluid factors.[21] Messenger RNA encoding 20,000 MW protein believed to be α-lactalbumin,[41] was most abundant in caput but also present in initial segment. Acidic epididymal glycoprotein (AEG) was identified previously by immunoperoxidase staining in epithelial cells of caput, corpus, and cauda.[25] AEG was not readily identified on electrophoresis of total translated proteins, but when concentrated by immunoprecipitation with purified AEG antibody prior to electrophoresis, AEG appeared in both caput plus corpus, and in cauda poly(A)RNA translations.

REFERENCES

1. BEDFORD, J. M. 1963. Changes in the electrophoretic properties of the rabbit spermatozoa during passage through the epididymis. Nature **200:** 1178–1180.
2. HAMILTON, D. W. 1975. Structure and function of the epithelium lining the ductuli efferentes, ductus epididymis and ductus deferens in the rat. *In* Handbook of Physiology. Endocrinology. Vol. 5. Male Reproductive System. D. W. Hamilton & R. O. Greep, Eds.: 259–301. American Physiological Society. Bethesda, MD.
3. ORGEBIN-CRIST, M. C., B. J. DANZO & J. DAVIES. 1975. Endocrine control of the development and maintenance of sperm fertilizing ability in the epididymis. *In* Handbook of Physiology. Endocrinology. Vol. 5. Male Reproductive System. D. W. Hamilton & R. O. Greep, Eds.: 319–338. American Physiological Society. Bethesda, MD.
4. BARKER, L. D. S. & R. P. AMANN. 1971. Epididymal physiology II immunofluorescence analyses of epithelial secretion and absorption, and of bovine sperm maturation. J. Reprod. Fert. **26:** 319–332.
5. JOHNSON, W. L. & A. G. HUNTER. 1972. Immunofluorescence evaluation of the male rabbit reproductive tract for sites of secretion and absorption of seminal antigens. Biol. Reprod. **6:** 13–22.
6. KILLIAN, G. J., R. P. AMANN & R. H. HAMMERSTEDT. 1973. Immuno-electrophoretic characterization of fluid and sperm entering and leaving bovine epididymis. Biol. Reprod. **9:** 489–499.
7. SCHELLPFEFFER, D. A. & A. G. HUNTER. 1976. Specific proteins of the male reproduction tract. *In* Regulatory Mechanisms of Male Reproductive Physiology. C. H. Spilman, T. J. Lobl & K. T. Kirton, Eds.: 115–132. Excerpta Medica. Amsterdam.
8. HAMMERSTEDT, R. H., A. D. KEITH, D. HAY, N. DELUCA & R. P. AMANN. 1979. Changes in ram sperm membranes during epididymal transit. Arch. Biochem. Biophys. **196:** 7–12.
9. EDELMAN, G. M. & C. F. MILLETTE. 1971. Molecular probes of spermatozoan structures. Proc. Natl. Acad. Sci. USA **68:** 2436–2440.
10. FOURNIER-DELPECH, S., B. J. DANZO & M. C. ORGEBIN-CRIST. 1977. Extraction of concanavalin A affinity material from rat testicular and epididymal spermatozoa. Anal. Biol. Anim. Biochim. Biophys. **17:** 207–213.
11. NICOLSON, G. L., N. USUI, R. YANAGIMACHI, H. YANAGIMACHI & J. R. SMITH. 1977. Lectin binding sites on the plasma membranes of rabbit spermatozoa. Changes in surface receptors during epididymal maturation and after ejaculation. J. Cell Biol. **74:** 950–962.
12. OLSON, G. E. & B. DANZO. 1981. Surface changes in rat spermatozoa during epididymal transit. Biol. Reprod. **24:** 431–443.
13. LAVON, U., R. VOLCANI & D. DANON. 1971. The proteins of bovine spermatozoa from caput and cauda epididymis. J. Reprod. Fert. **24:** 219–232.
14. FOURNIER-DELPECH, S., F. BAYARD & C. BOULARD. 1973. Contribution a l'etude de la maturation du sperme Etude d'une proteine acide de l'epididyme chez la rat. Dependence androgene, relation avec l'acide sialique. Biol. C. R. **167:** 1989–2000.
15. JONES, R., C. PHALPRAMOOL, B. SETCHELL & C. R. BROWN. 1981 Labelling of membrane glycoproteins on rat spermatozoa collected from different regions of the epididymis. Biochem. J. **200:** 457–460.
16. KOHANE, A. C., M. S. CAMEO, L. PINEIRO, J. C. GARBERI & J. A. BLAQUIER. 1980. Distribution and site of production of specific proteins in the rat epididymis. Biol. Reprod. **23:** 181–187.
17. ORGEBIN-CRIST, M. S. & N. JAHAD. 1978. Maturation of rabbit epididymal spermatozoa in organ culture-inhibition by antiandrogens and inhibitors of ribonucleic acid and protein synthesis. Endocrinology **103:** 46–53.
18. CAMEO, M. S. & J. A. BLAQUIER. 1976. Androgen-controlled specific proteins in rat epididymis. J. Endocrinol. **69:** 47–55.
19. FLICKINGER, C. J. 1981. Regional differences in synthesis, intracellular transport, and secretion of protein in the mouse epididymis. Biol. Reprod. **25:** 871–883.

20. GARBERI, J. C., A. C. KOHANE, M. S. CAMEO & J. A. BLAQUIER. 1979. Isolation and characterization of specific rat epididymal proteins. Mol. Cell. Endocr. **13:** 73–82.
21. JONES, R., C. R. BROWN, K. I. VON GLOS & M. G. PARKER. 1980. Hormonal regulation of protein synthesis in the rat epididymis. Characterization of androgen-dependent and testicular fluid-dependent proteins. Biochem. J. **188:** 667–676.
22. JONES, R., K. I. VON GLOS & C. R. BROWN. 1981. Characterization of hormonally regulated secretory proteins from the caput epididymis of the rabbit. Biochem. J. **196:** 105–114.
23. KLEINFELTER, G. R., R. P. AMANN & R. H. HAMMERSTEDT. 1982. Culture of principal cells from the rat caput epididymis. Biol. Reprod. **26:** 885–901.
24. KOPECNY, V. & V. PECH. 1977. An autoradiographic study of macromolecular synthesis in the epithelium of the ductus epididymis in the mouse. Histochemistry **50:** 229–238.
25. LEA, O. A., P. PETRUSZ & F. S. FRENCH. 1978. Purification and localization of acid epididymal glycoprotein (AEG): A sperm coating protein secreted by the rat epididymis. Int. J. Andro. Suppl **2:** 592–605.
26. MOORE, H. D. M. 1980. Localization of specific glycoproteins secreted by the rabbit and hamster epididymis. Biol. Reprod. **22:** 705–718.
27. ACOTT, T. C. & D. D. HOSKINS. 1981. Bovine sperm forward motility protein: Binding to epididymal spermatozoa. Biol. Reprod. **24:** 234–240.
28. LEA, O. A. & F. S. FRENCH. 1981. Characterization of an acid glycoprotein secreted by principal cells of the rat epididymis. Biochim. Biophys. Acta **668:** 370–376.
29. KIERSZENBAUM, A. L., O. A. LEA, P. PETRUSZ, F. S. FRENCH & L. L. TRES. 1981. Isolation, culture and immunocytological characterization of epididymal epithelial cells from pubertal and adult rats. Proc. Natl. Acad. Sci. USA **78:** 1675–1679.
30. KIERSZENBAUM, A. L., P. PETRUSZ, O. A. LEA, F. S. FRENCH & L. L. TRES. 1981. Acidic epididymal glycoprotein in primary epithelial cell cultures of caput, corpus and cauda epididymis. J. Cell Biol. **91:** 190a.
31. DEPHILIP, R. M., L. L. TRES & A. L. KIERSZENBAUM. 1984. Secretory proteins in short-term incubated tubular segments and epithelial cell cultures of rat epididymis. J. Reprod. Fertility. (In press.)
32. MURPHY, E. C. & R. B. ARLINGHAUS. 1978. Cell-free synthesis of Rauscher murine leukemia virus "gag" and "gag-pol" precursor polyproteins from virion 35S RNA in a mRNA dependent translation system from mouse tissue culture cells. Virology **86:** 329.
33. BROOKS, D. W., D. W. HAMILTON & A. H. MALLEK. 1974. Anatomical segments of the rat epididymis. J. Reprod. Fertility **36:** 141–160.
34. DEELEY, R. G., J. I. GORDON, A. T. H. BURNS, K. P. MULLINIX, M. BINA-STEIN & R. F. GOLDBERGER. 1977. Primary activation of the vitellogenin gene in the rooster. J. Biol. Chem. **252:** 8310.
35. AVIV, H. & P. LEDER. 1972. Purification of biologically active globin messenger RNA by chromatography on oligo thymidylic acid-cellulose. Proc. Natl. Acad. Sci. USA **69:** 1408.
36. MURPHY, E. C., D. CAMPOSE & R. B. ARLINGHAUS. 1979. Cell-free synthesis of Rauscher murine leukemia virus "gag" and "env" gene products from separate cellular mRNA species. Virology **93:** 293.
37. EAST, J. L., L. S. NELL, J. E. KNESEK, J. C. CHAN & L. DROSCHOWSKI 1977. Nucleotide sequence homology of mammalian RNA tumor viruses. *In* Advances in Comparative Leukemia Research. P. Bentvelsen, J. Hilgers & D. S. Yohn, Eds.: 141–143. Elsevier/North-Holland Biomedical Press. New York.
38. WILSON, E. M., D. H. VISKOCHIL, R. J. BARTLETT, O. A. LEA, C. M. NOYES, P. PETRUSZ, D. W. STAFFORD & F. S. FRENCH. 1981. Model systems for studies on androgen dependent gene expression in the rat prostate. *In* The Prostatic Cell: Structure and Function. G. P. Murphy, A. A. Sandberg & J. P. Karr, Eds.: 351–380. Alan R. Liss, Inc. New York.
39. D'AGOSTINO A., R. JONES, R. WHITE & M. G. PARKER. 1980. Androgenic regulation of messenger RNA in rat epididymis. Biochem. J. **190:** 505–512.

40. BROOKS, D. E. & S. J. HIGGINS. 1980. Characterization and androgen-dependence of proteins associated with luminal fluid and spermatozoa in rat epididymis. J. Reprod. Fertility 59: 363–375.
41. HAMILTON, D. W. 1981. Evidence for α-lactalbumin-like activity in reproductive tract fluids of the male rat. Biol. Reprod. 25: 385–392.
42. BROOKS, D. E. 1981. Secretion of proteins and glycoproteins by the rat epididymis: Regional differences, androgen-dependence, and effects of protease inhibitor, procaine and tunicamycin. Biol. Reprod. 25: 1099–1117.

Molecular Properties of the Androgen Receptor in Rat Ventral Prostate[a]

DONALD J. TINDALL, CHING H. CHANG, THOMAS J. LOBL,[b] and DAVID R. ROWLEY

Department of Cell Biology
Baylor College of Medicine
Houston, Texas

[b]The Upjohn Company
Kalamazoo, Michigan 49001

INTRODUCTION

Receptor proteins are essential for the biological function of androgens in male accessory sex organs.[1-3] By defining the molecular properties of these proteins, we further our understanding of the mechanism by which receptors mediate biological events within target tissues. Recently, we developed a procedure to purify an androgen receptor from steer seminal vesicle to apparent homogeneity as determined by sodium dodecyl sulfate gel electrophoresis.[4] This procedure combined two techniques, differential DNA chromatography and steroid affinity chromatography, which had been used for purifying other steroid hormone receptors.[5-10] Because the rat prostate has been one of the most widely studied male accessory glands,[11-16] the purification of the prostate receptor would represent an important step in our efforts to understand the mechanism of androgen action in this target tissue. This report describes the purification of the androgen receptor from rat ventral prostate cytosol and the characterization of a number of its physicochemical and steroid binding properties.

PURIFICATION OF THE RECEPTOR

The rat ventral prostate contains many proteolytic enzymes. Therefore, before any progress could be made in purifying the androgen receptor it was first necessary to stabilize the receptor against proteolytic degradation. FIGURE 1 shows the effects of leupeptin, a specific inhibitor of serine and sulfhydryl proteases, in preserving a large molecular weight component of the receptor protein. In the absence of leupeptin (FIGURE 1A), binding activity eluted from an agarose A-1.5 m column as small molecular weight species immediately in front of the unbound steroid (Vi). These small molecular weight species probably represent proteolytic fragments of the receptor protein. Leupeptin (10 μg/ml) prevented this proteolysis, and the receptor eluted as a single peak of binding activity with a Stoke's radius of 42 Å (FIGURE 1B). Thus, we were able to prevent most of the proteolytic

[a] This research was supported in part by grants HD-12788 and CA-32387, from the National Institutes of Health. D. J. T. is the recipient of a Research Career Development Award (HD-00318) from the National Institutes of Health. C. H. C. is the recipient of a Postdoctoral Fellowship from the Muscular Dystrophy Association. D. R. R. is the recipient of a Postdoctoral Fellowship from the National Institutes of Health.

cleavage of the receptor molecule by.including leupeptin in the homogenization buffer.

Two affinity resins containing either calf thymus DNA or testosterone 17β-hemisuccinate were tested for the receptor purification. First, a testosterone 17β-hemisuccinate affinity resin was synthesized and tested for its ability to retain the androgen receptor. Saturation analysis revealed that the resin had a capacity of 10 pmol of androgen receptor per ml of packed resin. The dissociation constant of the receptor-resin complex obtained by this analysis was 2.5 nM (FIGURE 2), which was identical to the dissociation constant of the [³H]testosterone-receptor complex (2.5 nM) obtained by Scatchard analysis. Moreover, the receptor could be eluted specifically from the resin with testosterone and 5α-dihydrotestosterone but not with progesterone, estradiol-17β, or cortisol (TABLE 1). These findings indicate that the receptor was bound to the affinity resin via the hormone binding site.

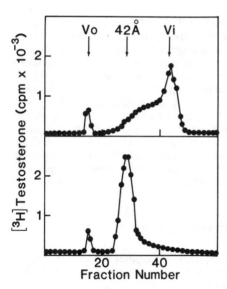

FIGURE 1. Effect of leupeptin on gel filtration profile of the androgen receptor. Rat ventral prostates from 24 hr castrated rats were homogenized in 50 mM Tris-HCl buffer (pH 7.4 at 22°C) containing 1.5 mM EDTA, 1.5 mM dithiothreitol, and 20% glycerol either in the absence (*upper panel*) or presence (*lower panel*) of 10 μg/ml leupeptin. After incubation with 16 nM [³H]dihydrotestosterone for 4 hr at 4°C and charcoal treatment, the samples were applied to an agarose A-1.5 m column (1.8 × 50 cm) pre-equilibrated with buffer containing 0.4 M KCl. Vo refers to the void volume and Vi refers to the volume required to elute the unbound steroid.

One of the hallmarks of steroid receptor proteins is their ability to be transformed to a state in which they will bind to polyanionic resins such as DNA- or phosphocellulose. We therefore tested the prostate receptor for this transforming property. FIGURE 3A demonstrates that very little receptor (~10–20%) bound to phosphocellulose prior to transformation. However, after transformation by heat treatment at 22°C for 30 min, more than 80% of the receptor was bound to the polyanionic resin (FIGURE 3B). This unique property of the receptor has been utilized as a powerful purification step, whereby an initial DNA-Sepharose column was used to remove polyanionic binding proteins prior to receptor transformation, and then a second DNA-Sepharose column was used to separate receptor from non-polyanionic binding of proteins after transformation.

FIGURE 2. Lineweaver-Burk plot of receptor-affinity resin interaction. Prostate cytosol was precipitated with 40% ammonium sulfate and the pellet was resuspended in one-sixth the original volume of buffer. Increasing amounts of receptor in a constant volume of 3 ml were incubated with 0.5 ml of testosterone-17β-hemisuccinyl-3,3'-diamino-dipropylamine-Sepharose 4B affinity resin for 2 hr at 4°C. The resin was removed by centrifugation and 0.25 ml aliquots were labeled with 16 nM [³H]dihydrotestosterone ± 100-fold excess dihydrotestosterone. The amount of specific binding activity remaining in solution was determined by charcoal adsorption assay. Lineweaver-Burk plot analysis was used to calculate the binding kinetics of the receptor protein-affinity resin interaction (K_d = 2.5 nM, binding capacity = 10 pmol receptor/ml packed resin).

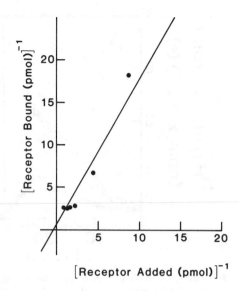

Another unique property of the androgen receptor that was used in its purification was its high affinity for pyridoxal 5'-phosphate. FIGURE 4 demonstrates this property of the prostate receptor. Transformed receptor was applied to a DNA-Sepharose column and then eluted with a gradient of pyridoxal 5'-phosphate (0–20 mM). A major peak of receptor binding activity eluted from the column with 10 mM pyridoxal 5'-phosphate. Very little protein co-eluted at this concentration of pyridoxal 5'-phosphate, whereas the majority of proteins were eluted with 1.0 M NaCl following the pyridoxal phosphate gradient. A small amount of androgen binding activity eluted with the salt wash.

TABLE 1. Steroid Specificity of Receptor Elution from Affinity Resin

Steroid	Concentration[a] (μM)	Receptor Eluted[b] (%)
Testosterone	345.0	24
	34.5	6
	3.4	4
	0.3	<3
Progesterone	345.0	<1
Estradiol-17β	345.0	<1
Cortisol	345.0	<1

[a] A partially purified receptor preparation was incubated with 17β-hemisuccinyl-3,3'-diaminodipropylamine-Sepharose 4B affinity resin for 75 min at 0°C. After thoroughly washing the resin with buffer the receptor was eluted from the resin with the indicated concentration of steroid.

[b] Receptor eluted indicates the percent of receptor eluted relative to specific binding activity applied to the resin.

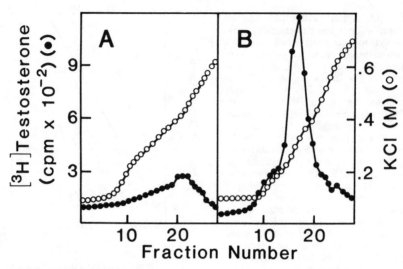

FIGURE 3. Transformation of receptor to polyanionic binding state. Cytosol from rat ventral prostate was incubated with 16 nM [³H]dihydrotestosterone for 4 hr at 0°C and aliquots were either (A) maintained at 0°C or (B) warmed at 22°C for 30 min before application to a phosphocellulose column. Closed circles represent radioactivity. Open circles represent the KCl gradient.

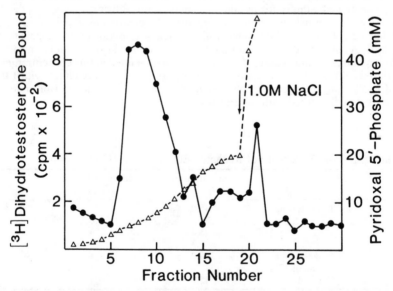

FIGURE 4. Pyridoxal 5'-phosphate elution of receptor from DNA-Sepharose. Cytosol from rat ventral prostate was incubated with 16 nM [³H]dihydrotestosterone for 4 hr at 0°C, precipitated with 40% ammonium sulfate, and applied to a DNA-Sepharose column. After washing with buffer the column was eluted with a gradient of pyridoxal 5'-phosphate (0–20 mM). Following this gradient the column was step-eluted with 1 M NaCl. The closed circles represent the radioactivity. The open triangles represent the ionic concentration.

Using a combination of the techniques characterized above, we developed the following protocol for purifying the androgen receptor from rat ventral prostate. Cytosol prepared from 38 g of rat ventral prostate was passed through a DNA column (DNA-I). This step resulted in a 0.8-fold purification and a 78% recovery of binding activity. The DNA-I flow-through fractions were precipitated with ammonium sulfate at 40% saturation. This step resulted in an overall purification of 16.5-fold and a recovery of approximately 100%. Ammonium sulfate precipitation also served to transform the receptor to a DNA-binding state. Testosterone

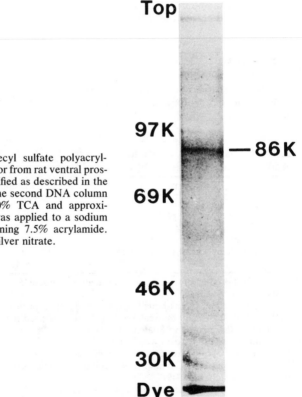

FIGURE 5. Sodium dodecyl sulfate polyacrylamide gel of purified receptor from rat ventral prostate. The receptor was purified as described in the text. Peak fractions from the second DNA column were precipitated with 10% TCA and approximately 0.5 μg of protein was applied to a sodium dodecyl sulfate gel containing 7.5% acrylamide. The gel was stained with silver nitrate.

affinity chromatography was next performed. The overall purification at this point was 460-fold, and a 30% yield of binding activity was obtained. Binding activity of the purified receptor at this stage of purification may have been underestimated due to the presence of a large excess of testosterone. The testosterone affinity resin eluate was applied to a second DNA column (DNA-II) and eluted with 10 mM pryidoxal 5'-phosphate in sodium borate buffer. This purification step resulted in an overall purification of 120,000-fold and a yield of 24%. This unusually large purification resulted from the selective elution of receptor by pyridoxal 5'-phosphate. In contrast, elution with sodium chloride resulted in only a 5,000-fold purification. Approximately 8 μg of purified protein was obtained by using this protocol. The purified receptor was stable for more than two weeks when stored at 2°C.

When the purified material was electrophoresed through a sodium dodecyl sulfate gel, a major polypeptide band corresponding to a molecular weight of 86,000 was observed by a silver nitrate staining procedure (FIGURE 5). Earlier studies by Bruchovsky et al.[17] demonstrated that the rat prostate androgen receptor in crude cytosol had a Stokes radius of 48 Å and a sedimentation coefficient of 4.4 S, which was calculated to be a molecular weight of 86,000. This would suggest that the 86,000 dalton protein band observed by sodium dodecyl sulfate gel electrophoresis is the receptor protein.

PHYSICOCHEMICAL PROPERTIES OF THE PURIFIED RECEPTOR

We examined the binding properties of the purified receptor. Scatchard analysis of the purified receptor revealed a high affinity binding component with a K_d of 6.5 nM (TABLE 2), which was slightly higher than that found for the receptor in

TABLE 2. Dissociation Constant, Isoelectric Point, and Molecular Size of the Androgen Receptor from Rat Prostate Cytosol

Property	Purified Receptor[a]	Cytosol
Dissociation constant (nM)	6.5[b]	3.6[c]
Isoelectric point (pI)[d]	6.3	6.5
Stokes radius (Å)[e]	42	42
Sedimentation coefficient (S)[e]	4.5	4.5
Molecular weight (M_r)[f]	85,000	85,000
Frictional ratio(f/f$_o$)[f]	1.41	1.41

[a] The final product of the receptor purification protocol, as described in the text, was used in these experiments.

[b] Purified receptor plus boiled cytosol, which had been proven to have no binding to [^{3}H]dihydrotestosterone by Scatchard analysis, was used for determining the dissociation constant by the method of Scatchard (1949).

[c] Ventral prostate cytosol was incubated with various concentrations of [^{3}H]dihydrotestosterone ± 100-fold excess unlabeled dihydrotestosterone for 4 h. Bound activity was determined by a charcoal binding assay and the dissociation constant was determined by the method of Scatchard (1949).

[d] Chromatofocusing, as described previously,[4] was used to determine the isoelectric point of the receptor.

[e] These parameters were determined as described in EXPERIMENTAL PROCEDURES (Chang et al.[4])

[f] Calculated from the combined values of Stokes radius and sedimentation coefficient.

cytosol (K_d = 3.6 nM) (TABLE 2). The higher K_d value may have resulted from the removal of some factor during the purification procedure since a similar change in K_d was noted following ammonium sulfate precipitation. Based on the receptor concentration (~0.14 nM) taken from the abscissa intercept of the Scatchard plot and a molecular weight of 86,000 determined from sodium dodecyl sulfate gel electrophoresis, it was estimated that there is 0.8 mole binding site per mole protein. These data suggest that there is one hormone binding site per receptor molecule. The specificity of steroid binding to the purified receptor was also studied. Testosterone exhibited less binding affinity (84%) than that of dihydrotestosterone (100%). Progesterone was not very effective in competing with [³H]dihydrotestosterone for receptor binding (24%). Even less affinity was found for 5α-androstane-3α17β-diol (17%), estradiol-17β (7%), and cortisol (1%). The relative affinities of each of these steroids for the purified receptor were similar to those for receptor in crude cytosol.

The molecular charge of the purified androgen receptor was studied. Purified receptor was labeled with 16 nM [³H]dihydrotestosterone by the steroid exchange assay procedure described in the EXPERIMENTAL PROCEDURES (Chang *et al.*[4]) and applied to a chromatofocusing column. The column was eluted with a buffer gradient of pH 7.4 to 4. The purified receptor eluted at a pH of 6.3, which is similar to that found for the receptor in crude cytosol (pI = 6.5) (TABLE 2). This isoelectric point was similar to that found for the purified receptor (6.6) from steer seminal vesicle cytosol (4). This is also in agreement with the findings of Mainwaring and Irving[13] that the heat-activated receptor or nuclear receptor complex has an isoelectric point of 6.5. In contrast, the unactivated androgen receptor has an isoelectric point of 5.8 as determined by sucrose gradient focusing[13] and polyacrylamide gel electrofocusing.[14] However, chromatofocusing of the activated or unactivated androgen receptors revealed no differences in pI values.

The M_r of 86,000 was verified by the hydrodynamic properties of the nondenatured receptor (TABLE 2). A major peak of binding activity with Stokes' radius of 42 Å was observed on a Sephacryl S-200 column and a major binding peak with sedimendation coefficient of 4.5 S was observed on a 5–20% glycerol gradient. These data were used to calculate a M_r of 85,000 and a frictional ratio of 1.41 for the nondenatured protein. Although 0.02% heparin was added to prevent extensive receptor aggregation, two small peaks of binding activity with higher Stokes' radii and sedimentation coefficients were also observed. Similar peaks of binding activity were observed by gel-exclusion high performance liquid chromatography. The receptor protein detected at A_{210} corresponded with the peaks of binding activity, suggesting that both the 85,000 dalton component and its aggregate forms were present under these experimental conditions. When the purified receptor was applied to a nondenaturing 5% polyacrylamide gel, we observed one band of silver-stained protein, which corresponded to one peak of radioactivity at the very top of a parallel lane. Addition of 0.01% heparin in the upper electrophoretic buffer did not facilitate the migration of the receptor into the gel. It therefore appeared that the purified receptor was aggregated under these conditions and could not enter the gel.

CHARACTERIZATION OF THE RECEPTOR WITH THE ELECTROPHILIC AFFINITY LABEL, DIHYDROTESTOSTERONE-17β-BROMOACETATE

The molecular weight of the receptor was examined by the use of affinity labeling techniques. Electrophilic steroid affinity labels have been used extensively to characterize a number of steroid-metabolizing enzymes[18–22] and more recently, steroid receptor proteins.[23–26] These compounds usually possess a good "leaving" group, such as a bromine atom or a methanesulfonyloxy (mesylate) moiety, that is

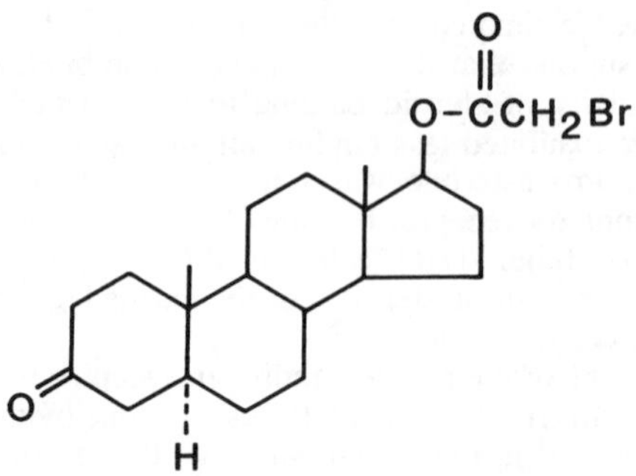

FIGURE 6. The molecular structure of 17β-[(bromoacetyl)oxy]-5α-androstan-3-one.

displaced, thus allowing the steroid to bind covalently to the active site of the protein. Preliminary results suggested that we could use an electrophilic affinity label, dihydrotestosterone-17β-bromoacetate, to covalently tag this receptor protein and identify its molecular weight by polyacrylamide gel electrophoresis under denaturing conditions. In order to more fully define the properties of this affinity label, we have further studied the conditions for this reaction. The chemical structure of 17β-[(bromoacetyl)oxy]-5α-androstan-3-one is shown in FIGURE 6.

The unlabeled dihydrotestosterone-17β-bromoacetate, which we synthesized, was pure as judged by nuclear magnetic resonance spectroscopy, mass spectroscopy, infrared spectroscopy, and elemental analysis. Chromatography of the tritium-labeled compound on a thin-layer plate showed only one peak of radioactivity, which co-migrated with the nonradioactive material. A similar protocol was used to synthesize the tritiated compound from [³H]dihydrotestosterone. A radiochromatogram of the thin layer chromatograph showed only one peak of radioactive material (FIGURE 7) that co-migrated with dihydrotestosterone-17β-bromoacetate.

BINDING OF DIHYDROTESTERONE-BROMOACETATE TO THE RECEPTOR

In order to determine whether the nonradioactive affinity label would compete with dihydrotestosterone for the active binding site on the androgen receptor, we incubated rat prostate cytosol with [³H]dihydrotestosterone and increasing concentrations of either dihydrotestosterone or dihydrotestosterone-17β-bromoacetate. Dihydrotestosterone competed with [³H]dihydrotestosterone for the binding site in a dose-dependent manner. Fifty percent of the binding activity was competed with 0.5 nM dihydrotestosterone (TABLE 3), which is consistent with the dissociation constant of the dihydrotestosterone-receptor complex.[27] Dihydrotestosterone-17β-bromoacetate also competed with [³H]dihydrotestosterone in a dose-dependent manner. Approximately 15 nM of dihydrotestosterone-17β-bromoacetate was required to compete for 50% of the binding sites (TABLE 3), indicating that dihydrotestosterone-17β-bromoacetate has less affinity than dihydrotestosterone for the binding site. Nonetheless, 100% of the [³H]dihydrotestosterone was displaced by the affinity label at higher concentrations (4 μM).

The time course of [³H]dihydrotestosterone-17β-bromoacetate binding in prostate cytosol was measured over a period of 3 hr at 0°C. Half-maximum binding was achieved at approximately 4 min after initial incubation. Maximum binding was obtained at approximately 60 min and thereafter a plateau was reached. The rate of association (K_a) during the initial 30 min was determined by the following equation[28]:

$$1 - \frac{[RS] \, (K_a \, [S] + K_i)}{R_1 \, K_a \, [S]} = e^{-(K_a[S]+K_d)t}$$

where [RS] is receptor-steroid complex concentration, [S] is steroid concentration, K_i is the rate of inactivation, R_t is total receptor sites determined from Scatchard analysis, K_d is the dissociation rate, and t is time. Both dissociation and inactivation of the steroid-receptor complex were assumed to be negligible during this time period, and therefore, K_d and K_i were made zero. The rate of association was 0.05×10^9 M^{-1}hr^{-1} for [³H]dihydrotestosterone-17β-bromoacetate and 0.3×10^9 M^{-1}hr^{-1} for [³H]dihydrotestosterone (TABLE 3). The faster rate of association with [³H]dihydrotestosterone than with [³H]dihydrotestosterone-17β-bromoacetate is consistent with the higher affinity of [³H]dihydrotestosterone for the receptor.

The steroid specificity of the [³H]dihydrotestosterone-17β-bromoacetate binding was investigated. Both dihydrotestosterone-17β-bromoacetate and dihydro-

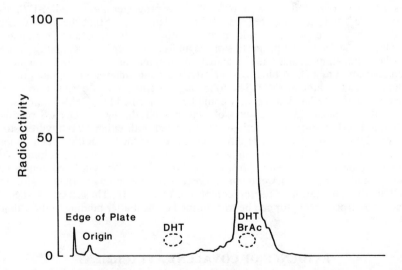

FIGURE 7. Thin layer chromatogram of 17β-[(bromoacetyl)oxy]-[1,2,4,5,6,7,16,17-³H₈]-5α-androstan-3-one. The radioactive compound was chromatographed over a silica gel thin layer plate, developed with hexane/ethyl acetate (6:4) and scanned for radioactivity. DHT, dihydrotestosterone; DHT-BrAc, 17β-[(bromoacetyl)oxy]-5α-androstan-3-one.

TABLE 3. Comparison of Receptor Properties after Labeling with either Dihydrotestosterone-17β-Bromoacetate or Dihydrotestosterone

Property	Dihydrotestosterone-17β-bromoacetate	Dihydrotestosterone
ID$_{50}$ (nM)[a]	15	0.5
Rate of association (M^{-1} hr^{-1})[b]	0.05	0.3
DNA binding[c]	+	+
Transformation[d]	+	+
Stokes radius (Å)[e]	42	42
Sedimentation coefficient (S)[f]		
high salt	4.5, 9.0	4.5
low salt	9.0	9.0
Molecular weight (M_r)[g]	85,000	85,000

[a] Concentration of unlabeled steroid required to compete for 50% of [³H]dihydrotestosterone binding to receptor.

[b] Determined from the time required to fill 50% of the binding sites with the radioactive ligand.

[c] Determined with DNA-Sepharose.

[d] Transformed to DNA binding state by precipitation with 40% ammonium sulfate.

[e] Determined by gel filtration over an agarose A-1.5 column in buffer containing 0.4 M KCl.

[f] Determined by sucrose gradient sedimentation in buffer containing 0.4 M KCl (High salt) or no KCl (Low salt).

[g] Calculated from the Stokes radius and sedimentation coefficient in high salt.

testosterone competed with 100% of the radioactive dihydrotestosterone-17β-bromoacetate for the receptor binding site at the concentrations tested. Testosterone competed less well (69%). Neither progesterone, estradiol-17β, nor cortisol were able to compete (< 1%). These data suggest that the affinity label binds to the active site of the androgen receptor in a structure-specific manner.

One of the functional properties of the androgen receptor is its ability to bind to DNA after transformation. The androgen receptor has been shown to undergo transformation to a DNA binding state after warming, ammonium sulfate precipitation, or salt treatment.[27,29,30] The following experiment was designed to determine if the affinity-labeled receptor could be transformed to a DNA binding state by heat treatment. Prostate cytosol was passed through a DNA-Sepharose column. The flow-through fractions were labeled with either [³H]dihydrotestosterone-17β-bromoacetate or [³H]dihydrotestosterone for 1 hr at 0°C. Each sample was incubated at 23°C for 30 min and applied to a DNA-Sepharose column. The bound radioactivity was eluted from the column. The affinity-labeled complexes were eluted from the DNA column in a region corresponding to the transformed [³H]dihydrotestosterone-receptor complexes (TABLE 3). These results suggest that the androgen receptor can be transformed by heat after binding to the affinity label.

EVIDENCE OF COVALENT ATTACHMENT

Two criteria were chosen to test whether covalent attachment existed between [³H]dihydrotestosterone-17β-bromoacetate and the androgen receptor: resistance to treatment with organic solvent and irreversible binding under nondenaturing conditions.

Experiments were performed to determine if specific covalent binding remains after trichloroacetate precipitation and treatment with organic solvents. One set of tubes containing either [³H]dihydrotestosterone-17β-bromoacetate or [³H]dihydrotestosterone were incubated at 0°C for 3 hr while another set was incubated at 0°C for 2.5 hr and then 23°C for 0.5 hr. Half of each set was subjected to a charcoal binding assay, while the other half was precipitated with trichloroacetate and then extracted with ether. Results from the charcoal binding assay of the nondenatured receptor revealed a 40% reduction in specific affinity-labeled binding activity after 0.5 hr incubation at 23°C. This reduction in specific binding was due to increased nonspecific binding during incubation. In contrast, when the same affinity labeled-receptor complexes were treated with trichloroacetate and ether, this additional 30 min incubation at 23°C increased the specific covalent binding by 31%. Control experiments using [³H]dihydrotestosterone exhibited a 16% increase in specific binding activity by the charcoal binding assay of the nondenatured receptor. However, only background radioactivity was observed after treatments with trichloroacetate and ether, indicating that no covalent bonds were formed between [³H]dihydrotestosterone and the receptor. Covalent binding was linear up to 64 nM of [³H]dihydrotestosterone-17β-bromoacetate indicating that binding of the affinity label was concentration dependent as well. This agrees with the binding study, which showed that approximately 4 μM of the affinity label is needed to saturate all the [³H]dihydrotestosterone binding sites.

If the [³H]dihydrotestosterone-17β-bromoacetate is binding covalently to the active site of the receptor molecule, then it should be possible to saturate the available binding sites with non-radioactive affinity label and prevent further binding of [³H]dihydrotestosterone to the receptor under exchange conditions. We therefore incubated a receptor preparation with 4 μM dihydrotestosterone-17β-bromoacetate overnight at 0°C and then attempted to exchange [³H]dihydrotestosterone onto the receptor at 30°C after removing excess unlabeled affinity label by charcoal treatment. It can be seen in TABLE 4 that little or no [³H]dihydrotestosterone could be exchanged onto the affinity-labeled receptor for up to 120 min at 30°C. In contrast, [³H]dihydrotestosterone could easily be exchanged at 30°C onto receptor in samples that had been labeled with saturating amounts of dihydrotes-

TABLE 4. Inhibition of [³H]dihydrotestosterone Binding to Receptor by Dihydrotestosterone-17β-bromoacetate

	Preincubation Conditions[a]	
Exchange Time (min)	Dihydrotestosterone-17β-Bromoacetate (cpm)	Dihydrotestosterone
0	310	300
30	250	1,200
60	275	1,800
120	350	2,300

[a] Prostate cytosol was precipitated with 40% ammonium sulfate. After centrifugation the pellet was resuspended in buffer and divided into two fractions: One fraction was treated with saturating amounts of either dihydrotestosterone or dihydrotestosterone-17β-bromoacetate at 0°C for 16 hr. At the end of the incubation, both groups were treated with dextran-coated charcoal and incubated with [³H]dihydrotestosterone at 30°C for the indicated times. Specifically bound activity was determined by charcoal binding assay and is listed as cpm.

tosterone overnight. Control samples maintained at 0°C exhibited no exchangeable binding activity, either when preincubated with the affinity label or dihydrotestosterone. These results add further evidence that dihydrotestosterone-17β-bromoacetate is binding covalently to the active site of the nondenatured receptor.

MOLECULAR PROPERTIES OF THE
DIHYDROTESTOSTERONE-17β-BROMOACETATE RECEPTOR
COMPLEX

In order to determine if the protein that bound the affinity label was in fact the androgen receptor, we examined a number of physicochemical properties of the binding complex and compared them with the dihydrotestosterone-receptor complex. First, the Stokes radius of the receptor was examined. Cytosol from rat prostate was precipitated with 40% ammonium sulfate, incubated with [³H]dihydrotestosterone-17β-bromoacetate, and applied to a gel filtration column. Each fraction was assayed for covalent binding by precipitation with trichloroacetate and extraction with methanol. Two major peaks of radioactivity were eluted from the column. One peak, which may represent an aggregated form of the receptor, co-eluted with blue dextran (void volume) and a second peak eluted at a Stokes radius of 42 Å (TABLE 3). The same Stokes radius was found when rat prostate cytosol was labeled with [³H]dihydrotestosterone.[30]

We next investigated the sedimentation properties of the affinity-labeled complex. A partially purified receptor preparation was labeled with [³H]dihydrotestosterone-17β-bromoacetate and centrifuged through a 2–20% sucrose gradient. The gradient tubes were fractionated, and each fraction was precipitated with trichloroacetate and extracted with methanol. The receptor complexes sedimented as a major component at 4.5 S and a minor component at 9 S (TABLE 3). Under these conditions, specific [³H]dihydrotestosterone-labeled receptor complexes sedimented as one peak at 4.5 S. When salt was removed from the gradient only one peak of activity sedimenting at 9 S was observed (TABLE 3). These hydrodynamic properties (Stokes radius and sedimentation coefficient) were used to calculate a M_r of 85,000 for the affinity-labeled receptor.

In order to confirm the M_r of the receptor we analyzed an affinity-labeled receptor preparation by gel electrophoresis under denaturing conditions. Due to the relatively low concentration of receptor binding sites in cytosol, a partially purified preparation was used for gel electrophoresis. The receptor preparation was equilibrated with [³H]dihydrotestosterone-17β-bromoacetate for 2.5 hr at 0°C and then warmed at 23°C for 30 min. The incubate was cooled in an ice bath (0°C) and precipitated with 10% trichloroacetate. The precipitant was resuspended in sample buffer and electrophoresed through a sodium dodecyl sulfate gel. After sequential washing of the gel with 40% methanol and 7% acetic acid, the gel was dried and subjected to fluorographic analysis and densitometer scanning. FIGURE 8A shows a peak of specific radioactivity corresponding to a M_r of 86,000 that was similar to the M_r (85,000) determined under non-denaturing conditions. Nonradioactive dihydrotestosterone-17β-bromoacetate competed for this binding component (FIGURE 8B). Several labeled bands of smaller M_r (45,000 to 30,000) were also observed. However, these bands were variable among preparations in both intensity and displacement by nonradioactive ligand. When [³H]dihydrotes-

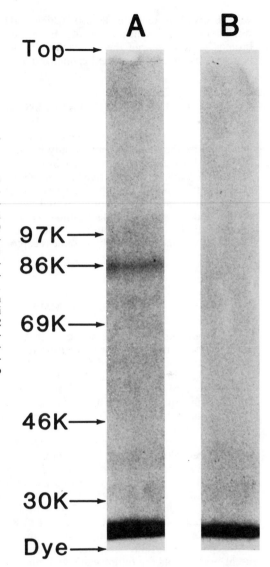

FIGURE 8. Sodium dodecyl sulfate polyacrylamide gel of affinity-labeled androgen receptor. A partially purified receptor preparation (approximately 5,000-fold purified) was labeled with 10 nM [^{3}H]dihydrotestosterone-17β-bromoacetate in either the absence (A) or presence (B) of 2 μM unlabeled dihydrotestosterone-17β-bromoacetate. The samples were precipitated with 10% TCA, resuspended in Laemmli sample buffer, heated at 90°C for 2 min and applied to a sodium dodecyl sulfate gel. After electrophoresis the gel was treated with EN-HANCE, dried, and exposed to X-ray film.

tosterone-17β-bromoacetate alone was electrophoresed in a similar gel, radioactivity was only observed at the dye front. When receptor preparations were incubated with [^{3}H]dihydrotestosterone, no radioactive bands were detected in the gel, indicating that this steroid dissociated when the receptor was denatured.

Previous studies[31,32] have shown that the androgen receptor in rat seminal vesicle has physicochemical properties that are similar to those of the rat prostate receptor. We therefore compared the binding proteins of seminal vesicle and prostate. A specific peak of radioactive dihydrotestosterone-17β-bromoacetate was observed at an M_r of 86,000, which corresponded to the same molecular weight species found in rat prostate. Excess unlabeled dihydrotestosterone-17β-bromoacetate displaced the radioactive ligand from this band. Specific bound activity was also found at the beginning and bottom of the running gel.

PHOTOAFFINITY LABELING OF THE RECEPTOR

The molecular weight of the receptor under denaturing conditions was further confirmed by the use of a photoaffinity label. We have reported previously that [³H]R1881 binds covalently to the androgen receptor from steer seminal vesicle.[4] In order to demonstrate selective binding of this ligand to the prostate receptor we used a partially purified receptor preparation. [³H]R1881 was incubated with this receptor preparation and photoactivated with ultraviolet irradiation. Following sodium dodecyl sulfate gel electrophoresis, fluorography demonstrated one band of radioactivity at 86,000 daltons.[30] When excess unlabeled R1881 together with [³H]R1881 was incubated with the same receptor preparation, binding activity was displaced.

SUMMARY

Results from these studies demonstrate that we have purified a protein from rat prostate cytosol that is similar to the β-protein (complex II) but different from the α-protein (complex I) reported by Liao et al.[1] The purified receptor was different from androgen binding protein (ABP) in that ABP has a faster dissociation rate (6 min), a lower pI value (4.6), and requires higher concentrations of ammonium sulfate for precipitation (40–50%) than the prostatic androgen receptor.[14,33,34] It is not likely that we have purified a serum sex-steroid binding protein since no such protein is found in rat serum.[3]

This report presents a rapid and efficient procedure for the purification of androgen receptor from rat ventral prostate. However, the present procedure only allowed us to obtain a limited quantity of purified receptor from each preparation. It is obvious that we need to scale up the purification of the receptor in order to study in detail its physicochemical properties and to produce monospecific antibodies against the protein. This work is in progress. In addition, we have demonstrated that two affinity labels can be used to bind covalently to the androgen receptor. Most importantly, these compounds can be used to characterize androgen receptors under both nondenaturing and denaturing conditions and represent useful tools for future work with androgen receptor proteins and androphilic proteins in general.

ACKNOWLEDGMENTS

We thank Dr. C. March for performing the gel-exclusion high performance liquid chromatography. We thank Mr. L. Graham and Mrs. T. Raiford for their assistance in the preparation of this manuscript.

REFERENCES

1. Liao, S., J. L. Tymoczko, E. Castaneda & T. Liang. 1975. Vitam. Horm. **33**: 297–317.
2. Mainwaring, W. I. P. 1978. *In* Receptors and Hormone Action II. B. W. O'Malley & L. Birnbaumer, Eds.: 105–120. Academic Press. New York.
3. Chan, L. & D. J. Tindall. 1981. *In* Pediatric Endocrinology. R. Collu, J. R. Ducharme & H. Guyda, Eds.: 63–97. Raven Press. New York.
4. Chang, C. H., D. R. Rowley, T. J. Lobl & D. J. Tindall. 1982. Biochemistry **21**: 4102–4109.
5. Coty, W. A., W. T. Schrader & B. W. O'Malley. 1979. J. Steroid Biochem. **10**: 1–12.
6. Wrange, Ö., J. Carlstedt-Duke & J.-Å Gustafsson. 1979. J. Biol. Chem. **254**: 9284–9290.
7. Westphal, H. M. & M. Beato. 1980. Eur. J. Biochem. **106**: 395–403.
8. Kuhn, R. W., W. T. Schrader, R. G. Smith & B. W. O'Malley. 1975. J. Biol. Chem. **250**: 4220–4228.
9. Govindan, M. V. & C. E. Sekeris. 1978. Eur. J. Biochem. **89**: 95–104.
10. Sica, V. & F. Bresciani. 1979. Biochemistry **18**: 2369–2378.
11. Baulieu, E.-E. & I. Jung. 1970. Biochem. Biophys. Res. Commun. **38**: 599–606.
12. Fang, S. & S. Liao. 1971. J. Biol. Chem. **246**: 16–24.
13. Mainwaring, W. I. P. & R. Irving. 1973. Biochem. J. **134**: 113–127.
14. Tindall, D. J., V. Hansson, W. S. McLean, E. M. Ritzen, S. N. Nayfeh & F. S. French. 1975. Mol. Cell. Endocrinol. **3**: 83–101.
15. Wilson, E. M. & F. S. French. 1976. J. Biol. Chem. **251**: 5620–5629.
16. Wilson, E. M. & F. S. French. 1979. J. Biol. Chem. **254**: 6310–6319.
17. Bruchovsky, N., P. S. Rennie & A. Vanson. 1975. Biochim. Biophys. Acta **394**: 248–266.
18. Ganguly, M. & J. C. Warren. 1971. J. Biol. Chem. **246**: 3646–3652.
19. Sweet, F., F. Arias & J. C. Warren. 1972. J. Biol. Chem. **247**: 3424–3433.
20. Strickler, R. C., F. Sweet & J. C. Warren. 1975. J. Biol. Chem. **250**: 7656–7662.
21. Sweet, F. & B. R. Samant. 1980. Biochemistry **19**: 978–986.
22. Thomas, J. L. & R. C. Strickler. 1983. J. Biol. Chem. **258**: 1587–1590.
23. Simons, S. S., Jr., R. E. Schleenbaker & H. J. Eisen. 1983. J. Biol. Chem. **258**: 2229–2238.
24. Katzenellenbogen, J. A., K. E. Carlson, D. F. Heiman, D. W. Robertson, L. L. Wei & B. S. Katzenellenbogen. 1983. J. Biol. Chem. **258**: 3487–3495.
25. Weisz, A., R. L. Buzard, D. Horn, M. P. Li, L. V. Dukerton & F. S. Markland, jr., 1983. J. Steroid Biochem. **18**: 375–382.
26. Holmes, S. D. & R. G. Smith. 1983. Biochemistry **22**: 1729–1734.
27. Liao, S., J. L. Tymoczko, E. Castaneda & T. Liang. 1975. Vitam. Horm. **33**: 297–317.
28. Nakahara, T. & L. Birnbaumer. 1974. J. Biol. Chem. **249**: 7886–7891.
29. Chang, C. H. & D. J. Tindall. 1983. Endocrinology **113**: 1486–1493.
30. Chang, C. H., D. R. Rowley & D. J. Tindall. 1983. Biochemistry. (In press.)
31. Wilson, E. M. & F. S. French. 1976. J. Biol. Chem. **251**: 5620–5629.
32. Wilson, E. M. & F. S. French. 1979. J. Biol. Chem. **254**: 6310–6319.
33. Tindall, D. J., D. A. Miller & A. R. Means. 1977. Endocrinology **101**: 13–23.
34. Tindall, D. J., G. R. Cunningham & A. R. Means. 1978. J. Biol. Chem. **253**: 166–169.

Modulation of Androgen Receptor Activity in the Rat Ventral Prostate

RICHARD A. HIIPAKKA and SHUTSUNG LIAO[a]

The University of Chicago
Ben May Laboratory for Cancer Research
Chicago, Illinois 60637

One of the major effects of androgens on a target tissue, such as the rat ventral prostate, is increased synthesis of specific proteins.[1-4] Several steps are believed to be necessary before an androgen can exert its effects. A hypothetical scheme representing this process is shown in FIGURE 1.

Testosterone, the major testicular androgen in blood, enters prostatic tissue and is reduced to 5α-dihydrotestosterone (DHT) by a 5α-steroid reductase.[5,6] Formation of DHT appears to be critical for prostatic development and function. A deficiency or defect in 5α-reductase leads to incomplete sexual differentiation, including abnormal prostatic development from the urogenital sinus.[7,8] Inhibitors of α-reductase, such as DMAA (17β-N,N-diethylcarbamoyl-4-methyl-4-aza-5α-androstan-3-one, FIGURE 2) block formation of DHT from testosterone and limit growth of the rat prostate.[9,10] Testosterone may be responsible for androgenic effects in tissues having low levels of 5α-reductase, such as muscle[11] and kidney[12] or high levels of testosterone, such as testis.[13] The development of certain androgen-regulated tissues, like the epididymis and seminal vesicle, is not impaired in some individuals who are deficient in 5α-reductase.[7,8] Testosterone therefore, may be the active androgen in some tissues without being converted to DHT.

DHT binds with high affinity and specificity to a protein (receptor) in prostate cells.[14,15] The importance of the receptor for DHT function is emphasized by the observations that antiandrogens (FIGURE 2) like cyproterone[16] and flutamide[17,18] compete with DHT for binding to the receptor and inhibit androgen-dependent effects. Also, hereditary defects that are characterized by a diminished or total absence of receptor binding activity result in an insensitivity to androgens.[8,12]

The ability of the receptor to bind DHT is regulated or influenced by various factors. When tissue from the rat ventral prostate is incubated with inhibitors or uncouplers of cellular energy production, such as cyanide, azide or 2,4-dinitrophenol, DHT binding to receptor is inhibited.[19] The energy state of the cell may affect steroid receptor modifications, such as protein phosphorylation, which has been proposed to regulate steroid binding activity of glucocorticoid[20] and estrogen[21] receptors. The steroid binding activity of androgen receptor is sensitive to low concentrations (10 μM) of certain metal ions. $ZnCl_2$, $CuSO_4$, $CdSO_4$, $HgCl_2$, and $AgNO_3$ inhibit androgen binding to unoccupied androgen receptor from rat ventral prostate. $CaCl_2$, $CoCl_2$, $MgCl_2$, and $MnCl_2$ are much less active or are not inhibitors at similar concentrations. Occupied receptor is less sensitive to the inhibitory effects of these metals.[22,23] Zn^{2+} is a competitive inhibitor of DHT binding and at a concentration of 10 μM inhibits androgen binding by 50%. Dithiothreitol and the metal chelator EDTA reverse the effects of these metals. A

---

[a] Address correspondence to S. L.

sulfhydryl group on the receptor, sensitive to metal ions, may be responsible for some of these effects. The receptor may also be a metalloprotein whose function is regulated by cellular metal ions, such as Zn^{2+}. Zn^{2+} also modifies the sedimentation properties of the androgen receptor complex from rat ventral prostate.[24]

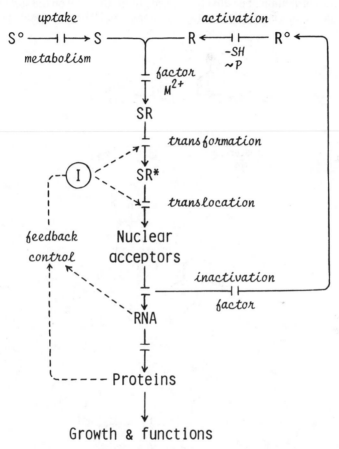

FIGURE 1. A hypothetical scheme describing the steps involved in recycling of androgen receptor of rat ventral prostate. A receptor protein ($R°$) is activated to a steroid binding form (R) by a step sensitive to the energy state of the cell (i.e., inhibited by respiratory poisons such as CN^-, N_3^-, and 2,4-dinitrophenol). The activated receptor (R) then binds an active androgen such as DHT (S), which is produced by the action of a 5α-reductase on testosterone ($S°$). The androgen-receptor complex is transformed and binds to nuclear acceptors. Interaction of androgen-receptor complex with chromatin leads to production of specific RNAs and ultimately proteins. RNA and protein induced by this mechanism may have a role in regulating the response to androgen.

After the DHT-receptor complex is formed changes in the complex take place (transformation or activation) that increase the affinity of the receptor for certain nuclear components (acceptor). The exact nature of the nuclear acceptor is unknown. DHT-receptor complex interacts with many nuclear components, such as the nuclear membrane,[25] non-histone proteins,[26-29] RNA and ribonucleoprotein particles,[30,31] nuclear matrix,[32,33] and DNA.[34,35] Many of these nuclear components may interact and provide structural and functional prerequisites for the response to steroids. Transformation of receptor may increase the number or change the distribution of positively charged groups (lysines) on the surface of the receptor promoting interactions with polyanions, like DNA. Pyridoxal phosphate,

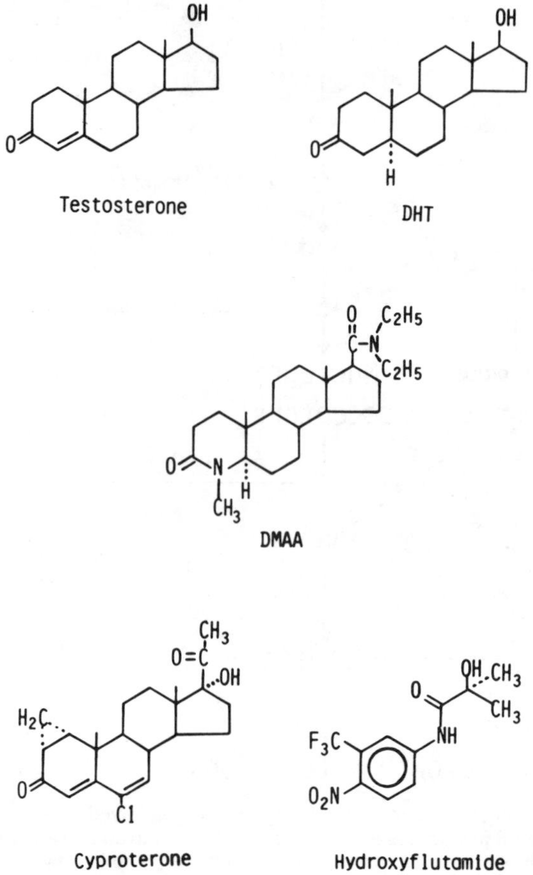

Testosterone

DHT

DMAA

Cyproterone

Hydroxyflutamide

FIGURE 2. Structures of androgens, antiandrogens, and 17β-N,N-diethylcarbamoyl-4-methyl-4-aza-5α-androstan-3-one (DMAA), an inhibitor of 5α-steroid reductase.

which modifies the ε-amino of lysine residues on proteins, blocks receptor binding to prostate nuclei.[36]

Transformation leads to a redistribution of receptor within the cell (translocation). After exposure to steroids the amount of receptor found in the cytosol fraction of tissue homogenates is decreased and the amount found in the nuclear fraction is increased compared to tissue not exposed to steroid. The location of these receptors before homogenization of the tissue may be altered upon destruction of the cell membrane and dilution of cell contents with buffer.[37] Therefore, some caution must be exercised when interpreting the apparent cytosol to nuclear translocation.[38]

The association of the androgen-receptor complex with the nuclear acceptor ultimately leads to enhanced transcription and increased production of certain proteins. How receptor enhances specific gene transcription is not clear. However, certain steroid receptors interact with potential regulatory sequences on genes regulated by steroid hormones.[39–41]

The fate of the androgen-receptor complex after stimulating gene transcription is unknown. There is some indication that steroid receptors may be degraded and thus, *de novo* synthesis of receptor required before the process can be reinitiated.[42,43] There is also evidence that steroid receptors may be recycled.[19,44] Recycling of the androgen receptor of the rat ventral prostate was observed using pulse-chase techniques in conjunction with inhibitors of cellular energy production.[19] These studies demonstrated an active recycling process for the androgen receptor even in the presence of saturating levels of steroid. The data were consistent with a slow release of the steroid-receptor complex ($t_{1/2} \sim 70$ min) from nuclei, followed by a rapid inactivation/reactivation process ($t_{1/2} \sim 2$ min), which was dependent upon the energy state of the cell. Reactivation of the receptor was achieved by removal of the inhibitors even in the presence of cycloheximide, which should inhibit *de novo* synthesis of receptor. Once reactivated to a steroid-binding form, the receptor would repeat the cycle upon combining with steroid.[19] The androgen-receptor complex was maintained at a constant level for at least two hours after exposure to steroid even in the absence of new protein synthesis. Early effects of androgens on RNA synthesis, therefore, do not require a loss of a major portion of cellular receptors as observed for certain estrogen receptors.[46]

The long half-life of the nuclear androgen receptor may reflect a complex process essential for the hormonal response. Such a process may involve interaction of the androgen-receptor complex with different nuclear components. An orderly sequence of events, involving more than the interaction of the androgen receptor with a few specific genes, may be required before all aspects of the hormonal response are complete.

The mechanism of release of androgen receptor from the nuclear acceptor has not been determined. Evidence for a mechanism based on dephosphorylation of the estrogen-receptor complex has been presented.[47] The possibility that certain steroid-induced gene products (RNA and/or protein) regulate the interaction of the steroid-receptor complex with the nuclear acceptor has also been investigated by our laboratory. In the rat ventral prostate, a subunit of a major androgen-induced protein can release the androgen-receptor complex bound to nuclei *in vitro*.[48] Whether this process occurs *in vivo* is not known; however, feedback inhibition is a common biological control mechanism.

We have characterized the interaction of the androgen-receptor complex of rat ventral prostate with RNA using competition studies based on DNA-cellulose chromatography, gradient centrifugation of phage DNA, and cell-free incubations with isolated prostate nuclei.[30] Only single-stranded polyribonucleotides of certain size and composition competed well with DNA for binding to androgen-receptor complex. Naturally occurring RNAs, such as mRNA and rRNA, were also active. However, the highest activity was found with synthetic polymers containing uracil and/or guanine. Polymers containing only adenine or cytosine were poor competitors. This specificity was maintained with heterologous systems, such as calf thymus DNA–cellulose and prostate androgen receptor as well

TABLE 1. Percent Inhibition of Binding of [³H]Dihydrotestosterone Receptor Complex

	DNA-Cellulose	Prostate Nuclei
Poly G	77	35
Poly U	54	25
Poly C	6	5
Poly A	6	5

All polymers were at a monomer concentration of 150 μM.

as with homologous systems, such as prostate nuclei and prostate androgen receptor. A significant difference in the result using these two systems was a requirement for higher concentrations of polyribonucleotides for inhibition of receptor binding to prostate nuclei (TABLE 1). The reason for this difference was not apparent but may reflect a higher affinity of the prostate androgen receptor for its nuclear acceptor than for calf thymus DNA.

Interaction of steroid-receptor complexes with RNA has been observed with many different classes of receptors. The association of rat liver glucocorticoid,[49] mouse kidney androgen,[50] and rat mammary tumor estrogen[51] receptors with synthetic polyribonucleotides had specificity similar to our studies with rat ventral prostate androgen receptor.[30] Also, treatment of estrogen[51,52] and glucocorticoid[52,53] receptors with ribonuclease increased DNA-cellulose binding activity. The binding of rat ventral prostate androgen receptor to the nuclear matrix of prostate nuclei,[32,33] a possible site of synthesis and processing of heterogeneous nuclear RNA,[54] may indicate a potential role for receptors in maturation of RNA. The interaction of steroid receptors with RNA *in vivo* may facilitate release of steroid-receptor complexes from nuclear acceptors (FIGURE 3). Binding of newly transcribed RNA to receptor may facilitate reuse of the DNA template. Continued association of receptor with newly transcribed RNA may also influence transport of RNA out of the nucleus. Although such a role has not been directly demonstrated, steroid receptors do interact with ribonucleoprotein particles.[31,55] Steroid receptors may also have a role in the utilization of RNA in the cytoplasm. Certain mRNAs are transcribed more efficiently than others[56]; receptors may promote such a selective process.

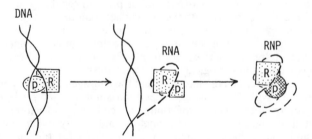

FIGURE 3. A scheme showing a possible role for RNA in receptor function. Receptor may bind to RNA after or during transcription of DNA. Removal of RNA makes the DNA template available for another round of synthesis. Continued association of receptor with RNA may facilitate maturation and utilization of RNA. R, steroid-receptor complexes and P, other protein complexes. Simplified from Liao and Fang.[57]

Interaction of androgen and other steroid receptors with certain RNAs may be used as a form of control. Receptors may bind with high affinity and specificity to RNA induced by the steroid-receptor complex. Once bound to the RNA, receptor would be unavailable for stimulation of specific gene transcription especially if the receptor accompanies RNA out of the nucleus. Only those receptors not bound to RNA or ribonucleoprotein particles would be available to interact with the nuclear acceptor.

REFERENCES

1. MEZZETTI, G., R. LOOR & S. LIAO. 1979. Biochem. J. **184:** 431–440.
2. HEYNS, W., B. PEETERS, J. MOUS, W. ROMBAUTS & P. DE MOOR. 1979. J. Steroid Biochem. **11:** 209–213.
3. PARKER, M. G., G. T. SCRACE & W. I. P. MAINWARING. 1978. Biochem. J. **170:** 115–121.
4. CHAMBERLIN, L. L., O. D. MPANIAS & T. Y. WANG. 1983. Biochemistry **22:** 3072–3077.
5. ANDERSON, K. M. & S. LIAO. 1968. Nature (London) **219:** 277–279.
6. BRUCHOVSKY, N. & J. D. WILSON. 1968. J. Biol. Chem. **243:** 2012–2021.
7. IMPERATO-MCGINLEY, J., L. GUERRO, T. GAUTIER & R. E. PETERSON. 1974. Science **186:** 1213–1215.
8. WILSON, J. D., J. E. GRIFFIN & F. W. GEORGE. 1980. Biol. Reprod. **22:** 9–17.
9. BROOKS, J. R., E. M. BAPTISTA, C. BERMAN, E. A. HAM, M. HICHENS, D. B. R. JOHNSTON, R. L. PRIMKA, G. H. RASMUSSON, G. F. REYNOLDS, S. M. SCHMITT & G. E. ARTH. 1981. Endocrinology **109:** 830–836.
10. LIANG, T. & C. E. HEISS. 1981. J. Biol. Chem. **256:** 7998–8005.
11. KREIG, M. & K. D. VOIGT. 1976. J. Steroid Biochem. **7:** 1005–1012.
12. BARDIN, C. W. & J. F. CATTERALL. 1981. Science **211:** 1285–1294.
13. BAKER, H. W. G., D. J. BAILEY, P. D. FEIL, L. S. JEFFERSON, R. J. SANTEN & C. W. BARDIN. 1977. Endocrinology **100:** 709–721.
14. FANG, S., K. M. ANDERSON & S. LIAO. 1969. J. Biol. Chem. **244:** 6584–6595.
15. MAINWARING, W. I. P. 1969. J. Endocrinol. **45:** 531–541.
16. FANG, S. & S. LIAO. 1969. Mol. Pharmacol. **5:** 428–431.
17. PEETS, E. A., M. F. HENSON & R. NERI. 1974. Endocrinology **94:** 532–540.
18. LIAO, S., D. K. HOWELL & T.-M. CHANG. 1974. Endocrinology **94:** 1205–1209.
19. ROSSINI, G. P. & S. LIAO. 1982. Biochem. J. **208:** 383–392.
20. SANDO, J. J., A. C. LaFOREST & W. B. PRATT. 1979. J. Biol. Chem. **254:** 4772–4778.
21. AURICCHIO, F., A. MIGLIACCIO, G. CASTORIA, S. LASTORIA & E. SCHIAVONE. 1981. Biochem. Biophys. Res. Commun. **101:** 1171–1178.
22. DONOVAN, M. P., L. G. SCHEIN & J. A. THOMAS. 1980. Mol. Pharmacol. **17:** 156–162.
23. LIAO, S., D. WITTE, K. SCHILLING & C. CHANG. 1984. J. Steroid Biochem. **20:** 11–17.
24. LIAO, S., J. L. TYMOCZKO, E. CASTANEDA & T. LIANG. 1975. Vitam. Horm. **33:** 297–317.
25. LEFEBVRE, Y. A. & Z. NOVOSAD. 1980. Biochem. J. **186:** 641–647.
26. MAINWARING, W. I. P., E. K. SYMES & S. J. HIGGINS. 1976. Biochem. J. **156:** 129–141.
27. WANG, T. Y. 1978. Biochim. Biophys. Acta **518:** 81–88.
28. KLYZSEJKO-STEFANOWICZ, L., J.-F. CHIU, Y.-H. TASI & L. S. HNILICA. 1976. Proc. Natl. Acad. Sci. USA **73:** 1954–1958.
29. TYMOCZKO, J. L. & S. LIAO. 1971. Biochim. Biophys. Acta **252:** 607–611.
30. LIAO, S., S. SMYTHE, J. L. TYMOCZKO, G. P. ROSSINI, C. CHEN & R. A. HIIPAKKA. 1980. J. Biol. Chem. **255:** 5545–5551.
31. LIAO, S., T. LIANG & J. L. TYMOCZKO. 1973. Nature (London) New Biol. **241:** 211–213.
32. BARRACK, E. R. 1983. Endocrinology **113:** 430–432.

33. BARRACK, E. R. & D. S. COFFEY. 1980. J. Biol. Chem. **255:** 7265–7275.
34. RENNIE, P. S. 1979. J. Biol. Chem. **254:** 3947–3952.
35. MAINWARING, W. I. P. & R. IRVING. 1973. Biochem. J. **134:** 113–127.
36. HIIPAKKA, R. A. & S. LIAO. 1980. J. Steroid Biochem. **12:** 841–846.
37. SHERIDAN, P. J., J. M. BUCHANAN, V. C. ANSELMO & P. M. MARTIN. 1979. Nature (London) **282:** 579–582.
38. JENSEN, E. V., G. L. GREENE, L. E. CLOSS, E. R. DESOMBRE & M. NADJI. 1983. Rec. Prog. Horm. Res. **38:** 1–40.
39. MULVIHILL, E. R., J. P. LEPENNEC & CHAMBON. 1982. Cell **28:** 621–632.
40. COMPTON, J. G., W. T. SCHRADER & B. W. O'MALLEY. 1983. Proc. Natl. Acad. Sci. USA **80:** 16–20.
41. PAYVAR, F., O WRANGE, J. CARLSTEDT-DUKE, S. OKRET, J. GUSTAFSSON & K. R. YAMAMOTO. 1981. Proc. Natl. Acad. Sci. USA **78:** 6628–6632.
42. BLONDEAU, J.-P., E.-E. BAULIEU & P. ROBEL. 1982. Endocrinology **110:** 1926–1932.
43. BAUDENDISTEL, L. J., M. F. RUH, E. M. NADEL & T. S. RUH. 1978. Acta Endocrinol. **89:** 599–611.
44. KASSIS, J. A. & J. GORSKI. 1981. J. Biol. Chem. **256:** 7378–7382.
45. LIAO, S., K. R. LEININGER, E. SAGHER & R. W. BARTON. 1965. Endocrinology **77:** 763–765.
46. HORWITZ, K. B. & W. L. MCGUIRE. 1980. J. Biol. Chem. **255:** 9699–9705.
47. AURICCHIO, F., A. MIGLIACCIO & A. ROTONDI. 1981. Biochem. J. **194:** 569–574.
48. SHYR, C. & S. LIAO. 1978. Proc. Natl. Acad. Sci. USA **75:** 5969–5973.
49. TYMOCZKO, J. L., J. SHAPIRO, D. J. SIMENSTAD & A. D. NISH. 1982. J. Steroid Biochem. **16:** 595–598.
50. LIN, S. & S. OHNO. 1982. Eur. J. Biochem. **124:** 283–287.
51. FELDMAN, M., J. KALLOS & V. P. HOLLANDER. 1981. J. Biol. Chem. **256:** 1145–1148.
52. CHONG, M. T. & M. E. LIPPMAN. 1982. J. Biol. Chem. **257:** 2996–3002.
53. TYMOCZKO, J. L. & M. M. PHILLIPS. 1983. Endocrinology **112:** 142–149.
54. CIEJEK, E. M., J. L. NORDSTROM, M.-J. TSAI & B. W. O'MALLEY. 1982. Biochemistry **21:** 4945–4953.
55. LIANG, T. & S. LIAO. 1974. J. Biol. Chem. **249:** 4671–4678.
56. HERSON, D., A. SCHMIDT, S. SEAL. A. MARCUS & L. VAN VOLTEN-DOTING. 1979. J. Biol. Chem. **254:** 8245–8249.
57. LIAO, S. & S. FANG. 1969. Vitam. Horm. **27:** 17–90.

Disorders of Androgen Receptor Function

JAMES E. GRIFFIN and JEAN D. WILSON

Department of Internal Medicine
The University of Texas Health Science Center at Dallas
Southwestern Medical School
Dallas, Texas 75235

INTRODUCTION

Resistance to androgen action was first recognized in the syndrome of testicular feminization.[1] Subsequently, additional syndromes of androgen resistance have been delineated, so that the phenotypic spectrum ranges from normal-appearing women with testicular feminization to otherwise normal men with infertility. This review will describe some aspects of normal androgen physiology, the clinical syndromes associated with disorders of the androgen receptor, and the studies of the nature of the abnormalities identified to date.

NORMAL ANDROGEN PHYSIOLOGY

Testosterone, formed by the testes under control of luteinizing hormone (LH) from the pituitary, is the principal androgen in the circulation. In peripheral tissues it can be converted to two types of active metabolites: 5α-dihydrotestosterone and 17β-estradiol (FIGURE 1).[2] Dihydrotestosterone formed from testosterone by the 5α-reductase enzyme mediates androgen action in many target tissues. Estradiol, formed from testosterone by the aromatase enzyme complex, acts in some instances in concert with androgens and in others has independent or opposite effects to those of androgens. The 5α-reduced metabolites are formed primarily in androgen target tissues (e.g. the prostate). Adipose tissue is the major site for extraglandular estrogen formation. In normal men about 85% of the estradiol formed each day is the result of extraglandular aromatization of androgen and only about 15% of estradiol production is directly secreted by the testes.[3] However, when plasma LH concentration is increased, direct secretion of estradiol by the testes increases.[4]

Inside target cells testosterone and dihydrotestosterone bind to the same high affinity androgen receptor in the cytosol (FIGURE 1). The hormone receptor complexes diffuse into the nuclei and interact with sites on the chromosomes to result in the generation of new messenger RNA and ultimately new protein synthesis in the cytoplasm of the cell.[5] The final result can be viewed as effecting the major functions of androgens in men: regulation of gonadotropin secretion by the hypothalamic-pituitary system, initiation and maintenance of spermatogenesis, formation of the male phenotype during sexual differentiation, and promotion of sexual maturation at puberty. The testosterone-receptor complex is thought to regulate gonadotropin secretion and the virilization of wolffian ducts during male sexual differentiation.[6] The dihydrotestosterone-receptor complex is responsible for external virilization during embryogenesis and most aspects of sexual maturation at puberty.[6] The hormonal control of spermatogenesis is not completely resolved. Initially, it was felt that testosterone was not converted to dihydrotestosterone in rodent testes and that testosterone thus controlled spermatogenesis. However, dihydrotestosterone is formed in human testes, and men with 5α-reductase deficiency have impaired spermatogenesis.[7] The reason that dihydrotestosterone formation is required for some androgen actions is not entirely clear; however, because testosterone binds less avidly to the receptor than does dihydrotestosterone, its formation may serve as a magnifier of androgen action.[8] The mechanisms by which estrogens act to augment or block androgen action are also unclear (FIGURE 1). In prostatic hyperplasia estrogens appear to enhance androgen action by increasing the level of androgen receptor,[9] whereas in the breast estrogens and androgens appear to be antagonists.[10]

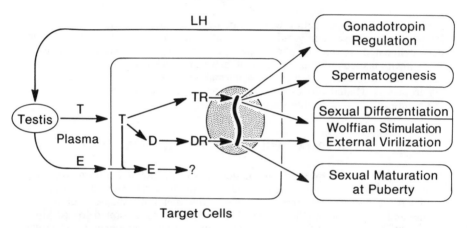

FIGURE 1. A schematic diagram of normal androgen physiology. LH, luteinizing hormone; T, testosterone; D, dihydrotestosterone; E, estradiol; R, androgen receptor. Major functions of androgen in men are shown on right with those mediated by testosterone-receptor complex (TR) and dihydrotestosterone-receptor complex (DR) indicated by arrows. (From Griffin & Wilson.[11] With permission from *New England Journal of Medicine*.)

CHARACTERISTICS OF ANDROGEN RESISTANCE SYNDROMES

The androgen resistance syndromes comprise one category of disorders of phenotypic sex in which 46, XY males with bilateral testes fail to develop as completely normal men. By definition, testosterone synthesis and mullerian regression are normal in androgen resistance, and the abnormality resides in some aspect of androgen action. These disorders were originally delineated by studying patients with male pseudohermaphroditism, i.e. defective virilization of the external genitalia in individuals with bilateral testes. Subsequently, men with infertility alone as the clinical manifestation of androgen resistance have been identified, extending the clinical spectrum recognized. The molecular defects responsible for androgen resistance may occur at any of the three major sites in the pathway of androgen action: abnormalities in the 5α-reductase, defects in the androgen receptor, or abnormalities in the subsequent phases of androgen action (so-called receptor-positive resistance).[11]

RECEPTOR DISORDERS

Disorders of the androgen receptor may result in several distinct phenotypes. Despite differences in clinical presentation and molecular pathology these disorders are similar in regard to endocrinology, genetics, and basic pathophysiology. The major clinical features of each of the four disorders will be followed by a combined discussion of the similar endocrinology and pathophysiology.

Complete Testicular Feminization

Complete testicular feminization is an X-linked recessive disorder characterized by a uniform clinical presentation.[1] The phenotype is that of a normal woman except for decreased or absent axillary and pubic hair. Breast development and distribution of body fat are truly feminine. The external genitalia are unambiguously female, and the clitoris is normal. The vagina is short and blind-ending. Internal genitalia are absent except for the testes which may be in the abdomen, the inguinal canal, or the labia majora. Histology of the testes reveals incomplete or absent spermatogenesis and normal or hyperplastic Leydig cells. Patients either come to medical attention because of an inguinal hernia or primary amenorrhea. There is often a family history of similarly affected family members, compatible with X-linkage, but about a third of patients have negative family histories and are presumed to represent new mutations.

Incomplete Testicular Feminization

Incomplete testicular feminization is about a tenth as common as the complete form and resembles it except that there is some ambiguity of the external genitalia, normal pubic hair, and some virilization as well as feminization at the time of expected puberty.[1] There is usually partial fusion of the labioscrotal folds and some degree of clitoromegaly. The vagina is short and blind-ending. In contrast to the complete form of the disorder, the wolffian-duct derivatives are usually present but not completely normal. The family history in most cases is uninformative. However, in several instances multiple family members are affected, and in at least one family the pattern of inheritance is compatible with X-linkage.

Reifenstein Syndrome

Reifenstein syndrome is the term now applied to a variety of forms of incomplete male pseudohermaphroditism initially described by Reifenstein, Rosewater, Gilbert-Dreyfus, and Lubs and their colleagues.[12] Each of these disorders was originally assumed to be a distinct entity and was designated by a separate eponym. Since several pedigrees compatible with X-linkage have now been described in which affected members of the same family exhibit variable defects that span the phenotypes described by these authors, it is now believed that these syndromes constitute variable manifestations of a similar mutation. The predominant phenotype is male, and the spectrum of defective virilization ranges from gynecomastia and azoospermia to more severe defects such as hypospadias and even to the presence of a pseudovagina. The most common phenotype is that of men with perineoscrotal hypospadias and gynecomastia. Axillary and pubic hair is normal, but chest and facial hair is minimal. Cryptorchidism is common, and the testes are often smaller than normal. Spermatogenesis is incomplete. Some subjects have defects in wolffian-duct derivatives such as absence or hypoplasia of the vas deferens. The psychological development in most subjects is unequivocally male.

Infertile Male Syndrome

The infertile male syndrome is the most recently recognized form of androgen resistance and in contrast to the other disorders is not a form of male pseudohermaphroditism.[13] Although some of the least severely affected patients in families with Reifenstein syndrome were noted to have azoospermia alone as the presenting manifestation of a receptor abnormality, it was not anticipated that individuals with idiopathic infertility and negative family histories might have androgen resistance. However, evaluation of men with normal external genitalia, apparently normal wolffian-duct structures, and infertility due to azoospermia has suggested that a receptor disorder may be present in a fourth or more.[14]

Endocrinology and Pathophysiology

The endocrine pattern is similar in all forms of androgen receptor disorders but has been best characterized in complete testicular feminization. Plasma testosterone levels and rates of production by the testes are those of normal men (or higher). The elevated rate of testosterone production is secondary to a high mean plasma level of LH, which in turn is the consequence of defective feedback regulation caused by resistance to the action of androgen at the hypothalamic-pituitary level. Elevations in LH are also believed to be responsible for the increased estrogen secretion by the testes.[3] Thus, variable degrees of androgen resistance coupled with enhanced production of estradiol results in both varying degrees of defective virilization and variable feminization in the four clinical syndromes. In complete testicular feminization the defective virilization is most severe and the full feminizing effect of the increased estrogen is expressed. In incomplete testicular feminization an almost complete feminizing effect of estrogen is expressed together with slight virilization. Estrogen production in Reifenstein syndrome is increased to an extent similar to or greater than that in testicular feminization. However, a less severe androgen resistance results in a predominantly male phenotype and less pronounced feminization. Only a few men with the infertile male syndrome have had evaluation of androgen-estrogen dynamics. The hormonal changes seem similar to those in the other receptor disorders but less marked, e.g. some men do not have an elevation of plasma LH, at least when assessed by single plasma samples.[14]

RECEPTOR STUDIES IN FIBROBLASTS

Androgen resistance in testicular feminization is due to abnormalities of the androgen receptor. Keenan and co-workers documented that a specific dihydrotestosterone receptor protein is present in fibroblasts cultured from the skin of normal subjects.[15] The receptor level is greater in fibroblasts cultured from genital skin sites (foreskin, scrotum, labia majora) than from non-genital sites.[16] The receptor has a dissociation constant of approximately 1 nM and is believed to be the same intracellular receptor protein as in androgen target tissues. Furthermore, Keenan *et al.* established that fibroblasts grown from some patients with complete testicular feminization showed no detectable dihydrotestosterone binding,[15] a

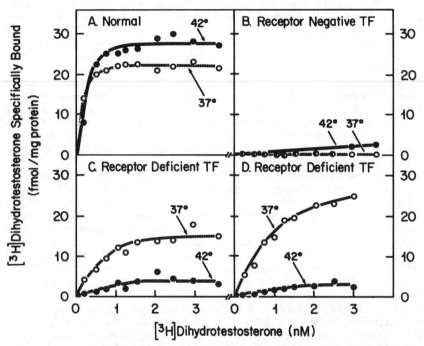

FIGURE 2. Dihydrotestosterone binding at 37°C and 42°C in genital skin fibroblasts derived from a normal subject, one patient with receptor-negative testicular feminization (TF), and two subjects with receptor-deficient testicular feminization. Specific binding of [³H]dihydrotestosterone is plotted as a function of dihydrotestosterone concentration. The amount of high-affinity binding in cells from the normal subject (A) increases slightly at 42°C compared with the usual binding condition of 37°C. The specific binding in the cells from the patient with receptor-negative testicular feminization (B) is virtually undetectable at both temperatures. The high-affinity dihydrotestosterone binding in the cells from the two patients with receptor-deficient testicular feminization (C and D) is clearly measurable at 37°C but decreases at the higher temperature to a level that is similar to that seen in the cells from the patient with the receptor-negative disorder. (From Griffin.[18] With permission from *Journal of Clinical Investigation.*)

finding that has been confirmed in other laboratories.[16,17] The finding that binding is absent in fibroblasts from some patients with testicular feminization provides an explanation for the profound resistance to all androgen actions in this disorder. Whether absence of binding of dihydrotestosterone in such cases is due to true absence of the androgen receptor protein or to the presence of a mutant protein that cannot bind the ligand is not known.

Other subjects with complete testicular feminization have a demonstrable qualitative abnormality in the receptor protein. Identification of such a phenomenon came first from studies of thermolability of binding[18] and subsequently from studies of stabilization of the receptor by sodium molybdate.[19] The initial studies involved fibroblasts from two sisters with complete testicular feminization which had about half normal levels of binding under the usual assay conditions at 37°C. When the assay was performed at an elevated temperature (42°C) dihydrotestosterone binding decreased to less that one-fifth of that seen at 37°C (FIGURE 2). The binding was rapidly restored on lowering the assay temperature to 37°C, suggesting that the alteration of the structure at elevated temperatures is reversible. Similar receptor thermolability has been observed by others.[20,21] Clones of skin fibroblasts were used by Meyer et al. to establish X-linkage of human testicular feminization associated with absent dihydrotestosterone binding.[22] A significant portion of fibroblast clones derived from skin of an obligate heterozygote was shown to have deficient binding, as would be predicted if random inactivation of the locus occurs in the X chromosome of females.[22] We have used genital skin fibroblast clones from the obligate heterozygote carrier of the original family identified as having testicular feminization associated with a thermolabile androgen receptor to confirm that this receptor defect is also X-linked.[23] A significant fraction of the clones derived from the heterozygous carrier was shown to exhibit thermolability of androgen binding (FIGURE 3).[23]

Qualitative abnormalities of the receptor in subsequent experiments have also been identified by examining the ultracentrifugation characteristics of the cytosol receptor in the presence of molybdate, a compound that stabilizes the normal 8S androgen receptor but not the receptor from many subjects with androgen resistance (FIGURE 4).[19] The characteristics of the androgen receptor in fibroblasts grown from skin biopsies of individuals from 35 families that fulfill the phenotypic and endocrine requirements to be designated androgen resistance, including 15 families with complete testicular feminization, are summarized in FIGURE 5.[19] The receptor has been designated as qualitatively abnormal when it is measurable in intact cells at 37°C and exhibits thermolability or inability to form an 8S complex in the presence of molybdate or both. In nine such families binding was virtually undetectable in fibroblast monolayers at any temperature and was designated as absent; these families are representative of the receptor-negative category of testicular feminization identified in the early studies of the problem. However, such a defect could not be the explanation for the androgen resistance in the remaining families with complete testicular feminization. In five families with complete testicular feminization, the receptor was measurable but was thermolabile in monolayers or unstable in fibroblast cytosol preparations or both. In one family the receptor was qualitatively and quantitatively normal. Likewise, in the initial studies in fibroblasts grown from a subject with incomplete testicular feminization, binding was about half-normal:[16] however, when binding in fibroblasts from affected individuals from seven families with incomplete testicular feminization was compared, a qualitative abnormality was demonstrated in four families, a diminished amount of binding was present in one family, and no defect could be identified in the other two families. Similarly, in our initial studies of the Reifenstein syndrome and the infertile male syndrome the only defect identified was a diminished amount of binding. When this residual binding was re-examined and additional patients were studied, the androgen receptor was found to be qualitatively abnormal in two families exhibiting Reifenstein syndrome and in three infertile men and was diminished in amount in three Reifenstein syndrome families and four unrelated infertile men. In affected subjects of four families (one with complete testicular feminization, two with incomplete testicular feminization, and one with the infertile male syndrome), no abnormality of the androgen receptor was demonstrable, despite endocrine evidence of androgen resistance.

One of the most interesting observations made from the studies of disorders of

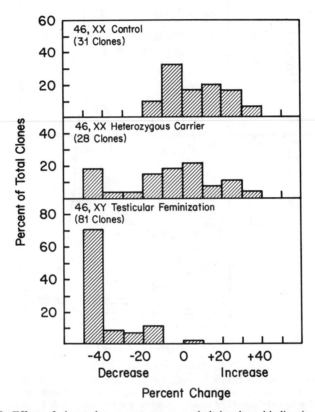

FIGURE 3. Effect of elevated temperature on methyltrienolone binding in genital skin fibroblast clones. On the day of assay, medium was replaced with medium prewarmed to either 30°C or 41°C for a 1-hr preincubation at the appropriate temperature. Medium containing 1 nM [³H]methyltrienolone with or without 250 nM nonradioactive methyltrienolone that also had been prewarmed to 30°C or 41°C was then incubated with the monolayers for 1 hr at the appropriate temperature. The monolayers were rinsed and harvested with trypsin-EDTA, and the specific binding at each temperature was calculated. Specific binding at 41°C was compared with that at 30°C and expressed as a percent decrease or increase. Percentage of total clones for each cell strain exhibiting a given magnitude of increase or decrease in binding is plotted. (From Elawady et al.[23] With permission from *American Journal of Human Genetics.*)

the human androgen receptor concerns the implication that defects in the androgen receptor can be manifested solely as male infertility and that such defects are a common cause of infertility in men. It is possible that the defects identified in cultured skin fibroblasts are not the cause of the infertility but rather secondary

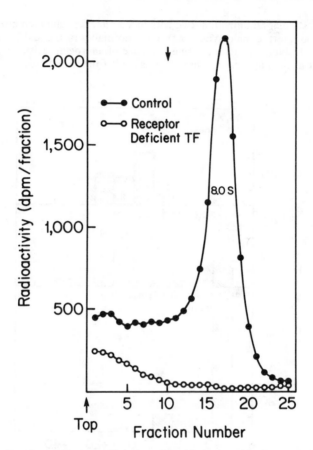

FIGURE 4. Density-gradient centrifugation of fibroblast cytosol from a control subject and a patient with complete testicular feminization associated with thermolability of androgen binding in the monolayer assay. Fibroblasts from a control subject and a patient with complete testicular feminization (TF) whose cells had partial receptor deficiency in whole cell binding (receptor-deficient TF) were grown under standard conditions, harvested, ultrasonically disrupted in the presence of sodium molybdate, and centrifuged at 100,000 g. The resultant supernatants were incubated with 1 nM [³H]dihydrotestosterone for 3 hr. Following dextran-coated charcoal treatment the supernatants were layered on the top of 5–20% sucrose density gradients, centrifuged, and frationated. The vertical arrow indicates the position of the [¹⁴C]albumin marker. (●) Control, (○) Testicular feminization. (Adapted from Griffin & Durrant.[19])

consequences of some other lesion. However, several features of the disorder suggest that this is not the case and that the abnormality in the androgen receptor is, in fact, the primary gene defect. First, androgen action is required for normal sperm production. Spermatogenesis normally takes place in the presence of very high concentration of androgen within the testes, perhaps 100-fold greater than in other androgen target tissues. Thus it is reasonable to assume that a class of subtle defects in the receptor may exist in which the principal or only manifestation is impaired sperm production. Second, some men with infertility have a qualitatively abnormal receptor, indicating that in these individuals the abnormal androgen receptor is the cause rather than the consequence of the infertility. Third, in some of the families, male infertility associated with the abnormal receptor is inherited in a fashion compatible with X-linkage, as would be predicted if the primary gene defect involved the androgen receptor. Fourth, as indicated above, the fact that the defect in some affected individuals in Reifenstein syndrome families is manifested primarily as male infertility suggests that new mutations that affect the androgen receptor could have similar manifestations.

To summarize, absent binding appears to be associated with the syndrome of complete testicular feminization. Qualitatively abnormal receptors and decreased amount of receptors are associated with a spectrum of phenotypes from female to male. We assume that those qualitative defects associated with complete testicular feminization are the result of mutations that impair the function of the receptor more severely than do those mutations that cause the infertile male syndrome. The category designated "decreased amount of receptor" is almost certainly a mixture of quantitative defects and qualitative abnormalities not yet identified. As more subtle tests of receptor function become available, it will be possible to assess structure-function relationships more completely.

The four families designated as "abnormality unidentified" in FIGURE 5 may represent a category of androgen resistance that does not involve the receptor. This possibility was originally suggested by the report of three affected members of one family with the phenotype of testicular feminization and who have normal 5α-reductase, normal amounts of androgen receptor, and normal nuclear localization of dihydrotestosterone.[24] Subsequent subjects with variable phenotypes have been reported to have a similar lack of abnormality in fibroblast studies in spite of a clinical presentation suggestive of an androgen receptor disorder.[25–27] This cate-

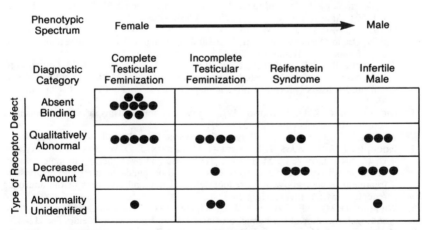

FIGURE 5. Androgen receptor assays in subjects from 35 families with androgen resistance and putative defects in androgen receptor. The 35 families include 31 families with established defects of androgen receptor and 4 with no abnormality identified (receptor-positive resistance). Absent binding is associated with the phenotype of complete testicular feminization, but qualitative and quantitative defects in receptor can be associated with a spectrum of phenotypes from complete testicular feminization to infertile men. (Data from Griffin & Durrant.[19])

gory has been termed receptor-positive resistance.[11] The site of the molecular abnormality in these patients and our four subjects is unclear. It is possible that a qualitative abnormality of the receptor is present but that the defect is too subtle to be detected by current methods. Indeed, subsequent studies of the first family reported to have receptor-positive resistance indicate that a qualitative defect in the receptor is the cause of the androgen resistance in these subjects.[21] Alternatively, the defect may reside at some step in androgen action distal to the receptor, such as the site of generation of specific messenger RNA. Indeed it is not established that a uniform defect is present; this group is probably due to a heterogeneous set of molecular abnormalities. Potential markers of post-receptor abnormalities in androgen action are under investigation.[28,29] It is interesting that this category appears to account for only a small fraction of the families we have studied (FIGURE 5).[19] This relative infrequency of potential post-receptor defects is similar to that reported in abnormalities of the glucocorticoid receptor in glucocorticoid-resistant lymphoma cells.[30–32] It is likely that even fewer of the "abnormality unidentified" group in the androgen resistance disorders than now indicated will prove to have true post-receptor resistance as more refined techniques of assessing subtle qualitative receptor defects are developed.

REFERENCES

1. WILSON, J. D., J. E. GRIFFIN, M. LESHIN & P. C. MACDONALD. 1983. The androgen resistance syndromes: 5α-reductase deficiency, testicular feminization, and related disorders. *In* Metabolic Basis of Inherited Disease. J. B. Stanbury, J. B. Wyngaarden, J. L. Goldstein, M. S. Brown & D. S. Fredrickson, Eds.: 1001–1026. McGraw-Hill. New York.

2. WILSON, J. D. 1975. Metabolism of testicular androgens. *In* Handbook of Physiology. Endocrinology. Male Reproductive System. R. O. Greep & E. B. Astwood, Eds. **5:** 491–508. American Physiology Society. Washington D.C.

3. MACDONALD, P. C., J. D. MADDEN, P. F. BRENNER, J. D. WILSON & P. K. SIITERI. 1979. Origin of estrogen in normal men and in women with testicular feminization. J. Clin. Endocrinol. Metab. **49:** 905–916.

4. WEINSTEIN, R. L., R. P. KELCH, M. R. JENNER, S. L. KAPLAN & M. M. GRUMBACH. 1974. Secretion of unconjugated androgens and estrogens by the normal and abnormal human testis before and after human chorionic gonadotropin. J. Clin. Invest. **53:** 1–6.

5. HIGGINS, S. J. & U. GEHRING. 1978. Molecular mechanisms of steroid hormone action. Adv. Cancer Res. **28:** 313–397.

6. WILSON, J. D. 1978. Sexual differentiation. Annu. Rev. Physiol. **40:** 279–306.

7. PRICE, P., J. A. H. WASS, J. E. GRIFFIN, M. LESHIN, J. D. WILSON, M. O. SAVAGE, D. C. ANDERSON & G. M. BESSER. High dose androgen therapy in male pseudohermaphroditism due to androgen resistance: Biochemical features and response to treatment in subjects with 5α-reductase deficiency and disorders of the androgen receptor. J. Clin. Invest. (In press).

8. WILBERT, D. M., J. E. GRIFFIN & J. D. WILSON. 1983. Characterization of the cytosol androgen receptor of the human prostate. J. Clin. Endocrinol. Metab. **56:** 113–120.

9. MOORE, R. J., J. M. GAZAK & J. D. WILSON. 1979. Regulation of cytoplasmic dihydrotestosterone binding in dog prostate by 17β-estradiol. J. Clin. Invest. **63:** 351–357.

10. WILSON, J. D., J. E. AIMAN & P. C. MACDONALD. 1980. The pathogenesis of gynecomastia. Adv. Intern. Med. **25:** 1–31.

11. GRIFFIN, J. E. & J. D. WILSON. 1980. The syndromes of androgen resistance. N. Engl. J. Med. **302:** 198–209.

12. WILSON, J. D., M. J. HARROD, J. L. GOLDSTEIN, D. L. HEMSELL & P. C. MAC-

DONALD. 1974. Familial incomplete male pseudohermaphroditism, type 1: evidence for androgen resistance and variable clinical manifestations in a family with the Reifenstein syndrome. N. Engl. J. Med. **290:** 1097–1103.

13. AIMAN, J., J. E. GRIFFIN, J. M. GAZAK, J. D. WILSON & P. C MACDONALD. 1979. Androgen insensitivity as a cause of infertility in otherwise normal men. N. Engl. J. Med. **300:** 223–227.

14. AIMAN, J. & J. E. GRIFFIN. 1982. The frequency of androgen receptor deficiency in fertile men. J. Clin. Endocrinol. Metab. **54:** 725–732.

15. KEENAN, B. S., W. J. MEYER III, A. J. HADJIAN, H. W. JONES & C. J. MIGEON. 1974. Syndrome of androgen insensitivity in man: absence of 5α-dihydrotestosterone binding protein in skin fibroblasts. J. Clin. Endocrinol. Metab. **38:** 1143–1146.

16. GRIFFIN, J. E., K. PUNYASHTHITI & J. D. WILSON. 1976. Dihydrotestosterone binding by cultured human fibroblasts: comparison of cells from control subjects and from patients with hereditary male pseudohermaphroditism due to androgen resistance. J. Clin. Invest. **57:** 1342–1351.

17. KAUFMAN, M., C. STRAISFELD & L. PINSKY. 1976. Male pseudohermaphroditism presumably due to target organ unresponsiveness to androgens. Deficient 5α-dihydrotestosterone binding in cultured skin fibroblasts. J. Clin. Invest. **58:** 345–350.

18. GRIFFIN, J. E. 1979. Testicular feminization associated with a thermolabile androgen receptor in cultured human fibroblasts. J. Clin. Invest. **64:** 1624–1631.

19. GRIFFIN, J. E. & J. L. DURRANT. 1982. Qualitative receptor defects in families with androgen resistance: failure of stabilization of the fibroblast cytosol androgen receptor. J. Clin. Endocrinol. Metab. **55:** 465–474.

20. PINSKY, L., M. KAUFMAN & R. L. SUMMIT. 1981. Congenital androgen insensitivity due to a qualitatively abnormal androgen receptor. Am. J. Med. Genet. **10:** 91–99.

21. BROWN, T. R., M. MAES, S. W. ROTHWELL & C. J. MIGEON. 1982. Human complete androgen insensitivity with normal dihydrotestosterone receptor binding capacity in cultured genital skin fibroblasts: evidence for a qualitative abnormality of the receptor. J. Clin. Endocrinol. Metab. **55:** 61–69.

22. MEYER, W. J. III, B. R. MIGEON & C. J. MIGEON. 1975. Locus on human X-chromosome for dihydrotestosterone receptor and androgen insensitivity. Proc. Natl. Acad. Sci. USA **72:** 1469–1472.

23. ELAWADY, M. K., D. R. ALLMAN, J. E. GRIFFIN & J. D. WILSON. 1983. Expression of a mutant androgen receptor in cloned fibroblast derived from a heterozygous carrier for the syndrome of testicular feminization. Am. J. Hum. Genet. **35:** 376–384.

24. AMRHEIN, J. A., W. J. MEYER III, H. W. JONES. JR. & C. J. MIGEON. 1976. Androgen insensitivity in man: evidence for genetic heterogeneity. Proc. Natl. Acad. Sci. USA **73:** 891–894.

25. AMRHEIN, J. A., G. J. KLINGENSMITH, P. C. WALSH, V. A. MCKUSICK & C. J. MIGEON. 1977. Partial androgen insensitivity: the Reifenstein syndrome revisited. N. Engl. J. Med. **297:** 350–356.

26. KEENAN, B. S., J. L. KIRKLAND, R. T. KIRKLAND & G. W. CLAYTON. 1977. Male pseudohermaphroditism with partial insensitivity. Pediatrics **59:** 224–231.

27. COLLIER, M. G., J. E. GRIFFIN & J. D. WILSON. 1978. Intranuclear binding of [³H]dihydrotestosterone by cultured human fibroblasts. Endocrinology **103:** 1499–1505.

28. KAUFMAN, M., L. PINSKY, R. HOLLANDER & J. D. BAILEY. 1983. Regulation of the androgen receptor by androgen in normal and androgen-resistant genital skin fibroblasts. J. Steroid Biochem. **18:** 383–390.

29. GYORKI, S., G. L. WARNE, B. A. K. KHALID & J. W. FUNDER. 1983. Defective nuclear accumulation of androgen receptors in disorders of sexual differentiation. J. Clin. Invest. **72:** 819–825.

30. YAMAMOTO, K. R., U. GEHRING, M. R. STAMPFER & C. H. SIBLEY. 1976. Genetic approaches to steroid hormone action. Rec. Prog. Horm. Res. **32:** 3–32.

31. BOURGEOIS, S., R. F. NEWBY & M. HUET. 1978. Glucocorticoid resistance in murine lymphoma and thymoma lines. Cancer Res. **38:** 4279–4284.

32. GEHRING, U. 1980. Cell genetics of glucocorticoid responsiveness. *In* Biochemical Actions of Hormones. G. Litwack, Ed. **7:** 205–232. Academic Press. New York.

Ornithine Decarboxylase mRNA in Mouse Kidney: A Low Abundancy Gene Product Regulated by Androgens with Rapid Kinetics[a]

OLLI A. JÄNNE, KIMMO K. KONTULA, VELI V. ISOMAA, and C. WAYNE BARDIN

The Population Council
The Rockefeller University
New York, New York 10021

INTRODUCTION

Sexual dimorphism of the kidney is known to exist in many species, and has been extensively studied in the mouse. The cells of Bowman's capsule and proximal convoluted tubule are larger in males than females,[1,2] and enlargement of these tubules in females can be produced by administration of androgens.[2,3] Testosterone-induced increase in the size of the kidneys is secondary to cellular hypertrophy rather than to hyperplasia,[2,3] in contrast to the situation in the male reproductive tract where androgens produce an increase in both the number and size of the cells. In association with the morphological changes in mouse kidney, testosterone and other androgenic steroids facilitate the synthesis of several defined gene products.[2,4-9] Recent studies in our own[10-13] and other laboratories[14-18] have indicated that ornithine decarboxylase (ODC), the first and rate-controlling enzyme in polyamine biosynthesis,[19-21] is one of the renal gene products that is markedly induced by androgens. The induction of ODC in mouse kidney occurs within a few hours, which has allowed us to correlate early changes in androgen receptor dynamics with the expression of a well-characterized gene product.[10,12,22] To further understand androgenic regulation of ODC synthesis and turnover, we prepared DNA sequences complementary to ODC mRNA and showed that ODC concentration is regulated, at least in part, by androgen-induced accumulation of mRNA encoding this protein.[13] We will describe how testosterone-regulated changes in ODC mRNA accumulation relate to the synthesis and turnover of ODC protein in mouse kidney.

STEROID SPECIFICITY OF ODC INDUCTION

In order to demonstrate which classes of steroids were involved in the regulation of ODC in mouse kidney, castrated male animals were treated for five days with pharmacological doses of 5α-dihydrotestosterone, estradiol, progesterone, dex-

[a] Supported by National Institutes of Health Grants HD-13541 and 3 FO5 TW3192-0151.

72

amethosone, and cortisol (FIGURE 1A). 5α-Dihydrotestosterone administration elicited a 400- to 600-fold increase in renal ODC activity, while other classes of steroids produced little or no effect.[10] Additional studies indicated that testosterone was as potent as 5α-dihydrotestosterone in stimulating the enzyme activity. Since testosterone is the physiologically active androgen in mouse renal tissue, this steroid was used in most of the subsequent experiments. These specificity

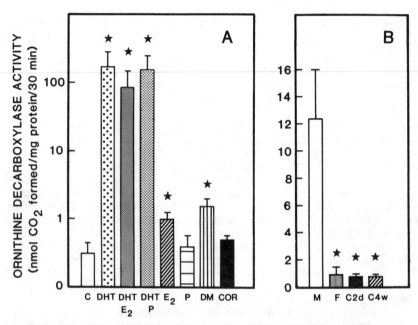

FIGURE 1. Regulation of renal ornithine decarboxylase is specific for androgens and occurs with physiological steroid concentrations. (A) Castrated male mice were treated for 5 days with daily doses of 5α-dihydrotestosterone (DHT, 1 mg/day), estradiol-17β (E_2, 20 μg/day), progesterone (P, 1 mg/day), dexamethasone (DM, 100 μg/day), and cortisol (COR, 1 mg/day). The effects of administration of DHT plus E_2 and DHT plus P were also examined using the same doses. The animals were killed 24 hr after the last steroid dose. Each bar shows the mean ± S.E. for 6–10 animals ($\star p<0.05$, compared to vehicle-treated, castrated control mice). (B) Renal ornithine decarboxylase activity in intact and castrated mice. M, intact males; F, intact females; C2d, male mice 2 days after orchiectomy; and C4w, male mice 4 weeks after orchiectomy. Each bar shows the mean ± S.D. for 6 animals ($\star p<0.05$, compared to intact male animals).

studies led us to conclude that androgens were the dominant steroidal regulators of ODC gene expression in mouse kidney, rather than glucocorticoids and estrogens as is the case in rat kidney.[23,24] The fact that physiological concentrations of androgens were capable of regulating ODC activity was shown by measurements of the enzyme activity in kidneys of intact female and male animals: the enzyme activity was 12-fold higher in males than females (FIGURE 1B). In addition, ODC

TABLE 1. Immunoreactive Ornithine Decarboxylase Concentration in Mouse Kidney

Animal Group	Immunoreactive ODC Concentration (ng/mg soluble protein)
Intact females	2.78 ± 0.20 (14)
Intact males	36.2 ± 2.7 (20)
Castrated males	2.0 ± 0.6 (7)
Tfm/Y animals	3.0[a]
Androgen-treated males[b]	522.0 ± 66.0 (12)

The enzyme protein was measured by radioimmunoassay from soluble cytosol fraction as described by Isomaa et al.[11] The values are mean ± S.E. for the number of animals given in parentheses.

[a] Mean of three animals.

[b] Treated with testosterone-releasing implants for 5–7 days.

activity in the males declined to that of the females as early as two days after orchiectomy (FIGURE 1B). These changes in ODC activity were not due to androgen-controlled alterations in the enzyme's catalytic site, since parallel changes were also measured in the ODC protein concentration (TABLE 1).

These observations strongly suggested that androgen receptors were involved in the regulation of ODC gene expression. To confirm this possibility we studied androgen-insensitive (Tfm/Y) mice with defective androgen receptors.[25] The results of this study showed that Tfm/Y animals had basal ODC activities similar to those of untreated females but failed to respond to androgen administration.[10] The basal immunoreactive ODC concentrations in renal cytosol of Tfm/Y animals were also similar to those in intact female or castrated male animals (TABLE 1). No significant increase in enzyme content occurred during androgen treatment (3.0 and 2.64 ng of immunoreactive ODC protein/mg of cytosol protein before and after androgen administration, respectively).

In addition to studies of Tfm/Y animals, the androgen receptor requirement for the regulation of ODC gene expression was further supported by experiments in which changes in nuclear androgen receptor concentration were related to stimulation of ODC activity. In these studies, groups of castrated male mice received a single injection of testosterone at four different doses (0.3, 1, 3, and 10 mg). Two interesting correlations between the nuclear receptor concentrations and induction of ODC activity emerged in these experiments. First, a prolonged residence of androgen receptors in renal cell nuclei was accompanied with a pronounced and sustained stimulation of the ODC gene.[10] This was exemplified by comparison of the smallest and largest doses of testosterone. The residence time of the nuclear androgen receptor was less than 6 hr after treatment with 0.3 mg testosterone and this was associated with fourfold stimulation of ODC activity that returned to the control level by 24 hr. By contrast, treatment with 10 mg testosterone resulted in accumulation of nuclear receptors for over 120 hr, which was associated with a 150-fold increased ODC concentration that remained elevated for at least 120 hr. The second parameter that correlated with receptor number was the lag between hormone treatment and the first rise in enzyme activity. Sustained nuclear accumulation of the androgen receptors resulted in a shorter lag period prior to the increase in ODC activity in mouse kidney.[10]

PURIFICATION OF ODC mRNA AND CLONING OF DNA SEQUENCES COMPLEMENTARY TO ODC mRNA

ODC mRNA Purification

Despite its 400- to 600-fold increase following androgen treatment, ODC is still a minor component of mouse kidney in that it represents about 0.03–0.05% of total soluble protein after a maximal induction.[11,16,17] Assuming that the relative abundance of ODC mRNA sequences was similar to the enzyme protein concentration, it was clear that the cloning of DNA sequences complementary for ODC mRNA would be greatly facilitated if an enriched message preparation were available. To accomplish this, we used a modification of the protein A-Sepharose immunoadsorbent technique (FIGURE 2) described by Shapiro and Young[26,27] and routinely achieved at least 300-fold purification of ODC mRNA by this method (TABLE 2). The additional steps we introduced to the procedure, such as passage of polysomes through protein A-Sepharose column prior to antibody addition, use of human placental ribonuclease inhibitor, and inclusion of high heparin concentrations in the buffers, increased the purity of ODC mRNA.[13] The final purity of the mRNA in different preparations ranged from 5 to 15%, as judged by immuno-precipitation of peptides from cell-free translation reactions with monospecific ODC antiserum.[13] The purity of the mRNA preparation used for cDNA synthesis and cloning was about 5%.

Analysis of the cell-free translation products by sodium dodecylsulfate-poly-acrylamide gel electrophoresis (SDS-PAGE) after immunoprecipitation with ODC antiseurm revealed the presence of three peptides with molecular weights of about 54,000, 37,500, and 33,000. Although only the largest peptide co-migrated with the homogeneous ODC subunit,[11,13] additional peptides seemed to be derived from ODC, as inclusion of excess non-radioactive ODC protein in the reaction mixture prevented immunoprecipitation of all three peptides.[13]

Cloning of DNA Sequences Complementary to ODC mRNA

Synthesis of double-stranded complementary DNA (ds-cDNA) from the purified ODC mRNA, insertion of the tailed ds-cDNA into the *Pst* I site of plasmid pBR 322, and propagation of the chimeric plasmids in *E. coli* were performed using standard techniques.[13,28] The initial screening of about 1,600 tetracycline-resistant, ampicillin-sensitive colonies was performed by differential colony hybridization, in which the (+)probe was prepared by reverse transcription from the

TABLE 2. Purification of Ornithine Decarboxylase mRNA from Kidneys of Androgen-treated Mice

Step	Total Amount of RNA (mg)	Purity of ODC mRNA (%)[a]
Polysomal RNA	48.6	0.05
Protein A-Sepharose	0.16	n.d.[b]
Oligo(dT)-cellulose	0.0026	15

[a] As judged by cell-free translation and immunoprecipitation.
[b] Not determined.

Renal tissue (50–75 g)

Isolation of total polysome fraction

Passage through protein A–Sepharose column

Collection of the flow–through fraction

Incubation with ODC–antibodies
(1 mg IgG per 7 mg RNA, 2 h)

Adsorption of immune complexes to
protein A–Sepharose column

Elution of RNA with 20 mM EDTA

Oligo(dT)–cellulose chromatography

FIGURE 2. Flow-sheet for the purification of ornithine decarboxylase mRNA. Kidneys of 100–150 mice were homogenized in a buffer containing 20 mM Tris/HCl, 10 mM Mg(OAc)$_2$, 75 mM KCl, 7 mM mercaptoethanol, 0.25 M sucrose, 5 mg/ml heparin, and 5 μg/ml cycloheximide (pH 7.6). Polysomes were isolated by centrifugation through discontinuous gradients of 24 and 60% (w/vol) sucrose and suspended in polysome buffer [25 mM Tris/HCl, 150 mM NaCl, 5 mM MgCl$_2$, 0.1% (vol/vol) Nonidet P-40, 1 μg/ml cycloheximide, 100 U/ml human placental ribonuclease inhibitor, and 5 mg/ml heparin, pH 7.6] to yield RNA concentration of 1 mg/ml. This suspension was passed through a protein A-Sepharose column (bed volume: 5 ml) equilibrated with the polysome buffer, and the flow-through fraction collected. The eluate was incubated for 2 hr with an IgG fraction of monospecific ODC-antiserum and then adsorbed to the protein A-Sepharose column equilibrated with the polysome buffer. After washing the matrix with 30 column volumes of the buffer, bound RNA was eluted with 20 mM EDTA in 25 mM Tris/HCl, 1 mg/ml heparin (pH 7.5). The released RNA was adjusted to 0.5 M KCl and 0.1% (w/vol) sodium dodecylsulfate and enriched for poly(A)-containing RNA by two cycles of oligo(dT)-cellulose chromatography.[38]

mRNA used for cloning and the (−)probe from the poly(A)-containing RNA that failed to bind to protein A-Sepharose during the purification of ODC mRNA.[12] Additional screening procedures involved colony hybridization with a [^{32}P]cDNA prepared from an ODC mRNA sample of the highest purity, radioimmunological determination of ODC-like antigens (fusion proteins between β-lactamase and ODC sequences) from culture media of selected colonies, and finally, hybridization selection of mRNA from renal polysomal RNA with four different plasmid DNAs that gave positive signals in the preceding screening studies.[13] In all four cases, the hybridization-selected mRNA directed the synthesis of peptides which, after immunoprecipitation, had electrophoretic mobilities identical with those of the cell-free translation products of the ODC mRNA purified by the immunoadsorption method. FIGURE 3 shows analysis by SDS-PAGE of the immunoprecipi-

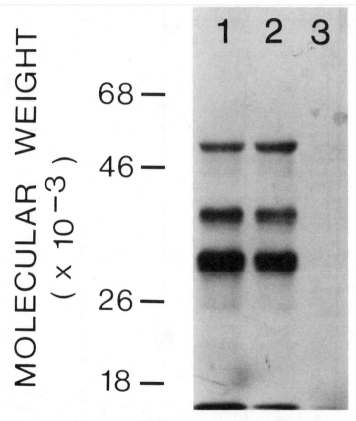

FIGURE 3. SDS-PAGE analysis of L-[^{35}S]methionine-labeled peptides immunoprecipitated with monospecific ornithine decarboxylase antiserum from the cell-free translation of hybrid selected RNA preparations. Lanes 1 and 2, immunoprecipitated translation products of the mRNAs selected by plasmids pODC54 and pODC152, respectively; lane 3, immunoprecipitated translation products of the material eluted from an empty nitrocellulose filter used for hybridization selection. The mobility of reference proteins (albumin, ovalbumin, α-chymotrypsinogen, and β-lactoglobulin) are shown on the left.

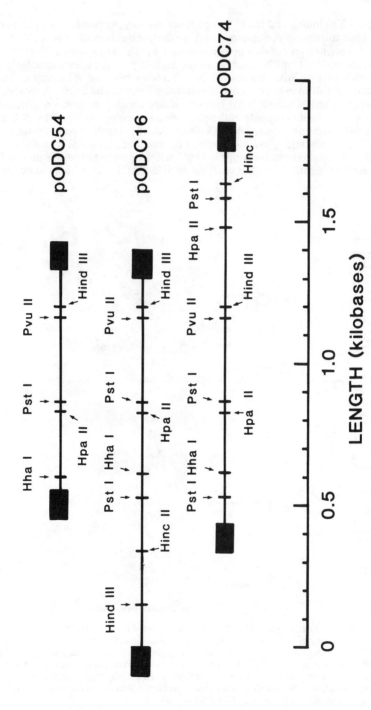

FIGURE 4. Cleavage sites of selected restriction enzymes in three cDNA clones (plasmids pODC54, pODC16, and pODC74) for ornithine decarboxylase mRNA. (━━) pBR322 DNA; (——) clones DNA. The orientation of the cloned DNAs corresponds to 5′- (*left*) and 3′-regions (*right*) of the mRNA.

tated products from cell-free translations directed by two of these hybrid-selected mRNAs (clones pODC54 and pODC152); the three peptides had molecular weights of 54,000, 37,500, and 33,000. Also in this case, the immunoprecipitation of the labeled peptides was abolished by the presence of excess of homogeneous ODC in the reaction mixture (not shown).

One of the clones (pODC54) that contained a 730-base pair (bp) insert was used to further screen the cDNA library prepared from the purified ODC mRNA. For this purpose, we used a 330-bp long internal *Pst* I/*Hin*d III fragment of pODC54 (FIGURE 4) and detected about 130 additional clones with DNA sequences complementary to ODC mRNA. Two of these clones (designated pODC16 and pODC74) had much longer inserts than pODC54 (FIGURE 4). Interestingly, one of them (pODC74) was about 450 bp longer at the 3'-end than the other two clones. It is not currently known whether this heterogeneity at the 3'-end of the isolated cDNAs is a reflection of a similar situation in mature ODC mRNAs. It is tempting to suggest, however, that this is the case, since two ODC mRNA species can be detected by Northern blot analysis (see below).

ANDROGENIC REGULATION OF ODC mRNA CONCENTRATION IN MOUSE KIDNEY

The clear sexual dimorphism in both ODC activity and immunoreactive enzyme protein concentration suggested that physiological testosterone concentrations might influence ODC mRNA concentration. This postulate was confirmed in experiments showing that intact male animals had about five times higher ODC mRNA concentrations than females (FIGURE 5). In keeping with the observations on enzyme concentration (TABLE 1), ODC mRNA content in castrated male animals was low and indistinguishable from that in intact female mice (FIGURE 5).

Two different mRNA species with molecular sizes of 2.15 and 2.7 kilobases (kb) hybridized to the *Pst* I/*Hin*d III internal fragment of the plasmid pODC54 that was used as the hybridization probe in the Northern blot analyses. This was true for all the RNA samples analyzed regardless of the previous treatment of the animals. The molecular size of the major mRNA species (2.15 kb) was compatible with that of intact ODC mRNA, assuming that the mature mRNA contains about 500 nucleotides in the non-translated regions. The size heterogeneity observed in this study for ODC mRNA does not seem to be an uncommon phenomenon for eukaryotic mRNAs.[7,29,30] One of the possible reasons is that there is a different degree of post-transcriptional processing of the primary transcript, as can occur with alternative polyadenylation sites.[30]

Prolonged androgen treatment for four to five days with implants releasing about 200 μg testosterone daily increased ODC mRNA accumulation 10- to 20-fold over the values in intact females or castrated males, and about threefold over those in intact male animals (FIGURES 5 and 6). Although the ODC mRNA measurements were only semiquantitative, it looks as if the increases in the enzyme activity and immunoreactive ODC protein concentration were relatively greater than those in the mRNA accumulation (*cf.* TABLE 1, and FIGURES 1, 5, and 6). In contrast to the wild-type animals, androgen-insensitive (Tfm/Y) mice showed no response in ODC mRNA concentration during prolonged testosterone treatment, although the basal level of this mRNA in kidneys of Tfm/Y animals was not markedly different from that in intact females (FIGURE 6). In this regard, the results were similar to those in the catalytic activity or enzyme protein concentration (TABLE 1).[11] Thus, our inability to stimulate ODC gene activity by androgen

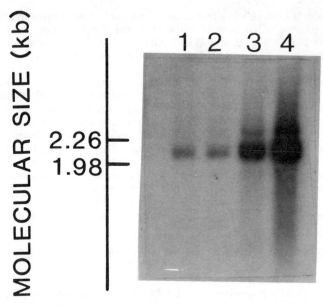

FIGURE 5. Northern blot hybridization analysis of poly(A)-RNA from kidneys of intact females (lane 1), castrated males (lane 2), intact males (lane 3), and androgen-treated males (lane 4). Total RNA was isolated from mouse renal tissue by LiCl/urea extraction method[39] and enriched for poly(A)-containing RNA by oligo(dT)-cellulose chromatography.[38] Androgen treatment of male mice lasted for 5 days. Identical amounts of each RNA (8 μg/sample) were first denatured with glyoxal, fractionated by gel electrophoresis on 1.1% agarose, and transferred to nitrocellulose filter.[40] Hybridization of the filter-bound RNA was carried out with the *Pst* I/*Hin*d III internal fragment of pODC54 labeled by nick translation. Molecular size markers shown on the left represent mobilities of two *Eco* RI/*Hin*d III fragments of bacteriophage λ.

administration in Tfm/Y animals further substantiated the notion[2] that even though androgen receptors may be present in low concentrations in these animals,[31,32] the receptors are defective and/or biologically inactive. It is of interest to note that basal ODC activities, immunoreactive enzyme concentrations, and ODC mRNA levels were all very similar in kidneys of intact females, castrated males, and Tfm/Y animals. Therefore, they seem to represent constitutive values rather than levels regulated by low circulating androgen concentrations (females and castrated males) or by a low target cell receptor concentration (Tfm/Y animals). On the basis of these and other findings, we hypothesize that, at least in the mouse kidney, a certain threshold concentration of nuclear androgen receptors (over 100 receptors/cell present in females[21]) must be exceeded and should be present for an extended period of time before stimulation of androgen-responsive genes occurs. On the basis of available information from other hormone-regulated systems, there is no reason to assume *a priori* that constitutive and androgen-induced ODCs would not be products of the same gene, although this should be demonstrated directly.

A typical feature of androgenic regulation of ODC activity is the rapid induction kinetics that seems to represent *de novo* synthesis of the enzyme.[11,12,14] It was therefore pertinent to determine how rapidly ODC mRNA begins to accumulate in mouse renal cells after administration of a single pharmacological dose of testosterone (10 mg/animal). These studies were performed in intact female animals whose renal ODC concentration is stimulated rapidly at 8 hr after steroid administration.[11] As illustrated in FIGURE 7, ODC mRNA concentration started to increase between 2 and 6 hr, with a maximal accumulation occurring by 24 hr after testosterone administration. These data clearly illustrated that there is reasonable agreement between changes in enzyme concentration and mRNA accumulation and suggest that androgens stimulate transcription of the ODC gene. However, this postulate has to be proven directly by studies indicating that androgens indeed facilitate the rate of ODC gene transcription.

In an attempt to find out whether androgens regulate directly ODC gene activity, we carried out experiments in which animals were treated with cycloheximide to inhibit protein synthesis *in vivo* prior to and during an androgen challenge that lasted for eight hours. Under these conditions, there was no increase in the catalytic enzyme activity (0.4 and 0.5 nmoles of CO_2 released/mg protein/30 min without and with androgen stimulation, respectively) or ODC protein concentration (1.3 versus 1.1 ng immunoreactive ODC/mg protein) indicating that *de novo* protein synthesis is required for testosterone-stimulated increase in ODC concentration. Inhibition of protein synthesis, however, also decreased the androgen-elicited accumulation of ODC mRNA measured 8 hr after testosterone administration

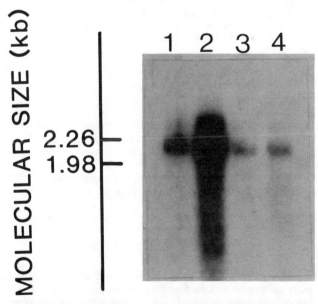

FIGURE 6. Northern blot hybridization analysis of poly(A)-RNA from kidneys of androgen-treated castrated male mice and of androgen-insensitive (Tfm/Y) mice. The experimental protocol was as in legend to FIGURE 5. Lane 1, untreated castrated male mice; lane 2, castrated male mice treated for 4 days with testosterone-releasing implants; lane 3, untreated Tfm/Y mice; and lane 4, Tfm/Y mice treated for 4 days with testosterone-releasing implants.

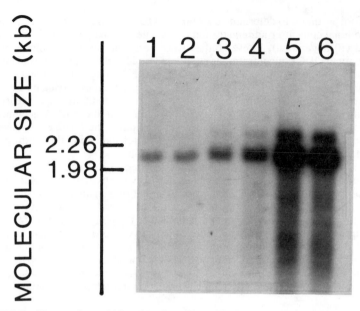

FIGURE 7. Changes in ornithine decarboxylase mRNA concentration in mouse kidney after administration of a single dose of testosterone (10 mg/animal). RNA isolation and Northern blot analysis were performed as described in the legend to FIGURE 5. Lane 1, intact non-treated female mice; lanes 2, 3, 4, 5, and 6, renal RNA from animals killed 2, 6, 12, 24, and 48 hr after steroid administration.

(FIGURE 8). Although this result could indicate that androgens regulate ODC gene expression indirectly via induction of intermediate regulatory protein(s), other explanations are also possible. A similar dependency on continuous protein synthesis has also been observed for stimulation of a number of other hormone-regulated mRNAs,[33-35] as judged by measurements of mature mRNA sequences. It may well be that continuous protein synthesis is required for proper splicing and processing of the primary transcript and/or for factors maintaining an undisturbed rate of general cellular transcription. More direct experiments, such as measurements of the rate of transcription of the ODC gene, are required to address this question.

SUMMARY AND CONCLUSIONS

We have used ODC gene expression in mouse kidney as the biological marker for studies of early androgen action. Some of the characteristics of this regulation involve its strict androgen specificity, the dependency on functional androgen receptors, the lack of requirement for pituitary hormones, and the ability of physiological androgens to bring about activation of the ODC gene. Some recent findings have revealed an additional intriguing feature in the regulation of ODC gene expression in that androgen sensitivity of ODC stimulation is genetically regulated in the mouse kidney (unpublished observations).[36]

One of the mechanisms by which androgens regulate renal ODC synthesis is to increase the concentration of ODC mRNA. Increased accumulation of this mRNA was seen as soon as 6 hr after testosterone administration, and it peaked 24 hr posttreatment. In general, acute changes in immunoreactive ODC concentration and ODC mRNA accumulation had very similar kinetics, suggesting that androgens induced *de novo* synthesis of ODC by increasing the rate of ODC gene transcription. In addition, there was always a highly significant correlation between the catalytic enzyme activity and immunoreactive enzyme protein concentration indicating that androgens do not specifically regulate the active site of ODC by either activating or inhibiting the enzyme by posttranslational modifications.

A typical feature of ODC in virtually all eukaryotic tissues is the extremely rapid turnover rate of the enzyme with a biological half-life of 10–30 min.[19–21] However, no direct information on the turnover rate of ODC mRNA is currently available, although indirect experiments have assigned a half-life of about seven hours for this mRNA.[37] The availability of cDNA clones for ODC mRNA measurements will now permit us to address this question more directly, and also to investigate a possible role of androgens in the stabilization of ODC mRNA. In this regard it is of interest to note that chronic treatment of mice with pharmacological doses of testosterone prolongs the half-life of ODC protein four- to tenfold.[11,18]

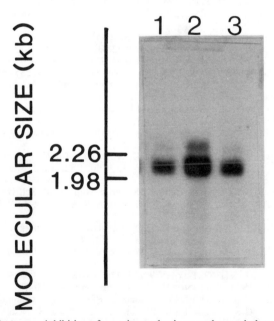

FIGURE 8. Influence on inhibition of protein synthesis on androgen-induced accumulation of ornithine decarboxylase mRNA. Castrated male mice were given two doses of cycloheximide, 1 hr before and 3 hr after androgen administration (100 μg and 50 μg cycloheximide/g body weight, respectively), and the animals were killed 8 hr after the steroid dose (10 mg testosterone/animal). Lane 1, cycloheximide alone; lane 2, testosterone alone; and lane 3, combined cycloheximide and testosterone. RNA isolation and Northern blot analysis were carried out as described in the legend to FIGURE 5.

REFERENCES

1. DUNN, T. B. 1949. J. Natl. Cancer Inst. **9:** 285–293.
2. BARDIN, C. W. & J. F. CATTERALL. 1981. Science **211:** 1285–1294.
3. KOCHAKIAN, C. P. 1975. Pharmacol. Ther. Sect. **B1:** 149–177.
4. SWANK, R. T., R. DAVEY, L. JOYCE, P. REID & M. R. MACEY. 1977. Endocrinology **100:** 473–480.
5. SWANK, R. T., K. PAIGEN, R. R. DAVEY, V. CHAPMAN, C. LABARCA, G. WATSON, R. GANSHOW, E. J. BRANDT & E. NOVAK. 1978. Rec. Prog. Horm. Res. **34:** 401–436.
6. TOOLE, J. J., N. D. HASTIE & W. A. HELD. 1979. Cell **17:** 441–448.
7. BERGER, F. G., K. W. GROSS & G. WATSON. 1981. J. Biol. Chem. **256:** 7006–7013.
8. CATTERALL, J. F. & S. L. LEARY. 1983. Biochemistry **22:** 6049–6053.
9. WATSON, C. S., D. SALOMON & J. F. CATTERALL. 1984. Ann. N.Y. Acad Sci. (This volume.)
10. PAJUNEN, A. E. I., V. V. ISOMAA, O. A. JÄNNE & C. W. BARDIN. 1982. J. Biol. Chem. **257:** 8190–8198.
11. ISOMAA, V. V., A. E. I. PAJUNEN, C. W. BARDIN & O. A. JÄNNE. 1983. J. Biol. Chem. **258:** 6735–6740.
12. JÄNNE, O. A., K. K. KONTULA, V. V. ISOMAA, T. K. TORKKELI & C. W. BARDIN. 1983. Androgen receptor-dependent regulation of ornithine decarboxylase gene expression. *In* Steroid Hormone Receptors: Structure and Function. H. Eriksson & J.-Å. Gustafsson, Eds.: 461–476. Elsevier Science Publishers B. V. Amsterdam.
13. KONTULA, K. K., T. K. TORKKELI, C. W. BARDIN & O. A. JÄNNE. 1984. Proc. Natl. Acad. Sci. USA. **81:** 731–735.
14. SEELY, J. E. & A. E. PEGG. 1983. J. Biol. Chem. **258:** 2496–2500.
15. HENNINGSSON, S., L. PERSSON & E. ROSENGREN. 1978. Acta Physiol. Scand. **102:** 385–393.
16. PERSSON, L. 1981. Acta Chem. Scand. **B35:** 451–459.
17. SEELY, J. E., H. PÖSÖ & A. E. PEGG. 1982. Biochemistry **21:** 3394–3399.
18. SEELY, J. E., H. PÖSÖ & A. E. PEGG. 1982. J. Biol. Chem. **257:** 7549–7553.
19. TABOR, C. W. & H. TABOR. 1976. Annu. Rev. Biochem. **45:** 285–306.
20. JÄNNE, J., H. PÖSÖ & A. RAINA. 1978. Biochim. Biophys. Acta **473:** 241–293.
21. PEGG, A. E. & P. P. MCCANN. 1982. Am. J. Physiol. **243:** C212–C221.
22. ISOMAA, V., A. E. I. PAJUNEN, C. W. BARDIN & O. A. JÄNNE. 1982. Endocrinology **111:** 833–843.
23. BRANDT, J. T., D. A. PIERCE & N. FAUSTO. 1972. Biochim. Biophys. Acta **279:** 184–193.
24. NICHOLSON, W. E., J. H. LEVINE & D. N. ORTH. 1976. Endocrinology **98:** 123–128.
25. BULLOCK, L. P. & C. W. BARDIN. 1972. J. Clin. Endocrinol. Metab. **35:** 935–937.
26. SHAPIRO. S. Z. & J. R. YOUNG. 1981. J. Biol. Chem. **256:** 1495–1498.
27. KRAUS, J. P. & L. E. ROSENBERG. 1982. Proc. Natl. Acad. Sci. USA **79:** 4015–4019.
28. STEIN, J. P., J. F. CATTERALL, S. L. C. WOO, A. R. MEANS & B. W. O'MALLEY. 1978. Biochemistry **17:** 5763–5772.
29. SETZER, D. R., M. McGROGAN, J. H. NUNBERG & R. T. SCHIMKE. 1980. Cell **22:** 361–370.
30. LAGACE, L., T. CHANDRA, S. L. C. WOO & A. R. MEANS. 1983. J. Biol. Chem. **258:** 1684–1688.
31. WIELAND, S. J. & T. O. FOX. 1979. Cell **17:** 781–787.
32. FOX, T. O. & S. J. WIELAND. 1981. Endocrinology **109:** 790–797.
33. DELAP, L. & P. FEIGELSON. 1978. Biochem. Biophys. Res. Commun. **82:** 142–149.
34. CHEN, C.-L. C.& P. FEIGELSON. 1979. Proc. Natl. Acad. Sci. USA **76:** 2669–2673.
35. LOOSFELT, H., F. FRIDLANSKY, J.-F. SAVOURET, M. ATGER & E. MILGROM. 1981. J. Biol. Chem. **256:** 3465–3470.
36. BULLOCK, L. P. 1983. Endocrinology **112:** 1903–1909.
37. KALLIO, A., H. PÖSÖ, G. SCALABRINO & J. JÄNNE. 1977. FEBS Lett. **79:** 195–199.
38. AVIV, H. & P. LEDER. 1972. Proc. Natl. Acad. Sci. USA **69:** 1408–1412.
39. AUFFRAY, C. & F. ROUGEON. 1980. Eur. J. Biochem. **107:** 303–314.
40. THOMAS, P. J. 1980. Proc. Natl. Acad. Sci USA **77:** 5201–5205.

Factors That Influence the Interaction of Androgen Receptors with Nuclei and Nuclear Matrix[a]

ELIZABETH M. WILSON[b] and DOUGLAS S. COLVARD

Departments of Pediatrics and Biochemistry
The Laboratories for Reproductive Biology
University of North Carolina School of Medicine
Chapel Hill, North Carolina 27514

INTRODUCTION

Steroid hormone receptors interact with nuclei to potentiate gene transcription. The search for nuclear sites for steroid hormone receptors has yielded evidence that binding sites are present in nonhistone chromosomal proteins,[1-3] DNA,[4] ribonucleoproteins,[5] or nuclear matrix.[6] In this report, we present further evidence that the matrix is a major nuclear binding site for the androgen receptor. The nuclear matrix provides a structural framework for the nucleus and is becoming recognized as a focal point for several vital functions of the cell including gene transcription,[7] RNA processing,[8,9] and DNA synthesis.[10] Studies presented here suggest that androgen receptor interaction with nuclear matrix is dependent on zinc.

It is well known that steroid hormone receptors are generally observed in two distinct forms, a 4–5S form and the larger 8–9S receptor. In its native form, the androgen receptor has a sedimentation coefficient of 4.5S. Smaller receptor fragments that retain high steroid binding affinity of 3.6S and 3.0S have been shown to be proteolytic products of the native androgen receptor.[11] Their appearance in tissue extracts results from cleavage of the 4.5S receptor by endogenous proteases. The 8 to 9S form of the androgen receptor can be observed on sucrose gradients of low ionic strength. Our recent work suggests that this 8S form of the androgen receptor is a complex of the native 4.5S receptor with a protein different from the receptor.[12] This protein, which we refer to as the 8S androgen receptor–promoting factor, has been partially purified and found to markedly inhibit binding of the 4.5S androgen receptor to nuclei and nuclear matrix.

METHODS OF PROCEDURE

Materials

[1,2,4,5,6,7-³H]Dihydrotestosterone (~120 Ci/mmol) was purchased from New England Nuclear; diisopropyl fluorophosphate from Calbiochem; cellulose

[a] Supported by U.S. Public Health Service Research Grants HD16910 and HD04466 and the American Cancer Society Institutional Grant IN-15V.
[b] Correspondence to: Elizabeth M. Wilson, Department of Pediatrics, Clinical Sciences Building 229H, University of North Carolina, Chapel Hill, NC 27514.

phosphate P11 from Whatman; pyridoxal 5'-phosphate from Aldrich Chemical Co.; mercaptoethanol from Eastman; Trizma base (Tris buffer) and ovalbumin from Sigma; DEAE-Sepharose from Pharmacia Fine Chemicals; hydroxylapatite from Bio-Rad; reagent-grade chemicals from Fisher Scientific Co.

Animals

Copenhagen rats (3 to 8 months of age) obtained from Charles River received subcutaneous transplantations of the Dunning R3327H tumor. Following 4 to 6 months of tumor growth to ~3 cm diameter, rats were castrated under ether anesthesia through an abdominal incision. After 24 hr, rats were decapitated, and their tumors excised, rinsed in saline (0.9% NaCl), frozen in liquid N_2, and stored at −70°C.

Subcellular Fractionation

Nuclei from tumors and other tissues were isolated through 1.9 M sucrose, 0.025 M KCl, 3 mM $MgCl_2$, and 50 mM Tris, pH 7.5 as previously described.[16,17] The 100,000 × g supernatant (cytosol) fractions of tumor were prepared as previously described[12] and used as the source of androgen receptor. The 4.5S receptor was labeled with [3H]dihydrotestosterone and partially purified[12] resulting in its separation from the 8S androgen receptor–promoting factor. Nuclear matrix was isolated as previously described.[18,19]

In Vitro Binding Assays

The phosphocellulose-purified [3H]dihydrotestosterone receptor was dialyzed for 2 hr at 4°C against a large volume of 0.025 M KCl, 10% glycerol, 0.25 M sucrose, 5 mM mercaptoethanol, 3 mM $MgCl_2$, and 50 mM Tris, pH 7.5. Aliquots of isolated nuclei (20–750 μg DNA) or nuclear matrix (100 to 300 μg protein) were incubated with the dialyzed 4.5S [3H]dihydrotestosterone receptor (10 to 330 pM). Unless otherwise indicated, nuclear incubations were for 30 min at 25°C in a total volume of 0.3 ml of 0.25 M sucrose, 0.15 M KCl, 5 mM mercaptoethanol, 300 μM $ZnCl_2$, 3 mM $MgCl_2$, and 50 mM Tris, pH 7.5. Sucrose was omitted in matrix incubations. In this buffer, a total Zn^{2+} concentration of 300 μM corresponds to 0.5 μM free Zn^{2+} due to complexing of Zn^{2+} with mercaptoethanol. Free zinc concentrations were estimated by proton release.[20] After incubation, nuclei or nuclear matrix were centrifuged at 4,000 rpm in an HB-4 Sorvall rotor for 5 min. Supernatants were aspirated, nuclear pellets suspended in 0.3 ml of the same buffer, but without $ZnCl_2$ or mercaptoethanol, and centrifuged as before. The combined supernatant fractions were assayed for radioactivity in 6 ml of Scintiverse : toluene (1 : 1) with a counting efficiency of 45%. Nuclear and matrix pellets were extracted with 0.25 ml ethanol for 10 min at 0°C, unless indicated otherwise and radioactivity determined as above. Longer periods of extraction released no further radioactivity. Receptor association with nuclei is expressed as the difference in radioactive counts sedimented in the presence and absence of nuclei. Under standard assay conditions, sedimentation of receptor alone ranges from 5 to 15%, where the lower limit represents binding of [3H]steroid to glass.

Partial Purification of 8S Androgen Receptor–Promoting Factor

The 8S-promoting factor was partially purified from rat serum as previously described.[12] An additional purification step is chromatography on ATP-Sepharose, prepared as previously described.[21] Partially purified 8S-promoting factor was applied to ATP-Sepharose, equilibrated in 1 mM EDTA (disodium ethylenediamine tetraacetate), 50 mM Tris, pH 7.5, and the column was washed in the same buffer and sequentially step-eluted with 0.05, 0.1, and 0.2 M KCl. The 8S-promoting factor activity elutes in 0.1 M KCl.

Assay for 8S Androgen Receptor–Promoting Factor

The presence of 8S-promoting factor activity was determined in sucrose gradients containing 0.025 M KCl as previously described.[12] One unit of 8S-promoting factor activity is defined as that amount of protein required to shift 60 fmol of 4.5S [^{3}H]dihydrotestosterone-labeled androgen receptor to 8S in a sucrose gradient containing 25 mM KCl.

Protein and DNA Assays

Protein concentration was estimated by the method of Lowry[22] using ovalbumin as standard. DNA was assayed by the method of Burton[23] using calf thymus DNA as standard.

RESULTS

An important consideration when studying the effects of zinc on androgen receptor binding to nuclei is the careful control for nonspecific co-sedimentation of receptor with nuclei or nuclear matrix. Our initial attempts to study zinc effects were carried out in the absence of mercaptoethanol and resulted in aggregation of receptor. We found that the addition of salt (0.15 M KCl) and mercaptoethanol (5 mM) in the presence of micromolar amounts of Zn^{2+} minimized receptor aggregation. In the absence of mercaptoethanol, the androgen receptor sediments to the bottom of sucrose gradients containing 0.15 M KCl and 300 μM Zn^{2+};[17] addition of 5 mM mercaptoethanol causes the receptor to sediment in the 4.5S form. That mercaptoethanol eliminated Zn^{2+}-induced aggregation of receptor raised the possibility that mercaptoethanol binds Zn^{2+}.

The extent of Zn^{2+} binding to mercaptoethanol was measured by proton release[20,24] with a pH electrode at varying concentrations of Zn^{2+} and mercaptoethanol. Modified Scatchard analysis[a] (FIGURE 1) indicated three apparent binding constants: $K_1 = 1.4 \times 10^3$ M^{-1}, $K_2 = 6.0 \times 10^3$ M^{-1}, and $K_3 = 0.08 \times 10^3$ M^{-1}. Cooperative binding of the second molecule of mercaptoethanol to Zn^{2+} is reflected in the concave downward curve. The computed curve (dotted line) derived from the equation in the legend of FIGURE 1 is in excellent agreement with the experimental data (solid points). The product of the three binding constants of 6.7×10^9 M^{-3} differs substantially from that previously reported.[24]

Addition of Zn^{2+} to the *in vitro* binding buffer, which consisted of 0.25 M sucrose, 0.15 M KCl, 3 mM $MgCl_2$, 5 mM mercaptoethanol, and 50 mM Tris, pH

[a] L. Pedersen, Department of Chemistry, University of North Carolina, Chapel Hill, NC, unpublished studies.

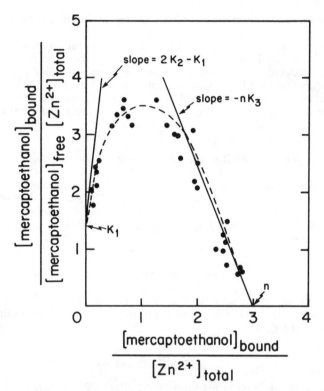

FIGURE 1. Modified Scatchard analysis of the binding of Zn^{2+} and mercaptoethanol. To 20 ml of buffer containing 0.15 M KCl, 0.1 mM HEPES, pH 7.5, and mercaptoethanol up to 5 mM, sequential aliquots of 0.1 M $ZnCl_2$, pH 5, were added, resulting in a drop in pH proportional to the amount of mercaptoethanol bound to Zn^{2+}. After each addition of $ZnCl_2$ to make a total Zn^{2+} concentration of 0.01, 0.025, 0.05 mM, a measured amount of a fresh solution of NaOH (0.01 M) was added to back-titrate to pH 7.5. At mercaptoethanol concentrations in excess of 1 mM, total Zn^{2+} concentrations of 0.1, 0.2, and 0.3 mM were used as well. The molar amount of NaOH required to neutralize released H^+ indicates the extent of binding of mercaptoethanol to Zn^{2+}. Addition of $ZnCl_2$ to buffer without mercaptoethanol lowered the pH by up to 0.05 pH units and was subtracted from values measured in the presence of mercaptoethanol. Treatment of the data was based on unpublished studies of L. Pederson[a] and that of Klotz and Hunston,[48–50] where the apparent K_1 is estimated from the y intercept, K_2 from the slope of the tangent extrapolated to the y intercept (slope = $2K_2 - K_1$), n (the number of mercaptoethanol molecules bound per Zn^{2+} atom at saturation), and K_3 from the slope of the line extrapolated to the x intercept (slope = $-nK_3$). The points are experimentally derived. The dotted line represents the function described by the following equation using the three experimentally determined binding constants ($K_1 = 1.4 \times 10^3$ M^{-1}, $K_2 = 6.0 \times 10^3$ M^{-1}, and $K_3 = 0.8 \times 10^3$ M^{-1}).

$$M_b = Zn_T \cdot \frac{K_1[M]_{free} + 2K_1K_2[M]_{free}^2 + 3K_1K_2K_3[M]_{free}^3}{1 + K_1[M]_{free} + K_1K_2[M]_{free}^2 + K_1K_2K_3[M]_{free}^3},$$

where M_b is bound mercaptoethanol, Zn_T is the total $ZnCl_2$ concentration, $[M]_{free}$ is free mercaptoethanol (i.e., the difference between total and bound mercaptoethanol), and K_1, K_2, and K_3 are the three binding constants.

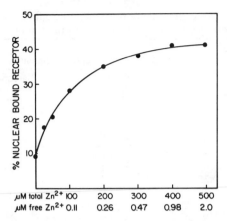

μM total Zn²⁺ 100   200   300   400   500
μM free Zn²⁺ 0.11   0.26   0.47   0.98   2.0

FIGURE 2. Zinc dependence of androgen receptor binding to nuclei. Prostate tumor nuclei (400 μg) were incubated with the 4.5S [³H]dihydrotestosterone receptor partially purified by phosphocellulose chromatography. Incubation was for 30 min at 25°C in a total volume of 0.3 ml of 0.25 M sucrose, 0.15 M KCl, 3 mM MgCl₂, 5 mM mercaptoethanol, and 50 mM Tris, pH 7.5, as described in METHODS. Receptor aggregation in the absence of nuclei and adhesion of [³H]steroid to glass totaled 5–8% of total radioactivity and was subtracted from each point. Free Zn²⁺ concentration was estimated using the three Zn²⁺-mercaptoethanol binding constants, K_1 (1.4×10^3 M⁻¹), K_2 (6.0×10^3 M⁻¹), and K_3 (0.8×10^3 M⁻¹), determined from the modified Scatchard analysis shown in FIGURE 1. Free Zn²⁺ was calculated using the equation: $Zn_{total} = Zn_{free} (1 + K_1[M]_{free} + K_1K_2[M]^2_{free} + K_1K_2K_3[M]^3_{free}$, where M is mercaptoethanol and $[M]_{free} = [M]_{total} - [M]_{bound}$.

7.5, results in a concentration-dependent increase in binding of the 4.5S androgen receptor to nuclei (FIGURE 2). Receptor sedimentation in the absence of nuclei over this range of Zn²⁺ ranged from 5 to 8% and was subtracted from each experimental point. Free Zn²⁺ concentrations were estimated from experimentally determined concentrations of free mercaptoethanol ($[M]_{free} = [M]_{total} - [M]_{bound}$), the total Zn²⁺ concentration, and the three apparent binding constants derived by the modified Scatchard analysis using the following equation:

$$Zn_{total} = Zn_{free} (1 + K_1 [M]_{free} + K_1K_2 [M]^2_{free} + K_1K_2K_3 [M]^3_{free}).$$

Half-maximal binding of receptor to nuclei observed at 50 μM total Zn²⁺ corresponds to approximately 0.05 μM free Zn²⁺. Although direct measurements of intracellular free Zn²⁺ are not available, this amount of free Zn²⁺ is likely within the physiological range in the prostate. The optimum concentration of ZnCl₂ (200 to 300 μM total) for receptor binding to nuclei corresponds to a range from 0.3 to 0.5 μM free Zn²⁺.

The nuclear matrix, a structure that forms a lattice framework for the nucleus, was isolated using a conventional technique that includes treatment of nuclei with DNase, 2 M NaCl, and 1% Triton X-100.[18] Androgen receptor binding to intact nuclei and isolated nuclear matrix are similar in that binding is potentiated by Zn²⁺. The concentration of total Zn²⁺ required for half-maximal binding to matrix is 20 μM, which corresponds to 20 nM free Zn²⁺ (not shown). This amount of Zn²⁺ is about 25-fold lower than that required for receptor binding to intact nuclei, which may reflect binding of Zn²⁺ to nuclei independent of the receptor. The extent to which nuclei lower the free Zn²⁺ concentration was not assessed.

TABLE 1. Effects of Mercaptoethanol on Receptor Sedimentation in the Presence and Absence of a Control Membrane Fraction or Nuclei

[Mercaptoethanol] (mM)	% Receptor Sedimentation[a]	
	− Sarcoplasmic Reticulum[a]	+ Sarcoplasmic Reticulum
0	55	75
1	45	55
5	19	23
10	16	14
	− Nuclei[c]	+ Nuclei
0	21	53
0.25	16	53
1	9	52
5	7	45
10	6	37

[a] Percent of total added 4.5S [³H]dihydrotestosterone receptor that sedimented following centrifugation.

[b] The 4.5S [³H]dihydrotestosterone receptor (22 fmol) was incubated for 30 min at 25°C in the presence or absence of rabbit skeletal sarcoplasmic reticulum vesicles (0.6 mg protein) in 0.3 ml of 0.25 M sucrose, 300 μM $ZnCl_2$, 0.15 M KCl, 3 mM $MgCl_2$, and 50 mM Tris, pH 7.5 with increasing concentrations of mercaptoethanol. Following incubation, samples were centrifuged at 30,000 rpm in a Beckman type 40 rotor for 10 min at 4°C. Pellets were extracted with ethanol and the radioactivity determined as described in METHODS.

[c] The 4.5S [³H]dihydrotestosterone receptor (22 fmol) was incubated as above except in the presence or absence of prostate tumor nuclei (860 μg DNA). Following incubation, samples were centrifuged at 2,600 × g for 5 min at 4°C. Radioactivity in supernatants and ethanol extracts of pellets were determined.

In order to test the specificity of the receptor-nuclear interaction, a control membrane fraction, sarcoplasmic reticulum, was isolated from rabbit skeletal muscle.[25] As expected at low mercaptoethanol concentrations, receptor sedimentation was high due to aggregation. Addition of mercaptoethanol to 5 to 10 mM greatly diminished receptor aggregation, and revealed no receptor association with sarcoplasmic reticulum (TABLE 1). In contrast, receptor sedimentation with nuclei remained elevated in 5 and 10 mM mercaptoethanol. The higher receptor sedimentation in the absence of sarcoplasmic reticulum than in the absence of nuclei is due to the greater centrifugal force required to sediment sarcoplasmic reticulum membrane vesicles. Thus, the amount of receptor associated with nuclei (six- to sevenfold greater than background) indicates binding of the 4.5S androgen receptor with nuclei. The concentration of free Zn^{2+} is estimated to be as low as 0.5 μM. Other divalent cations that had little or no potentiating effect include Ca^{2+}, Mg^{2+}, Mn^{2+}, Co^{2+}, Cu^{2+}, and Cd^{2+}. Ni^{2+} was about one half as effective as Zn^{2+}.[17] Of these ions, only Cd^{2+}, Cu^{2+}, Ni^{2+}, and Zn^{2+} form complexes with mercaptoethanol. The relative effects of Zn^{2+} and other divalent cations on binding of receptor to nuclear matrix were nearly identical to those observed with intact nuclei.

Saturability and Tissue Differences in Nuclear and Nuclear Matrix Binding of Receptor

Incubation of increasing amounts of 4.5S [³H]dihydrotestosterone receptor with a constant amount of nuclei resulted in saturation of binding at a receptor concentration of 200 pM (FIGURE 3). In order to minimize loss of receptor steroid binding activity (*see below*), incubations were carried out for 30 min at 25°C. It can be estimated that there are approximately 10^{-13} mol nuclear receptor binding sites/mg DNA. If it is assumed that there are 12 pg DNA/rat cell nucleus,[26] then there are approximately 1200 sites/nucleus. The apparent binding constant of 10^{13} M^{-1} is higher than previously reported for nuclear binding of other steroid receptors.[1,27,28]

Binding of androgen receptor to nuclear matrix of the Dunning prostate tumor is saturable at 300 fmol/mg matrix protein, which is equivalent to ~80 fmol/mg DNA equivalent (FIGURE 4). Since matrix accounts for 10 to 15% of nuclear protein, it is estimated there are 1400 receptor binding sites/nucleus. The similarity in the number of sites for intact nuclei and nuclear matrix suggests that matrix binding of receptor accounts for the majority of nuclear binding sites under *in vitro* assay conditions.

The tissue specificity of receptor binding was investigated using nuclear matrix isolated from the Dunning R3327H prostate tumor, ventral prostate, and liver of rats sacrificed 18 hr after castration. Increasing amounts of 4.5S [³H]dihydrotestosterone receptor were incubated with a constant amount of nuclear matrix resulting in an apparent saturation of matrix binding sites (FIGURE 4). When expressed relative to mg DNA equivalents, Dunning tumor matrix contained the highest number of sites, followed by ventral prostate, with liver matrix containing the lowest number of sites. The apparent binding constants ranged from 5×10^{12} to 3×10^{13} M^{-1}. The lower number of binding sites in liver is consistent with its lower degree of androgen responsiveness. It is conceivable that the higher number of sites in the prostate tumor may reflect an alteration related to its neoplastic state.

Effects of Temperature

The effects of increased temperature on androgen receptor binding in nuclei and nuclear matrix were similar. As shown in FIGURE 5A, binding to nuclear matrix is enhanced by raising the temperature from 0 to 15°C and is slightly faster at 25°C. With the faster rate of binding there occurs a more rapid degradation of receptor as indicated by the decrease in binding after 2 hr at 25°C. Association rate constants were as follows: 2.7×10^5 M^{-1} min^{-1} at 0°C; 1.2×10^6 M^{-1} min^{-1}

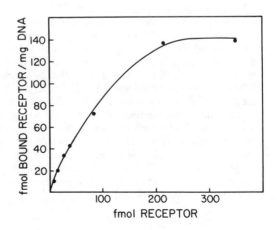

FIGURE 3. Saturation of androgen receptor binding sites in nuclei. Increasing amounts of the phosphocellulose-purified [³H]dihydrotestosterone receptor complex were incubated with prostate tumor nuclei (430 µg DNA) as described in METHODS, except in a final volume of 0.9 ml.

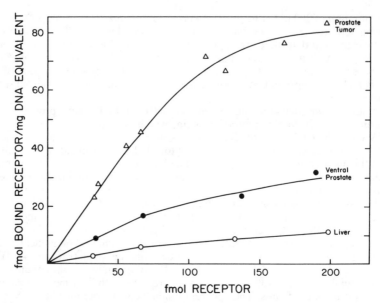

FIGURE 4. Tissue specificity of androgen receptor binding to nuclear matrix. Increasing amounts of the phosphocellulose-purified 4.5S [³H]dihydrotestosterone receptor were incubated with 120 μg of nuclear matrix protein isolated from the Dunning prostate tumor (△; 0.47 mg protein/mg DNA equivalent), ventral prostate (●; 0.11 mg protein/mg DNA equivalent), and liver (○; 0.05 mg protein/mg DNA equivalent) as described in METHODS except that the total volume was 0.7 ml.

at 15°C; and $2.4 \times 10^6 \, M^{-1} \, min^{-1}$ at 25°C. The energy of activation determined from an Arrhenius plot (FIGURE 5B) is 15 kcal/mole.

Effects of Ionic Strength and Pyridoxal 5'-phosphate

The effect of ionic strength on receptor-nuclear binding was investigated at concentrations of KCl ranging from 0.025 M to 0.5 M. Receptor binding to nuclei was unaltered by salt concentrations from 0.15 to 0.5 M KCl (FIGURE 6). As mentioned previously, the use of salt concentrations lower than 0.15 M KCl was complicated by aggregation of the receptor. In accordance with these observations, addition of 0.4 M KCl to nuclei or nuclear matrix following receptor binding in the presence of Zn^{2+} caused only 20 to 30% of bound receptor to be extracted.[17] When Zn^{2+} was omitted and EDTA (3 mM) added to the extraction buffer, receptor extraction was increased up to 60% of the total bound receptor.

A similar potentiating effect of EDTA was noted when receptor bound to nuclei or nuclear matrix was extracted with pyridoxal 5'-phosphate. In the presence of 3 mM EDTA, and in the absence of Zn^{2+}, 60% of bound receptor could be extracted from nuclei. The effectiveness of EDTA in enhancing receptor release supports the role of Zn^{2+} in the binding reaction. Pyridoxal 5'-phosphate was also found to inhibit receptor binding to nuclei and nuclear matrix in a concentration-dependent manner (not shown).

Inhibition by the 8S Androgen Receptor–Promoting Factor

The addition of the 8S androgen receptor–promoting factor to the partially purified 4.5S [³H]dihydrotestosterone receptor causes a shift in sedimentation to an 8S form.[12] The 8S-promoting factor has been purified 100-fold from serum. Following chromatography on ATP-Sepharose, the 8S-promoting factor retains its ability to shift the 4.5S receptor to the 8S form (FIGURE 7).

The 3.6S proteolytic fragment of the rat androgen receptor has a molecular weight of 62,000,[11] which is one half that of the 4.5S native receptor (MW 117,000). The 3.6S form is generated in rat ventral prostate cytosol prepared in the presence of diisopropyl fluorophosphate, due to the action of a prostate-specific non-serine protease.[11] As shown in FIGURE 8A, the 3.6S receptor fragment retains the ability of the native receptor to form an 8S complex upon addition of the partially purified 8S-promoting factor. However, further cleavage of the receptor with trypsin to the 3S receptor fragment (MW 29,000) results in loss of its ability to reform the 8S complex (FIGURE 8B). These results suggest that the recognition site on the receptor for the 8S-promoting factor is lost when the receptor is

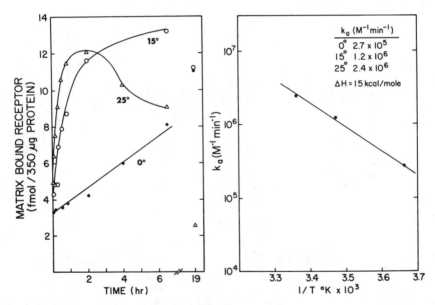

FIGURE 5. Temperature dependence and an Arrhenius plot of androgen receptor binding to nuclear matrix. (*Left*) The 4.5S [³H]dihydrotestosterone-receptor (21.3 fmol) was incubated with nuclear matrix (350 μg protein) at 0°C (●), 15°C (○), and 25°C (△) for increasing times up to 19 hr, and assayed for binding as described in METHODS. Maximal binding achieved at 15°C for 6 hr represented 61% of the total added receptor. (*Right*) Arrhenius plot of temperature-dependent androgen receptor binding to nuclear matrix. Association rate constants (k_a) were calculated using the equation $[t\ k_a\ (b-a)]/2.303 = \log\ (a/b) + \log[(b-x)/(a-x)]$ where a is the maximal number of matrix receptor binding sites (817 fmol/ml), b is the total amount of [³H]dihydrotestosterone-receptor added to the binding reaction (71 fmol/ml), and x is the amount of matrix-bound receptor (fmol/ml) at a given time t (min). The activation energy (+15 kcal/mol) was calculated from the slope of the Arrhenius plot: $\Delta H = \log k_1/\log k_2\ [2.303\ R/(T_1 - T_2)]$ where $R = 1.987$ cal/mol/degree.

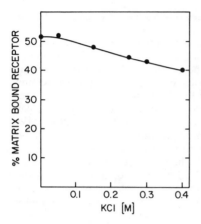

FIGURE 6. Effect of increasing KCl concentration on androgen receptor binding to nuclear matrix. The 4.5S [³H]dihydrotestosterone receptor partially purified on phosphocellulose (31 fmol) was incubated with nuclear matrix (154 μg protein) for 40 min at 25°C as described in METHODS at increasing concentrations of KCl up to 0.4 M. Radioactive steroid was extracted with ethanol as described.

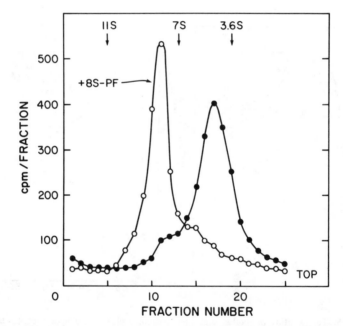

FIGURE 7. Sucrose gradient centrifugation of the 4.5S [³H]dihydrotestosterone-receptor in the presence or absence of 8S androgen receptor-promoting factor. The 4.5S [³H]dihydrotestosterone receptor was obtained by chromatography on phosphocellulose as previously described.[12] The 8S-promoting factor (8S-PF) was partially purified by fractionation of adult male rat serum with (NH₄)₂SO₄, followed by sequential chromatography on DEAE-Sepharose, hydroxylapatite, and ATP-Sepharose. Receptor fractions (62 fmol each) dialyzed with (○) or without (●) the 8S-promoting factor fraction (62 μg protein eluted from ATP-Sepharose at 0.1 M KCl) against 250 ml of 25 mM KCl, 10% glycerol, 1 mM EDTA, 10 mM 2-mercaptoethanol, and 50 mM Tris, pH 7.5 for 2 hr at 4°C. Aliquots (0.3 ml) were layered onto 2 to 20% sucrose gradients prepared in the same buffer and analyzed as described previously.[12]

cleaved to 29,000 MW, even though it retains its high affinity androgen binding site.

The presence of 8S-promoting factor in serum of the adult male rat appears to result from secretion by androgen-responsive cells. Serum of immature male rats of age 16 days or less have no detectable 8S-promoting factor in serum, yet the 8S factor is present in tissues that contain androgen receptor.[12] The spleen was found to lack both androgen receptor and 8S-promoting factor. Previous studies indicate the 8S-promoting factor is a protein of MW ~170,000 that does not bind [^{3}H]androgens.

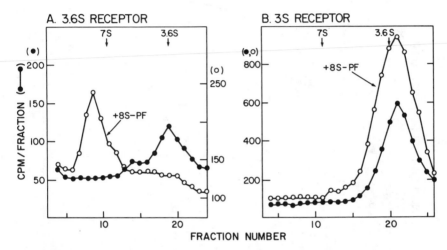

FIGURE 8. Sucrose gradients of the 3.6S and 3.0S proteolytic fragments of the androgen receptor with and without the 8S androgen receptor-promoting factor (A) Ventral prostate cytosol was prepared in the presence of 2 mM diisopropyl fluorophosphate. The 3.6S [^{3}H]dihydrotestosterone-labeled receptor was partially purified by phosphocellulose chromatography and incubated alone (●) or with (○) the 8S-promoting factor (3 mg protein). The 8S-factor (8S-PF) was partially purified by ($NH_4)_2SO_4$ fractionation and DEAE-Sepharose chromatography as described. (B) The Dunning prostate tumor [^{3}H]dihydrotestosterone-labeled receptor was partially purified by phosphocellulose chromatography and treated with bovine pancreatic trypsin (200 μg/0.2 ml receptor) for 5 min at 25°C followed by the addition of 5 mM diisopropyl fluorophosphate and incubated in the presence (○) or absence (●) of the 8S-promoting factor partially purified as described above. Sucrose gradient centrifugation was as described using the marker proteins, ovalbumin (3.6S) and bovine γ-globulin (7S).

The partially purified 8S-promoting factor markedly inhibits Zn^{2+}-potentiated binding of 4.5S [^{3}H]dihydrotestosterone receptor to nuclei and to nuclear matrix as shown in FIGURE 9, where binding is assayed at increasing amounts of DNA. Inhibition of receptor binding to nuclei or nuclear matrix is dependent on the concentration of the 8S-promoting factor. From 40 to 100 μg of partially purified 8S factor are required to inhibit binding by 50%.

The amount of 8S-promoting factor required to inhibit nuclear binding by 50% is approximately one half the minimum required to convert an equivalent amount of 4.5S receptor to 8S on low salt sucrose gradients. These findings suggest that the

8S-promoting factor, in addition to promoting formation of the 8S complex, causes inhibition of the receptor-nuclear matrix interaction.

A question that arises is whether one protein has both 8S reconstituting activity and inhibitory activity, or if two proteins of differing activities have been co-purified. The reconstituted 8S receptor is stable in buffer containing 0.025 M KCl, yet is dissociates to the 4.5S form during centrifugation for 21 hr through sucrose gradients containing 0.15 M KCl. Nuclear inhibitory activity of the 8S-promoting

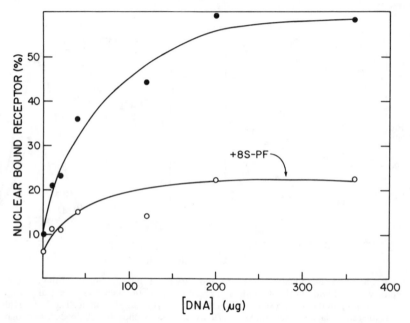

FIGURE 9. Inhibition of Zn^{2+}-dependent 4.5S androgen receptor binding to nuclei by the 8S androgen receptor–promoting factor at increasing concentrations of nuclei. Increasing amounts of nuclei from the Dunning prostate tumor were incubated under standard conditions with the [^{3}H]dihydrotestosterone-labeled 4.5S androgen receptor (33 fmol in 0.3 ml) in the presence (○) or absence (●) of 130 μg partially purified 8S androgen receptor–promoting factor. The 8S-promoting factor (8S-PF) was isolated as described in METHODS by $(NH_4)_2SO_4$ fractionation, followed by sequential chromatography on DEAE-Sepharose, hydroxylapatite, and phosphocellulose. The 8S-promoting factor fraction was added at the beginning of the 30 min incubation at 25°C. Radioactivity in nuclear pellets was extracted and is expressed at the percent of total radioactivity added in the form of the 4.5S [^{3}H]dihydrotestosterone receptor.

factor is detected in an assay buffer containing 0.15 M KCl. A possible explanation for this apparent discrepancy is that the dilution effect and long centrifugation time result in dissociation of the 8S complex that does not occur under conditions of the nuclear binding assay. In agreement with this hypothesis, dilution of the receptor-nuclear binding assay by two- to fourfold results in loss of inhibitory activity of the 8S-promoting factor. Dilution has been shown to transform the progesterone receptor,[29] and may explain the instability of the 8S complex in sucrose gradients containing 0.15 M KCl. Heat inactivation of 8S-promoting factor (60°C for 30 min) assayed by loss of its ability to shift the 4.5S receptor to 8S, likewise destroys inhibiting activity of receptor-nuclear binding. Since the 8S-promoting factor has not been purified to homogeneity, we cannot rule out the possibility that the partially purified fraction contains two distinct components, one that reconstitutes the 8S steroid receptor, and another that inhibits nuclear binding of the 4.5S receptor. That both activities are inherent in one protein is in agreement with the hypothesis that 8S steroid receptors are incapable of binding in nuclei, and represent the nontransformed receptor, while the 4S to 5S forms are transformed to bind in nuclei.

DISCUSSION

Evidence is presented that zinc potentiates binding of the 4.5S androgen receptor to nuclei and nuclear matrix. The binding is temperature dependent, saturable, tissue specific, and of high affinity. The presence of mercaptoethanol in the binding buffer lowers the free Zn^{2+} concentration by about 1000-fold; thus optimum matrix binding occurs at 20 nM free zinc. The similarity in the number of sites for receptor in intact nuclei and in nuclear matrix (1000–1500 sites/nucleus) suggests that nuclear binding of receptor is accounted for primarily by its binding to matrix.

The importance of Zn^{2+} in steroid receptor-nuclear interactions is supported by previous indirect evidence suggesting that steroid receptors may be metalloproteins, e.g. the mouse mammary gland estrogen receptor[30] and the chick oviduct progesterone receptor.[31] The metal chelator 1,10-phenanthroline caused inhibition of binding of the activated glucocorticoid receptor to DNA-cellulose[32] and progesterone receptor binding to nuclei, ATP-Sepharose, and DNA-cellulose.[31,32] It was speculated that inhibition results from chelation of metal ions associated directly with the glucocorticoid receptor.[32]

Zn^{2+} has an important, though poorly defined, role in male sexual development and fertility.[15] Radio-tracer techniques have shown that the rat testis and male accessory sex organs accumulate $^{65}Zn^{2+}$ from blood.[13,14] It was suggested that a total concentration of 2 mM Zn^{2+} corresponds to a free Zn^{2+} concentration of 20 μM in the prostate.[34] Spermatozoa within the testis bind Zn^{2+} and are maintained in a high Zn^{2+} environment within the seminal fluid.[14] Dietary Zn^{2+} deficiency leads to degeneration of the testis, reduction in spermatozoa, and decrease in the weight of the male accessory sex organs.[15] Uptake of Zn^{2+} by rat prostate is androgen dependent; castration causes a decrease in Zn^{2+} levels that can be restored by administration of testosterone.[34] Whether the physiological effects of Zn^{2+} in the male reproductive system are directly related to a requirement for Zn^{2+} in androgen receptor action remains to be established.

The data presented suggest that a non-steroid binding protein associates with the high affinity 4.5S androgen receptor, and that this protein must dissociate in order for the receptor to bind in nuclei. Proteins that do not bind steroids have been shown by Murayama et al. to interact with the estrogen receptor of cow uterus[35] and the progesterone receptor of hen oviduct.[36] One of these, an "8S estrogen receptor-forming factor," could be dissociated in 0.4 M NaSCN and fractionated by gel filtration into two components (Stokes' radius 37Å and 18.5Å) that bind in various ratios to form 5S, 6S, and 8S forms of the estrogen receptor.[37,38] Furthermore, the 37Å component, when added to an in vitro nuclear binding assay, showed a dramatic inhibition of nuclear binding of the 4.5S estrogen receptor derived from porcine uterus.[39]

Others[40] have demonstrated a heat-sensitive macromolecular factor in mature rat uterus, but not rat liver cytosol, that causes loss of estrogen receptor binding in nuclei. This factor appeared to be specific for the estrogen receptor since the effect occurred neither with the liver glucocorticoid receptor nor with rat prostate androgen receptor.

More recently, monoclonal and polyclonal antibodies raised against the avian 8S progesterone receptor have been shown to bind to a 90,000 molecular weight non-progesterone binding component of the 8S receptor. Antibodies against this component cross-react with the 8S glucocorticoid, estrogen, and androgen receptors[41] suggesting that these nontransformed receptor complexes share a similar

ANDROGEN TARGET CELL

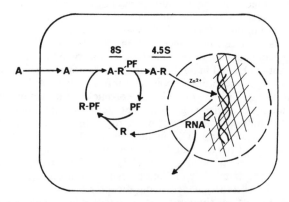

FIGURE 10. Schematic diagram of a proposed mechanism for androgen receptor action in target cells. The binding of androgen (A) to the 8S receptor (R-PF) may shift the equilibrium toward the 4.5S receptor form (AR). Release of the 8S androgen receptor–promoting factor (PF) enables the "transformed" 4.5S androgen receptor to bind to nuclear matrix in a manner that is dependent on low levels of Zn^{2+}. Following binding to matrix and perhaps DNA, the receptor may recycle to the cytoplasmic fraction or remain within the nuclear compartment where it again associates with the 8S-promoting factor. Whether the 8S-promoting factor independently associates with a component of the nucleus has not been determined. Abbreviations are 8S androgen receptor–promoting factor, PF; androgen receptor, R; androgen (e.g., dihydrotestosterone), A. The 8S form of the androgen receptor is represented by R-PF or AR-PF, while the 4.5S form is R or AR.

non-steroid binding component. Monoclonal antibodies to the estrogen receptor indicate also that the 8S complex is not a dimer of identical subunits but consists of receptor associated with another protein.[42]

Evidence that argues against another protein associating with 4–5S steroid receptors is that the purified molybdate-stabilized 8S form of the chick oviduct progesterone receptor (MW ~280,000) consisted of a single band on SDS polyacrylamide gels, indicating a protein composed of only ~85,000 MW polypeptide chains.[43]

A schematic diagram shown in FIGURE 10 illustrates how the 8S-promoting factor and Zn^{2+} might influence binding of the androgen receptor to nuclei. An equilibrium exists between the native 4.5S receptor and the 8S receptor complex formed by association with the 8S androgen receptor-promoting factor. When associated with 8S-promoting factor, the receptor has a low binding affinity for nuclei. Upon dissociation from the 8S-promoting factor, which may be favored by receptor binding of androgen, the 4.5S receptor binds with high affinity to nuclear matrix in a manner that is dependent on zinc. Receptor association with matrix might facilitate subsequent interaction with hormone-dependent genes preferentially associated with matix.[10] Zn^{2+}-dependent receptor binding to nuclear matrix is reversible, thus the receptor may be released in its original 4.5S form. Receptor forms smaller than 4.5S, i.e. 3.6S and 3.0S, have been shown to be proteolytic artifacts generated during isolation.[11,44] We know little as yet about the steriod-free form of the androgen receptor, due to the lability of the ligand-free steroid binding site.[45] It is conceivable that phosphorylation is a crucial factor in maintaining the activity of its binding site, as has been suggested for glucocorticoid[46] and progesterone[47] receptors.

ACKNOWLEDGMENTS

We would like to thank Dr. Lee Pedersen, Department of Chemistry, University of North Carolina at Chapel Hill, who kindly provided the mathematical formulation to determine the mercaptoethanol-Zn^{2+} binding constants. We are grateful to the Papanicolaou Cancer Research Institute, Inc., for providing Copenhagen-Fischer rats bearing the R3327H Dunning tumor.

REFERENCES

1. KON, O. L. & T. C. SPELSBERG. 1982. Endocrinology **111:** 1925–1935.
2. KLYZSEJKO-STEFANOWICZ, L., J. F. CHIU, Y. H. TSAI & L. S. HNILICA. 1976. Proc. Natl. Acad. Sci. USA **73:** 1954–1958.
3. MAINWARING, W. I. P., E. K. SYMES & S. J. HIGGINS. 1976. Biochem. J. **156:** 129–141.
4. RENNIE, P. S. 1979. J. Biol. Chem. **254:** 3947–3952.
5. LIAO, S., G. MEZZETTI & C. CHEN. 1979. *In* The Cell Nucleus. H. Busch, Ed. **7:** 201–227. Academic Press. New York.
6. BARRACK, E. R. & D. S. COFFEY. 1980. J. Biol. Chem. **255:** 7265–7275.
7. ROBINSON, S. I., B. D. NELKIN & B. VOGELSTEIN. 1982. Cell **28:** 99–106.
8. MILLER, T. E., C. Y. HUANG & A. O. POGO. 1978. J. Cell Biol. **76:** 675–691.
9. HERMAN, R., L. WEYMOUTH & S. PENMAN. 1978. J. Cell Biol. **78:** 663–674.
10. PARDOLL, D. M., B. VOGELSTEIN & D. S. COFFEY. 1980. Cell **19:** 527–536.
11. WILSON, E. M. & F. S. FRENCH. 1979. J. Biol. Chem. **254:** 6310–6319.
12. COLVARD, D. S. & E. M. WILSON. 1981. Endocrinology **109:** 496–504.
13. MANN, T. 1964. *In* The Biochemistry of Semen and of the Male Reproductive Tract. Methuen. London.
14. WETTERDAL, B. 1958. Acta Radiologica Suppl. **156:** 3–83.
15. SANDSTEAD, H. H., A. S. PRASAD, A. R. SCHULERT, Z. FARID, A. MIALE, S. BASSILLY & W. J. DARBY. 1967. Am. J. Clin. Nutr. **20:** 422–442.
16. SPELSBERG, T. C., A. W. STEGGLES & B. W. O'MALLEY. 1971. J. Biol. Chem. **246:** 4188–4197.
17. COLVARD, D. S. & E. M. WILSON. 1983. Endocrinology Abst. 228. 65th Endocrine Society Meeting. San Antonio, Texas.
18. BEREZNEY, R. & D. S. COFFEY. 1977. J. Cell Biol. **73:** 616–637.
19. ROSS, D. A., R. W. YEN & C. B. CHAE. 1982. Biochemistry **21:** 764–771.

20. ARMANET, J. P. & J. C. MERLIN. 1961. Bull. Soc. Chim. France 440.
21. MOUDGIL, V. K. & D. O. TOFT. 1975. Proc. Natl. Acad. Sci. USA 72: 901–905.
22. LOWRY, O. H., N. J. ROSEBROUGH, A. L. FARR & R. J. RANDALL. 1951. J. Biol. Chem. 193: 265–275.
23. BURTON, K. 1956. Biochem. J. 62: 315–323.
24. SILLEN, L. G. & A. E. MARTELL. 1971. Stability constants of metal-ion complexes. Special publication of the Chemical Society No. 25. Supplement No. 1. Burlington House. London.
25. MEISSNER, G. 1974. Methods Enzymol. 31: 238–246.
26. BRUCHOVSKY, N., P. S. RENNIE & A. VANSON. 1975. Biochim. Biophys. Acta 394: 248–266.
27. KUHN, R. W., W. T. SCHRADER, W. A. COTY, P. M. CONN & B. W. O'MALLEY. 1977. J. Biol. Chem. 252: 308–317.
28. CLARK, J. H., H. A. ERIKSSON & J. W. HARDIN. 1976. J. Steroid Biochem. 7: 1039–1043.
29. BULLER, R. E., D. O. TOFT, W. T. SCHRADER & B. W. O'MALLEY. 1975. J. Biol. Chem. 250: 801–808.
30. SHYAMALA, G. & Y. F. YEH. 1975. Biochem. Biophys. Res. Commun. 64: 408–415.
31. LOHMAR, P. H. & D. O. TOFT. 1975. Biochem. Biophys. Res. Commun. 67: 8–15.
32. SCHMIDT, T. J., B. C. SEKULA & G. LITWACK. 1981. Endocrinology 109: 803–812.
33. TOFT, D., P. E. ROBERTS, H. NISHIGORI & V. K. MOUDGIL. 1979. Adv. Exp. Med. Biol. 117: 329–341.
34. GUNN, S. A., T. C. GOULD & W. A. D. ANDERSON. 1961. J. Endocrinol. 23: 37–45.
35. MURAYAMA, A., F. FUKAI, T. HAZATO & T. YAMAMOTO. 1980. J. Biochem. 88: 963–968.
36. MURAYAMA, A., F. FUKAI & T. YAMAMOTO. 1980. J. Biochem. 88: 1305–1315.
37. MURAYAMA, A., F. FUKAI & T. YAMAMOTO. 1980. J. Biochem. 88: 969–976.
38. MURAYAMA, A., F. FUKAI & T. YAMAMOTO. 1980. J. Biochem. 88: 1457–1466.
39. MURAYAMA, A. & F. FUKAI. 1982. J. Biochem. 92: 2039–2042.
40. NISHIZAWA, Y., Y. MAEDA, K. NOMA, B. SATO, K. MATSUMOTO & Y. YAMAMURA. 1981. Endocrinology 109: 1463–1472.
41. JOAB, I., J. M. RENOIR, J. MESTER, N. BINART, C. RADANYI, T. BUCHOU, R. ZOOROB & M. G. CATELLI. 1983. Endocrinology Abst. 577. 65th Endocrine Society Meeting. San Antonio, Texas.
42. MONCHARMONT, B., J. L. SU & I. PARIKH. 1982. Biochemistry 21: 6916–6921.
43. RENOIR, J. M., C. R. YANG, P. FORMSTECHER, P. LUSTENBERGER, A. WOLFSON, G. REDEUILH, J. MESTER, H. RICHARD-FOY & E. E. BAULIEU. 1982. Eur. J. Biochem. 127: 71–79.
44. WILSON, E. M., O. A. LEA & F. S. FRENCH. 1980. In Testicular Development, Structure and Function. A. Steinberger & E. Steinberger, Eds.: 201–209. Raven Press. New York.
45. WILSON, E. M. & F. S. FRENCH. 1976. J. Biol. Chem. 251: 5620–5629.
46. HOUSLEY, P. R. & W. B. PRATT. 1983. J. Biol. Chem. 258: 4630–4635.
47. DOUGHERTY, J. J., R. K. PURI & D. O. TOFT. 1982. J. Biol. Chem. 257: 14226–14230.
48. KLOTZ, I. M. & D. L. HUNSTON. 1971. Biochemistry 10: 3065–3069.
49. KLOTZ, I. M. & D. L. HUNSTON. 1975. J. Biol. Chem. 250: 3001–3009.
50. KLOTZ, I. M. & D. L. HUNSTON. 1979. Arch. Biochem. Biophys. 193: 314–328.

Structure and Expression of Androgen-regulated Genes in Mouse Kidney[a]

CHERYL S. WATSON, DANIELA SALOMON,[b]
and JAMES F. CATTERALL[c]

The Population Council
The Rockefeller University
New York, New York, 10021

INTRODUCTION

Testosterone and other androgenic steroids induce the synthesis of several enzymes in the proximal tubules of the mouse kidney[1] and these responses are dependent on the presence of androgen receptor.[2,3] A major advantage of the mouse kidney model for the study of androgen action over other androgen-dependent tissues is the absence of cell division in the proximal tubule in response to androgens.[4] In addition, these cells lack 5α-reductase, which converts testosterone into its more active metabolite 5α-dihydrotestosterone.[2]

The best characterized of the androgen-inducible mouse renal enzymes is β-glucuronidase.[3,5] Its unique response to testosterone includes a lag period of approximately two days[6] and slow kinetics of enzyme activity induction reaching maximal level after about three weeks of chronic hormone treatment. The rate of enzyme synthesis increases 300-fold over this induction period while the specific activity of the enzyme increases 20–50-fold,[5] the difference being due to secretion of the enzyme into urine.

The activities of several other enzymes are under androgenic control in mouse kidney including ornithine decarboxylase,[6] alcohol dehydrogenase,[7] arginase,[8] and 3-ketoreductase.[9] However, it is clear that androgens do not cause major changes in overall protein concentration as occurs in some other steroid hormone–responsive tissues.

Recently, a different approach to the identification of androgen-regulated gene products has been taken.[10,11] Translation of mouse renal mRNA *in vitro* before and after testosterone treatment revealed a relatively abundant androgen-inducible mRNA that coded for a 20,000 dalton peptide.[10] This peptide was designated kidney androgen–regulated protein or KAP. The native structure and function of this protein is unknown, but its synthesis is specific for kidney cells. Another androgen-regulated mRNA was identified from mouse kidney and designated

[a] Supported by National Institutes of Health Grant HD-13541.

[b] Present address: Department of Biochemistry, Weizmann Institute of Science, Rehovot, Israel.

[c] Correspondence to: J. F. C., The Population Council, 1230 York Avenue, Box 273, New York, NY 10021.

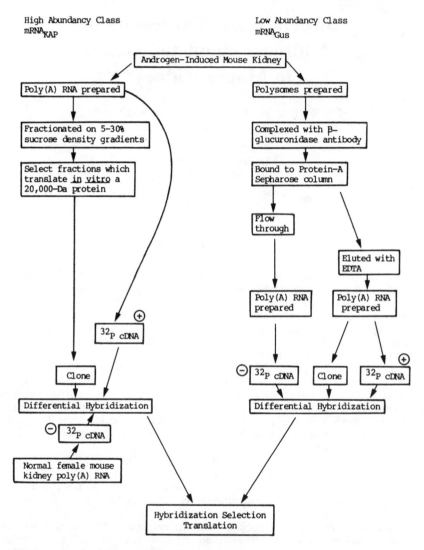

FIGURE 1. Purification of mRNAs, cloning strategies, and selection of specific sequences for KAP and β-glucuronidase. See text for details.

mRNA 908.[11] This mRNA codes for a 43,000 dalton polypeptide *in vitro* but again its identity and function are unknown. Determination of the subcellular localization and function of the proteins coded for by these induced mRNAs awaits further investigation.

While much is known about these distal events in the androgen response, the underlying genetic parameters responsible for the induction of specific genes by androgens are not well understood. Again, the β-glucuronidase model system provides unique features for such studies. The response of the β-glucuronidase gene is under the control of a *cis*-acting regulatory site designated Gus-r.[12] The alleles of this genetic locus determine the extent to which structural gene (Gus-s) responds to hormone treatment. In this report, complementary DNA (cDNA) clones have been used to analyze the structure and expression of KAP mRNA and β-glucuronidase mRNA (mRNA$_{Gus}$). These two gene products are representative of different classes of mRNA and also differ in their androgenic response. KAP is an abundant gene product that exhibits a relatively rapid response to the hormone. On the other hand, β-glucuronidase mRNA is non-abundant, representing less than 0.04% of the poly(A)-mRNA in fully induced tissue and displays an unusually slow response to hormone treatment.

PURIFICATION OF KAP AND β-GLUCURONIDASE mRNAs

Diagrammatic representations of the purification of mRNAs and the cloning and selection of specific sequences are shown in FIGURE 1. In order to obtain DNA complementary to specific mRNAs from androgen-induced mouse kidney, we purified total poly(A)-mRNA from animals treated for 21 days with 5α-dihydrotestosterone (DHT)-containing Silastic® implants, which release ~120 μg steroid/day. Since KAP mRNA was known to be the most abundant androgen-responsive mRNA in this tissue,[10] it was purified simply by sucrose density gradient centrifugation. Aliquots of sucrose gradient fractions were analyzed by cell-free translation using nuclease-treated rabbit reticulocyte lysate (Bethesda Research Laboratories, Gaithersburg, MD) in the presence of L-[^{35}S]methionine and the other 19 L-amino acids. Three fractions, sedimenting at approximately 10S, coded for a 20,000 dalton peptide, which was consistent with the published molecular size of KAP (FIGURE 2).[10] Aliquots of gradient fractions at higher sedimentation coefficient values were similarly assayed and the products immunoprecipitated with β-glucuronidase antiserum. However, no β-glucuronidase-specific peptides were detected in these assays.

β-Glucuronidase mRNA (mRNA$_{Gus}$) was purified from total polysomes from kidneys of androgen-treated mice according to the method of Kraus & Rosenberg[13] as described previously.[14] Briefly, protein A-Sepharose (Pharmacia, Uppsala, Sweden) purified β-glucuronidase antibody was incubated with the polysome preparation. The resulting immune complexes were bound to a second protein A-Sepharose column and RNA was eluted with EDTA. Enrichment of β-glucuronidase mRNA was then confirmed by *in vitro* translation yielding an immunoprecipitable 69,000 dalton protein.[14] The purification of mRNA$_{Gus}$ by this method was at least 100-fold as determined by translation *in vitro* (TABLE 1).

TABLE 1. Purification of mRNA$_{Gus}$ from Kidneys of Androgen-treated Mice

	RNA (μg)	Purity of mRNA$_{Gus}$ (%)
Polysomal RNA	18,000	0.02
Protein A-Sepharose	45	—
Poly(A) RNA	4	2.0[a]

[a] Estimated by translation *in vitro*.

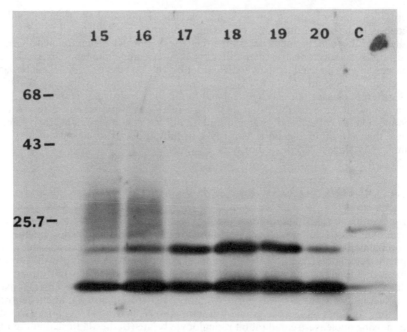

FIGURE 2. SDS-Polyacrylamide gel electrophoresis (SDS-PAGE) of cell-free translation products of sucrose density gradient–purified kidney mRNA. Poly(A)-containing kidney RNA from androgen-induced mice was centrifuged in a 5–30% sucrose density gradient (11.5 ml) at 35,000 rpm for 18 hr in a Beckman SW 41 rotor. Fractions (0.35 ml) were collected and analyzed by cell-free translation followed by SDS-PAGE (10%) as previously described.[14] Fractions 17–19 were pooled and used for subsequent cDNA synthesis and cloning into the *Pst* I site of pBR322 according to Stein *et al.*[36] Lane C contained the product of a viral mRNA used as a positive control. Protein molecular weight markers shown at the left of the figure were bovine serum albumin (68,000), ovalbumin (43,000), and α-chymotrypsinogen (25,700).

IDENTIFICATION OF cDNA CLONES FROM ANDROGEN-INDUCED mRNA

Groups of cDNA clones prepared from DHT-treated mouse kidney tissue were analyzed for androgen-responsiveness of the mRNA from which they were derived by differential colony hybridization.[15] Clones that hybridized to [^{32}P]cDNA from an androgen-induced mRNA preparation but to a lesser extent to labeled cDNA from uninduced mRNA preparations were scored as positive for androgen responsiveness. A quantitative modification of this assay was used to identify clones for mRNA 908 by Berger *et al.*[11] Using the direct *in situ* colony hybridization method in combination with hybrid selected translation (*see below*) we identified cDNA clones for KAP mRNA.

This assay was modified for selecting clones containing β-glucuronidase cDNA. In selecting cDNA clones to androgen-responsive mRNA (*above*) the "minus" tracer cDNA was prepared from normal female animals. This is not a true minus tracer as androgen-regulated mRNAs are present in this tissue but in lower concentrations than after androgen treatment. However, in the case of mRNA$_{Gus}$, a truly minus probe could be prepared from mRNA in the flow-through fraction of the protein A-Sepharose column, which was depleted of β-glucuronidase mRNA. Therefore, differential hybridization for selection of β-glucuronidase cDNA clones was carried out using [^{32}P]cDNA from mRNA enriched for (positive) or depleted of (negative) mRNA$_{Gus}$ (FIGURE 1.)

SELECTION OF KAP AND β-GLUCURONIDASE cDNA CLONES

Final identification of a cDNA clone required direct correlation of the cloned sequence with mRNA biological activity (i.e. its peptide product). Hybrid selection followed by cell-free translation was used as a means of making the necessary correlation. Plasmid DNA was prepared by the simple and rapid method described by Ish-Horwicz and Burke,[16] attached to nitrocellulose filters, and hybridized to kidney mRNA according to Parnes *et al.*[17] KAP clones were identified by selection of mRNA coding for a 20,000 dalton peptide (FIGURE 3) and one of

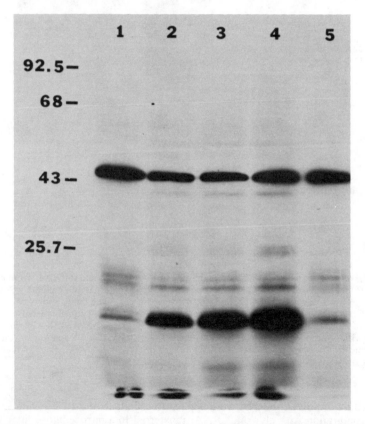

FIGURE 3. Hybrid-selected cell-free translation showing the ^{35}S-labeled products of mRNA that hybridized to three KAP cDNA clones. Each lane represents the total peptide products of mRNA selected by hybridization to: lane 1, a cDNA plasmid that was positive in the differential hybridization assay (*see text*): lanes 2–4, three KAP cDNA clones; lane 5, pBR322. Conditions for SDS-PAGE were as described in the legend to FIGURE 2.

these, designated pKAP11 (lane 3), was used in further studies. The β-glucuronidase cDNA plasmid was identified by selection of a mRNA that coded for a 69,000
dalton peptide that was immunoprecipitated by a monospecific antibody.[14]

The length of KAP mRNA was determined to be 0.85 kilobases (kb) and that
for mRNA$_{Gus}$ to be 2.6 kb by Northern blot analysis (FIGURE 4). In this experi-

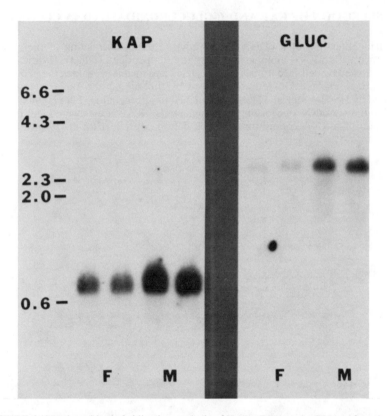

FIGURE 4. Northern blot hybridization analysis of KAP mRNA and mRNA$_{Gus}$ from intact
male (M) and female (F) NCS mice. RNA was isolated by the LiCl-urea method.[37] Poly(A)
RNA (8 μg) was denatured and applied to a 1% agarose gel.[18] The figure shows two exposures of the same nitrocellulose filter, which had been hybridized to ^{32}P-labeled pGUS 7
(GLUC) followed by washing and rehybridization to ^{32}P-labeled pKAP11 (KAP). The specific activities of the hybridization probes were approximately 5.0×10^7 cpm/μg and autoradiographic exposures were 5 days (GLUC) and 20 hr (KAP) at −70°C. Size markers (in
kilobases) were λ-Hind III fragments labeled by 3' end labeling.[38]

ment 8.0 μg of poly(A)-mRNA were applied to each lane of a 1.0% agaraose gel
after denaturation with glyoxal.[18] RNA transferred to a nitrocellulose filter was
hybridized to ^{32}P-labeled pGUS7 DNA[14] and exposed to X-ray film (Kodak XAR)
for five days at −70°C in the presence of a CaWO$_4$ intensifying screen (FIGURE 4,
GLUC). The pGUS7 probe was then washed off the nitrocellulose[18] and replaced

in a second hybridization reaction by ^{32}P-labeled pKAP11. The result of this second hybridization is shown in Figure 4 (KAP) after a 20-hr exposure as described above. Thus, the sex differences (*see legend to* Figure 4) in the concentration of these mRNAs are directly comparable, males containing 1.8- and 5.7-fold higher levels of mRNA$_{KAP}$ and mRNA$_{Gus}$, respectively than females. However, the relative amounts of mRNA$_{KAP}$ and mRNA$_{Gus}$ cannot be compared in Figure 4 because of the difference in length of exposure time. We have found the successive hybridization of Northern filters with different probes to be very useful and generally applicable as long as the less abundant mRNA is analyzed first. In our experience if mRNA$_{KAP}$ was detected first, even the most stringent washing procedures could not remove the labeled KAP probe so that it was not detected in the long exposures required for mRNA$_{Gus}$ detection.

Unequivocal identification of cDNA clones can be achieved by direct comparison of amino acid sequence data with similar data derived from DNA sequencing of cloned cDNA. This was not possible in the case of KAP as the protein has yet to be identified *in vivo*. However, the amino acid sequences of six cysteine-containing fragments of rat β-glucuronidase have been reported.[19] The cDNA sequence determined from the clones shown in Figure 5A contained a long reading frame by computer analysis of the three possible codon phases.[20] The sequences surrounding the two cysteine residues in this inferred sequence were compared to the six published cysteine-containing peptides. A perfect match was found for one of these peptides (Figure 6) and the position of this region on the cDNA map is shown in Figure 5A (*marked by solid bar*). The only differences in the sequences are derived from the difficulty in differentiating between the acid and amide forms of aspartic acid by peptide sequence analysis.

The identity of the sequences from mouse and rat suggests an important function of this site in the protein. This may simply reflect the importance of the cysteine residue to the secondary structure of the protein, or it may indicate that this sequence is at or near the active site of the enzyme. Comparison of the complete sequences of β-glucuronidase cDNA from rat[21] and mouse[14] will help to reveal conserved sequences that may function in enzyme activity and structure as well as protein secretion and sorting. It is interesting to note in this regard that mouse β-glucuronidase has two subcellular locations, in the lysosome and on the microsomal membrane.[22] Erickson *et al.*[23] have shown that the lysosomal protease cathepsin D is secreted using the same cellular machinery as that described for secretory proteins. Thus, the mechanism by which the cell differentiates between these two types of proteins must involve steps distal to membrane translocation into the lumen of the endoplasmic reticulum. Recent evidence suggests that this sorting function involves the cleavage of a peptide from the C-terminus of some lysosomal enzymes.[24] The determination of amino acid sequences for lysosomal enzymes like β-glucuronidase will be required for the identification of the sequences for protein sorting.

STRUCTURAL MAPS FOR cDNAs

Restriction endonuclease maps of the cDNA segments for the two mRNAs are shown in Figure 5. The KAP cDNA sequencing studies (not shown) indicate that this fragment codes for the C-terminal 40 amino acids of the putative KAP protein and the 3' non-coding region that contains 200 nucleotides excluding the poly(A) tail. The restriction map of β-glucuronidase cDNA was derived from four individual clones. Three of these (pGUS 5, 7, and 48) were isolated in the original

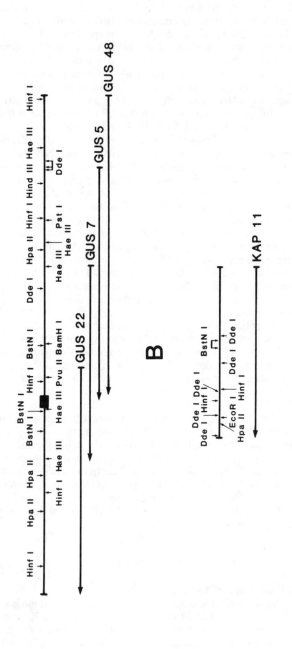

FIGURE 5. Composite restriction maps of the cloned regions of mRNA$_{Gus}$ (A) and mRNA$_{KAP}$ (B). Arrows point toward the 5' end of the mRNA. The solid bar in A indicates the positions of nucleotides that correspond to a known peptide sequence of rat β-glucuronidase (FIGURE 6). All cleavage sites for the enzymes listed in either (A) or (B) are shown for both cDNA segments. Enzymes that do not cleave either of these regions include: *Hha* I, *Bgl* II, *Hinc* II, *Kpn* I, and *Xba* I.

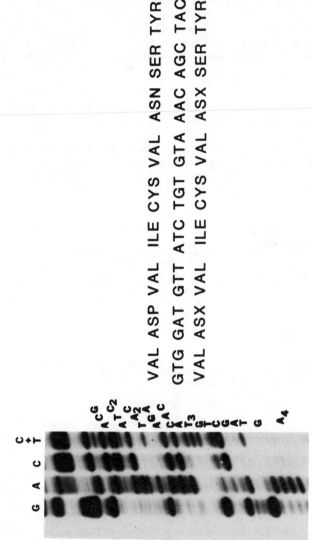

VAL ASP VAL ILE CYS VAL ASN SER TYR
GTG GAT GTT ATC TGT GTA AAC AGC TAC
VAL ASX VAL ILE CYS VAL ASX SER TYR

FIGURE 6. Amino acid sequence derived from the nucleotide sequence of a fragment of pGUS7 matches the sequence of a peptide from rat β-glucuronidase. DNA sequencing reactions[39] were carried out as previously described[38] and the products separated on a 10% polyacrylamide gel containing 7 M urea at 40 W constant power for 1 hr and 50 min. The data shown were derived from a 5' end-labeled *Hinf* I fragment of pGUS7 recut with *Hpa* II and represent the cDNA equivalent strand. The sequence at right is the reverse complement (mRNA equivalent strand) of the data shown. The derived amino acid sequence is shown above the nucleotide sequence and that determined by peptide sequence analysis[19] is shown below.

screening after polysome immunoadsorption of mRNA$_{Gus}$.[14] The fourth segment (contained in pGUS22) was obtained by internally primed synthesis of cDNA from the PvuII-DdeI 240 bp fragment of pGUS7. The overall length of the combined cDNA segments is 1.3 kb. This represents one half of the complete mRNA$_{Gus}$ sequence and includes the 310 C-terminal codons of the β-glucuronidase coding region and 345 nucleotides of the non-coding region. The 3′ end is apparently not included in any of the original three clones as neither the poly-adenylation signal AAUAAA[25] nor the poly(A) tail itself are found in these clones. This may be due to loss of the 5′ end of the cDNA strand during second strand synthesis in the presence of the Klenow fragment of E. coli DNA polymerase I.

EXPRESSION OF KAP AND β-GLUCURONIDASE mRNAs AFTER ACUTE TESTOSTERONE ADMINISTRATION

β-Glucuronidase exhibits an initial lag in the androgenic induction of enzyme activity and synthesis. In the NCS Swiss mouse used in the studies described here, the lag period is approximately two days when a single injection of testosterone (10 mg) is administered.[6] Similar kinetics of induction have been reported for

TABLE 2. Accumulation of mRNAs for KAP and β-Glucuronidase after Acute Testosterone Administration

Hr after Treatment	Fold Induction[a]	
	mRNA$_{KAP}$	mRNA$_{Gus}$
0	1.0	1.0
2	0.8	0.9
6	1.6	1.0
12	1.5	1.0
24	1.9	1.5
48	2.0	1.7

[a] Determined by densitometer scanning of autoradiographic bands after Northern blot analysis using a Shimadzu model CS-910 scanner.

mRNA$_{Gus}$ activity using an assay that involved injection of frog oocytes followed by enzyme assay.[26] However, this assay cannot measure mRNA$_{Gus}$ in the absence of biological activity and is not sensitive enough to detect mRNA$_{Gus}$ prior to three days after hormone implantation.

TABLE 2 presents a comparison of the initial induction of the accumulation of mRNA$_{KAP}$ and mRNA$_{Gus}$. KAP mRNA concentration begins to increase within 6 hr of hormone injection. In contrast, mRNA$_{Gus}$ remains at basal level until 24 hr after hormone injection. This precedes the increase in enzyme activity by about 24 hr in this mouse strain.[6] The fact that the accumulation of KAP mRNA, as well as other androgen-regulated kidney mRNAs,[11,27] is induced 2–6 hr after treatment indicates that the androgen receptor is not limiting the induction of the β-glucuronidase gene. It has been suggested that the association of androgen receptors with chromatin is the limiting step in the induction of the β-glucuronidase gene by testosterone.[28] Alternatively, the activity of another androgen-induced early gene may be required for increased β-glucuronidase gene activity. In this regard, it is interesting to note that androgen-inducible ornithine decarboxylase (ODC) mRNA accumulation can be detected 2–6 hr after administration of testosterone.[27] ODC is the rate-limiting enzyme in polyamine biosynthesis and polyamines have been shown to have an essential role in macromolecular synthesis.[29] During testosterone treatment, inhibition of ODC blocked secretion of β-glucuronidase into the urine while enzyme activity in the kidney was changed only by a delay in achieving the maximal level.[30] However, blockage of secretion of the enzyme could produce an androgen-independent accumulation in enzyme activity in kidney cells. Measurement of β-glucuronidase and KAP mRNA concentration under conditions that inhibit ODC activity and hence accumulation of polyamines would resolve the question of any specific effect of polyamine biosynthesis on β-glucuronidase gene induction by androgens.

DEPENDENCE OF KAP AND β-GLUCURONIDASE GENE EXPRESSION ON THE ANDROGEN RECEPTOR

The androgen-insensitive Tfm/Y mouse has been shown to contain little or no androgen receptor in what are considered to be the classically androgen-dependent tissues.[2] Therefore we analyzed poly(A) RNA prepared from the kidneys of such mice to determine whether the induction of both KAP and β-glucuronidase was dependent upon the presence of androgen receptor. As shown by Northern blot analysis (FIGURE 7), androgen administration to Tfm mice does not induce β-glucuronidase-specific RNA, thus confirming the androgen-receptor dependence in this induction. However, when the same nitrocellulose filter is hybridized to nick-translated KAP cDNA, an induction by androgens is evident. This is in contrast to a negative result published by Toole *et al.*[10] These data suggest that KAP mRNA can be induced by androgens via a mechanism that is independent of androgen receptors binding testosterone or its 5α-reduced metabolite 5α-DHT. We are currently testing the possible dependence of this induction of the β-steroid receptor, which has greater affinity for β-epimeric forms of testosterone,[31] but to which Tfm/Y animals respond normally.[32] It is also possible that KAP mRNA induction is dependent on more general tissue growth-promoting effects of testosterone or other compounds.

An alternative interpretation of these data is that the KAP gene can be regulated and maximally stimulated by very low concentrations of occupied androgen receptors. In the presence of pharmacological doses of androgen, enough occupied receptors would be produced in Tfm/Y animals to induce the KAP mRNA accumulation although not to the same extent as in normal castrated males (FIGURE 7A). In addition, intact males are maximally stimulated for KAP mRNA accumulation and do not respond further to pharmacological doses of hormone (unpublished results). In contrast, β-glucuronidase (unpublished data) and ODC (O. A. Jänne, personal communication) mRNAs were stimulated by androgen treatment of intact males. Similar variance in sensitivity to steroid hormone–receptor complexes has been reported for hormonally regulated genes in chick oviduct.[33]

SUMMARY AND PROJECTIONS

In this report we describe the physical characterization and expression of mRNAs representing two classes of androgen-inducible mouse kidney proteins. KAP

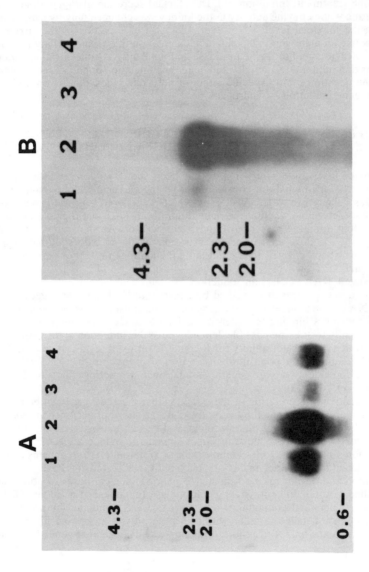

FIGURE 7. Northern blot hybridization analysis of mRNA$_{KAP}$ (A) and mRNA$_{Gus}$ (B) induction by androgens in castrate NCS (lanes 1 and 2) and Tfm/Y (lanes 3 and 4) male mice. Lanes 2 and 4, animals were treated for 4 days with Silastic® implants containing testosterone as described in text. Hybridization, autoradiography, and size markers were the same as described in the legend to FIGURE 4.

mRNA is relatively abundant (4.0% of poly(A) mRNA) and may not rely completely on androgen receptor–mediated events for its enhancement. In contrast, β-glucuronidase is representative of the low abundancy class of messages (0.02% of poly(A) RNA) and appears to be totally dependent on androgen receptor for its induction. In addition, these two gene products exhibit quite different kinetics of induction of mRNA accumulation.

The mouse kidney is a particularly interesting model for androgen action due to the availability of genetic mutants that affect the androgen response; an example reported in this paper is the correlation of Tfm/Y receptor–deficient animals with the loss of response in the case of $mRNA_{Gus}$ but not KAP mRNA induction. Our future studies will focus on mutants of another type—the *cis*-acting regulatory alleles of the β-glucuronidase genetic complex (Gus-r). Preliminary evidence has already suggested that these regulatory alleles can be correlated with different levels of accumulation of β-glucuronidase mRNA in genetically inbred mouse strains (data not shown). Eventual isolation of genomic clones containing the regulatory loci should further elucidate the molecular basis of these regulatory differences.

β-Glucuronidase is a well-characterized lysosomal enzyme that is apparently under sex steroid control only in the mouse kidney although it is produced in many other tissues. KAP mRNA is not found in tissues other than the mouse kidney,[10] but little is known about its biochemical role or its localization *in vitro*. It is not clear why the androgenic regulation of either one of these proteins is of importance in this non-reproductive tissue. Perhaps it is only a reflection of the overlap in early development history that causes renal tissues to share sex steroid hormone regulation with reproductive tissues. On the other hand, it has long been known that pheromones transmitted via the mouse urine have profound effects on reproductive behavior. Recent reports suggest that there are some behavioral consequences of tampering with certain constituents of rodent urine such as polyamines[34] and β-glucuronidase.[35] This leads us to speculate that androgenic control of mouse urinary pheromal elements may be one of the coordinating links between steroid hormone action in the kidney and mouse reproductive behavior.

ACKNOWLEDGMENTS

The authors would like to acknowledge the excellent technical assistance of Susan L. Leary and the help of Jean E. Schweis and Susan Richman in the preparation of the manuscript.

REFERENCES

1. BARDIN, C. W. & J. F. CATTERALL. 1981. Science **211:** 2185–2194.
2. BULLOCK, L. P. & C. W. BARDIN. 1974. Endocrinology **94:** 746–756.
3. BARDIN, C. W., T. R. BROWN, N. C. MILLS, C. GUPTA & L. P. BULLOCK. 1978. Biol. Reprod. **18:** 74–83.
4. KOCHAKIAN, C. D. & D. G. HARRISON. 1962. Endocrinology **70:** 99–108.
5. SWANK, R. T., K. PAIGEN, R. DAVEY, V. CHAPMAN, C. LABARCA, G. WATSON, R. GANSCHOW, E. J. BRANDT & E. NOVAK. 1978. Rec. Progr. Horm. Res. **34:** 401–436.
6. PAJUNEN, A. E. I., V. V. ISOMAA, O. A. JÄNNE & C. W. BARDIN. 1982. J. Biol. Chem. **257:** 8190–8198.

7. OHNO, S., C. STENIUS, L. CHRISTIAN, C. HARRIS & C. IVEY. 1970. Biochem. Genet. 4: 565–577.
8. SWANK, R. T., K. PAIGEN & R. GANSCHOW. 1973. J. Molec. Biol. 81: 225–243.
9. MOWSZOWICZ, I. & C. W. BARDIN. 1974. Steroids 23: 793–807.
10. TOOLE, J. J., N. D. HASTIE & W. A. HELD. 1979. Cell 17: 441–448.
11. BERGER, F. G., K. W. GROSS & G. WATSON. 1981. J. Biol. Chem. 256: 7006–7013.
12. PAIGEN, K. 1979. Annu. Rev. Genet. 13: 417–466.
13. KRAUS, J. P. & L. E. ROSENBERG. 1982. Proc. Natl. Acad. Sci. USA 79: 4015–4019.
14. CATTERALL, J. F. & S. L. LEARY. 1983. Biochemistry 22: 6049–6053.
15. ST. JOHN, T. P. & R. W. DAVIS. 1979. Cell 16: 443–452.
16. ISH-HOROWICZ, D. & J. F. BURKE. 1981. Nuc. Acids Res. 9: 2989–2998.
17. PARNES, J. R., B. VELAN, A. FELSENFELD, L. RAMANATHAN, V. FERRINI, E. APPELLA & J. G. SEIDMAN. 1981. Proc. Natl. Acad. Sci. USA 78: 2253–2257.
18. THOMAS, P. S. 1980. Proc. Natl. Acad. Sci. USA 77: 5201–5205.
19. LEIGHTON, P. H., W. K. FISHER, K. E. MOON & E. O. P. THOMPSON. 1980. Aust. J. Biol. Sci. 33: 513–520.
20. STADEN, R. 1977. Nuc. Acids Res. 4: 4037–4051.
21. NISHIMURA, Y., M. ROSENFELD, G. KREIBICH, M. ADESNIK & D. D. SABATINI. 1983. J. Cell Biol. 97: 103a.
22. LUSIS, A. J. & K. PAIGEN. 1977. Curr. Top. Biol. Med. Res. 2: 63–106.
23. ERICKSON, A. H., P. WALTER & G. BLOBEL. 1983. Biochem. Biophys. Res. Commun. 115: 275–280.
24. ERICKSON, A. H. & G. BLOBEL. 1983. Biochemistry 22: 5201–5205.
25. FITZGERALD, M. & T. SHENK. 1981. Cell 24: 251–260.
26. LABARCA, C. & K. PAIGEN. 1977. Proc. Natl. Acad. Sci. USA 74: 4462–4465.
27. KONTULA, K., J. K. TORKKELI, C. W. BARDIN & O. A. JÄNNE. 1983. Proc. Natl. Acad. Sci. USA 81: 731–735.
28. WATSON, G., R. A. DAVEY, C. LABARCA & K. PAIGEN. 1981. J. Biol. Chem. 256: 3005–3011.
29. JÄNNE, J., H. PÖSO & A. RAINA. 1978. Biochim. Biophys. Acta 473: 241–293.
30. LAITENEN, S. I. & A. E. I. PAJUNEN. 1983. Biochem. Biophys. Res. Commun. 112: 770–777.
31. URABE, A., S. SASSA & A. KAPPAS. 1979. J. Exp. Med. 149: 1314–1325.
32. BESA, E. C. & L. P. BULLOCK. 1981. Endocrinology 109: 1983–1989.
33. PALMITER, R. D., E. R. MULVIHILL, J. H. SHEPPARD & G. S. MCKNIGHT. 1981. J. Biol. Chem. 256: 7910–7916.
34. PINEL, J. P. J., B. B. GORZALKA & F. LADAK. 1981. Physiol. Behav. 27: 819–824.
35. INGERSOLL, D. W., G. BOBOTAS, C.-T. LEE & A. LUKTON. 1982. Physiol. Behav. 29: 789–793.
36. STEIN, J. P., J. F. CATTERALL, S. L. C. WOO, A. R. MEANS & B. W. O'MALLEY. 1978. Biochemistry 17: 5763–5772.
37. AUFFRAY, C. & F. ROUGEON. 1980. Eur. J. Biochem. 107: 303–314.
38. CATTERALL, J. F., J. P. STEIN, P. KRISTO, A. R. MEANS & B. W. O'MALLEY. 1980. J. Cell Biol. 87: 480–487.
39. MAXAM, A. M. & W. GILBERT. 1977. Proc. Natl. Acad. Sci. USA 74: 560–564.

Organization and Expression of Genes Encoding Prostatic Steroid Binding Protein

MALCOLM PARKER, HELEN HURST, and MARTIN PAGE

Imperial Cancer Research Fund
Lincoln's Inn Fields
London WC2A 3PX
United Kingdom

INTRODUCTION

In common with other classes of steroid hormone,[1,2] androgens bind to receptors in target cells to form a steroid receptor complex that is translocated into the cell nucleus. To investigate the regulatory role played by testosterone we are studying the mechanism by which it stimulates the rate of synthesis of prostatic steroid binding protein, the predominant protein secreted into rat prostatic fluid.[3] The protein is tetrameric, consisting of two subunits, one subunit containing the polypeptides C1 and C3 and the other containing the polypeptides C2 and C3.[4] We have shown that testosterone acts via effects on transcription rate and RNA turnover to markedly affect steady-state levels of mRNAs specific for the C1, C2, and C3 polypeptides.[5,6]

Recent work with certain other hormone-responsive genes such as the mouse mammary tumor virus genome, whose transcription is stimulated by glucocorticoids, suggests that the steroid receptor complex interacts directly with the viral genome at a limited number of sites including specific DNA sequences adjacent to the viral promoter.[7–11] The functional significance of these binding sites has been investigated by gene transfer experiments that enable DNA required to confer hormone sensitivity on gene expression to be identified. Thus far it appears that the glucocorticoid binding region associated with the viral promoter is both necessary and sufficient to stimulate viral transcription.[12–16]

Our approach to study androgen action has been to introduce the rat C3 genes into a tumor cell line from mouse mammary gland (S115 cells). This cell line was selected because its growth is stimulated by testosterone[17] showing that S115 cells have functional androgen receptors. Selection of transformed cells containing the gene was achieved by using SV2-gpt vectors[18] that contain the gene for the bacterial enzyme xanthine-guanine phosphoribosyl-transferase (gpt). There is no equivalent mammalian enzyme so that wild type cells will not grow in HAT medium (250 μg/ml hypoxanthine, 2 μg/ml aminopterin, and 10 μg/ml thymidine) containing mycophenolic acid and xanthine because the *de novo* and salvage pathways for purine biosynthesis are inhibited. However, transformed cells expressing the gpt gene will grow providing the medium is supplemented with xanthine. The C3 genes have been introduced into S115 cells either intact or as chimeric genes. The chimeric gene consists of putative C3 promoters and the marker gene interferon (IF), whose expression depends on the C3 promoter. Interferon is secreted from mammalian cells and can be measured in culture medium using a cytopathic effect assay because it confers resistance on cells to viral infection. Thus it is possible to analyze the effect of different C3 promoters on interferon production and thereby investigate promoter and regulatory DNA function.

MATERIALS AND METHODS

Reagents

The following materials were gifts: reverse transcriptase (J. Beard, Life Sciences Inc., U.S.A.); mycophenolic acid (V. Mason, Lilly Research Centre, U.K.); pSV2-gpt (P. Berg, Stanford University, U.S.A.); mouse S115 cells (R. King, I.C.R.F., London); cyproterone acetate (Schering AG, Berlin); human β-interferon cDNA (W. Fiers, State University of Ghent, Belgium); polyoma MboI DNA fragment that contains poly(A) addition sites (M. Fried, I.C.R.F., London).

Isolation and Characterization of Genomic DNA Clones

Genomic DNA clones were isolated from Sprague-Dawley rat DNA that had been cloned in bacteriophage λ.[19,20] The clones are designated as follows: λ11A contains the C1 gene, λ21B contains the C2 gene, λ6 contains the C3(1) gene, and λ11B contains the C3(2) gene. The organization of the four genes was determined by restriction enzyme mapping. The DNA sequence of the genes for C3 was obtained by subcloning restriction enzyme fragments into the bacteriophage M13 followed by dideoxy sequencing.[21]

Construction of Vectors

The intact C3(1) and C3(2) genes were inserted into SV2-gpt[18] by digesting λ6 and λ11B with Eco RI and Bam HI, respectively, and ligating the genes into the unique Eco RI and Bam HI sites in SV2-gpt as previously described.[22] After transformation of *E. coli* HB101, plasmid DNA was isolated using lysozyme and SDS treatment in alkaline conditions.[23]

The chimeric gene was constructed by ligating a MboI polyoma DNA fragment that contains early and late poly(A) addition sites[24] to human β-interferon cDNA.[25] This DNA was then ligated in both orientations to λ6 DNA from nucleotide −800 to +20 in the C3(1) gene. The chimeric gene was then inserted between the Bam HI and Eco RI sites in SV2-gpt. Full details of the constructions will be published elsewhere.

Cell Cultures and Transfection Procedures

S115 cells maintained and transfected using the calcium phosphate coprecipitation method as previously described.[22] Interferon was quantitated using a cytopathic effect bioassay (CPE). Media, which contained interferon, was serially diluted onto 10^4 human embryo fibroblast cells in 96-well dishes for 6 hr at 37°C and then infected with 10^4 plaque-forming units (pfu) of encephalomyocarditis (EMC) virus. After approximately 30 hr cells were stained with crystal violet.

RNA Analysis

Cytoplasmic RNA was isolated using phenol/chloroform.[5] C3 mRNA transcripts were mapped by primer extension using a 70 base-pair (bp) Xba I-Alu I DNA fragment from the 5' end of pA34 a cDNA clone specific for C3 mRNA.[21]

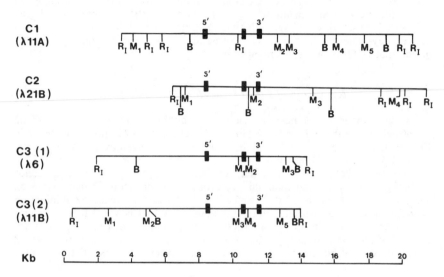

FIGURE 1. Restriction enzyme maps of genes encoding prostatic steroid binding protein. The maps were constructed on the basis of restriction enzyme analysis and R-loop analysis of genomic clones: λ11A for C1, λ21B for C2, λ6 for C3(1), and λ11B for C3(2). Solid blocks represent exons. The following restriction enzymes are presented: Bam HI (B), EcoRI (R_I), and Msp I (M).

RESULTS

Gene Organization

The organization of the genes that code for prostatic steroid binding protein was determined by analysis of genomic DNA clones λ11A for C1, λ21B for C2, λ6 for C3(1), and λ11B for C3(2). Restriction enzyme mapping of the recombinant clones indicated that all four genes were 3.0 to 3.2 kilobases (kb) and consisted of three exons separated by two introns (FIGURE 1). The genes for C1 and C2 share 76% DNA sequence homology[19] and the two genes for C3 share 97% DNA sequence homology,[21] suggesting that these two pairs of genes were derived by gene duplication. The DNA sequence homology between the genes for C1 and C3 and between the genes for C2 and C3 is less striking, being approximately 35%. However, in view of the similarity in their organization it is quite conceivable that all four genes have arisen by a series of gene duplications from a single ancestral gene followed by divergent evolution.

Analysis of prostate RNA by primer extension and S1 mapping[21] indicates that C3(1) is transcribed *in vivo* to produce approximately 2×10^5 C3 RNA molecules per epithelial cell whereas C3(2) transcripts could not be detected and must represent less than 20 molecules per cell. To understand the basis for such differences in expression we have analyzed the structure of the C3 genes and found distinct differences in the state of DNA methylation associated with the two genes. Both genes are hypermethylated at CCGG sites in all rat tissues that were analyzed except for the ventral prostate where C3(1) but not C3(2) is demethylated during the period 14–28 days of age (FIGURE 2). Since there is a strong correlation between hypomethylation and gene expression[26,27] our observation supports the notion that C3(2) is not transcribed *in vivo*.

Expression of Intact Genes for C3 in S115 Cells

We have investigated the expression of C3 and the role played by testosterone by introducing both C3(1) and C3(2) into S115 cells using SV2-gpt vector shown in FIGURE 3. The amount of DNA upstream of the genes ranged from 6,000 bp to 800 bp for C3(1) and was 4,000 bp for C3(2).

Transformed clones were isolated, checked for the presence of intact C3 genes by Southern blotting, and then analyzed for gene expression. Primer extension analysis was used to map C3 RNA since it both assesses the accuracy of initiation of transcription and also quantitates the abundance of RNA. C3 RNA from rat ventral prostate results in major products of 130 nucleotides (T_1) and a minor product of 170 nucleotides (T_2). Both C3(1) and C3(2) were accurately transcribed in S115 cells resulting in a major T_1 transcript and in certain cases a T_2 transcript is

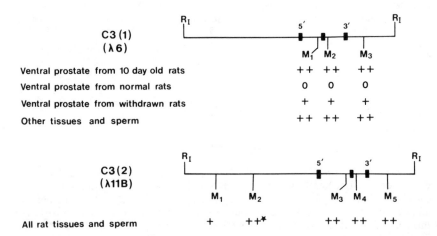

FIGURE 2. Summary of state of DNA methylation associated with the genes for C3. DNA methylation was examined at CCGG sites in ventral prostate from 10-day-old rats, mature normal rats, and rats withdrawn from androgen for 6 days, in other tissues (seminal vesicle, coagulating gland, heart, liver, kidney, and spleen), and in sperm. The extent of DNA methylation is shown by 0 (approximately 0%), + (approximately 50%), and ++ (approximately 100%). A star indicates that the site was resistant to digestion by both Msp I and Hpa II. M represents Msp I sites and R_1 represents Eco RI sites.

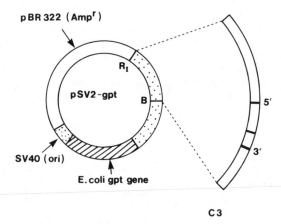

FIGURE 3. Construction of DNA vectors that contain the rat C3 gene. The genomic clones λ6 and λ11B were digested with Bam HI or Eco RI and the C3(1) and C3(2) genes, respectively, were cloned into the appropriate sites in pSV2-gpt.[18] The recombinant clones consist of rat C3 exons (solid blocks), rat C3 introns or flanking DNA (open blocks), plasmid DNA labeled, pBR322, SV40 DNA (stippled blocks), and *E. coli* guanine phosphorinosyl transferase (hatched blocks).

just visible (FIGURE 4). We estimate that there are 100–1,000 RNA copies per integrated gene per cell, which represents 0.1–1.0% of the *in vivo* concentration.

The effect of testosterone on C3 gene expression was investigated by growing the clones in the absence or presence of 10^{-8} M testosterone using 2% fetal calf serum that had been stripped of endogenous steroids with dextran-charcoal treatment (FIGURE 5). Individual clones varied in their response to testosterone irrespective of the amount of DNA upstream of the C3 gene. About one third of the clones produced up to fivefold more C3 mRNA in the presence of testosterone than in its absence. Thus in certain clones 800 bp DNA upstream of the C3 gene was sufficient to confer a small androgenic response. The possibility that nonresponsive clones had lost androgen receptors was ruled out because their rate of proliferation was still stimulated by testosterone.

Expression of Chimeric Gene in S115 Cells

We have investigated whether the effect of testosterone on C3 gene expression was directly on the promoter by analyzing the expression of chimeric genes. A C3 DNA fragment from the start of transcription to 800 nucleotides upstream was ligated to a marker gene, interferon (FIGURE 5). The putative C3 promoter was inserted in a 5'-3' and 3'-5' orientation relative to the interferon gene and then ligated into the SV2-gpt vector.[18] After translation into S115 cells, transformed clones were isolated in HAT medium containing mycophenolic acid plus xanthine. Six clones contained the promoter in a 5'-3' orientation and five clones contained the promoter in a 3'-5' orientation. Interferon gene expression was examined for each clone by testing for interferon production in the medium using a cytopathic effect bioassay. Human interferon confers resistance on human embryo fibroblasts to EMC viral infection and can be quantitated by serial dilution.

Interferon was produced by five of six clones in which the promoter was inserted in a 5'-3' orientation but not by clones in which the promoter was inserted in the opposite orientation. This result indicates that the rat C3 promoter is being used to transcribe interferon mRNA. Androgen sensitivity was tested as above by growing clones in the presence or absence of testosterone. None of the clones consistently produced more than twofold more interferon in the presence of testosterone than in its absence and is considered insignificant.

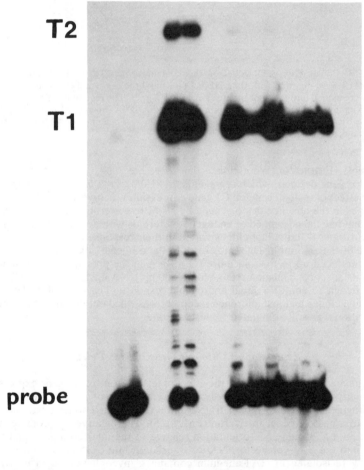

FIGURE 4. Primer extension analysis of C3 RNA expressed in mouse S115 cells. Primer extension analysis was carried out with RNA from individual mouse S115 clones expressing the C3 gene. The major extension product of 130–131 nucleotide is labeled T_1 and the minor extension product of 170 nucleotides is labeled T_2.

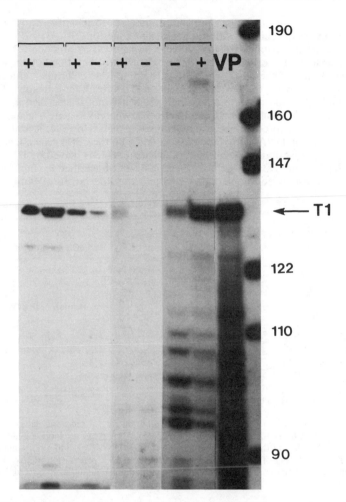

FIGURE 5. Effect of testosterone on C3 gene expression. Primer extension analysis was carried out with RNA from rat ventral prostate (VP) and four individual mouse S115 clones that expressed the C3 gene. The clones were grown in absence (−) or presence (+) of 10^{-8} M testosterone for 3 days prior to the analysis. The major extension product of 130–131 nucleotides is labeled T_1 and a minor extension product of 170 nucleotides is just visible. DNA size markers are shown on the right-hand side.

DISCUSSION

Gene transfer provides an approach for studying what is required, in the form of DNA, for various steps in gene expression. By this means, there has been considerable progress in identifying hormone-responsive regions associated with the gene promoter of the mouse mammary tumor virus[12–16] and certain egg white genes.[28-30] This paper describes our initial attempts to identify testosterone-responsive regions associated with the genes that code for C3.

In rat ventral prostate C3(1) is actively transcribed to produce C3 whereas C3(2) is transcribed poorly if at all. Our first observation was that both genes were expressed similarly when they were introduced into S115 cells albeit at a concentration of less than 1% that in ventral prostate. This result indicates that C3(2) is not a pseudogene and raises the possibility that it is not transcribed *in vivo* because it is methylated at certain CG dinucleotide whereas in gene transfer experiments the gene is expressed because it is unmethylated. However it is also possible that changes in DNA methylation associated with the C3(1) gene occur *in vivo* as a result of transcription. Nevertheless, whatever role is played by DNA methylation, it is still not clear why the C3(2) gene is not transcribed *in vivo*. Since the DNA sequence between nucleotide −235 and the first intron of both genes is

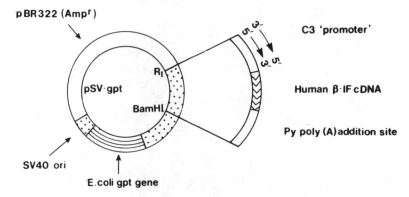

FIGURE 6. Construction of DNA vectors that contain rat C3 chimeric genes. Chimeric genes were constructed that consisted of rat C3(1) DNA from nucleotide −800 to +20 (relative to the 5′ end of the gene), human β-interferon cDNA (IF), and a polyoma poly(A) addition DNA fragment. The rat DNA was inserted in a 5′-3′ orientation relative to the β-interferon cDNA. The chimeric genes were then cloned between in the Eco RI and Bam HI sites in pSV2-gpt.[18]

identical with the exception of one nucleotide, we conclude that the promoter for each gene is similar but that the DNA signals involved in gene activation and perhaps DNA methylation are different in C3(1) and C3(2) and do not reside within the proximal 5′ flanking DNA.

We have demonstrated that testosterone stimulated the expression of both C3 genes in certain transformed cell lines when the intact gene was used. However, the hormone does not appear to stimulate transcription by interacting with DNA upstream of the gene, at least in these heterologous mouse cells. This result contrasts with that for several glucocorticoid-responsive genes such as mouse mammary tumor virus[12-16] or tryptophan oxygenase[29] but resembles that found for the chicken ovalbumin and lysozyme genes. These latter genes respond to dexamethasone and progesterone in chick oviduct cells but not heterologous cells that contain glucocorticoid receptors.[28-30] Therefore it is possible that hormone regulation of certain genes requires tissue-specific factors in addition to the steroid receptor complex. To investigate this further, we are analyzing the expression of the C3 gene, as a chimeric gene, in primary cultures of rat ventral prostate.

SUMMARY

We have cloned the genes for prostatic steroid binding protein to study the mechanism whereby their expression is regulated by testosterone. The genes for the C1 and C2 polypeptides are probably unique whereas there are two genes C3(1) and C3(2) for the C3 polypeptide of which only the former is transcribed *in vivo*. The state of DNA methylation associated with the two genes for C3 also differ, insofar as C3(1) is demethylated in ventral prostate from 14–28 days of age, whereas the C3(2) gene remains hypermethylated. The organization of all four genes is similar and appreciable DNA sequence homologies suggest that they may have arisen from a single ancestral gene. To study C3 expression and its hormonal regulation we have introduced the cloned genes into mouse S115 cells, an androgen-responsive cell line. Both genes were accurately transcribed and their expression was stimulated up to fivefold by 10^{-8} M testosterone in approximately one third of the clones tested. To delineate the site of action of the hormone we have constructed chimeric genes consisting of putative C3 promoters and regulatory sequences together with a marker gene, interferon. This chimeric gene resulted in interferon production but its expression was stimulated by less than twofold in all clones tested. Therefore, these results indicate that, in mouse cells, testosterone does not interact directly with the rat C3 promoter but, in certain clones, may act post-transcriptionally.

ACKNOWLEDGMENTS

We should like to thank Dr. M. Fried for his advice, Mr. R. White and Mr. M. Needham for their technical assistance, and Mrs. M. Barker for typing the manuscript.

REFERENCES

1. GORSKI, J. & F. GANNON. 1976. Annu. Rev. Physiol. **38:** 425–450.
2. HIGGINS, S. J. & U. GEHRING. 1978. Adv. Cancer Res. **28:** 313–393.
3. HEYNS, W. & P. DE MOOR. 1977. Eur. J. Biochem. **78:** 221–230.
4. HEYNS, W., B. PEETERS, J. MOUS, W. ROMBAUTS & P. DE MOOR. 1978. Eur. J. Biochem. **89:** 181–186.
5. PARKER, M. G. & W. I. P. MAINWARING. 1977. Cell **12:** 401–407.
6. PAGE, M. J. & M. G. PARKER. 1982. Mol. Cell. Endocrinology **27:** 343–355.
7. PAYVAR, F., O. WRANGE, J. CARLSTEDT-DUKE, S. OKRET, J.-A. GUSTAFSSON & K. R. YAMAMOTO. 1981. Proc. Natl. Acad. Sci. USA **78:** 6628–6632.
8. GOVINDAN, M. V., E. SPIESS & J. MAJORS. 1982. Proc. Natl. Acad. Sci. USA **79:** 5157–5161.
9. PFAHL, M. 1982. Cell **31:** 475–482.
10. GEISSE, S., C. SCHEIDERET, H. M. WESTPHAL, N. E. HYNES, B. GRONER & M. BEATO. 1982. EMBO J. **1:** 1613–1619.
11. SCHEIDERET, C., S. GEISSE, H. M. WESTPHAL & M. BEATO. 1983. Nature **304:** 749–752.

12. HUANG, A. L., M. C. OSTROWSKI, D. BERARD & G. L. HAGER. 1981. Cell **27:** 245–255.
13. LEE, F., R. MULLIGAN, P. BERG & G. RINGOLD. 1981. Nature **294:** 228–232.
14. HYNES, N. E., A. J. J. VAN OOYEN, N. KENNEDY, P. HERLICH, H. PONTA & B. GRONER. 1983. Proc. Natl. Acad. Sci. USA **80:** 3637–3641.
15. CHANDLER, V. L., B. A. MALEV & K. R. YAMAMOTO. 1983. Cell **33:** 489–499.
16. BUETTI, E. &. & H. DIGGELMANN. 1983. EMBO J. **2:** 1423–1429.
17. YATES, J. & R. J. B. KING. 1981. J. Steroid Biochem. **14:** 819–822.
18. MULLIGAN, R. C. & P. BERG. 1981. Proc. Natl. Acad. Sci. USA **78:** 2072–2076.
19. PARKER, M. G., M. NEEDHAM, R. WHITE, H. HURST & M. PAGE. 1982. Nucleic Acids Res. **10:** 5121–5132.
20. PARKER, M. G., R. WHITE, H. HURST, M. NEEDHAM & R. TILLY. 1983. J. Biol. Chem. **258:** 12–15.
21. HURST, H. & M. G. PARKER. 1983. EMBO J. **2:** 769–774.
22. PAGE, M. J. & M. G. PARKER. 1983. Cell **32:** 495–502.
23. BIRNBOIM, H. C. & J. DOLY. 1979. Nucleic Acids Res. **7:** 1513–1523.
24. SOEDA, E., J. R. ARRAND, N. SMOLAR, J. E. WALSH & B. E. GRIFFIN. 1980. Nature (London) **283:** 445–453.
25. DERYNCK, R., J. CONTENT, E. DECLERCQ, G. VOLCKAERT, J. TAVERNIER, R. DEVOS & W. FIERS. 1980. Nature **285:** 542–547.
26. RAZIN, A. & J. FRIEDMAN. 1981. Prog. Nuc. Acid. Res. Mol. Biol. **25:** 33–52.
27. FELSENFELD, G. & J. MCGHEE. 1982. Nature **296:** 602–603.
28. RENKAWITZ, R., H. BEUG, T. GRAF, P. MATTHIAS, M. GREZ & G. SCHÜTZ. 1982. Cell **31:** 167–176.
29. RENKAWITZ, R. U., DANESCH, P. MATTHIAS & G. SCHÜTZ. 1983. J. Steroid Biochem. (In press.)
30. DEAN, D. C., B. J. KNOLL, M. E. RISER & B. W. O'MALLEY. 1983. Nature. (In press.)

Characteristics of a Seminal Plasma Inhibitor of Sperm Motility

EVE DE LAMIRANDE,[a] MARTHE BELLES-ISLES, and
CLAUDE GAGNON

Unité de Biorégulation cellulaire et moléculaire
Le Centre hospitalier de l'Université Laval
Sainte-Foy (Québec) Canada G1V 4G2

and

Département de Pharmacologie
Faculté de Médecine, Université Laval
Québec, Canada G1K 7P4

INTRODUCTION

Mammalian spermatozoa, like sea urchin spermatozoa, can be immobilized by demembranation with Triton X-100 and their motility reinitiated by the addition of Mg·ATP.[1-5] This model system represents a useful tool to study the regulation of sperm movement at the axonemal level and to study the effects of substances directly affecting the axoneme, since it bypasses the problem of the rather impermeable sperm membrane.[6-8] This system was especially useful in the elucidation of the mechanism of action of *erythro*-9-[3-(2-hydroxynonyl)]-adenine (EHNA), a substance that blocks sperm motility by inhibiting the force-generating dynein ATPase on the axoneme.[9,10]

While attempting to reactivate ejaculated mammalian spematozoa (rabbit, man), it was observed that the presence of seminal plasma prevented the reinitiation of motility by Mg·ATP.[11] Ejaculated spermatozoa had to be carefully washed before demembranation to make possible the reinitiation of motility. Our present knowledge of the origin and the mode of action of this seminal plasma inhibitor of motility is presented here.

SPECIES AND TISSUE SPECIFICITIES

Originally found in human and rabbit seminal plasma, the motility inhibitor appears to be ubiquitous as it has been detected in all species investigated. The inhibitory potency of the seminal plasma from five species, when tested on rabbit demembranated reactivated spermatozoa, is shown in TABLE 1. Bull seminal plasma contained the highest concentration of motility inhibitor but the highest quantity was found in boar seminal plasma. When the same seminal plasma were tested with reactivated spermatozoa from another species, the inhibitory concentrations marginally varied from that in TABLE 1, but the order of inhibitory potencies remained the same: bull > boar > man > ram > rabbit.

[a] Address correspondence to: Dr. Eve de Lamirande, Urology Research Laboratory, Royal Victoria Hospital, 687 Pine Avenue West, Montreal, Quebec, Canada H3A 1A1.

In addition to the inhibition of reactivation observed with ejaculated spermatozoa, it was also noted that any of the seminal plasma could inhibit the reactivation of testicular or epididymal spermatozoa from the four species tested (bull, rat, rabbit, dog) (unpublished results).

From the data presented above, it is clear that seminal plasma inhibitor of motility is not species specific. However, it was found to be tissue specific since none of the tissues tested (liver, kidney, brain, and testes), up to a concentration of 10 mg protein per ml, had any inhibitory effect on rabbit reactivated spermatozoa.

TABLE 1. Inhibitory Potency of Seminal Plasma on Rabbit Demembranated Reactivated Spermatozoa

Source of Seminal Plasma	Inhibitory Concentration[a] (μg/ml)	Volume of Ejaculate[b] (ml)	Protein Concentration[b] (mg/ml)	Inhibitory Potency[c] (units/ml)	Total Inhibitory Capacity[c] (units/ejaculate)
Rabbit	662 ± 62	0.75	20	30	20
Ram	479 ± 32	1.5	35	70	100
Human	331 ± 29	3	45	136	400
Boar	65 ± 6	150	50	770	115000
Bull	8.6 ± 1.3	5	50	5800	29000

[a] These values represent the minimal protein concentration needed to inhibit completely and instantaneously the motility of rabbit demembranated spermatozoa reactivated with 0.5 mM Mg·ATP. They are expressed in μg of sample protein added per ml of reactivation medium. Values are means ± SEM for 4 to 20 samples.

[b] Volume and protein concentration of ejaculates are average values.

[c] Inhibitory potency is expressed in units/ml. One unit is the amount of protein needed to stop the movement of spermatozoa in 1 ml reactivation medium in the presence of 0.5 mM Mg·ATP.

ORIGIN OF THE MOTILITY INHIBITOR

The origin of the motility inhibitor was, therefore, looked for within the reproductive tract. In the bull, seminal vesicle and, to a much lesser extent, prostatic fluids contained a motility inhibitor (TABLE 2). However, considering the volumes of both fluids, the prostatic contribution was essentially negligible. It must be noted that the level of motility inhibitor found in seminal plasma was fourfold higher than that found in seminal vesicle fluid. These results were surprising since the seminal vesicle fluid is diluted with other fluids at the time of ejaculation; the level of inhibitor in seminal plasma ought to be lower than that of the seminal vesicle fluid. The possibility of a synergistic effect between seminal vesicle fluid and fluids from the prostate and the epididymidis was therefore tested. The maximal stimulatory effect obtained was about twofold with combinations of seminal vesicle and epididymal fluids or seminal vesicle and prostatic fluids at unphysiological ratios. The seminal vesicle : prostatic : epididymal fluid ratio of 2 : 1 : 2, a ratio close to that found in bull semen, only increased the inhibitory potency of seminal vesicle fluid by 77%.

TABLE 2. Concentration of Motility Inhibitor in Bull Tissues and Fluids

Sample		Protein Inhibitory Concentration (mg/ml)
Seminal plasma		0.0115 ± 0.0014
Seminal vesicles	Homogenate	0.375 ± 0.107
	Fluid	0.043 ± 0.008
Prostate	Homogenate	>13.4
	Fluid	0.564 ± 0.020
Testis	Homogenate	>12.4
Caput epididymis	Homogenate	>11.7
Cauda epididymis	Homogenate	>9.0
	Fluid	3.51 ± 0.43

These values represent the minimal protein concentration needed to inhibit completely and instantaneously the motility of rabbit spermatozoa reactivated with 0.5 mM Mg·ATP. Values are expressed in mg of sample protein added per ml of reactivation medium. Values are mean ± SEM for 3 to 6 experiments.

Dialysis experiments suggested an explanation for the fourfold higher inhibitory potency found in bull seminal plasma in comparison to that found in seminal vesicle fluid. When dialyzed at 4°C, pH 4 (water adjusted to pH 4 with acetic acid), the seminal plasma inhibitory activity was reduced by a factor of 3.3 (a 70% loss) while that of the seminal vesicle fluid remained unchanged (TABLE 3). Dialysis, therefore, lowered the inhibitory activity of the seminal plasma to the level found in seminal vesicle fluid. The experiment was repeated in a sequential fashion: the seminal plasma was first dialyzed against five volumes of water–acetic acid, pH 4 and 4°C, the dialysate was saved and the seminal plasma was redialyzed under the same conditions against a large volume of water–acetic acid. When the dialyzed seminal plasma was mixed with its dialysate in the 1 : 5 ratio, its original activity was restored. Furthermore, when the seminal vesicle fluid was mixed with seminal plasma dialysate in the same ratio, its activity was raised to a level similar to that found in seminal plasma. Dialysis of boar, human, and rabbit seminal plasma produced similar losses of activity (60% to 80%). Recovery of activity was always possible when the dialysate was added back to the corresponding dialyzed seminal plasma. The seminal plasma inhibitor of motility,

TABLE 3. Effect of Dialysis, pH 4.0, 4°C, on Bull Seminal Plasma and Seminal Vesicle Fluid Motility Inhibitor

Treatment	Seminal Plasma (units/mg protein)[a]	Seminal Vesicles (units/mg protein)[a]
Undialyzed	87	23
Dialyzed	26	23
Dialyzed and diluted with H₂O-CH₃COOH, pH 4.0	26	23
Dialyzed and diluted with seminal plasma dialysate	87	88

[a] One inhibitory unit is the amount of protein needed to stop the motility of spermatozoa in 1 ml of reactivation medium in the presence of 0.5 mM Mg·ATP.

therefore, appeared to be composed of a macromolecular portion with a low intrinsic activity and of a dialyzable activator with no intrinsic activity, but capable of potentiating the former up to fourfold. The macromolecular component, at least in bull, seemed to originate from the seminal vesicles whereas the dialyzable factor still has an unknown origin.

PHYSICOCHEMICAL PROPERTIES

The physicochemical properties of the motility inhibitor were investigated (TABLE 4). Boar seminal plasma was used because of the large volume available. The inhibitor was found to be stable to moderate heat (no loss of activity after 20 min at 60°C) but not to boiling (100% loss after 5 min at 100°C). It was also stable at pH 1 for at least 30 min but a progressive loss of activity was observed above pH 8.5 with a total loss at pH 12. It was precipitated with 5% trichloroacetic acid with no loss of activity but not by acetone (30%). It was also stable to lyophilization. Preliminary results on chromatofocusing indicated a basic pI for the inhibitor. Its molecular weight was estimated at 10,000–12,000 by molecular sieving on Ultrogel ACA-54. Since these physicochemical properties were quite similar to those of the aprotinin-like protease inhibitors normally present in seminal plasma,[12,13] the motility inhibitor was partially purified in order to determine its relationship with these aprotinin-like protease inhibitors. Acetone-treated seminal plasma was loaded on SP-Sephadex C-25 equilibrated in 20 mM Tris-HCl, pH 7.9, and eluted by a salt gradient. The active fractions were pooled, dialyzed against water, and lyophilized. Thereafter, the capacities of acetone-treated seminal plasma, partially purified seminal plasma factor, and aprotinin to inhibit trypsin activity and to block motility of reactivated spermatozoa were compared. Aprotinin and acetone-treated seminal plasma were respectively five- and eight fold more potent in inhibiting trypsin than in blocking sperm motility. To the contrary, the partially purified preparation of the inhibitor was 100-fold more potent in inhibiting motility than in blocking trypsin activity. The purification procedure specifically selected the product responsible for the inhibition of reactivation rather than the products responsible for trypsin inhibition. Therefore, the seminal plasma inhibitor of motility did not appear to be an aprotinin-like trypsin inhibitor.

TABLE 4. Physicochemical Properties of the Boar Seminal Plasma Inhibitor

Treatment	Inhibitory Activity[a]
None	100
60°C, 20 min	93
100°C, 5 min	4
TCA precipitation (5%)	
supernatant	4
solubilized pellet	94
NaOH, pH 12, 20 min	0
Acetone (30%) precipitation	
supernatant	98
solubilized pellet	0
Lyophilization	94

[a] Percentage of the initial inhibitory activity remaining after treatment. Demembranated reactivated rabbit spermatozoa were used for these experiments.

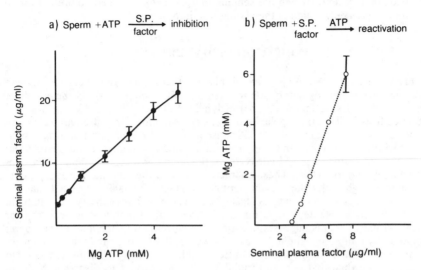

FIGURE 1. Competition between the partially purified seminal plasma factor and Mg · ATP. (a) Spermatozoa were demembranated and reactivated with different concentrations of Mg·ATP and then the amount of seminal plasma factor necessary to inhibit motility was determined for each Mg·ATP concentration. (b) After demembranation, different concentrations of seminal plasma factor were immediately added to spermatozoa and the amount of Mg·ATP required to reinitiate sperm motility was determined. Each point represents the mean ± SEM ($N = 4$).

REVERSIBILITY OF THE INHIBITION

It was noted that when seminal plasma was added initially to the reactivation medium and incubated for a few seconds with the demembranated spermatozoa before the addition of Mg·ATP, the minimal quantity of seminal plasma required to prevent any reactivation was one third to one half of that needed to stop the movement of already motile spermatozoa. These results suggested the possibility of a competition between ATP and the inhibitor for a site on demembranated spermatozoa. This possibility was investigated by the following experiments. In the first series of experiments, spermatozoa were demembranated and reactivated with various Mg·ATP concentrations and then, for each Mg·ATP concentration, the minimal amount of seminal plasma factor required to inhibit the motility instantaneously and completely was determined (FIGURE 1a). As the concentration of Mg·ATP used for reactivation increased from 0.1 to 5 mM the inhibitory amount of seminal plasma factor increased. In the second series of experiments, demembranated spermatozoa were incubated with various amounts of seminal plasma factor and, shortly after, the minimal Mg·ATP concentration needed for reactivation of motility was determined (FIGURE 1b). As the concentration of seminal plasma factor was increased, the concentration of Mg·ATP needed to reinitiate the movement increased rapidly. The data from FIGURE 1 suggest a competition between ATP and the seminal plasma factor for a common receptor on the demembranated spermatozoa. The data further suggest a higher affinity for the common receptor when the seminal plasma factor is added before the initiation of movement, which is the sliding of microtubules.

INHIBITION OF DYNEIN ATPase

This competition Mg·ATP–seminal plasma factor and the fact that dynein ATPase is a major regulatory site for sperm motility led us to study the effects of the seminal plasma factor on sperm dynein ATPase. Dynein ATPase was extracted from bull sperm flagella by dialysis against a low ionic strength buffer and purified by sucrose gradient. The ATPase activity of the preparation was associated with a 19S particle and was insensitive to both oligomycin and ouabain but sensitive to *erythro*-9-[3-(2-hydroxynonyl)]-adenine, a specific dynein ATPase inhibitor,[9,10] and to EDTA. These characteristics and the fact that the 19S particle contained high molecular weight peptides (400,000–500,000) suggested that the ATPase extracted was dynein ATPase. Bull dynein ATPase activity was inhibited up to 90% in a dose-dependent manner by the partially purified factor from boar seminal plasma. This suggests that the seminal plasma factor may block sperm motility by inhibiting dynein ATPase. However, it must be noted that the concentration of seminal plasma factor required to inhibit dynein ATPase was about ten times higher than that needed to inhibit sperm motility. This discrepancy could possibly be explained by the fact that dynein ATPase may be less sensitive to inhibition when dissociated from the axoneme. Differences between axonemal dynein ATPase and solubilized dynein ATPase have also been observed in sea urchin spermatozoa.[14]

CONCLUSION

The seminal plasma contains a factor that inhibits the movement of demembranated reactivated spermatozoa. We have shown that this inhibitor was not species specific. The seminal plasma inhibitor appeared, however, to be tissue specific and to originate, in bull, from seminal vesicles and to a much lower extent from the prostate.

Dialysis experiments suggest that the seminal plasma inhibitor is composed of a macromolecular portion with a low basic activity and of a dialyzable activator with no intrinsic activity, but capable of potentiating the former up to fourfold. The dialyzable activator can also potentiate up to fourfold the inhibitor present in seminal vesicle fluid. The macromolecular component of the inhibitor probably originates from the seminal vesicles whereas the dialyzable factor origin is still unknown. This small molecule could perhaps also be present in the seminal vesicles but not in a form that permits potentiation of the marcromolecular component of the inhibitor.

The mechanism by which the seminal plasma inhibits the motility of demembranated spermatozoa has been investigated. That higher concentrations of Mg·ATP can prevent or reverse the inhibition of motility and that a partially purified preparation of the boar seminal plasma inhibitor decreased, in a dose-dependent manner, the activity of isolated bull sperm dynein ATPase suggest that this seminal plasma inhibitor would block sperm motility by inhibiting the force-generating dynein ATPase on the axoneme.

The physiological importance of the motility inhibitor from seminal plasma is presently unknown. However, its effects on intact normal spermatozoa are probably not rapid since ejaculated spermatozoa in complete semen are motile. The possibility of slow and progressive action of the inhibitor on the motility of intact spermatozoa is supported by the observation that the level of inhibitor in a given semen appears to be inversely correlated with the length of time during which spermatozoa remain motile in their own seminal plasma. Definite proof of an action of the seminal plasma factor on intact spermatozoa must await the purification of the inhibitor.

REFERENCES

1. LINDEMANN, C. B. & I. R. GIBBONS. 1975. J. Cell Biol. **65:** 147–162.
2. LINDEMANN, C. B. 1978. Cell **13:** 8–18.
3. MOHRI, H. & R. YANAGIMACHI. 1980. Exp. Cell. Res. **127:** 191–196.
4. DE LAMIRANDE, E., C. W. BARDIN & C. GAGNON. 1983. Biol. Reprod. **28:** 788–796.
5. DE LAMIRANDE, E. & C. GAGNON. 1983. J. Submicro. Cytol. **15:** 83–87.
6. SUMMERS, K. E. & I. R. GIBBONS. 1973. J. Cell Biol. **58:** 618–629.
7. GIBBONS, B. H. & I. R. GIBBONS. 1973. J. Cell Sci. **13:** 337–357.
8. YANO, Y. & T. MIKI-NOUMURA. 1981. J. Cell Sci. **48:** 223–239.
9. BOUCHARD, P., S. M. PENNINGROTH, A. CHEUNG, C. GAGNON & C. W. BARDIN. 1981. Proc. Natl. Acad. Sci. USA **78:** 1033–1036.
10. PENNINGROTH, S. M., A. CHEUNG, P. BOUCHARD, C. GAGNON & C. W. BARDIN. 1982. Biochem. Biophys. Res. Commun. **104:** 234–240.
11. GAGNON, C., Y. LEE, L. BOURGET & C. W. BARDIN. 1981. Can. Fed. Biol. Soc. Abstract #73.
12. CECHOVA, D. & H. FRITZ. 1976. Hoppe-Seyler's Z. Physiol. Chem. **357:** 401–408.
13. VOGEL, R. 1979. *In* Handbook of Experimental Pharmacology. E. G. Erdos, Ed. Vol. 25 Suppl.: 163–225. Springer-Verlag. New York.
14. GIBBONS, I. R. & E. FRONK. 1979. J. Biol. Chem. **254:** 187–196.

Cyclic AMP-dependent Activation of Sea Urchin and Tunicate Sperm Motility[a]

CHARLES J. BROKAW

Division of Biology
California Institute of Technology
Pasadena, California 91125

INTRODUCTION

This report summarizes procedures that can be used to obtain high-quality reactivated motility of sperm flagella demembranated with Triton X-100. Although for years I have been reactivating sea urchin sperm flagella without exposing them to cyclic adenosine monophosphate (cAMP), the failure of these techniques to work with *Ciona* spermatozoa has led to the development of techniques involving incubation of demembranated spermatozoa with cAMP. This has led to the development of improved procedures for reactivating sea urchin spermatozoa, which give beat frequencies comparable to those of live spermatozoa. With both species, conditions can be found where a brief incubation with cAMP determines whether the spermatozoa are quiescent or fully motile when they are suspended in reactivation solution.

THE QUIESCENT STATE

In 1980, Barbara Gibbons reported on the intermittent swimming of spermatozoa from several species of sea urchins.[9] Normal swimming was interrupted by brief periods of quiescence, during which the sperm flagellum assumed a characteristic "cane-shaped" configuration. These quiescent periods were more frequent at high light intensities, required the presence of calcium in the sea water, and, in the presence of calcium, could be artificially induced by the calcium ionophore, A23187. Detailed examination of the flagellar bending patterns during the transitions between quiescence and swimming[14] revealed similarities with the characteristics of calcium-induced asymmetrical bending waves of demembranated and reactivated sperm flagella.[2] These findings suggested that quiescence was induced by an increase in internal calcium concentration.

Spermatozoa of the tunicate, *Ciona intestinalis,* also show intermittent swimming under some conditions, but the quiescent configuration is different. There is a sharp bend in the reverse bend direction near the sperm head, and a large bend in the principal bend direction that occupies most of the length of the flagellum.[3,21] This quiescent state can also be observed with demembranated spermatozoa, by using undiluted spermatozoa as collected from *Ciona* sperm ducts, demembranating in the presence of EGTA and suspending the demembranated spermatozoa in

[a] Supported by the National Institutes of Health (grant GM 18711).

132

reactivation solution containing 1 mM ATP.[3,21] FIGURE 1a illustrates the quiescent configuration obtained with demembranated *Ciona* spermatozoa. If the spermatozoa are collected carefully to avoid dilution it is easy to obtain 100% quiescence with *Ciona* spermatozoa. The bend angles of the quiescent configuration vary with the conditions used and are more extreme at higher pH values, in reactivation solutions containing Cl⁻ rather than acetate, or after brief exposure to cAMP.

Using similar conditions, quiescence can be obtained with demembranated spermatozoa from the sea urchin, *Lytechinus pictus*. FIGURE 1b illustrates the quiescent configuration of these spermatozoa. At best, 80–90% of the spermatozoa are quiescent; the remainder shows varying degrees of highly asymmetric movement. The conditions used to obtain this degree of quiescence with *Lytechinus* spermatozoa are different in several important respects from the conditions used in the past to study the reactivated movements of these spermatozoa. (1) Concentrated spermatozoa are used, without dilution with NaCl solution or sea water. (2) Demembranation is carried out under "potentially asymmetric"[11]

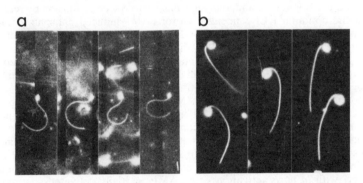

FIGURE 1. Photographs showing the quiescent configuration of sperm flagella of *Ciona* (a) and *Lytechinus* (b) after demembranation and suspension in reactivation solution.

conditions, with the demembranation solution containing EGTA to maintain a very low Ca^{2+} concentration. A relatively high salt concentration (0.25 M KCl) is also used in the demembranation solution. (3) The reactivation solution is made with 0.25 M potassium acetate, rather than with KCl. Gibbons, Evans, and Gibbons reported that substitution of chloride with acetate in reactivation solutions improved the motility of reactivated sea urchin sperm flagella.[13] (4) The reactivation solution contains 1 mM ATP, which in previous work appeared to be above the optimal concentration for reactivated motility.[1]

Quiescence has been reported previously in demembranated sea urchin spermatozoa,[11] but under the conditions used in that report, quiescence was only obtained by raising the Ca^{2+} concentration in the reactivation solution to approximately 10^{-4} M. The flagellar configuration obtained by this calcium-induced quiescence had a much more extreme basal bend than that seen with live spermatozoa, unless the pH was lowered. A similar quiescent configuration, sensitive to both pH and ATP concentration, was obtained by adding methanol or 2-propanol to the reactivation solutions.[10] Ishiguro, Murofushi, and Sakai obtained quiescence in several species of sea urchin spermatozoa by addition of a DEAE-absorbed fraction of the supernatant obtained during demembranation of spermatozoa with Triton X-100.[15] All of this previous work was performed using spermatozoa diluted with sea water before demembranation and reactivation solutions containing KCl.

ACTIVATION OF *CIONA* SPERM MOTILITY

Motility of reactivated *Ciona* spermatozoa can be obtained by two distinct procedures: (1) by activating motility of the live spermatozoa before demembranation[3] and (2) by exposing the spermatozoa to cAMP after demembranation. The *in vivo* activation requires considerable dilution and appears to be enhanced by addition of basic compounds such as histidine or theophylline. Good results were obtained by diluting spermatozoa 1:100 with a solution containing 10 mM theophylline in 10% sea water and 90% 0.5 M NaCl; this also reduces the amount of calcium carried over into the demembranation mixture. The *in vitro* activation with cAMP is favored by maintaining a high sperm concentration and by recognizing that the optimum KCl concentration for cAMP-induced phosphorylation of sperm proteins is less than 0.10 M.[22] Because of these factors, it is easy to terminate the incubation with cAMP by dilution into reactivation solution containing 0.25 M KCl or 0.25 M potassium acetate in order to measure the time required for activation. The need for a high sperm concentration can be partially eliminated by using an exogenous protein kinase (the catalytic subunit of the cAMP-dependent protein kinase).[22] Activation by cAMP can be completely abolished by raising the Ca^{2+} concentration of the cAMP incubation mixture. Only minimal activation of motility is obtained by incubation with trypsin instead of cAMP.[3]

Examination of *in vivo* activation under various conditions suggests that activation is an all-or-none process; varying proportions of spermatozoa are either quiescent or fully motile, with spermatozoa rarely showing intermediate motility. However, with *in vitro* activation with cAMP, partially activated spermatozoa can be obtained. FIGURE 2 illustrates some of these results. For these experiments, concentrated *Ciona* spermatozoa were diluted with demembranation solution containing 0.25 M KCl, 1 mM $MgSO_4$, 1 mM dithiothreitol (DTT), 0.4 mM EGTA, 0.04% Triton X-100, and 20 mM Tris-HCl buffer, pH 8.0. All work was done at 18°C. The dilution factor was determined by measuring the optical density of a 20 μl sample of sperm suspension diluted with 5.0 ml of 0.5 M NaCl. If the OD_{540} of this mixture was 0.40, a dilution factor of 1:50 was used. For other OD readings in the range of 0.30 to 0.50, the dilution factor was adjusted to maintain equivalent sperm concentrations, assuming a linear relationship between sperm concentration and OD in this range.

After 30 sec, one volume of this mixture of Triton X-100–demembranated spermatozoa was mixed with 1.5 volumes of solution containing 1 mM $MgSO_4$, 1 mM DTT, 0.2 mM EGTA, 1 mM ATP, 10 μM cAMP, and 20 mM Tris-HCl buffer, pH 8.0, in order to obtain a KCl concentration of 0.1 M during incubation with cAMP. After incubation for the desired time, a portion of this mixture was diluted 1:250 with reactivation solution containing 0.25 M potassium acetate, 1 mM $MgSO_4$, 1 mM DTT, 0.2 mM EGTA, 1 mM ATP, 0.5% polyethylene glycol, and 20 mM Tris-HCl buffer, pH 8.0. The $MgATP^{2-}$ concentration in this solution is 0.7 mM. Under these conditions, incubation with cAMP for 60 to 120 sec is sufficient to produce optimal motility, illustrated in FIGURE 2a, with mean beat frequencies

of about 32 Hz. FIGURE 2b illustrates the waveform of a partially activated spermatozoon observed after 30 sec incubation with cAMP. Such spermatozoa typically have more asymmetrical bending patterns and slightly lower beat frequencies. However, these parameters do not fully describe the differences between
partially and fully activated flagellar motility, and a more detailed analysis, similar
to that carried out by Gibbons,[12] will be required.

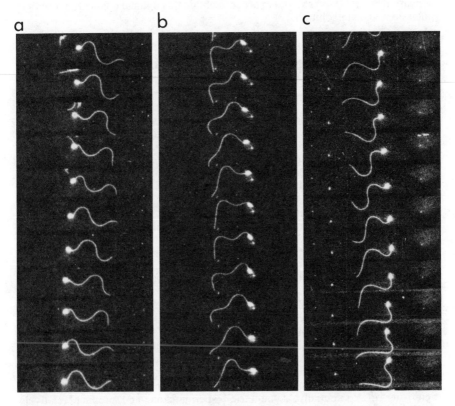

FIGURE 2. Photographs showing waveforms typical of reactivated sperm flagella of *Ciona*.
(a) After incubation for 120 sec with cAMP. (b) After incubation for 30 sec with cAMP. (c)
After incubation for 20 sec with cAMP, followed by 20 sec exposure to 0.35 M KCl.
Photographed on moving film (0.25 m sec^{-1}) with a flash frequency of 150 Hz. These are low-
resolution photographs of spermatozoa swimming at the upper surface of an open drop of
reactivation solution, using a 16× 0.40 na objective.

Spermatozoa diluted into the above reactivation solution after 20 sec incubation with cAMP are mostly quiesent, with configurations like those shown in
FIGURE 1a. However, they show active motility if diluted into reactivation solution containing 0.25 M KCl rather than 0.25 M potassium acetate. The activation
of partially phosphorylated sperm flagella by an increase in KCl concentration[22]
appears to be specific for Cl$^-$. FIGURE 2c illustrates the waveform of a spermato-

zoon in a suspension that was incubated for 20 sec with cAMP, and then mixed with an equal volume of a solution containing 0.6 M KCl. After 20 sec of exposure to 0.35 M KCl, the mixture was then diluted with reactivation solution. Although this procedure activates motility, unique waveforms are produced, and these will also require further, more detailed analysis. My preliminary conclusion is that more "normal" looking waveforms are obtained in reactivation solutions containing 0.25 M potassium acetate rather than 0.25 M KCl, but that a more complete activation by cAMP is required in order to obtain this optimal quality of motility in potassium acetate solutions.

ACTIVATION OF SEA URCHIN SPERM MOTILITY

Ishiguro et al. found that the motility of sea urchin spermatozoa made quiescent by addition of a DEAE fraction of Triton supernatant could be activated by addition of cAMP.[15] When *Lytechinus* spermatozoa are prepared by conditions that produce quiescence, as described above, they also can be activated by *in vitro* incubation with cAMP. The procedure originally described for activation of *Ciona* spermatozoa[11] gives good results with *Lytechinus* spermatozoa, probably because a higher initial sperm concentration can be obtained.

Concentrated spermatozoa are diluted 1:100 with demembranation solution containing 0.25 M KCl, 2 mM $MgSO_4$, 1 mM EGTA, 1 mM DTT, 0.04% Triton X-100, and 10 mM Tris-HCl buffer, at pH 8.2. After 30 sec, one volume of this mixture is diluted with three volumes of solution containing 0.05 M KCl, 2 mM $MgSO_4$, 1 mM DTT, 1 mM ATP, 10 μM cAMP, and 10 mM Tris-HCl buffer, pH 8.2. After incubation for the desired time, these spermatozoa are diluted 1:100 with reactivation solution containing 0.25 M potassium acetate, 3 mM $MgSO_4$, 0.2 mM EGTA, 1 mM DTT, 0.5% polyethylene glycol, 20 mM Tris-HCl buffer, pH 8.2, in addition to ATP.

FIGURE 3a illustrates flagellar bending patterns obtained with this procedure after 300 sec incubation with cAMP. Incubation for shorter periods (FIGURE 3b) gives slightly higher asymmetry and lower beat frequencies, but a more detailed analysis of these effects will be required. Even after optimal activation by cAMP, calcium-induced quiescence is obtained with these spermatozoa if 0.4 mM $CaCl_2$ is added to the reactivation solutions.

Even after 300 sec incubation with cAMP, these spermatozoa retain the characteristics of "potentially asymmetric" spermatozoa, and produce relatively asymmetric bending waves in reactivation solution containing very low Ca^{2+} concentrations. Symmetric waveforms have been obtained previously with sea urchin spermatozoa by exposure to millimolar Ca^{2+} concentrations either during demembranation[6] or subsequently.[20] To avoid inhibition of cAMP activation by Ca^{2+}, $CaCl_2$ can be added to the cAMP incubation mixture at the end of the incubation period, to bring the $CaCl_2$ concentration to 2.5 mM. After a further 20 sec incubation, the mixture is diluted with reactivation solution. The 0.2 mM EGTA in the reactivation solution is sufficient to bring the Ca^{2+} concentration back down to low levels (ca. 10^{-9} M). This brief exposure to millimolar Ca^{2+} is able to produce symmetrical bending waves, as illustrated by FIGURE 3c. As controls for these experiments, the time for incubation with cAMP before addition of $CaCl_2$ was reduced to zero, and the subsequent incubation with $CaCl_2$ was carried out with and without cAMP. In both cases, most of the spermatozoa became motile, but the beat frequencies averaged around 21 Hz, compared to

35–40 Hz after normal cAMP incubation. Therefore, these spermatozoa can be partially activated by Ca^{2+} alone, without exposure to cAMP. The presence of cAMP during Ca^{2+} activation has no significant effect, indicating that as in *Ciona* and dog spermatozoa[24] cAMP activation is inhibited by Ca^{2+}.

Since there is substantial activation by Ca^{2+}, the usual procedures for preparing "potentially symmetric" demembranated spermatozoa by demembranating in the presence of millimolar Ca^{2+} produce sperm preparations that show nearly 100% reactivation, even without incubation with cAMP. However, the properties

a   b   c

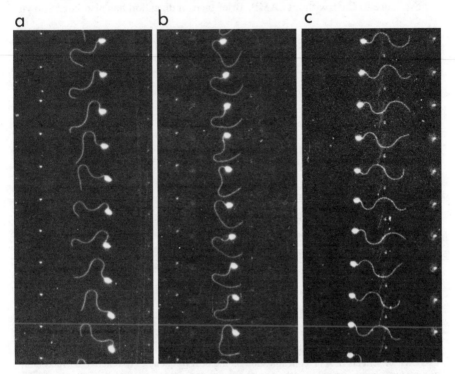

FIGURE 3. Photographs showing waveforms typical of reactivated sperm flagella of *Lytechinus*. (a) After incubation for 300 sec with cAMP. (b) After incubation for 10 sec with cAMP. (c) After incubation for 300 sec with cAMP, followed by 20 sec exposure to approximately 2 mM Ca^{2+}. Photographed as in FIGURE 2, with a flash frequency of 150 Hz.

of such spermatozoa differ significantly from those of spermatozoa activated by incubation with cAMP. This is illustrated by FIGURE 4, which compares the effects of ATP concentration on two types of sperm preparations: "potentially symmetric" spermatozoa prepared as in most of the previous work from my laboratory[1] and cAMP-activated spermatozoa prepared as described here, with 120 sec incubation with cAMP followed by 20 sec exposure to millimolar Ca^{2+}. Both preparations have essentially the same K_m for beat frequency, but the cAMP-incubated spermatozoa have beat frequencies that are about 50% greater than the usual "potentially symmetric" spermatozoa.

Since brief trypsin digestion was found to release calcium-induced quiescence,[11] I was not surprised to find that motile spermatozoa can be obtained by incubating with trypsin instead of cAMP. Incubation for 30 sec in the usual cAMP incubation mixture containing 0.05 μg/ml trypsin and no cAMP is sufficient to activate most of the spermatozoa. However, the waveforms are very asymmetric, and the beat frequencies are low, about 21 Hz. Further digestion leads to a deterioration in the quality of the reactivation, with a very diverse assortment of waveforms.

The effect of trypsin digestion is rather similar to the activation that is obtained by exposure to Ca^{2+} without cAMP. Brief trypsin digestion has also been shown

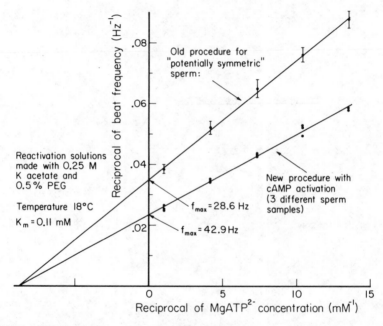

FIGURE 4. Effects of ATP concentration on the beat frequencies of reactivated spermatozoa of *Lytechnius,* prepared either by the usual procedure for "potentially symmetric" spermatozoa or the new procedure with cAMP incubation for 120 sec followed by 20 sec exposure to 2 mM Ca^{2+}.

previously to reduce the asymmetry of demembranated spermatozoa.[5,7] Trypsin activation and Ca activation can both be obtained with *Lytechinus* spermatozoa but not with *Ciona* spermatozoa. Correlations such as these suggest that the effects of Ca^{2+} might represent calcium activation of a protease normally present in the demembranated sperm preparations. Chun and Gibbons obtained evidence for such a conclusion by examining effects of protease inhibitors on production of "potentially symmetric" spermatozoa by exposure to Ca^{2+}.[8] However, I have had no success with attempts to inhibit calcium activation (or cAMP activation) of *Lytechnus* spermatozoa with protease inhibitors, using concentrations that completely block activation by trypsin. Inhibitors tried were aprotinin, benzamidine (at up to 5 mM), and chicken ovomucoid (at up to 4 mg/ml).

DISCUSSION

In addition to the two species discussed here, a requirement for cAMP for reactivation of demembranated sperm flagella has been observed in several other species (trout,[23] starfish,[18] and sand dollar[4]). Enhancement of reactivated motility of mammalian spermatozoa by cAMP has also been reported by several authors.[16,24] It is becoming reasonable to assume that a cAMP-dependent activation mechanism may be a general feature of sperm flagella.

Since it is usually easy to produce quiescent spermatozoa by demembranating spermatozoa taken directly from storage in the male with no *in vivo* activation, whereas spermatozoa activated *in vivo* have properties similar to cAMP-activated spermatozoa, it is commonly assumed that the quiescent state obtained with demembranated flagella is related to a quiescent state of stored spermatozoa. It then follows that the *in vitro* cAMP activation that enables the motility of demembranated sperm flagella may correspond to a cAMP-activation process that occurs during normal *in vivo* activation of sperm motility. However, the evidence for this conclusion is not absolute. Stored spermatozoa do not show the characteristic quiescent configurations, but this is not surprising since the low internal pH that is thought to be involved in maintaining the quiescence of stored spermatozoa would favor straighter configurations.

At least two interpretations of the quiescent state are possible. The quiescent state may be a state in which dynein-driven active sliding is completely disabled, with the characteristic quiescent configuration determined by other flagellar components. Alternatively, the quiescent state may correspond to a particular pattern of static, asymmetric activation of dynein arms, which produces the characteristic quiescent configuration.

The high sensitivity of the quiescent configuration to pH may support the first interpretation, but most other evidence favors the second interpretation. Relatively high ATP concentrations are in many cases required to maintain the quiescent configuration. The calcium-induced quiescence of sea urchin spermatozoa is an apparently unstable state that spontaneously disintegrates by sliding between axonemal tubules.[11] *Ciona* spermatozoa in the quiescent state show disintegration by sliding following digestion with trypsin.[3] Sea urchin sperm flagella, which have been relaxed by inhibiting dynein arm interactions with vanadate, do not assume the configuration typical of the quiescent state unless the Ca^{2+} concentration is increased to around 10^{-4} M.[17,19]

Since we still lack an adequate understanding of the control mechanisms in flagella that are responsible for converting the dynein-driven active sliding process into oscillation and bend propagation, situations in which the active sliding process is enabled but no oscillation occurs are particularly interesting to study. Understanding the role of cAMP in activating quiescent spermatozoa is therefore potentially valuable in understanding these mechanisms.

The role of cAMP in activation almost certainly involves activation of a cAMP-dependent protein kinase. Much of this kinase activity appears to be located in the Triton supernatant.[15,22] However, Ishiguro *et al.* presented evidence that the supernatant also contained an important substrate for phosphorylation,[15] and this is consistent with the observation that washed spermatozoa of *Ciona* could not be activated by exogenous protein kinase unless supernatant was added.[22] Examination of the phosphorylation of axonemal proteins of *Ciona*[22] revealed two interesting results that deserve further investigation: (1) cAMP-dependent phosphorylation of dynein heavy chains was observed during *in vitro* activation, but this phosphorylation was greatly reduced during incubation of spermatozoa that had already been activated *in vivo* and (2) one axonemal phosphoprotein with a molecular weight of about 150,000 appeared to be removed from the axoneme when the KCl concentration was increased from 0.1 M to 0.3 M, under conditions where this KCl concentration increase activates motility.

A complete understanding of the biochemical correlates of cAMP activation of sperm flagellar motility may provide some new insights into the mechanisms responsible for flagellar oscillation.

ACKNOWLEDGMENTS

I thank Sandra Nagayama and Scott Richman for assistance with recent experimental work, and Dr. Win Sale for sharing his unpublished work on quiescence in *Lytechinus* spermatozoa.

REFERENCES

1. BROKAW, C. J. 1975. Effects of viscosity and ATP concentration on the movement of reactivated sea urchin sperm flagella. J. Exp. Biol. **62:** 701–719.
2. BROKAW, C. J. 1979. Calcium-induced asymmetrical beating of Triton-demembranated sea urchin sperm flagella. J. Cell Biol. **82:** 401–411.
3. BROKAW, C. J. 1982. Activation and reactivation of *Ciona* sperm flagella. Cell Mot. Suppl. **1:** 185–189.
4. BROKAW, C. J. 1983. Unpublished observation.
5. BROKAW, C. J. & I. R. GIBBONS. 1975. Mechanisms of movement in flagella and cilia. *In* Swimming and Flying in Nature. T. Y.-T. Wu, C. J. Brokaw & C. Brennan, Eds.: 89–126. Plenum Publ. Corp. New York.
6. BROKAW, C. J., R. JOSSLIN & L. BOBROW. 1974. Calcium ion regulation of flagellar beat symmetry in reactivated sea urchin spermatozoa. Biochem. Biophys. Res. Commun. **58:** 795–800.
7. BROKAW, C. J. & T. F. SIMONICK. 1977. Motility of Triton-demembranated sea urchin sperm flagella during digestion by trypsin. J. Cell Biol. **75:** 650–665.
8. CHUN, J. J. M. & I. R. GIBBONS. 1980. Osmotic rupture of flagellar membranes provides a detergent-free method of exposing axonemes for reactivation studies. J. Cell Biol. **87:** 37a.
9. GIBBONS, B. H. 1980. Intermittent swimming in live sea urchin sperm. J. Cell Biol. **84:** 1–12.
10. GIBBONS, B. H. 1982. Effects of organic solvents on flagellar asymmetry and quiescence in sea urchin sperm. J. Cell Sci. **54:** 115–135.
11. GIBBONS, B. H. & I. R. GIBBONS. 1980. Calcium-induced quiescence in reactivated sea urchin sperm. J. Cell Biol. **84:** 13–27.
12. GIBBONS, I. R. 1982. Sliding and bending in sea urchin sperm flagella. Symp. Soc. Exp. Biol. **35:** 225–287.
13. GIBBONS, I. R., J. A. EVANS & B. H. GIBBONS. 1982. Acetate anions stabilize the latency of dynein 1 ATPase and increase the velocity of tubule sliding in reactivated sperm flagella. Cell Mot. Suppl. **1:** 181–184.
14. GIBBONS, I. R. & B. H. GIBBONS. 1980. Transient flagellar waveforms during intermittent swimming in sea urchin sperm. I. Wave parameters. J. Musc. Res. Cell Mot. **1:** 31–59.
15. ISHIGURO, K., H. MUROFUSHI & H. SAKAI. 1982. Evidence that cAMP-dependent protein kinase and a protein factor are involved in reactivation of Triton X-100 models of sea urchin and starfish spermatozoa. J. Cell Biol. **92:** 777–782.
16. LINDEMANN, C. B. 1978. A cAMP-induced increase in the motility of demembranated bull sperm models. Cell **13:** 9–18.

17. Okuno, M. 1980. Inhibition and relaxation of sea urchin sperm flagella by vanadate. J. Cell Biol. **85:** 712–725.
18. Okuno, M. 1981. Personal communication.
19. Okuno, M. & C. J. Brokaw. 1981. Calcium-induced change in form of demembranated sea urchin sperm flagella immobilized by vanadate. Cell Mot. **1:** 349–362.
20. Okuno, M. & C. J. Brokaw. 1981. Effects of Triton-extraction conditions on beat symmetry of sea urchin sperm flagella. Cell Mot. **1:** 363–370.
21. Omoto, C. K. & C. J. Brokaw. 1983. Quantitative analysis of axonemal bends and twists in the quiescent state of *Ciona* sperm flagella. Cell Mot. **3:** 247–259.
22. Opresko, L. K. & C. J. Brokaw. 1983. cAMP-dependent phosphorylation associated with activation of motility of *Ciona* sperm flagella. Gamete Res. **8:** 201–218.
23. Morisawa, M. & M. Okuno. 1982. Cyclic AMP induces maturation of trout sperm axonemes to initiate motility. Nature **295:** 703–704.
24. Tash, J. S. & A. R. Means. 1982. Regulation of protein phosphorylation and motility of sperm by cAMP and calcium. Biol. Reprod. **26:** 745–763.

The Modulation of Sperm Metabolism and Motility by Factors Associated with Eggs[a]

MARK P. BRADLEY,[b] NORIO SUZUKI,[c] and
DAVID L. GARBERS[d,e]

[b,c,d]*Departments of Pharmacology and* [d]*Physiology*
[c,d]*The Howard Hughes Medical Institute*
Vanderbilt University Medical Center
Nashville, Tennessee 37232

INTRODUCTION

The biochemical mechanisms by which gametes communicate with each other at the time of fertilization in either invertebrates or vertebrates are not clearly understood. However, within the last few years some of the potential chemical messengers have been isolated and characterized. By the use of these purified components and by the reconstitution of these purified factors it is anticipated that the gamete communication system will be eventually understood.

In the sea urchin, one isolated component, which we abbreviate FS-P (fucose-sulfate–rich factor from *Strongylocentrotus purpuratus*), is associated with the jelly coat of the egg.[1,2] FS-P is a large molecular weight complex consisting of fucose (32–45%), sulfate (36–44%), and protein (2.5–29%). It causes a large uptake of $^{45}Ca^{2+}$, marked increases in cyclic AMP concentrations, and the induction of an acrosome reaction in sea urchin spermatozoa.[2,3] FS-P causes these same effects in flagella-less sperm heads,[4] suggesting that the cyclic AMP elevations are related to the induction of an acrosome reaction or to a subsequent event related to fertilization. Support for this hypothesis is that other agents that induce an acrosome reaction in sea urchin spermatozoa (nigericin, A23187, high pH) also cause dramatic increases in sperm cyclic AMP concentrations.[2–4] FS-P does not appear to elevate cyclic GMP concentrations and does not stimulate, but inhibits sperm respiration rates.[5] It should be emphasized that added cyclic nucleotides or an elevation of cyclic AMP in the absence of extracellular Ca^{2+} does not result in an acrosome reaction. Work from the laboratory of Lennarz has demonstrated that the fucose-sulfate polymer shows a high degree of species specificity, suggesting the occurrence of unique receptor molecules.[5,6]

Based on the above as well as other data, Garbers and Kopf[3] have suggested

[a]Supported by the National Institutes of Health (grant HD 10254) and an Andrew W. Mellon Foundation grant.

[e] Address correspondence to David L. Garbers, Howard Hughes Medical Institute, Vanderbilt University Medical Center, 711 Light Hall, Nashville, TN 37232.

that Ca^{2+} is the key signal for the elevations of cyclic AMP. To date, no conclusive data showing direct or indirect Ca^{2+} regulation of the sea urchin sperm adenylate cyclase or of sperm cyclic nucleotide phosphodiesterases have appeared. Ca^{2+}-dependent regulation of adenylate cyclase[7] and of cyclic nucleotide phosphodiesterase[8,9] is established for other tissues. Since proteases or phospholipids[10] can in some cases activate these enzymes and destroy the Ca^{2+}-calmodulin regulation of enzyme activity, it is possible that in experiments designed to measure Ca^{2+} dependency protease activity or phospholipids present during the homogenization of sperm cells has already activated adenylate cyclase or phosphodiesterases in the sperm cell homogenate.

Lenz *et al.* recently demonstrated that chondroitin sulfate proteoglycan could induce the acrosome reaction of bovine spermatozoa.[11] In addition, heparin, chondroitin sulfate A, B, or C, and hyaluronic acid (but not dextran sulfate) could induce the acrosome reaction.[12] The potency depended on the degree of sulfation. The activity of chondroitin sulfate proteoglycan could be destroyed by chondroitinase ABC. In a later study the chondroitin sulfate A isomer was studied and was shown to induce acrosome reactions that resulted in an increased percentage of fertilization of matured bovine oocytes.[13] Since various glycosaminoglycans exist in the female reproductive tract, it is conceivable that the glycosaminoglycans have a functional role in the development of an acrosome reaction. If they do, the sea urchin system has served as a reasonable model since FS-P is also a highly sulfated complex.

The other purified component from the sea urchin system is a decapeptide that we have named speract.[14-16] The peptide isolated from *S. purpuratus* eggs has the amino acid sequence of Gly-Phe-Asp-Leu-Asn-Gly-Gly-Gly-Val-Gly and activates sperm motility and respiration in the 10^{-11} M range. Speract requires extracellular Na^+ but not Ca^{2+} for a biological response.[17] A primary effect of the peptide appears to be the induction of a net H^+ efflux from spermatozoa with a resultant elevation of intracellular pH;[18] it also elevates cyclic nucleotide concentrations. It has been demonstrated by our laboratory that sperm cells contain a receptor for speract[19] and a number of partial agonists have been synthesized.[18,19]

Although Holland and Cross[20] have questioned whether speract or its related analogues stimulates motility and metabolism of sea urchin sperm cells during fertilization, they failed to take into account the necessity of working under "artificial" conditions when assaying the biological activity of the pure material. Although Ohtake[21] suggested that the pH of egg jelly might be acidic and that this might explain the function of speract, the major point of his theory was that jelly would inhibit sperm respiration and that the peptide would relieve the inhibition. The eventual reconstitution of purified factors is obviously required to understand the biochemical regulation of a system and such reconsititution needs to be under appropriate physiological conditions. Here, we will show that if one uses jelly purified free of speract or, in some cases heterologous jelly, one inhibits sperm respiration rates. Reconstitution of the jelly with speract or other "activating peptides" results in a stimulation of sperm respiration rates.

Only limited evidence is available that indicates that the mammalian egg may have some effect on mammalian sperm motility. Gwatkin *et al.*[22] observed that bovine spermatozoa in the presence of cumulus intact eggs exhibited a greater percentage motility than sperm in control medium. Similarily Yanagimachi[23] showed that spermatozoa in the immediate environment of the cumulus oophorus cell swim in a vigorous manner.

This paper presents evidence that bovine cumulus oophorus cells are capable of releasing a factor(s) that stimulates bovine sperm motility.

EXPERIMENTAL PROCEDURES

Materials

Tyrode's medium was obtained from Gibco. Follicle-stimulating hormone (FSH) and bovine serum albumin (Fraction V) were obtained from Sigma. Sea urchins were obtained from Pacific Bio-Marine (Venice, CA) and the Marine Biological Laboratory (Woods Hole, MA). Speract was synthesized by Peninsula Laboratories, Inc. (San Carlos, CA).

Preparation of Gametes

Spermatozoa from the bovine caudal epididymis were washed twice with modified Tyrode's culture medium (TALPS)[24] containing 6 mg/ml bovine serum albumin and were then suspended to a final concentration of 1×10^8 cells/ml in the same buffer. Follicles from fresh bovine ovaries were aspirated with a 10 ml syringe fitted with an 18 gauge needle. The follicular contents were transferred to a 50 ml conical centrifuge tube containing 20 ml of phosphate-buffered saline and its contents were then placed in an incubator at 37°C, 100% humidity, 7% CO_2; the cellular contents were then allowed to settle out. After 15–30 min the cumulus oophorus–egg complexes were removed from the bottom of the tube and placed into phosphate-buffered saline, containing 3% bovine serum albumin. The cumulus oophorus–egg complexes were then individually collected using a screw action Hamilton syringe.

Isolated cumulus oophorus–egg complexes were placed into 50 μl droplets of TALPS medium supplemented with 6 mg/ml bovine serum albumin in the absence or presence of FSH (10 μg/ml). The cultures were maintained at 37°C in a 7% CO_2 atmosphere for 24 hr.

Sea urchin gametes were collected as described previously.[14]

Bovine Sperm–Egg Experiments **In Vitro**

Droplets (50 μl) of TALPS medium containing 6 mg/ml bovine serum albumin were placed under paraffin oil and pre-equilibrated to 37°C in a humidified incubator containing a 7% CO_2 atmosphere. Cultured cumulus oophorus–egg complexes (8–10) were then placed in each drop prior to the addition of 1×10^6 spermatozoa/50 μl. For control incubations, TALPS medium (50 μl) containing 6 mg/ml bovine serum albumin were added under paraffin oil instead of cumulus oophorus–egg complexes. In experiments where only the medium from the prior egg culture was tested, the medium was centrifuged at $13,000 \times g$ to remove egg debris and 50 μl of the medium were then used as described above. Controls used for these experiments were media ± FSH in which no eggs had been incubated. In all experiments a 30 min equilibration time period occurred prior to the initial motility measurement at time "zero."

Sperm Forward Motility and Respiration Rates

Bovine sperm forward motility was measured based on the method of Acott and Hoskins[25] with the modification of Stephens *et al.*[26] At defined time periods, 2

μl samples of spermatozoa were removed from the *in vitro* culture fluid and diluted into 50 μl culture medium that had been pre-equilibrated with 7% CO_2 at 37°C. From this, a 10 μl sample was removed and placed on a hemacytometer (at 37°C) and the motility assay was then performed.

Respiration rates of sea urchin spermatozoa were determined at 20°C using a Gilson-K-IC Table Top Oxygraph equipped with 2.2 ml capacity temperature control chamber fitted with a Clark type electrode and a semimicro pH electrode (Radiometer GK-2421C).

Isolation of Sea Urchin Egg Jelly

Sea urchin eggs collected in artificial sea water (ASW) were centrifuged at 1,500 $\times$ g for 10 min at 5°C. The pelleted eggs were suspended (10% vol/vol) in non-buffered ASW (pH 7.5–7.6). After 5–6 min, with occasional stirring, the eggs were centrifuged at 10,000 $\times$ g for 60 min and the resulting supernatant fluid was used as the egg jelly preparation.

L. pictus egg jelly was also treated in some cases with charcoal. The charcoal that had been extensively washed with Millipore-filtered H_2O and pre-equilibrated with ASW was then removed by centrifugation and subsequent filtration on Whatman No. 1 filter paper. The filtrate was dialyzed extensively at 25°C against ASW. The non-dialyzable fraction was centrifuged at 10,000 $\times$ g for 60 min at 4°C and the supernatant fluid was used for experiments.

RESULTS

Evidence for the Modulation of Mammalian Sperm Motility by Mammalian Egg Factors

During the establishment of an *in vitro* fertilization system for bovine gametes, it was observed that bovine spermatozoa incubated in the presence of cumulus oophorus–egg masses exhibited an enhanced motility compared to spermatozoa in culture medium alone. To quantitate these apparent differences in motility we used the forward motility index (FMI) assay of Acott and Hoskins *et al.*,[25] with the modification of Stephens *et al.*[26] Spermatozoa incubated in the presence of cumulus egg complexes previously cultured in the presence of FSH showed a significantly higher forward motility index than spermatozoa incubated in medium alone (TABLE 1). The sperm motility–stimulating factor appeared to be secreted by the cumulus oophorus–egg complexes during the 24 hr pre-culture period since when culture medium was separated from the cumulus–egg complexes and then tested for ability to stimulate sperm motility it had the effects described in TABLE 2. Again culture medium from FSH-treated eggs appeared to possess higher activity (TABLE 2). The cumulus oophorus cells appeared to be responsible for the secretion of the factor(s) since spermatozoa cultured with cumulus-free eggs did not show an increase in the forward motility index (TABLE 3), whereas spermatozoa cultured with cumulus oophorus cells (no eggs) showed a significant stimulation of the sperm motility forward motility index (TABLE 4). Thus, the site of release of the sperm motility activating factor(s) appears to be the cumulus oophorus cells and not the eggs. It is possible, however, that eggs also release a factor(s) when they are in contact with the cumulus oophorus cells. Identification

TABLE 1. The Effect of Cumulus Oophorus–Egg Complexes on Bovine Caudal Epididymal Spermatozoa in the Presence of the Antistick Agent Poly Glutamic-Lysine

	Forward Motility Index[a]		
	0 hr	6 hr	24 hr
Control	2532 ± 156	2805 ± 935	1987 ± 78
Cumulus oophorus–egg masses (−FSH)	3662 ± 935	4753 ± 702	2922 ± 117[b]
Cumulus oophorus–egg masses (+FSH)	5338 ± 468[b]	5571 ± 935[b]	3935 ± 584[b]

[a] Forward Motility Index $= \dfrac{n \cdot \bar{v}}{N} \times \dfrac{100}{1}$ n = Number of tracks/field
N = Total number of sperm in field
$\bar{v}$ = Average velocity

A 10 mg/ml solution of poly G-L was applied to the surface of the hemacytometer and dried prior to the initiation of the motility assays. Values are the mean ± SE of three separate experiments. Values that are significantly different ($p < 0.05$) from controls are represented by superscript b.

TABLE 2. The Stimulation of the Sperm Forward Motility Index by Supernatant Fluid from Cumulus Oophorus–Egg Masses Incubated in the Absence or Presence of FSH

	Forward Motility Index		
	0 hr	6 hr	24 hr
Control (−FSH)	1680 ± 273	2109 ± 430	1523 ± 273
Supernatant fluid (−FSH)	3398 ± 313[a]	2930 ± 391	2422 ± 703[a]
Control (+FSH)	2266 ± 547	1836 ± 508	1172 ± 469
Supernatant fluid (+FSH)	4609 ± 391[a]	4688 ± 547[a]	3789 ± 703[a]

For control incubations, 50 μl droplets of TALPS medium containing 6 mg/ml bovine serum albumin + 10 μg/ml FSH or −FSH were added under paraffin oil instead of the supernatant fluid. Values are the mean ±SE of three separate experiments. Differences ($p < 0.1$) from controls are represented by superscript a.

TABLE 3. The Effect of Eggs on the Sperm Forward Motility Index *in Vitro*

	Forward Motility Index		
	0 hr	6 hr	24 hr
Control	1948 ± 253	2260 ± 312	1636 ± 312
Eggs (−FSH)	2182 ± 351	2104 ± 702	1909 ± 351
Eggs (+FSH)	1948 ± 409	1792 ± 506	1812 ± 467

Spermatozoa were incubated in the following media containing (1) TALPS + 6 mg/ml bovine serum albumin (control); (2) cumulus oophorus–free eggs matured in the absence of FSH (Eggs − FSH); (3) cumulus oophorus–free eggs matured in TALPS + 6 mg/ml bovine serum albumin + 10 μg/ml FSH (Eggs + FSH). Values are the mean ±SE of three separate experiments.

TABLE 4. The Effect of Culture Medium from Isolated Cumulus Oophorus Cells on the Bovine Sperm Forward Motility Index *in Vitro*

	Forward Motility Index		
	0 hr	6 hr	24 hr
Control	2392 ± 275	2784 ± 627	3176 ± 314
Culture medium	4549 ± 667	5176 ± 1608	5098 ± 431

Spermatozoa were incubated in medium containing TALPS + 6 mg/ml bovine serum albumin (control) and culture medium from isolated cumulus oophorus cells, incubated with 10 μg/ml FSH. Values are the mean ±SE of three separate experiments. All values are different (p <0.1) from controls.

of the sperm motility stimulating factor(s) derived from the cumulus oophorus cells remains to be determined. However, when the supernatant fluid from cumulus cell culture fluid is added to a Bio-Gel A 0.5 m column and the collected fractions are pooled as shown in FIGURE 1, a motility-stimulating fraction can be identified.

Stimulation of Invertebrate Sperm Respiration and Motility

In the early 1900s, it was shown that soluble factors associated with the eggs of certain species of sea urchins could enhance the respiration and motility of sea urchin spermatozoa.[27–29] The factors were reported to be diffusible upon dialysis, heat stable, alcohol soluble, and non-volatile.[30] The factors also were shown to appear in the ovary in parallel with the progress of ovarian maturation;[31] they have been purified from several species of sea urchins and identified as peptides.[14–16]

Speract was first identified in *S. purpuratus* and *Hemicentrotus pulcherrimus* but we now know that natural analogues (Thr[5]-speract) and (Ser[5]-speract) also exist in *H. pulcherrimus*[15] and *Anthocidaris crassispina*[32] (TABLE 5).

TABLE 5. Structures of Identified Peptides that Activate Sea Urchin Spermatozoa

Source and Structure	
Strongylocentrotus purpuratus	
Gly-Phe-Asp-Leu-Asn-Gly-Gly-Gly-Val-Gly	(speract)
Hemicentrotus pulcherrimus	
Gly-Phe-Asp-Leu-Asn-Gly-Gly-Gly-Val-Gly	(speract)
Gly-Phe-Asp-Leu-Thr-Gly-Gly-Gly-Val-Gly	(Thr[5]-speract)
Anthocidaris crassispina	
Gly-Phe-Asp-Leu-Ser-Gly-Gly-Gly-Val-Gly	(Ser[5]-speract)
Gly-Phe-Asp-Leu-Thr-Gly-Gly-Gly-Val-Gly	(Thr[5]-speract)

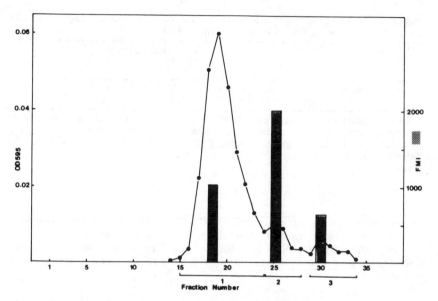

FIGURE 1. Biogel A 0.5 m gel chromatography of bovine cumulus oophorus cell culture supernatant fluid. Isolated bovine cumulus oophorus egg complexes were incubated in RPMI 1640 medium (leucine-free) containing 10% fetal calf serum and 10 μg/ml FSH for 24 hr as described in the text. The supernatant fluid (0.5 ml) was first applied to a Sephacryl S200 column (1 × 60 cm), and the fractions containing activity that elevated the forward motility index were pooled, dialyzed against Millipore-filtered H$_2$O, and lyophilized. The residue was then dissolved in 0.5 ml of a solution containing 0.5 M NaCl and 0.1 M Tris, pH 7.8. The 0.5 ml was applied to BioGel A 0.5m column (1 × 60 cm) equilibrated with the same buffer. Fractions of 0.85 ml were collected and protein was determined. Fractions were pooled as indicated and assayed for their effects on the forward motility index.

Stimulation of Sperm Respiration by Speract in the Presence of Egg Jelly

Speract and other egg-associated peptides (Thr⁵-speract; Ser⁵-speract) have been shown to stimulate the respiration of sea urchin spermatozoa at slightly acidic pH values. The physiological significance of this stimulation has been suggested to be due to a possible acidic pH of egg jelly[21,33] because of its high content of carboxyl- and ester-linked sulfate residues.[1,34,35] However, the pH of hydrated egg jelly is not very acidic (pH 7.4–7.7 in our measurements and pH 8.0 in the studies of Holland and Cross[20]) and thus may not represent the mechanism by which jelly can inhibit sperm respiration rates.

Because of the high potency of these peptides to stimulate sperm respiration and the binding affinity to receptor[16,19] it has been logical to expect that the peptides have a role in the normal fertilization process of the sea urchin. Since we had pure components from jelly we could now reconstitute the system and study physiological function at normal seawater pH. *A. punctulata* egg jelly has been reported to lack the agent capable of stimulating the respiration of *L. variegatus* spermatozoa[30] despite a similarity in the gross chemical composition of the egg jelly of both species.[1] No doubt the failure to stimulate will be shown to be due to peptide specificity between sea urchin species.

In initial studies we determined that the sea urchin, *A. punctulata,* contained a peptide that activated its own spermatozoa; this peptide did not, however, cross-react with *S. purpuratus* or *L. pictus* spermatozoa. Speract did not activate the *A. punctulata* spermatozoa but did activate *L. pictus* spermatozoa and a peptide from *L. pictus* cross-reacted with *S. purpuratus.* We have now initiated studies to purify and sequence the peptide from *A. punctulata.* FIGURE 2 demonstrates a high pressure liquid chromatographic profile of a crude mixture of peptides collected from the medium in which *A. punctulata* eggs had been incubated. Biologically active material (stimulation of respiration and motility) was observed at about 27 min. In other experiments, medium containing active peptide was first chromotographed on Sephadex G-10 and was then run on an octyl column (FIGURE 3). The active fraction was again found to elute at about 27 min; this fraction contains various amino acids but is particularly rich in glycine. Jelly has been

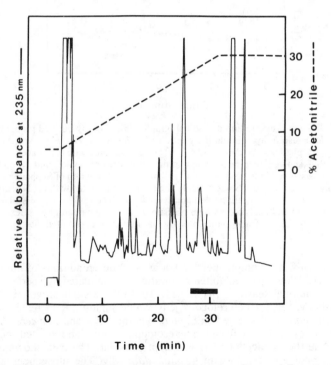

Time (min)

FIGURE 2. High pressure liquid chromatography of *A. punctulata* egg jelly extracts. About three liters of *A. punctulata* egg jelly were extracted with ethanol (final concentration of ethanol was 70%). The extracts were concentrated by a rotary evaporator to 120 ml and an aliquot (1 ml) was applied to an octyl column (4.6 × 250 mm) equilibrated with 5% acetonitrile in 0.1% trifluoroacetic acid. A program with a constant flow rate of 1.5 ml/min was initiated at 2 min to give the linear acetonitrile concentration shown. The column effluent was monitored for absorbance at 235 nm. Fractions (1.5 ml) were collected and 10 μl of a 1,000–10,000-fold dilution of each fraction were used to assay for respiratory stimulation of *A. punctulata* spermatozoa. The pooled fraction indicated by the solid area contained the activity that stimulated cell respiration.

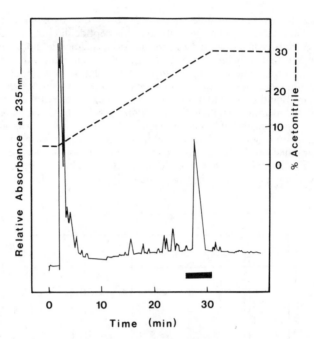

FIGURE 3. High pressure liquid chromatography of a partially purified preparation of the *A. punctulata* respiration-stimulating peptide. *A. punctulata* egg jelly extracts were first applied on a Sephadex G-10 column (2.5 × 90 cm) equilibrated with 0.1 M acetic acid and the fractions that showed respiratory-stimulating activity were pooled and lyophilized. The residue was dissolved in 0.1 N acetic acid and applied on a column of Sephadex G-15 (2.5 × 90 cm) equilibrated with 0.1 N acetic acid. The column was eluted with 0.1 N acetic acid and the active fractions were again pooled and lyophilized. The residue was dissolved in Milli-pore-filtered H$_2$O and analyzed by high pressure liquid chromatography as described in the legend to FIGURE 2. The fraction indicated by the solid area represented the stimulatory area of the effluent.

previously shown to inhibit sperm respiration under conditions of normal extra-cellular pH.[5] Would jelly-inhibited respiration be stimulated by speract or related peptides at normal seawater pH values? To do these studies, we initially deter-mined whether or not heterologous jelly would inhibit sperm respiration. Jelly from *A. punctulata* was tested on *L. pictus* spermatozoa and *vice versa*. As can be seen from FIGURE 4, jelly from the heterologous sea urchin inhibited sperm respi-ration while the extracellular pH was kept constant. The data shown are for *L. pictus* spermatozoa treated with *A. punctulata* jelly. The subsequent addition of the homologous (speract) peptide (FIGURE 4) greatly stimulated respiration. How-ever, the addition of the *Arbacia* peptide did not stimulate respiration (not shown). With *A. punctulata* spermatozoa inhibited by *L. pictus* jelly, the same effects are observed except speract does not whereas the *Arbacia* peptide does stimulate.

The factor(s) in jelly that was responsible for this respiratory decrease was non-dialyzable and was active at pH 6.6 to pH 7.8. Thus, respiratory inhibition was not necessarily correlated with the occurrence of an acrosome reaction. The activation of respiration by speract was dependent on the concentration of the peptide, and half-maximal stimulation of respiration occurred at about 10^{-9} M speract. When unfractionated, homologous egg jelly, which contains the activating peptide, was used respiration was not inhibited or inhibited only slightly in either *L. pictus* or *A. punctulata* spermatozoa. These results suggested that the function of speract and activating peptides from other sea urchins is to maintain sperm motility and metabolism while cells traverse the extracellular matrix around the egg. To determine this with more certainty, jelly was prepared to obtain fucose-sulfate polymer and other jelly components free of speract.[2] When the purified jelly (free of speract) was added to the spermatozoa, it inhibited respiration (FIGURE 5). The addition of speract to the *L. pictus* spermatozoa, however, stimulated sperm respiration. Since these studies were done at normal seawater pH values, these experiments strongly suggest that the peptide functions to maintain and/or stimulate sperm metabolism and motility under the natural condition of sperm traversing the jelly layer prior to coming in contact with the egg.

Whether or not speract still functions to elevate intracellular pH is not known, however, monensin A, an ionophore that catalyzes an electro-neutral Na^+/H^+ exchange and mimics speract at pH 6.6,[17] also mimics speract to overcome jelly-inhibited respiration (FIGURE 5). Thus, the mechanism of action of the peptide at normal extracellular pH may be identical to its effects at lower pH.

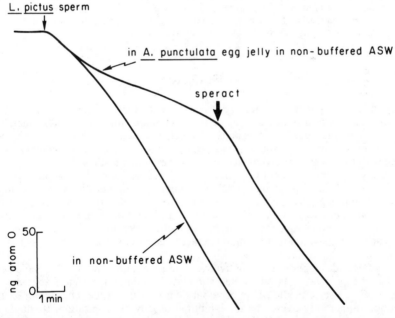

FIGURE 4. Respiration of *L. pictus* spermatozoa in the presence of *A. punctulata* egg jelly. The egg jelly was prepared as described in the text and was added to give 4.1 mg/ml protein and 135 μg/ml hexose. The pH of the unbuffered artificial seawater (ASW) with or without added jelly was 7.5–7.6. Sperm respiration was determined at 20°C using a Gilson K-IC Table Top Oxygraph equipped with a 2.2 ml capacity temperature control chamber. At the points indicated, spermatozoa and speract were added to give final concentrations of 4.5 mg wet weight/ml and 10^{-9} M, respectively.

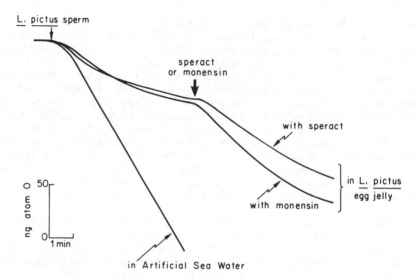

FIGURE 5. Respiration of *L. pictus* spermatozoa in the presence of *L. pictus* egg jelly. *L. pictus* egg jelly was purified through the charcoal step as described in the text. The egg jelly used was added to give 640 μg/ml protein and 137 μg/ml hexose. At the indicated points, *L. pictus* sperm, speract, and monensin were added to give final concentrations of 4.5 mg wet weight/ml, 10^{-9} M, and 2.5×10^{-5} M, respectively.

DISCUSSION

During fertilization spermatozoa appear to proceed through a series of activation processes, some of which appear to occur in the cellular or acellular matrices surrounding the egg. The biochemical mechanisms involved in the activation processes are not yet completely understood but the purification of factors associated with these egg-associated structures may eventually allow the reconstitution of the system and the identification of the importance of each component.

The sea urchin has become a valuable model system because various components of the egg jelly have now been purified. The effects of two components (FS-P and speract) are summarized in TABLE 6. These data summarize responses of *S. purpuratus* spermatozoa to these two factors. We now know that molecules similar in composition to FS-P and speract exist in other sea urchin species but that cross-reactivity may not occur.

The peptides (speract) that activate sperm respiration and motility have been and are being isolated based on their stimulation of these parameters at acidic pH values. The use of acidic pH is necessary since in the crude jelly mixtures, the peptides apparently overcome the inhibition of jelly on respiration. It should be emphasized, however, that the relief of inhibition may not be permanent (FIGURE 5). Under acidic pH conditions, the stimulatory effect of speract also often appears to be transient, lasting only a few minutes.

The component of jelly responsible for the inhibition of respiration in the studies reported here has not been identified. It is large in molecular weight (not dialyzable) and could be the fucose-sulfate polymer. Kinsey *et al.*[5] associated the respiratory decrease with the induction of an acrosome reaction since jelly from *A. punctulata* did not decrease the respiration nor induce the acrosome reaction of *S. purpuratus* spermatozoa, while A23187 induced an acrosome reaction and caused an inhibition of sperm respiration. The species specificity of the respiratory inhibition[5] is not the same as we report here. However, we tested *A. punctulata* and *L. pictus* in the heterologous system as opposed to *A. punctulata* and *S. purpuratus* in the previous study. Kinsey *et al.*[5] also found respiratory inhibition in the homologous system where crude egg jelly was used. As we mentioned above, it is possible that the peptide only delays the onset of respiratory inhibition as opposed to a permanent relief of such inhibition. Since the fertilizing capacity of sea urchin spermatozoa is decreased dramatically in less than 1 min after induction of an acrosome reaction,[5,36] the maintenance of motility and respiration for long periods of time is probably not necessary. In the homologous system monensin A, which catalyzes electrically neutral Na^+/H^+ exchange across cell membranes, reproduced the effect of speract on respiration; this suggests that jelly-inhibited sperm respiration may be relieved by the elevation of intracellular pH. The effect of speract on intracellular pH in the presence of jelly remains to be determined.

In the mammalian system, it also should be possible to eventually reconstitute components of the matrices surrounding the egg. However, components remain to be purified. In this paper, we show that the cumulus oophorus–egg complexes possess the ability to produce factor(s) that are capable of increasing the sperm forward motility index. The physiological significance of these observations is not yet clear especially since fowl, ram, and bull spermatozoal motility is maintained by the culture of these sperm cells with HeLa of BHK-21 cells.[37] Although motility of mammalian spermatozoa has been reportedly stimulated by various reproductive tract secretions[38] the responsible component(s) has not been isolated and thus specificity of the responses again remains to be determined. In recent years a motility stimulating factor has been identified in the hamster model[39-41] and a "hyperactivated" form of motility has been described for the sperm cells of various animals.[42] It remains to be determined whether or not the increase in the forward motility index of bovine sperm cells in response to cumulus cell factor(s) resulted in an altered pattern of motility.

TABLE 6. Biochemical Effects of Purified Egg Jelly Components on *S. Purpuratus* Spermatozoa

	Speract	FS-P
Cyclic AMP	↑	↑
Cyclic GMP	↑	—
$^{45}Ca^{2+}$ uptake	—	↑
$^{22}Na^+$ uptake	↑	nm[a]
Net H^+ efflux	↑	↑
Respiration rate	↑	↓
Motility	↑	↓
Fatty acid oxidation rates	↑	nm[a]
Acrosome reaction	—	↑

[a] nm, not measured.

ACKNOWLEDGMENTS

We wish to thank Drs. N. L. First and G. D. Ball, Department of Meat and Animal Sciences, University of Wisconsin, Madison, WI, for their help in establishing the *in vitro* fertilization procedures used in this study. We are also grateful to D. Janette Tubb for technical assistance, Helen Davis Watkins and Donna B. Hilliburton for drawing the figures, and Diane Smithson for typing the manuscript.

REFERENCES

1. SEGALL, G. K. & W. J. LENNARZ. 1979. Dev. Biol. **71:** 33–48.
2. KOPF, G. S. & D. L. GARBERS. 1980. Biol Reprod. **22:** 1118–1126.
3. GARBERS, D. L. & G. S. KOPF. 1980. Adv. Cyclic Nucleotide Res. **13:** 251–306.
4. GARBERS, D. L. 1981. J. Biol. Chem. **256:** 620–624.
5. KINSEY, W. H., G. K. SEGALL & W. J. LENNARZ. 1979. Dev. Biol. **71:** 49–59
6. SEGALL, G. K. & W. J. LENNARZ. 1981. Dev. Biol. **86:** 87–93.
7. BROSTROM, C. O., Y. C. HUANG, B. M. L. BRENKENRIDGE & D. J. WOLFF. 1975. Proc. Natl. Acad. Sci. USA **72:** 64–68
8. CHEUNG, W. Y. 1970. Biochem. Biophys. Res. Commun. **38:** 533–538.
9. KAKIUCHI, S. & R. YAMAZAKI. 1970. Biochem. Biophys. Res. Commun. **41:** 1104–1110.
10. LIN, Y. M. & W. Y. CHEUNG. 1980. *In* Calcium and Cell Function. W. Y. Cheung, Ed.:79–107. Academic Press. New York.
11. LENZ, R. W., R. L. AX, H. J. GRIMEK & N. L. FIRST. 1982. Biochem. Biophys. Res. Commun. **106:** 1092–1098.
12. HANDROW, R. R., R. W. LENZ & R. L. AX. 1982. Biochem. Biophys. Res. Commun. **107:** 1320–1332.
13. LENZ, R. W., G. D. BALL, J. K. LOHSE, N. L. FIRST & R. L. AX. 1983. Biol. Reprod. **28:** 683–690.
14. HANSBROUGH, J. R. & D. L. GARBERS. 1981. J. Biol. Chem. **256:** 1447–1452.
15. SUZUKI, N., K. NOMURA, H. OHTAKE & S. ISAKA. 1981. Biochem. Biophys. Res. Commun. **99:** 1238–1244.
16. GARBERS, D. L., H. D. WATKINS, J. R. HANSBROUGH, A. SMITH & K. S. MISONO. 1982. J. Biol. Chem. **257:** 2734–2737.
17. HANSBROUGH, J. R. & D. L. GARBERS. 1981. J. Biol. Chem. **256:** 2235–2241.
18. REPASKE, D. R. & D. L. GARBERS. 1983. J. Biol. Chem. **258:** 6025–6029.
19. SMITH, A. & D. L. GARBERS. 1983. *In* Biochemistry of Metabolic Process. D. L. H. Lennon, F. W. Stratman & R. N. Zahlten, Eds.: 15–28. Elsevier Science Publishing Co., Inc. New York.
20. HOLLAND, L. Z. & N. L. CROSS. 1983. Dev. Biol. **99:** 258–260.
21. OHTAKE, H. 1976. J. Exp. Biol. **198:** 303–312.
22. GWATKIN, R. B. L., O. F. ANDERSON & C. F. HUTCHINSON. 1972. J. Reprod. Fert. **30:** 389–394.
23. YANAGIMACHI, R. 1969. J. Reprod. Fert. **18:** 275–286.
24. BAVISTER, B. D. & R. YANAGIMACHI. 1977. Biol. Reprod. **16:** 228–237.
25. ACOTT, T. S. & D. D. HOSKINS. 1978. J. Biol. Chem. **253:** 6744–6750.
26. STEPHENS, D. T., T. S. ACOTT & D. D. HOSKINS. 1981. Biol. Reprod. **25:** 945–949.
27. LILLIE, F. R. 1913. J. Exp. Zool. **14:** 515–574.
28. COHN, E. J. 1918. Biol. Bull. **34:** 167–168.
29. GRAY, J. 1928. J. Exp. Biol. **5:** 337–344.
30. HATHAWAY, R. R. 1963. Biol. Bull. **125:** 486–498.
31. SUZUKI, N., K. KOBAYASHI & S. ISAKA. 1982. Experientia **38:** 1245–1246.
32. NOMURA, K., N. SUZUKI & S. ISAKA. 1983. Peptide Chemistry. (In press.)
33. VASSEUR, E. & B. HAGSTROM. 1946. Ark. Zool. **37A:** 1–17.

34. ISAKA, S., K. HOTTA & M. KUROKAWA. 1970. Exp. Cell Res. **59:** 37–42.
35. ISHIHARA, K., K. OGURI & H. TANIGUCHI. 1973. Biochim. Biophys. Acta **320:** 628–634.
36. VACQUIER, V. 1979. Develop. Growth Differ. **21:** 61–69.
37. ASHIZAWA, K., Y. TOKUDOME, K. OKAUCHI & H. NISHIYAMA. 1982. J. Reprod. Fert. **66:** 663–666.
38. HANSBROUGH, J. R. & D. L. GARBERS. 1981. Adv. Enzyme Reg. **19:** 351–376.
39. BAVISTER, B. D. 1981. J. Exp. Zool. **210:** 259–264.
40. MRSNY, R. J., L. WAXMAN & S. MEIZEL. 1979. J. Exp. Zool. **210:** 123–128.
41. MEIZEL, S., C. W. LUI, P. K. WORKING & R. J. MRSNY. 1980. Develop. Growth Differ. **22:** 483–494.
42. YANAGIMACHI, R. 1981. *In* Fertilization and Embryonic Development *in Vitro*. L. Mastroianni & J. D. Biggers, Eds.: 81–182. Plenum Publishing Co. New York.

Immunochemical Dissection of the Testes-specific Isozyme Lactate Dehydrogenase C_4[a]

THOMAS E. WHEAT and ERWIN GOLDBERG[b]

*Department of Biochemistry, Molecular
Biology and Cell Biology
Northwestern University
Evanston, Illinois 60201*

During spermatogenesis, genes are sequentially activated and inactivated in a complex developmental program to produce a highly differentiated cell with unique functional specializations. Many of these genes are activated only during this process. The properties of these testis-specific gene products must be well adapted to the physiological requirements of both spermatozoa and the differentiating germ cells. The C_4 isozyme of lactate dehydrogenase (LDH-C_4; LDH-X) is an excellent example of such a testis- and sperm-specific gene product. The biochemical properties, physiology, and biological specificity of this isozyme have been reviewed[1-3] and can be briefly summarized.

LDH-C_4 is observed only in mature testes and sperm. This isozyme is first detectable in the mid-pachytene primary spermatocyte,[3,4] and synthesis of LDH-C_4 continues into spermiogenesis.[5,6] This tissue specificity is consistent with adaptation of enzymic properties to metabolic requirements, and the kinetic properties of LDH-C_4 are different from LDH-A_4 and LDH-B_4.[2] However, no completely satisfying physiological rationale for a third LDH isozyme has emerged from numerous studies.[2,3,8] The high concentration of LDH-C_4 present during spermatogenesis is consistent with adaptation to the metabolic requirements of spermatocytes and spermatids as well as to those of sperm.[3] Since Sertoli cells provide lactate to round spermatids as an energy source[9] and since high concentrations of lactate are observed in both rete testis fluid[10] and oviductal fluid,[11] the relative insensitivity of LDH-C_4 to inhibition by lactate would seem physiologically relevant.[12-14]

For complete biochemical characterization, mouse LDH-C_4 has been purified to crystalline homogeneity.[15] The three-dimensional structure was determined to 2.9 Å resolution by X-ray crystallography,[16] and complete sequences for both mouse and rat LDH-C_4 have recently become available.[17] These structural studies confirm that LDH-C is homologous to the LDH-A and LDH-B subunits. However, LDH-C_4 displays extensive substitutions in amino acid sequence and some modifications in three-dimensional structure.

The immune response to LDH-C_4 reflects its chemical and biological specificity. This isozyme is a potent antigen, even in males of the species from which it was isolated.[18] Antibodies to LDH-C_4 do not react with LDH isozymes composed

[a] Research from this laboratory was supported by grants from the National Institutes of Health and by a contract with The Program for Applied Research on Fertility Regulation (PARFR/USAID).

[b] Address correspondence to: Dr. Erwin Goldberg.

of A and B subunits, but rabbit anti-mouse LDH-C$_4$ reacts with LDH-C$_4$ from all species tested.[18]

The specificity of the immune response to LDH-C$_4$ and the restriction of the isozyme to male gametes form the basis for investigations of an alternative contraceptive technology. Although LDH-C$_4$ is primarily an intracellular enzyme, it is present on the surface of sperm and does provide specific antibody binding sites.[2] Immunization with LDH-C$_4$ suppresses the fertility of female mice,[19] rabbits,[20] and baboons.[21] This effect is apparently mediated by circulating antibodies to LDH-C$_4$ that enter the oviduct as a transudate of serum[22] and interfere with sperm transport[23] by agglutinating sperm and by mediating complement-dependent cytolysis.[24] Thus, LDH-C$_4$ is a useful model system for investigating the potential utility and pitfalls of immunological approaches to contraception.

It is unlikely that LDH-C$_4$ or any antigen isolated from natural sources could form the basis of a widely used contraceptive vaccine. In addition to problems of supply, particularly if human LDH-C$_4$ is required, it would be difficult to ensure the homogeneity and antigenic specificity of such a mass-isolated preparation. Although recombinant DNA techniques and genetic engineering may eventually circumvent some of these problems, an antigen amenable to chemical synthesis would provide the greatest flexibility and would also ensure the specificity of the immune response. A small peptide bearing an antigenic domain of LDH-C$_4$ could be substituted for the natural product if it induced an immune response to the native protein.

The design of such peptides is based on a map of the immunological structure of LDH-C$_4$. For some proteins, the antigenic structure may be derived from the amino acid sequence by calculation of hydrophilicity indices,[25] but this approach[26] does not reveal the antigenic domains of LDH-C$_4$ that have been experimentally identified.[27-31] The ongoing immunological dissection of LDH-C$_4$ is proceeding by the parallel analysis of the antibody component using hybridoma technology and the antigen component using peptide chemistry. Four monoclonal antibodies to LDH-C$_4$ have been developed, and the binding site on LDH-C$_4$ has been identified for one of these.[29] Mapping of the antigenic surface of LDH-C$_4$ is being accomplished with small peptides that bear antigenic domains. These domains are identified by the binding of rabbit anti-mouse LDH-C$_4$ to the isolated peptide, and antigenicity is confirmed by immunization with the peptide to elicit antibodies to the native protein. The successful application of this approach with one tryptic peptide of LDH-C$_4$ has been reported.[28,30] A more complete antigenic map based on tryptic peptides has now been completed.

MONOCLONAL ANTIBODIES TO MOUSE LDH-C$_4$

A complete description of monoclonal antibodies to mouse LDH-C$_4$ has been presented.[29] Hybridomas were obtained by the fusion[32] of myeloma cells with spleen cells from SJL/J mice immunized with mouse LDH-C$_4$. Four stable clones, designated RG-1 to RG-4, producing useful amounts of antibodies, were prepared. The affinities of these antibodies range from 1.7×10^9 M^{-1} to 16.4×10^9 M^{-1}. RG-4 is an IgM while the other three are of the IgG$_2$ subclass. The monoclonal origin of these antibodies was confirmed by the analysis of binding data by Sips plots[33] that yielded a heterogeneity index of 1.0 in each case.

The specificity of these monoclonal antibodies was analyzed by the ability of one antibody to inhibit the binding of another to mouse LDH-C$_4$ and by their reaction with LDH-C$_4$ from different species. Monoclonal antibody RG-3 does not interfere with the binding of either RG-1 or RG-2 to mouse LDH-C_4, indicating that RG-3 recognizes a distinct domain. In contrast, mutual inhibition between RG-1 and RG-2 suggests that they recognize identical or overlapping domains.[29]

The ability of homologous LDH-C_4 isozymes from several species to inhibit binding of each antibody to mouse LDH-C_4 was measured. Binding was also directly demonstrated by the alteration of electrophoretic mobility of LDH-C_4 in the presence of the antibody. Each of the four monoclonal antibodies has a unique pattern of cross-reactivity among the LDH-C_4 isozymes tested.[29] This indicates that each antibody recognizes a distinct set of amino acids, or antigenic domain, on mouse LDH-C_4. Thus, the domains recognized by RG-1 and RG-2 must be overlapping or so closely spaced that simultaneous binding is sterically hindered.

The binding of each monoclonal antibody to peptides bearing sequential determinants was measured with the solid matrix radioimmunoassay (smRIA).[39] Mouse anti-mouse LDH-C_4 binds to each peptide. Among the monoclonal antibodies, there is appreciable binding of RG-4 to peptide MC_{97-110}. The specificity of this binding was confirmed by the ability of the free peptide MC_{97-110} to inhibit the binding of RG-4 to mouse LDH-C_4. The antigenic domain recognized by RG-4 is thus identified as the coenzyme binding loop.[29] Since the molecular site of RG-4 binding is known, the species specificity of this monoclonal antibody has been examined.

Antibody RG-4 has a high affinity for mouse LDH-C_4 and binds with lower affinity to rat LDH-C_4. Low levels of binding to human and rabbit LDH-C_4 are observed, and no reaction with hamster LDH-C_4 can be detected.[29] This pattern can only result from differences in structure among the LDH-C_4 isozymes. Therefore, monoclonal antibody RG-4 distinguishes four alternative structures of the coenzyme binding loop. Such structural changes reflect substitutions in the amino acid sequence. Two antigens that differ in affinity for a monoclonal antibody must differ by at least one residue. Such a substitution must be either in the amino acid sequence of the antigenic domain or, if not directly involved in binding, alter the conformation of the reactive amino acid side chains. This region of the molecule is a flexible loop, terminating at each end in a rigid helix.[16,37] Thus, the differences detected by antibody RG-4 probably reflect alternative sequences of the domain itself rather than a conformational change due to substitution elsewhere in the molecule.

The number of substitutions inferred from the binding of RG-4 to LDH-C_4 from different species is remarkable.[29] The evolutionary conservation of the coenzyme binding loop of the somatic LDH isozymes is well known. No variation has been observed in either A or B subunits of mammals, birds, and fish.[36,37] Thus, at least the coenzyme binding loop of LDH-C_4 is evolving more rapidly than the homologous region of other LDH isozymes. A similar analysis with additional monoclonal antibodies will reveal whether the whole *Ldh-c* gene has evolved at a similar rate.

The differences in reactivity can also reveal more precisely the exact combining site for this antibody. The coenzyme binding loop of rat LDH-C_4 differs from that of mouse at residues 103 and 106.[34,35] The change from the negatively charged aspartic acid-106 of mouse LDH-C_4 to the non-polar alanine-106 of the rat isozyme would probably eliminate binding. On the other hand, the observed reduction in affinity is consistent with the change from the larger side chain of threonine-103 of the mouse to the smaller serine-103 of the rat. In addition, no binding can be detected with peptides MC_{98-104} or $MC_{105-110}$ suggesting that the combining site extends past arginine-104. Removal of the first two residues from MC_{97-110} does not affect binding. These data are consistent with the localization of the binding site of antibody RG-4 to no more than residues 99–106. Studies are in progress to define whether this site can be narrowed further or whether these eight residues are the complete domain.

These studies exemplify the use of hybridoma technology in analyzing the antigenic structure of LDH-C_4. As the panel of monoclonal antibodies is expanded and more binding sites are identified, both functional analyses of LDH-C_4 and a survey of its evolutionary history can progress.

ISOLATION OF ANTIGENIC PEPTIDES

The tryptic peptides of mouse LDH-C_4 were separated using reverse-phase high pressure liquid chromatography (HPLC) on a Waters μBondapak C_{18} Column in the presence of 0.1% aqueous trifluoroacetic acid, pH 2.1. Elution was effected

TABLE 1. Immunologically Active Tryptic Peptides of LDH-C_4

Antibody Binding (cpm)	Position in Sequence (Residue No.)
1360	5–15
960	41–55
918	58–74
1032	176–210
1706	211–220
1478	231–243
1811	283–303
1140	304–315
1110	Unknown mixture of three peptides
1280	Not determined—approx. 15 residues
1935	Not determined—approx. 18 residues
1354	Not determined—approx. 9 residues
1329	Not determined—approx. 9 residues
0–478	Inactive peptides

Peptides that bind rabbit anti-mouse LDH-C_4 were identified by amino acid composition and partial or complete sequence determination. Antibody binding was determined with a solid matrix radioimmunoassay.[39]

with a complex gradient of increasing acetonitrile.[27] Peaks were collected separately, and final purification was achieved under isocratic conditions in the same chromatographic system. The amino acid composition was determined for each purified peptide, using an HPLC separation of o-phthalaldehyde derivatives.[38] The activity of each peptide in binding rabbit anti-mouse LDH-C_4 was measured with a solid matrix RIA.[39] Partial and complete amino acid sequences were determined by the Edman degradation[40-42] for those immunologically active peptides obtained in high yield.[31] The tryptic peptides of LDH-C_4 that bind relatively little rabbit anti-mouse LDH-C_4 do not contain intact antigenic domains. Those peptides that react with antibody directed against the native protein include antibody combining sites of the native protein. Eight peptides containing antigenic domains were identified in the overall structure of murine LDH-C_4 (TABLE 1). Four additional peptides were not obtained in sufficient yield for further analysis. One peptide warrants more detailed examination because it forms the basis of further studies and because the published sequence was not confirmed.

TABLE 2. Amino Acid Sequence of Peptide MC$_{5-15}$

Edman Cycle [a]	Amino Acid	Yield[b]	Edman Cycle	Amino Acid	Yield
1 (5)	Glu	Qual.[c] (FIG. 1)	7(11)	Leu	1.8
2 (6)	Gln	Qual.[c] (FIG. 2)	8(12)	Val	2.9
3 (7)	Leu	3.6	9(13)	Pro	1.9
4 (8)	Ile	2.3	10(14a)	Glu	1.2[c] (FIG. 3)
5 (9)	Gln	0.8	11(14b)	Asp	1.1[c] (FIG. 4)
6(10)	Asn	1.7	12	Lys	0.5

[a] Residue number in parentheses.
[b] Yield expressed in total nmoles.
[c] Qualitative identifications are shown in the designated figures.

The peptide corresponding to residues 5–15 was sequenced several times with careful adjustment of cleavage conditions at each cycle to maximize yield and minimize overlap. The quantitative results are presented in TABLE 2. FIGURES 1 and 2 show the HPLC identification of phenylthiohydantoin (PTH)-amino acids on cycles 1 and 2. This identification of residue 6 as glutamine is certain and in contrast to the glutamic acid previously reported.[17] Cycles 10 and 11 yield PTH-Glu and PTH-Asp respectively, as shown in FIGURES 3 and 4. The aspartic acid at position 15 is not present in the previous sequence.[17] The present sequence is

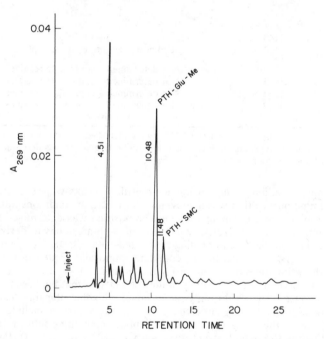

FIGURE 1. HPLC of PTH-amino acids; Edman cycle 1 of Peptide MC$_{5-15}$. Peak 1 (rt 4.51) is an unknown, probably salt, that appears in the first cycle of all peptides; Peak 2 (rt 10.48) is PTH-Glu-Me, residue 5 of LDH-C$_4$. Peak 3 (rt 11.48) is PTH-SMC, the internal standard.

unambiguous and agrees well with the composition. This insertion requires re-numbering of the sequence as Pro-13, Glu-14a, Asp-14b, Lys-15 to preserve the published residue identifications.

These data permit at least a partial description of the antigenic domains of mouse LDH-C₄. In addition to revealing the structural basis of the immunological specificity of this isozyme, this list of peptides can be used to define the distribution of domains in three-dimensional space.

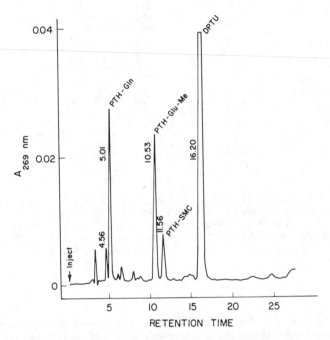

FIGURE 2. HPLC of PTH-amino acids; Edman cycle 2 of Peptide MC₅₋₁₅. Peak 1 (rt 4.56) is the unknown salt peak seen in FIGURE 1. Peak 2 (rt 5.01) is PTH-Gln, residue 6 of LDH-C₄. Peak 3 (rt 10.53) is PTH-Glu-Me, carryover from cycle 1, and deamidation of residue 6. Peak 4 (rt 11.56) is PTH-SMC, the internal standard. Diphenylthiourea (DPTU; rt 16.20) is a breakdown product of PITC.

ANTIGENIC DOMAINS

The antigenic domains of LDH-C₄ fit both the conformational and sequential models of protein immunogenicity and are consistent with the suggestion that any distinction between conformational and sequential determinants is artificial and no longer useful.[43] Indeed, it seems obvious that both the chemical nature of the amino acid side chains and their arrangement in space are essential in defining an antigenic determinant. These data fit best to the model of antigenic domains.[44,45] There are apparently numerous, perhaps partially overlapping antibody-binding

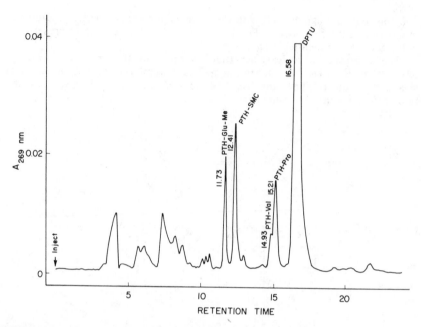

FIGURE 3. HPLC of PTH-amino acids; Edman cycle 10 of Peptide MC_{5-15}. Peak 1 (rt 11.73) is PTH-Glu-Me, residue 14a of LDH-C_4. Peak 2 (rt 12.41) is PTH-SMC, the internal standard. Peak 3 (rt 14.93) is PTH-Val, carryover from cycle 8. Peak 4 (rt 15.21) is PTH-Pro, carryover from cycle 9. Peak 5 (rt 16.58) is diphenylthiourea from PITC breakdown. Retention times are different from FIGURES 2 and 3 because of readjustment of chromatographic conditions.

sites on the surface of the LDH-C_4 molecule. The number, position, and precise boundaries of these domains are characteristic both of the protein structure and the antigen-host interaction.

The total antigenic structure of LDH-C_4 is most clearly revealed in a three-dimensional model (FIGURE 5). The model displays the surface features that serve as antibody-binding sites, for example, the carboxyl-terminal region of MC_{41-55} and the amino-terminal of MC_{58-74}. The constrained loop shapes of MC_{97-110} and $MC_{148-155}$ are readily apparent as are the more or less extended conformations of $MC_{231-243}$ and MC_{5-15}. Furthermore, surface regions formed by the close apposition of parallel secondary structures are revealed, for example, as between $MC_{316-329}$ and $MC_{274-283}$. An antigenic domain could include residues from both regions in a single combining site.

This analysis exemplifies the construction of an antigenic map of LDH-C_4 by the isolation of small peptides that bind rabbit anti-mouse LDH-C_4. Studies are in progress to extend this map by alternative proteolytic cleavages and by synthesis of selected sequences. In this way, it will be possible to define the antigenic status of every residue on the surface of LDH-C_4. Antigenicity is confirmed by active immunization with small peptides corresponding to antigenic domains.

ANTIGENICITY OF SYNTHETIC PEPTIDE MC$_{5-15}$

To demonstrate that MC$_{5-15}$ bears an antigenic domain of LDH-C$_4$, the synthetic peptide was purchased from Peninsula Laboratories (San Carlos, California). Cysteine was added to the amino-terminal to facilitate conjugation. This position is occupied by lysine in the native protein.

Bovine serum albumin (BSA; Sigma Chemical Co.) and diphtheria toxoid (DT; Connaught Laboratories) were used as carriers. Both proteins were activated with 6-maleimido caproic acyl N-hydroxysuccinimide (MCS).[46] The peptide was conjugated through its amino-terminal sulfhydryl group after reduction with dithiothreitol.

Rabbits were immunized with these conjugates, and serum anti-LDH-C$_4$ was measured at weekly intervals in the solid matrix radioimmunoassay.[39] The immune response profiles for the individual rabbits are shown in FIGURES 6 and 7. Every animal synthesized antibody specific for native LDH-C$_4$. In general, antibody titer increased following booster immunizations. Any differences in potency between DT-MC$_{5-15}$ and BSA-MC$_{5-15}$ are obscured by the variability among rabbits. DT-MC$_{5-15}$ appears to elicit a better response to the first immunization, and the best responder overall received this conjugate.

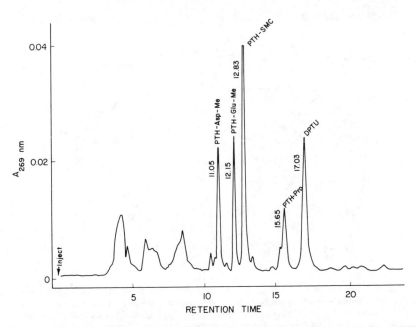

FIGURE 4. HPLC of PTH amino acids; Edman cycle 11 of Peptide MC$_{5-15}$. Peak 1 (rt 11.05) is PTH-Asp-Me, residue 14b of LDH-C$_4$. Peak 2 (rt 12.15) is PTH-Glu-Me, carryover from cycle 10. Peak 3 (rt 12.83) is PTH-SMC, the internal standard. Peak 4 (rt 15.65) is PTH-Pro, carryover from cycle 9. Peak 5 (rt 17.03) is diphenylthiourea from PITC breakdown.

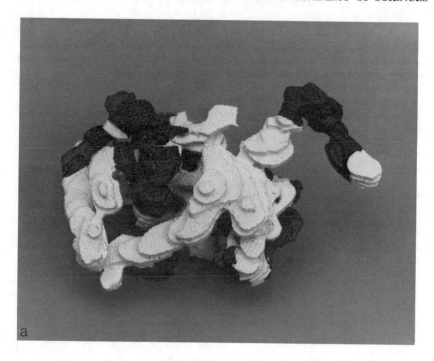

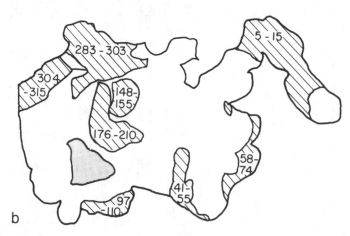

FIGURE 5. Three-dimensional model of antigenic structure of LDH-C$_4$. (A) Top view of one LDH-C subunit showing antibody-binding sequences in black. (B) Tracing of top view of LDH-C subunit. Antibody-binding sequences shaded and identified by residue numbers. (C) Front view of one LDH-C subunit showing antibody-binding sequences in black. (D) Tracing of front view of LDH-C subunit. Antibody-binding sequences shaded and identified by residue numbers.

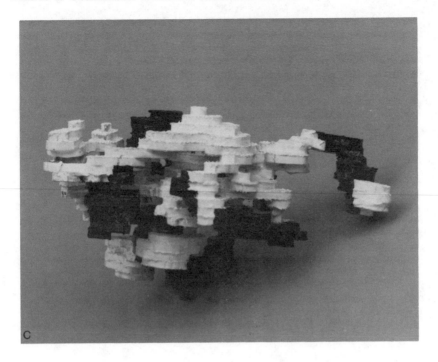

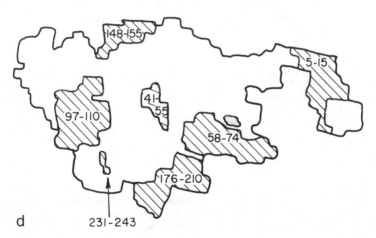

FIGURE 5 (*Continued*)

Similar results have been obtained with conjugates of MC_{97-105} and $MC_{211-220}$.[31] In addition to confirming that these sequences contain intact antigenic domains of LDH-C_4, the immune response to synthetic peptides reveals additional features of the molecular basis of antigenic specificity, particularly the importance of conformation.

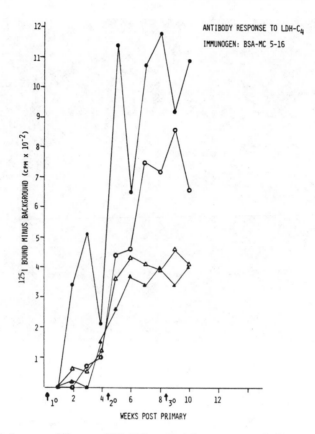

FIGURE 6. Immune response to BSA-MC$_{5-15}$. Each line represents the immune response of an individual rabbit that received a primary immunization of 2 mg BSA-MC$_{5-15}$ emulsified in Complete Freund's Adjuvant and booster immunizations of 1 mg peptide-carrier conjugate. Time of injection is indicated by arrows. The weekly serum samples were assayed simultaneously for anti–LDH-C$_4$ in the solid matrix radioimmunoassay.[39] Titer is expressed in cpm of ^{125}I-labeled goat anti-rabbit IgG bound. These samples were assayed in parallel to those shown in FIGURE 7 for purposes of comparison.

MC$_{97-110}$ is least effective in eliciting an immune response to the native protein.[31] This sequence forms the coenzyme binding loop of LDH-C$_4$. The conformation of these residues is constrained by the anchoring of the ends of the loop to the bulk of the protein such that the α-carbon of residue 97 is 14.7 Å from the α-carbon of residue 110.[16] This spacing is not maintained by the free peptide that can, therefore, assume other stable conformations. In contrast, both MC$_{5-15}$ and MC$_{211-220}$ contain proline residues that restrict the rotational freedom of the main polypeptide chain. In addition, residues 211–220 of the native protein form a bend that is partially folded back on itself,[16] suggesting that this sequence may have a tendency to self-stabilize in the native conformation. In peptide MC$_{5-15}$, Pro-13 should draw together residues 10 and 15 as it does in the native protein.[16] In addition, these residues of the native protein present an extended conformation lying across the surface of the LDH-C$_4$ tetramer.[16] Peptide MC$_{5-15}$ may tend to assume a similar shape across the surface of a carrier protein. Thus, the relative potencies of these three peptides are consistent with the degree of conformational stability. This suggests that the magnitude of the immune response to LDH-C$_4$ is a function, at least in part, of the fraction of the peptide immunogen in the same conformation that it has in the native protein.

The induction of an immune response to LDH-C$_4$ by synthetic peptides containing antigenic domains illustrates the general principle of eliciting an immune response to proteins with small peptide fragments. These synthetic antigens are also potentially useful in developing a contraceptive vaccine.

IMMUNOCONTRACEPTIVE POTENTIAL OF SYNTHETIC ANTIGENS

The immunosuppression of fertility by LDH-C$_4$ is apparently mediated by circulating antibodies entering the oviduct, binding to sperm, and preventing fertilization. A variety of *in vitro* experiments are available to test whether the anti-

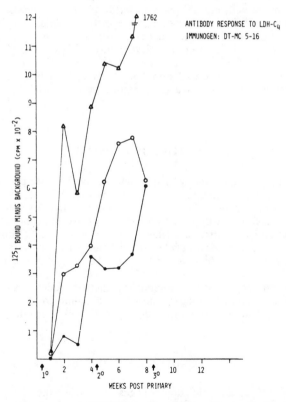

FIGURE 7. Immune response to DT-MC$_{5-15}$. For details of immunization and assay, see FIGURE 6. The serum samples shown in FIGURES 6 and 7 were assayed simultaneously for purposes of comparison.

peptide sera have sufficient affinity and appropriate specificity to interfere with fertilization.

The anti-peptide sera were assayed in a sperm radioimmunobinding assay. Mouse sperm were dried in the wells of a microtiter plate and incubated with test sera. The amount of antibody bound was quantitated with radioactively labeled second antibody. Rabbit anti-mouse LDH-C_4 clearly binds to mouse sperm, as do anti–DT-MC$_{5-15}$ and anti–DT-MC$_{211-220}$. Human sperm were tested in this assay, and significant reaction with both anti-peptide sera was demonstrated.[47]

The pattern of antibody binding to sperm was observed using immunofluorescence. Mouse sperm were dried on glass microscope slides and incubated with control serum or with the test antisera. Antibody binding sites were visualized with fluorescence microscopy after incubation with FITC-labeled second antibody. Mouse sperm incubated with rabbit anti-mouse LDH-C_4 displayed intense staining on the tail. This pattern was observed with anti–DT-MC$_{5-15}$ and with anti–DT-MC$_{211-220}$ but not with control serum. Similar results were obtained with human sperm. Thus, immunization with synthetic antigenic determinants of LDH-C_4 elicits antibodies that bind directly to mouse and to human sperm.[47]

The effect of these antibodies on fertilization was tested *in vitro*. Mouse sperm were incubated with either control serum or one of the test antisera. Treated sperm were mixed with mouse ova, and fertilization was identified by the presence of sperm inside the ovum, appearance of the second polar body, and the observation of pronuclei. The frequency of fertilization was significantly reduced in the presence of rabbit antisera to native mouse LDH-C_4, DT-MC$_{5-15}$, and DT-MC$_{211-220}$. When the sera were pre-absorbed with mouse LDH-C_4, they no longer reduced the frequency of fertilization. These findings confirm the principle of a synthetic peptide antigen to replace the natural product LDH-C_4 in a contraceptive vaccine.

FUTURE PROSPECTS

For many years, the antigenicity of spermatozoa has been suggested as the basis of an alternative contraceptive technology. The feasibility of this approach to fertility control and its long-term consequences remain to be established. Progress in this area is contingent upon the availability of a well-defined, biochemically characterized antigenic stimulus. LDH-C_4 was the first such antigen to be isolated, and it remains the best developed candidate for future studies. Immunization with LDH-C_4 does suppress fertility, and the complete biochemical characterization of this isozyme is well underway. The immunological map of this isozyme will provide a wealth of potential synthetic antigens to substitute for the natural product in studies to determine whether immunological contraception is appropriate and desirable for wide-scale application in human beings.

ACKNOWLEDGMENTS

The contents of this publication do not necessarily reflect the policy of the United States Agency for International Development. Helpful discussion with Dr. Joyce A. Shelton is gratefully acknowledged.

REFERENCES

1. WHEAT, T. E. & E. GOLDBERG. 1975. LDH-X: The sperm-specific C$_4$ isozyme of lactate dehydrogenase. *In* Isozymes. C. L. Markert, Ed. **3:** 325–346. Academic Press. New York.

2. GOLDBERG, E. 1977. Isozymes in testes and spermatozoa. *In* Isozymes: Current Topics in Biological and Medical Research. M. C. Rattazzi, J. G. Scandalios & G. S. Whitt, Eds. **1:** 79–124. Alan R. Liss, Inc. New York.

3. WHEAT, T. E. & E. GOLDBERG. 1983. Sperm-specific lactate dehydrogenase C$_4$: Antigenic structure and immunosuppression of fertility. *In* Isozymes: Current Topics in Biological and Medical Research, M. C. Rattazzi, J. G. Scandalios & G. S. Whitt, Eds. **7:** 113–130. Alan R. Liss, Inc. New York.

4. HINTZ, M. & E. GOLDBERG. 1977. Dev. Biol. **57:** 375–384.

5. WHEAT, T. E., M. HINTZ, E. GOLDBERG & E. MARGOLIASH. 1977. Differentiation **9:** 37–41.

6. MEISTRICH, M. L., P.K. TROSTLE, M. FRAPART & R. P. ERICKSON. 1977. Dev. Biol. **60:** 428–441.

7. WIEBEN, E. D. 1981. J. Cell Biol. **88:** 492–498.

8. BLANCO, A. 1980. The Johns Hopkins Med. J. **146:** 231–235.

9. MITA, M. & P. F. HALL. 1982. Biol. Reprod. **26:** 445–455.

10. EVANS, R. W. & B. P. SETCHELL. 1978. J. Reprod. Fertil. **52:** 15–19.

11. HOLMDAHL, T. H. & L. MASTROIANNI, JR. 1965. Fertil. Steril. **16:** 587–595.

12. GOLDBERG, E. 1964. Ann. N.Y. Acad. Sci. **127:** 560–570.

13. BATTELLINO, L. J., F. R. JAIME & A. BLANCO. 1968. J. Biol. Chem. **243:** 5185–5192.

14. HAWTREY, C. O. & E. GOLDBERG. 1970. J. Exp. Zool. **174:** 451–462.

15. GOLDBERG, E. 1972. J. Biol. Chem. **247:** 2044–2048.

16. MUSICK, W. D. L. & M. G. ROSSMANN. 1979. J. Biol. Chem. **254:** 7611–7620.

17. PAN, Y.-C. E., F. S. SHARIEF, M. OKABE, S. HUANG & S. S.-L. LI. 1983. J. Biol. Chem. **258:** 7005–7016.

18. GOLDBERG, E. 1971. Proc. Natl. Acad. Sci. USA **68:** 349–352.

19. LERUM, J. E. & E. GOLDBERG. 1974. Biol. Reprod. **11:** 108–115.

20. GOLDBERG, E. 1973. Science **181:** 458–459.

21. GOLDBERG, E., T. E. WHEAT, J. E. POWELL & V. C. STEVENS. 1981. Fertil. Steril. **35:** 214–217.

22. KILLE, J. W. & E. GOLDBERG. 1979. Biol. Reprod. **20:** 863–871.

23. KILLE, J. W. & E. GOLDBERG. 1980. J. Reprod. Immunol. **2:** 15–21.

24. GOLDBERG, E., V. GONZALES-PREVATT & T. E. WHEAT. 1981. Immunosuppression of fertility in females by injection of sperm-specific LDH-C$_4$ (LDH-X): Prospects for development of a contraceptive vaccine. *In* Human Reproduction, Proceedings of III World Congress. K. Semm & L. Mettler, Eds.: 360–364. Elsevier-North Holland. Amsterdam.

25. HOPP, T. P. & K. R. WOODS. 1981. Proc. Natl. Acad. Sci. USA **78:** 3824–3828.

26. LI, S. S.-L., R. J. FELDMANN, M. OKABE & Y.-C. E. PAN. 1983. J. Biol. Chem. **258:** 7017–7028.

27. WHEAT, T. E. & E. GOLDBERG. 1981. Immunologically active peptide fragments of the sperm-specific lactate dehydrogenase C$_4$ isozyme. *In* Peptides. Synthesis-Structure-Function. D. H. Rich & E. Gross, Eds.: 557–560. Pierce Chemical Company. Rockford, IL.

28. GONZALES-PREVATT, V., T. E. WHEAT & E. GOLDBERG. 1982. Molec. Immunol. **19:** 1579–1585.

29. GOLDMAN-LEIKIN, R. E. & E. GOLDBERG. 1983. Proc. Natl. Acad. Sci. USA **80:** 3774–3778.

30. GOLDBERG, E., T. E. WHEAT & V. GONZALES-PREVATT. 1983. Development of a contraceptive vaccine based on synthetic antigenic determinants of lactate dehydrogenase C$_4$. *In* Immunology of Reproduction, T. G. Wegmann, T. J. Gill III, C. D. Cummings & E. Nisbet-Brown, Eds.: 491–504. Oxford University Press. New York.

31. WHEAT, T. E. & E. GOLDBERG. 1984. Molec. Immunol. (In press.)
32. PIERRES, M., S. T. JU, C. WALTENBAUGH, M. E. DORF, B. BENACERRAF & R. N. GERMAIN. 1979. Proc. Natl. Acad. Sci. USA 76: 2425–2429.
33. STEWARD, M. W. 1978. Introduction to methods used to study antibody-antigen reactions. In Handbook of Experimental Immunology. D. M. Weir, Ed.: 16.1–16.20. Blackwell Scientific Publications. Oxford.
34. CHANG, S.-M. T., C.-Y. LEE & S. S.-L. LI. 1979. Biochem. Genet. 17: 715–729.
35. CHANG, S.-M. T., C.-Y. LEE & S. S.-L. LI. 1980. Int. J. Biochem. 11: 1–6.
36. TAYLOR, S. S. & S. S. OXLEY. 1976. Arch. Biochem. Biophys. 175: 373–383.
37. EVENTOFF, W., M. G. ROSSMANN, S. S. TAYLOR, H. J. TORFF, H. MEYER, W. KEIL & H. H. KILTZ. 1977. Proc. Natl. Acad. Sci. USA 74: 2677–2681.
38. HILL, D. W., F. H. WALTERS, T. D. WILSON & J. D. STUART. 1979. Anal. Chem. 51: 1338–1341.
39. PIERCE, S. K. & N. R. KLINMAN. 1976. J. Exp. Med. 144: 1254–1262.
40. TARR, G. E. 1975. Anal. Biochem. 63: 361–370.
41. TARR, G. E. 1977. Improved manual sequencing methods. In Methods in Enzymology. C. H. W. Hirs & S. Timasheff, Eds. 47: 335–357. Academic Press. New York.
42. TARR, G. E. 1981. Anal. Biochem. 111: 27–32.
43. SUTCLIFFE, J. G., T. M. SHINNICK, N. GREEN & R. A. LERNER. 1983. Science 219: 660–666.
44. EAST, I. J., J. G. R. HURRELL, P. E. E. TODD & S. J. LEACH. 1982. J. Biol. Chem. 257: 3199–3202.
45. TODD, P. E. E., I. J. EAST & S. J. LEACH. 1982. Trends Biochem. Sci. 7: 212–216.
46. LEE, A. C. J., J. E. POWELL, G. W. TREGEAR, H. D. NIALL & V. C. STEVENS. 1980. Molec. Immunol. 17: 749–756.
47. BEYLER, S. A., T. E. WHEAT & E. GOLDBERG. In preparation.

Factors that Regulate the Development of Testicular Autoimmune Diseases[a]

KENNETH S. K. TUNG, CORY TEUSCHER, and
SUZANNE SMITH

Department of Pathology
University of New Mexico
Albuquerque, New Mexico 87131

LEGRANDE ELLIS

Department of Physiology and Biochemistry
Utah State University
Logan, Utah 84322

MARIA L. DUFAU

Section on Molecular Endocrinology
Endocrinology and Reproduction Research Branch
National Institute of Child Health and Human Development
National Institutes of Health
Bethesda, Maryland 20205

INTRODUCTION

Over thirty years ago, experimental allergic orchitis (EAO), an autoimmune disease of the testis, was successfully induced in the guinea pig by immunization with homologous testis or sperm in complete Freund's adjuvant.[1,2] For many years that followed, the guinea pig model was studied exclusively as an experimental model of autoimmunity.[3] Amongst the findings of interest have been elucidation of the blood-testis barrier as an immunologic barrier,[4] evaluation of the relative importance between cell-mediated immunity and humoral antibody responses as pathogenetic mechanisms,[5,6] and isolation and characterization of antigens responsible for disease induction.[7-11] Testicular autoimmune diseases have since been described in vasectomized animals[12-14] and, as spontaneous diseases, found in association with infertility in the dog[15] and the mink.[16] Moreover, its clinical relevance has been suggested by the recent description of immune complex–like deposits of IgG and/or complement C3 in the tubular basement membrane of testes from infertile men.[17]

Recent work in our laboratories has provided evidence that testicular autoimmune disease is under complex but clearly definable genetic controls, and that there is evidence for an association between testicular autoimmunity and abnormal endocrinologic regulation of the testis. In this paper, we describe these findings in the context of two experimental models: murine experimental allergic orchitis and the infertile dark mink.

[a] Supported in part by National Institutes of Health Grant HD-14504 and Fellowship HD-06515.

MURINE EXPERIMENTAL ALLERGIC ORCHITIS

A highly reproducible model of experimental allergic orchitis (EAO) in the mouse will greatly facilitate our understanding of testicular autoimmunity since advantage can be taken of the numerous inbred congenic and mutant mouse strains for immunogenetic analysis. Furthermore, the well-characterized immune system, the readily available markers for the lymphocyte subsets, and the feasibility of producing autoreactive monoclonal antibodies and T cell clones should permit precise pathogenetic dissection of the disease in this species. Although several investigators have reported induction of murine EAO,[18-20] these studies were not followed by an incisive immunologic analysis. Recently, based on a modified protocol of Pokorna et al.,[18] severe orchitis has been consistently induced in the mouse.[21-23]

Induction and Immunopathology of Murine EAO

Murine EAO is induced in a susceptible mouse strain by a single injection of mouse testis homogenate, 10 mg dry weight, in complete Freund's adjuvant that contains 0.45 mg of *Mycobacterium tuberculosis* (H37Ra strain) on day 0, followed by injection(s) of an extract of *Bordetella pertussis*.[24] Pertussis is required for disease induction, and can be given as a single intravenous injection of 10 μg on day 0 or as two intraperitoneal injections (10 and 5 μg) on day 0 and day 1. It is unclear at present as to which of the many biologic properties of the pertussis extract are responsible for events leading to murine EAO. Murine EAO is an organ-specific autoimmune disease inasmuch as mice immunized with complete Freund's adjuvant and pertussis extract with another tissue antigen do not develop EAO; and mice with EAO do not exhibit histopathologic changes in organs outside the testis. Serum antisperm antibodies were detectable in 10 days, and histopathologic evidence of orchitis first appeared between 10–15 days after immunization. By day 20, maximum disease incidence was reached. Early signs of orchitis consisted of focal perivascular infiltration of mononuclear cells and eosinophils. These cells then surrounded and entered the lumen of seminiferous tubules. Orchitis severity was proportional to the sectional area of the testis with inflammatory infiltrates. In severe disease, necrosis was apparent (FIGURE 1). In contrast to EAO in the guinea pig, the ductus efferentes was rarely affected.

Murine EAO also manifested as vasitis: inflammation of the distal caudal epididymis and the proximal 1 cm of the vas deferens. Mild vasitis consisted of focal submucosal lymphoid infiltrates whereas severe vasitis was characterized by granulomatous inflammation with or without mucosal ulcerations (FIGURE 2). For the purpose of the immunogenetic study, we have semiquantitated the extent of orchitis and vasitis in grades ranging from 0 to 10 (FIGURES 1 and 2).

Concomitant to the development of orchitis, desquamation of germ cells was noted. This desquamation led to aspermatogenic tubules. Immunofluorescence study of testes with EAO demonstrated granular deposition of mouse C3 along tubular basement membrane, late in the disease.[23]

The histopathologic appearance of murine EAO is thus consistent with an immunologic disease mediated by cell-mediated immunity. Possible involvement of humoral antibodies is evidenced only late in the disease process. Indeed, murine EAO was transferred to syngeneic hypothymic nude mice by lymphoid cells but not by immune sera.[21]

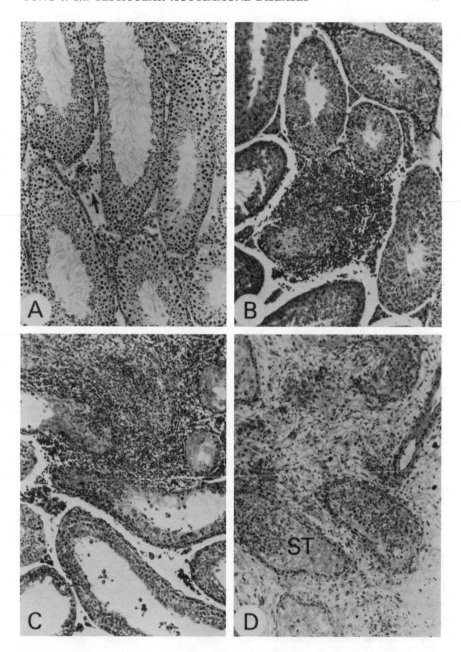

FIGURE 1. Histopathology or orchitis in murine EAO. (A) Focal perivascular infiltration of mononuclear cells (grade 1); (B) focal monocytic destruction of seminiferous tubules (grade 2); (C) extensive orchitis (grade 5); and (D) complete necrosis and interstitial fibrosis (grade 10). (PAS-hematoxylin, × 105).

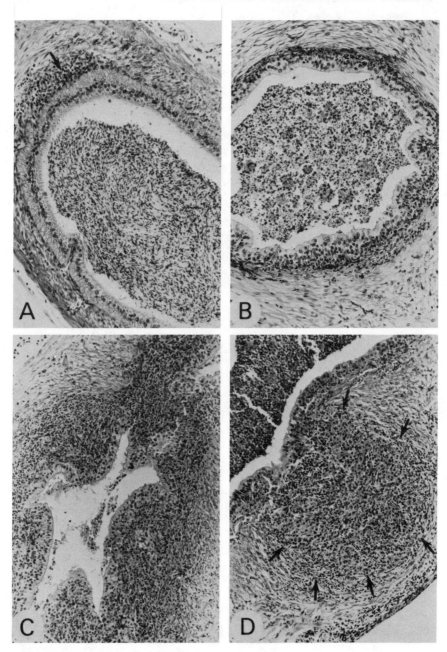

FIGURE 2. Histopathology of vasitis in murine EAO. (A) Focal submucosal lymphocytic infiltration (arrow) (grade 1); (B) circumferential submucosal inflammation with luminal cellular debris (grade 3); (C) heavy inflammatory infiltration (grade 8); and (D) well-defined submucosal granuloma (arrows), with mucosal ulceration and destruction of the muscularis. (PAS-hematoxylin, × 175).

Immunogenetic Analysis of Murine EAO

Rather than providing a detailed analysis of the genetic control of this experimental autoimmune disease, immunogenetic technique is employed by us as a means of dissecting the mechanisms of the autoimmune process. As the first step, the result of which will be described below, we attempt to identify gene loci that are associated with EAO susceptibility or resistance.[25] It is our intent in the future to search for associations between EAO susceptibility or resistance and other genetic traits among congenic and recombinant inbred mice.

Influence of Major Histocompatibility Complex Genes on Orchitis Development

Studies on the histocompatibility complex (H-2) congenics derived from the BALB/cBy and C57BL/10 mice provided clear evidence of an association between orchitis and the H-2^d haplotype (TABLE 1). Moreover, study on several BALB/cBy and C57BL/10 mice with intra-H-2 recombinance indicated that gene(s) coding for severe orchitis, a dominant trait in these mice, is mapped to the D end of H-2 (TABLE 1).

Influence of H-2 Gene on Orchitis Severity

The association of H-2^s haplotype with severe orchitis was evidenced in the study of EAO in the progeny between SJL (H-2^s), a responder mouse strain, and CBA/J (H-2^k), a nonresponder (TABLE 2). Both the (SJL × CBA/J) F1 and the (CBA/J × SJL) F1 developed severe orchitis, thus orchitis is an autosomal dominant trait. Since the backcross mice between (SJL × CBA/J) F1 and CBA/J segregated almost equally into those with severe orchitis (40%) and those with mild orchitis (60%), it was concluded that severe orchitis is governed in the SJL mice by a single gene. When the H-2 genotypes of the backcross mice were

TABLE 1. Demonstration of H-2 Linked Genetic Control of Orchitis in H-2 Congenic Mice and Mice with Intra–H-2 Recombinance

Study	Mouse	Non-H2 Genes	K	I–A	I–E	S	D	N	Orchitis
				Major Histocompatibility Complex					
H-2 congenic mice	B10·D2	C57BL/10	d	d	d	d	d	46	4.2 ± 3.6
	B10·BR	C57BL/10	k	k	k	k	k	33	0.4 ± 0.4
	C57BL/10	C57BL/10	b	b	b	b	b	17	1.7 ± 1.4
	BALB/cBy	BALB/c	d	d	d	d	d	29	5.6 ± 4.1
	BALB·K	BALB/c	k	k	k	k	k	28	0.3 ± 0.8
	BALB·B10	BALB/c	b	b	b	b	b	29	0.4 ± 0.7
Mice with intra–H-2 Recombinance	B10·A	C57BL/10	k	k	k	d	d	11	5.3 ± 3.3
	BALB·HTG	BALB/c	d	d	d	d	b	25	1.5 ± 2.3

Severity of orchitis is expressed as disease indices (means ± SEM), ranging from 1 to 10.

TABLE 2. Autosomal Dominant H-2 Linked Gene of the H-2^s Haplotype Is Associated with Severe Orchitis[a]

Mouse Strain	H-2	N	Orchitis[b]
AKR	k	25	0.3 ± 0.6
BALK·K	k	28	0.3 ± 0.8
C3H	k	27	0.2 ± 0.6
CBA	k	33	0.2 ± 0.7
SJL	s	31	3.6 ± 2.6
A·SW	s	31	4.4 ± 2.8
NFS/N	s	53	2.6 ± 3.6
SJL × CBA Fl	s/k	18	6.1 ± 3.4
CBA × SJL Fl	k/s	22	6.5 ± 3.3

[a] See text for additional evidence.
[b] Pathologic indices (means ± SEM).

determined serologically with anti–H-2^s and anti–H-2^k antiserum (generous gifts of Dr. Chris Kroco and Dr. Chella David, Mayo University, MN), severe orchitis was associated significantly ($x^2 = 8.82$, $p < 0.005$) with the H-2^s haplotype. This finding supports the conclusion that the gene in the SJL mice coding for severe orchitis is H-2 linked.

Effect of Non–H-2 Gene on Orchitis Resistance

The genetic trait of orchitis resistance was demonstrated in a study of the progeny of DBA/2 (H-2^d), a nonresponder, and BALB/cBy (H-2^d), a responder (TABLE 3). Orchitis resistance is clearly an autosomal dominant trait since only very mild disease developed in the (DBA/2 × BALB/cBy) Fl or the (BALB/cBy × DBA/2) Fl mice. Both parents are H-2^d, hence the gene(s) coding for disease resistance must be located outside the H-2. Moreover, it is clear that this non–H-2 genetic influence can override orchitis susceptibility, a trait already shown to be conferred by H-2^d. The backcross mice between (BALB/cBy × DBA/2) Fl and BALB/cBy also segregated into susceptible (60%) and resistance (40%) groups of comparable sizes, thus a single non–H-2 gene in the DBA/2 mice is responsible for orchitis resistance.

Orchitis and Vasitis Are under Separate Genetic Controls

Based on the disease profiles of mice with the different H-2 haplotypes, it was found that mice of H-2^s developed mainly orchitis with little or no vasitis, whereas

TABLE 3. Orchitis Resistance Is Controlled by Gene Locus Mapped Outside H-2 in the DBA/2 Mice

Mouse	H-2	N	Orchitis Indices[a]
BALB/cBy	d	26	5.6 ± 4.1
DBA/2	d	29	0.1 ± 0.2
BALB/cBy × DBA/2	d/d	20	0.5 ± 1.7
DBA/2 × BALB/cBy	d/d	17	0.9 ± 2.0

[a] Means ± SEM.

mice of the $H-2^k$ haplotypes developed mainly vasitis with little or no orchitis (TABLE 4). Further study compared two of the mouse strains, A.SW ($H-2^s$ on the A/J background genes) and BALB.K ($H-2^k$ on the BALB/cBy background genes), with their respective H-2 congenics, A/J ($H-2^a$) and BALB/cBy ($H-2^d$). The result revealed that $H-2^s$ was associated with absence of vasitis, and $H-2^k$, absence of orchitis. Further studies are necessary to clarify the interesting observation of an association between H-2 genotype and preferential tissue distributions of this autoimmune disease. Nevertheless, the available data indicate that orchitis and vasitis of murine EAO are under different genetic controls.

TABLE 4. Relative Severity of Orchitis and Vasitis in Mice with the $H-2^s$ or the $H-2^k$ Haplotype and in H-2 Congenic Mice

Study	Mouse	H-2 Haplotype	N	Orchitis	Vasitis
Mice with	A·SW/SnJ	s	31	4.4 ± 2.8	0.4 ± 0.8
$H-2^s$ or	NFS/N	s	53	2.6 ± 3.6	0.4 ± 0.8
$H-2^k$	SJL/J	s	31	3.6 ± 2.6	1.7 ± 1.5
haplotype	BALB·K	k	22	0.3 ± 0.8	2.7 ± 3.7
	AKR	k	25	0.3 ± 0.6	2.3 ± 1.7
	C3H	k	27	0.2 ± 0.6	1.2 ± 1.9
H-2 congenic	A/J	a	25	4.4 ± 3.7	3.3 ± 2.5
mice	A·SW	s	31	4.4 ± 2.8	0.4 ± 0.8
	BALB/cBy	d	29	5.6 ± 4.1	2.1 ± 2.2
	BALB·K	k	22	0.3 ± 0.8	2.7 ± 3.7

Disease severity of orchitis and vasitis is expressed as disease indices (means ± SEM) derived from a range of 1 to 10.

THE INFERTILE DARK MINK

Research on organ-specific disease is facilitated by the study of a natural model of the disease. This helps to explore immunologic and non-immunologic aberrations in the diseased individual, the physiologic and the pathologic tolerance states of the individual to the organ-specific autoantigens, and the genetic control of the disease. Furthermore, naturally occurring autoimmune diseases are probably more relevant to human diseases.

Breeding mink in Utah for a fine dark fur has selected for the undesirable phenotype of male infertility. Some mink are infertile soon after puberty (primary infertility), and others become infertile following a period of proven fertility (secondary infertility).[16] Autoimmune disease of the testis is a common finding and may account for the infertile state in mink with secondary infertility. In contrast, defects in the hypothalamic-pituitary-testicular axis are the main abnormality in mink with primary infertility. While testicular autoimmunity and abnormal endocrinologic control of the testis have been co-selected with the dark fur characteristics, it is not known at present whether the two traits are in any way related. Also, the endocrinologic status of mink with secondary infertility has not yet been explored.

Sexual Cycle and Sex Hormone Levels in the Male Mink

Mink, being seasonal breeders, mate in February and deliver their kits in May. Their testes regress at the end of March and by April and May, regression is complete. Seasonal development of spermatogenesis again occurs in December, and by February the male mink are sexually active. Mink plasma testosterone concentrations were reported to be low from July to September, with increases during November reaching maximal levels at the end of January.[26] In our recent study on a large group of animals, the mean testosterone levels were significantly higher in September than in December in 64% of dark, 50% of pastel, and 72% of

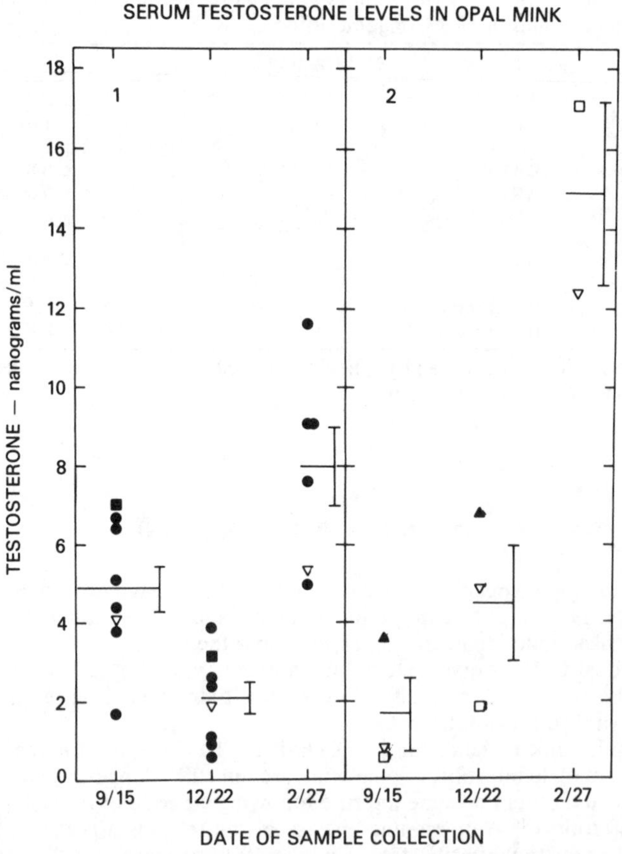

SERUM TESTOSTERONE LEVELS IN OPAL MINK

FIGURE 3. Serum testosterone levels of individual fertile opal mink studied in September (9/15), December (12/27), February (2/27). Each animal, denoted by the same symbol, was studied two to three times sequentially. A rise in hormone level occurred between December and February in all instances. Animals are divided into panels according to the profile of hormone changes they exhibit.

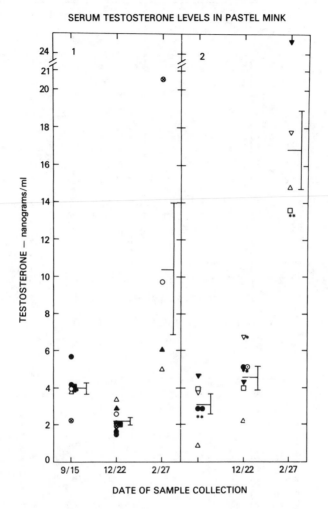

FIGURE 4. Serum testosterone levels of individual fertile pastel mink. See legend in FIGURE 3 for details.

opal milk (FIGURES 3–5). In the same animals, testosterone levels were significantly elevated in February over values observed in September and December in 100% of the opal and pastel mink and in 60% of dark mink. The 40% of dark mink that did not show increase in testosterone levels could be accounted for by animals with primary or secondary infertility—since this percentage is consistent with the prevalence of male infertility among dark mink in Utah. It is of further interest to note that the circulating testosterone and LH levels decreased abruptly close to mating of the fertile and the infertile mink (FIGURES 6 and 7, levels between February and March).

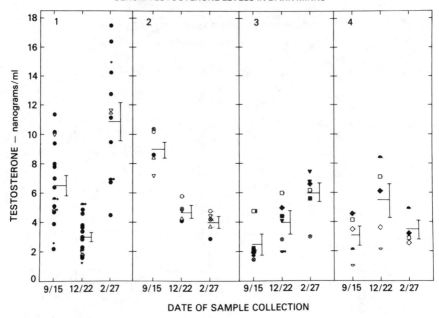

FIGURE 5. Serum testosterone levels of dark mink, fertile, and infertile. See legend in FIGURE 3 for details.

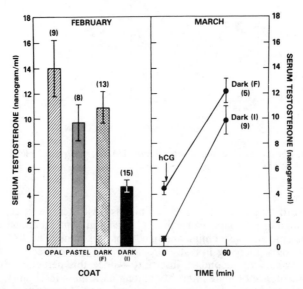

FIGURE 6. Serum testosterone levels in primary infertile mink and fertile mink of different fur colors (left panel). Testosterone response to hCG injection (100 μg) (*right panel*). Note that the testosterone levels of both fertile and infertile dark mink declined between February and March. (From Tung *et al.*[30] With permission from *Endocrinology*.)

The Hypothalamic-pituitary-testicular Axis of Mink with Primary Infertility

The testes in 62% of animals showed partial to complete aspermatogenesis without evidence of orchitis. In 27% of the animals, the testes were bilaterally or unilaterally cryptorchid. Diffuse orchitis occurred in less than 10% of the animals. Although most animals have serum antisperm antibodies detectable by indirect immunofluorescence, the antibodies were of low titer consistent with the so-called natural antisperm antibodies described in humans[27] and experimental animals.[28] The findings in the primary infertile mink are essentially those of idiopathic hypogonadism.

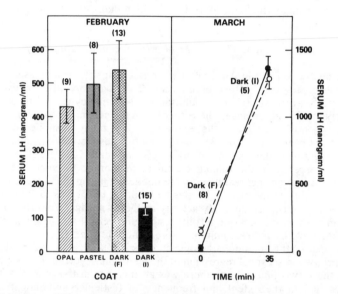

FIGURE 7. Serum LH measured by the rat Leydig cell testosterone bioassay. In the left panel, the LH levels of primary infertile mink were compared with that of fertile mink of different fur colors. The right panel illustrates changes in LH levels in primary infertile mink following GnRH injection. These animals were injected with GnRH, 10 μg, three times per week for two weeks. LH levels were then determined before and 30 minutes after 400 IU μg of GnRH, intramuscularly. Note that the LH levels in both fertile and infertile dark mink declined between February and March. (From Tung *et al.*[30] With permission from *Endocrinology*.)

To further analyze the hormonal status of the mink and to gain insight on the cause of hypogonadism in the primary infertile mink, we have applied the rat interstitial cell bioassay for the measurement of circulating luteinizing hormone (LH) essentially as previously optimized for determination of rat and human serum LH.[29] With this technique, we have determined that mink pituitaries contain equivalent concentrations of biologically active LH as rat pituitaries. Furthermore, mink LH was found to be a glycoprotein as judged by its chromatographic property on Sepharose–concanavalin A. The following hormone determinations on the primary infertile and fertile mink were conducted in March, at the peak of mink sexual activity.[30]

The serum levels of LH and testosterone in the primary infertile mink were significantly below that of the fertile dark mink or mink of other color phases (*left panels,* FIGURES 6 and 7). However, these animals responded to exogenous gonadotropin releasing hormones (GnRH) by a prompt elevation of serum LH (*right panel,* FIGURE 7). The hormonal response was corroborated by a parallel increase in the percentage and surface area of LH-positive gonadotropes in the anterior pituitaries (a study conducted by Dr. Gwen Child, University of Texas, Galveston, TX). Furthermore, the mink responded to exogenous human chorionic gonadotropin, or to endogenous LH following GnRH stimulation (data not shown), by prompt elevation of serum testosterone (*right panel,* FIGURE 6). These findings suggest that the primary defect lies with abnormal hypothalamic functions or defective neuroendocrinologic control of the hypothalamus.

Autoimmune Orchitis in Mink with Secondary Infertility

In a study conducted in April, after the onset of testicular regression, 47% of the animals had severe diffuse orchitis and 25% focal orchitis. In testes with severe orchitis (FIGURE 8), heavy infiltration of lymphocytes and macrophages completely or partially replaced the germ cells in the seminiferous tubules, sperm phagocytosis was common in the epididymis, and many seminiferous tubules were aspermatogenic. In testes where aspermatogenesis was the main abnormality, diffuse granular depositions of mink IgG and mink C3 were detectable by immunofluorescence in the tubular basement membrane throughout the organ (FIGURE 9). Although sperm antigens were not detectable in the immune deposits, IgG dissociated from the diseased testes with buffer, pH 3, was found to have 10 times as much antisperm antibody activity as the serum IgG from the same animal. All mink with secondary infertility had high levels of serum antisperm antibodies detectable by indirect immunofluorescence (FIGURE 10).

By comparing the immunopathologic findings in March, at peak sexual activity and in April, when seasonal regression of the testis has occurred, it was clear that between these two time points, there was an increase in the titer of antisperm antibodies and in the extent and frequency of testicular immunopathology.[30] Whether these findings are in any way related to the breakdown of the blood-testis barrier, which may occur during seasonal regression of mink testis, is worthy of exploration.

CONCLUSIONS AND SPECULATIONS

A reproducible model of murine EAO is now available for study of testicular autoimmunity. A study, based on appropriate congenic mice and progeny of high and low responder parents, has revealed that the disease is under complex genetic controls. Genes linked to the major histocompatibility complex influence the susceptibility and severity of orchitis, while genes mapped outside H-2 have been shown, in the DBA/2 mice, to code for orchitis resistance. Moreover, preliminary data have indicated that orchitis and vasitis, pathologic processes affecting two separate locations in murine EAO, are under different genetic controls.

The genetic control of a disease, unlike that of immune response to a simple antigen, is likely to be complex. Since crude antigens have been used to induce murine EAO, and it is known that multiple antigens capable of EAO induction in the guinea pig are present in the guinea pig testis,[7-11] the results obtained could

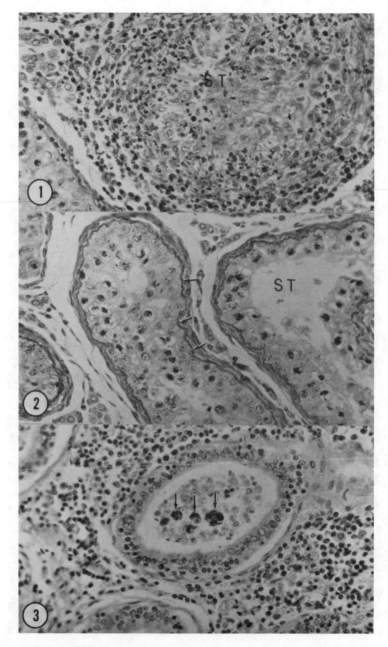

FIGURE 8. Histopathologic changes in the testis of mink with secondary infertility. (1) Severe orchitis completely destroyed seminiferous tubule (ST); (2) incomplete aspermatogenesis with tubular atrophy and wrinkling of the tubular basement membrane (arrows); and (3) sperm phagocytosis in the caput epididymis. (PAS-hematoxylin, ×250). (From Tung *et al.*[16] With permission from *Journal of Experimental Medicine*.)

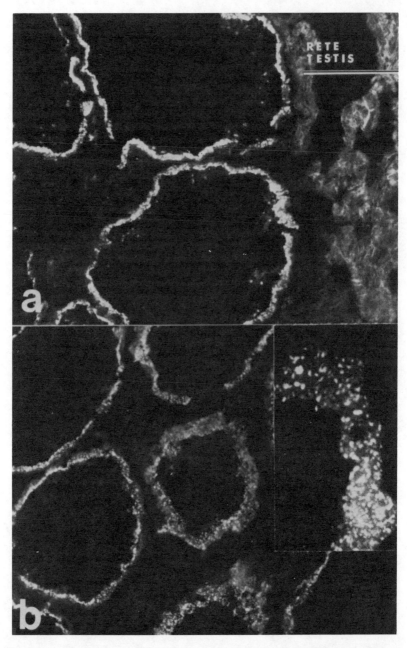

FIGURE 9. Immunofluorescence findings in the testis from mink with secondary infertility. Massive granular depositions of mink IgG (a) and mink C3 (b) in the basement membrane of seminiferous tubules but not of the rete testis. Insert in (b) illustrates the granularity of the immune deposits, typical of immune complexes. (× 250). (From Tung et al.[16] With permission from *Journal of Experimental Medicine*.)

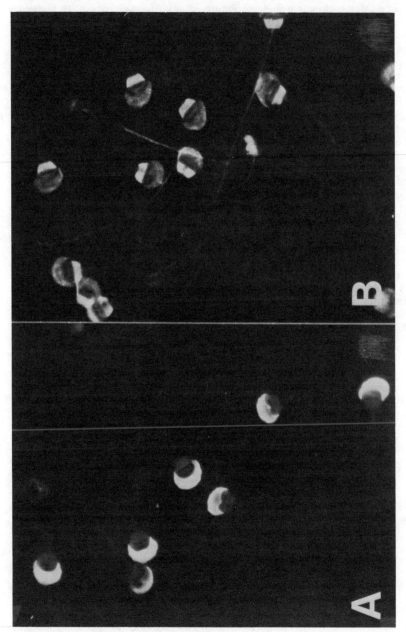

FIGURE 10. Antisperm antibodies in serum of secondary infertile mink detected by indirect immunofluorescence. Antibodies to the acrosome (A) and the postacrosomal region (B). (× 900). (From Tung *et al.*[31] With permission from *Immunological Reviews*.)

represent the summation of genetic control to several antigens or antigenic determinants. In addition, the complexity may reflect the multiple factors that must influence the development and the nature of any disease process. In testicular autoimmunity, such factors might include the quantity and quality of the immune responses and difference in response to adjuvant. In addition, nonimmunologic factors that govern the susceptibility of the testis to autoimmune disease, including the blood-testis barrier, Sertoli cell function, and any local immunosuppressive environment, might also be important. As a corollary, we anticipate that understanding the mechanisms of genetic control of EAO should elucidate the relative physiologic significance of these parameters.

The fact that abnormal hypothalamic function and testicular autoimmunity are co-inherited in the dark mink must raise the question of whether the two disease processes are somehow related. However, until more is known about the endocrinologic and immunologic controls of the annual testicular development and regression in the seasonal breeder, the possible association between these disease processes remains speculative. As a testable hypothesis, we suggest that hypothalamic control of the testis, influenced by duration of the light cycle and regulated via gonadotropins, normally leads to uneventful regression and development of spermatogenesis. Changes in the testis, which might involve the orderly formation and breakdown of the blood-testis barrier, must also assure that the highly immunogenic germ cell autoantigens are not in a position to induce testicular autoimmunity. In the dark mink, then, the primary defect may be abnormal hypothalamic function. In severe cases, testicular development fails to occur at puberty, leading to primary infertility, while in less severe cases, hypothalamic dysfunction manifests late and exerts its effect mainly at the critical period of testicular regression. Autostimulation by germ cell antigens at this stage can lead to testicular autoimmune disease.

ACKNOWLEDGMENTS

We thank the Utah mink Farmer's Coop. for providing animals in the study.

REFERENCES

1. VOISIN, G. A., A. DELAUNAY & M. BARBER. 1951. Lesions testiculaires provoquees chez le cobaye par injection d'estrait de testicule homologue. C. R. Hedb. Seances. Acad. Sci. **232:** 48–63.
2. FREUND, J., M. M. LIPTON & G. E. THOMPSON. 1953. Aspermatogenesis in the guinea pig induced by testicular tissue and adjuvant. J. Exp. Med. **97:** 711–725.
3. TUNG, K. S. K. 1980. Autoimmunity in the testis. In Immunological Aspects of Infertility and Fertility Regulation. D. S. Dhindsa & G. F. B. Schumacher, Eds.: 33–91. Elsevier-North Holland. New York.
4. JOHNSON M. H. 1973. Physiological mechanisms for the immunological isolation of spermatozoa. Adv. Reprod. **6:** 279–324.
5. TUNG, K. S. K., E. R. UNANUE & F. J. DIXON. 1971. Pathogenesis of experimental allergic orchitis. I. Transfer with immune lymph node cells. J. Immunol. **106:** 1453–1462.
6. TOULLET, F. & G. A. VOISIN. 1976. Passive transfer of autoimmune aspermatogenic orchiepididymitis (AIAO) by antispermatozoa sera. Influence of the type of autoantigen and of the class of antibody. Clin. Exp. Immunol. **26:** 549–562.

7. JACKSON, J. J., A. HAGOPIAN, D. J. CARLO, G. A. LIMJUCO & E. H. EYLAR. 1975. Experimental allergic aspermatogenic orchitis, III. Isolation of a spermatozoal protein (AP1) which induced allergic aspermatogenic orchitis. J. Biol. Chem. **250:** 6141–6150.

8. HAGOPIAN, A., T. JACKSON, D. J. CARLO, G. A. LIMJUCO & E. H. EYLAR. 1975. Experimental allergic aspermatogenic orchitis. III. Isolation of spermatozoal glycoproteins and their roles in allergic aspermatogenic orchitis. J. Immunol. **115:** 1731–1743.

9. TEUSCHER, C., G. C. WILD & K. S. K. TUNG. 1983. Acrosomal autoantigens of guinea pig sperm. I. The purification of an aspermatogenic protein, AP2. J. Immunol. **130:** 317–322.

10. TEUSCHER, C., G. C. WILD & K. S. K. TUNG. 1983. Experimental allergic orchitis: the isolation and partial characterization of an aspermatogenic polypeptide (AP3) with an apparent sequential disease-inducing determinant(s). J. Immunol. **130:**2683–2688.

11. TOULLET, F., G. A. VOISIN & G. NEMIROVSKY. 1973. Histochemical localization of three guinea pig spermatozoal autoantigens. Immunology **24:** 635–735.

12. BIGAZZI, P. E., L. L. KOSUDA, K. C. HSU & G. A. ANDRES. 1976. Immune complex orchitis in vasectomized rabbits. J. Exp. Med. **143:** 382–404.

13. TUNG, K. S. K. 1978. Allergic orchitis lesions are adoptively transferred from vasectomized guinea pigs to syngeneic recipients. Science **201:** 833–835.

14. TUNG, K. S. K. & N. J. ALEXANDER. 1980. Monocytic orchitis and aspermatogenesis in normal and vasectomized rhesus macaques (*Macaca mulatta*). Am. J. Pathol. **101:** 17–29.

15. FRITZ, T. E., L. S. LOMBARD, S. A. TYLER & W. P. NORRIS. 1976. Pathology and familial incidence of orchitis and its relation to thyroiditis in a closed Beagle colony. Exp. Mol. Pathol. **24:** 142–158.

16. TUNG, K. S. K., L. ELLIS, C. TEUSCHER, A. MENG, J. C. BLAUSTEIN, S. KOHNO & R. HOWELL. 1981. The black mink (*Mustela vison*). A natural model of immunologic male infertility. J. Exp. Med. **154:** 1016–1032.

17. SALOMON, F., P. SAREMASLANI, M. JAKOB & C. E. HEDINGER. 1982. Immune complex orchitis in infertile men. Immunoelectron microscopy of abnormal basement membrane structures. Lab. Invest. **47:** 555–567.

18. POKORNA, Z., M. VOJTISKOVA, M. RYCHLIKOVA & J. CHUTNA. 1963. An isologous model of experimental autoimmune aspermatogenesis in the mouse. Folia Biol. **9:** 203–209.

19. BOHME, D. 1965. Experimentelle allergische orchitis und reticuloendotheliales system. II. Histologische Veranderungen. Immun. Allerg. Forsch. **128:** 31–51.

20. HARGIS, B. J., S. MALKIEL & J. BERKEHA. 1968. Immunologically induced aspermatogenesis in the white mouse. J. Immunol. **101:** 374–376.

21. BERNARD, C. C. A., G. F. MITCHELL, J. LEYDON & A. BARGERBOS. 1978. Experimental autoimmune orchitis in T cell-deficient mice. Int. Arch. Allerg. Appl. Immunol. **56:** 256–263.

22. SATO, K., K. HIROKAWA & S. HATAKEYAMA. 1981. Experimental allergic orchitis in mice. Virchow/Arch. (Pathol. Anat.). **392:** 147–158.

23. KOHNO, S., J. A. MUNOZ, T. S. WILLIAMS, C. TEUSCHER, C. C. A. BERNARD & K. S. K. TUNG. 1983. Immunopathology of murine experimental allergic orchitis. J. Immunol. **130:** 2675–2682.

24. MUNOZ, J. J. & H. ARAI. 1982. Studies on crystalline pertussigen. *In* Seminars in Infectious Diseases. J. B. Robbins, J. C. Hill & J. C. Sadoff, Eds. **4:** 395–400. Thieme-Stratton. New York.

25. TEUSCHER, C., S. SMITH, E. H. GOLDBERG & K. S. K. TUNG. 1984. Genetic control of murine autoimmune orchitis. Fed. Proc. **43:** 2443.

26. PILBEAN, T. E., P. W. CONCANNON & H. F. TRAVIS. 1979. The annual reproductive cycle of mink (*Mustela vison*). J. Animal Sci. **48:** 578–584.

27. TUNG, K. S. K. 1975. Human sperm antigens and antisperm antibodies. I. Studies in vasectomy patients. Clin. Exp. Immunol. **20:** 93–104.

28. TUNG, K. S. K., R. BRYSON, E. GOLDBERG & L.-P. B. HAN. 1979. Antisperm antibody

in vasectomy: studies in human and guinea pig. *In* Vasectomy: Immunologic and Pathophysiologic Effects in Animals and Man. I. H. Lepow & R. Crozier, Eds.: 267–284. Academic Press. New York.

29. SOLANO, A. R., M. L. DUFAU & K. J. CATT. 1979. Bioassay and radioimmunoassay of serum LH in the male rat. Endocrinology **105:** 372–381.
30. TUNG, K. S. K., L. E. ELLIS, G. V. CHILD & M. DUFAU. 1984. The dark mink: a model of male infertility. Endocrinology **114:** 922–929.
31. TUNG, K. S. K., C. TEUSCHER & A. L. MENG. 1981. Autoimmunity to spermatozoa and the testis. Immunol. Rev. **55:** 217–255.

Cytometric Analysis of Shape and DNA Content in Mammalian Sperm[a]

BARTON L. GLEDHILL

Lawrence Livermore National Laboratory
Biomedical Sciences Division
University of California
Livermore, California 94550

INTRODUCTION

Concern over reproductive toxins in the environment has created a need for methods of testing for induced testicular damage. Sperm can serve as a biological dosimeter of induced alteration. The frequency of sperm with malformed heads in mice and humans increases after exposure to most mutagens, carcinogens, and teratogens. Increases of the frequency of abnormally shaped sperm may indicate induced genetic damage.[34,35] The usual methods for assessment of sperm defects, visual examination of morphological features of sperm mounted on microscope slides or estimation of sperm motility, are subjective. Individuals may score reproducibly, but substantial variability exists among technicians. Quantitative procedures are needed to provide objectivity and improve reproducibility. Automation would enhance speed, could provide standardization, and should lead to improved archival libraries and data exchange and retrieval systems.

Advances in interpreting induced abnormalities in sperm require an improved means to measure sperm characteristics. This report reviews the application of several methods for automated, quantitative detection of shape changes, methods that are faster and more sensitive than conventional visual techniques. Variability of sperm deoxyribonucleic acid (DNA) content as a bioassay of genotoxic damage has been explored by us, and limitations of the bioassay are discussed. New flow cytometric techniques that could lead to sexing mammalian sperm have been developed during the course of this work and are described.

The goal of our studies is development of sensitive, noninvasive, statistically robust, analytical tools that can detect and quantify the frequency of altered sperm. These methods would be applicable in screening protocols and in programs that monitor effects of environmental contaminants. This approach is promising because the high rate of analysis allows measurement of large numbers of sperm so that small changes of frequencies might be detected.

QUANTITATIVE MICROSCOPY OF SPERM SHAPE

Quantitative microscopy, employing the tools of image processing and pattern recognition, is that branch of analytical cytology dealing with measurement of immobilized, individual cells and subsequent characterization of populations of

[a] Work performed under the auspices of the U.S. Department of Energy by the Lawrence Livermore National Laboratory under contract number W-7405-ENG-48.

189

those cells through statistical modeling. Research in this field began in the 1930s with Caspersson's work on the nucleic acid content of cell nuclei and cytoplasm.[2] In the 1960s, with the availability of computers and a variety of sensitive, electro-optical transducers, a number of studies on the quantitative characterization of cell images were begun.[28] By the early 1970s automated systems based upon the techniques of quantitative microscopy had been developed to perform differential leukocyte counts and assess erythrocyte morphology.[12,36]

Radiation-induced Abnormalities in Sperm Head Shape

We have used quantitative microscopy to detect changes in sperm after varying doses of testicular x-irradiation.[37] Our goal was to reduce subjectivity in the assessment of sperm head morphology. We employed x-irradiation because of the relatively uncomplicated dose-to-target determinations as compared to chemical mutagens. In this study five groups of three mice received single testicular doses of x-irradiation at dosages ranging from 1 to 120 rads. A random sample of 100 mature sperm per mouse was analyzed five weeks later to quantitate abnormal sperm head morphology as a function of dosage. Cells were stained[16] with gallo-cyanin chrom alum (GCA) so that only the DNA in the sperm head was visible. The ACUity quantitative microscope system at Lawrence Livermore National Laboratory[37] was used to scan and digitize the sperm image at a sampling density of 16 points per linear micrometer and with 256 possible brightness levels per point. The contour of each cell was extracted by conventional thresholding techniques on high-contrast images. For each contour 10 shape features were computed to characterize the morphology of the cell.

With the control group's distribution of shape features determining the variability of a normal mouse sperm population, 95% limits on normal morphology were established. We found that as dose increased, surface area of cells became smaller and shape features indicated a significant trend toward circularity. With only the optimal 4 of the 10 shape features extracted from the sperm images, a doubling dose of approximately 39 rads was determined. That is, at 39 rads exposure the percentage of abnormal cells was twice the percentage in the control population. Comparison to a doubling dose of approximately 70 rads obtained from a concurrent conventional visual procedure may indicate a greater sensitivity of the image analysis method.

A companion study[19] also suggests that quantitative methods can improve the sensitivity of measuring the effects of x-irradiation on sperm morphology. Quantitative measurements made on enlarged photographs of mouse sperm heads were related to radiation dose. Using a Mahalanobis distance statistic to measure distance in a multivariate space from a control group of measurements reduced the doubling dose from approximately 70 rad to 10 to 15 rad while keeping the percentage of abnormal sperm in control mice at 3%, equal to the concurrent visual method.

Influence of Chromosomal Translocations on Sperm Morphology

Certain chromosomal translocations[33] influence the morphology of sperm heads of mice, e.g., T(14,15)6Ca. We used quantitative microscopy to determine whether we could distinguish mice with normal chromosomes from those carrying chromosomal rearrangements. We examined sperm from control mice and from mice heterozygous or homozygous for one of five chromosomal translocations. For each translocation a set of 100 sperm cells was chosen randomly from a heterozygote-bred mouse and from a homozygote-bred mouse. One hundred control sperm cells were selected randomly from each of two control mice. Cells were stained with GCA and the ACUity quantitative microscope system was used to scan the sperm cells at a spatial resolution and sampling density of four points per micrometer. Each cell contour was extracted by conventional thresholding techniques, and for each contour a variety of shape features was computed to characterize the morphology of that cell. Two features that reflect roundness, elliptical eccentricity, and perimeter^2 per area, yielded highly significant ($p < 0.0001$) separation of the groups of mice. These preliminary studies suggest that quantitative microscopy of sperm can be used to distinguish normal mice from certain translocation heterozygotes and translocation homozygotes.

ANALYSES OF SPERM BY FLOW CYTOMETRY

Accurate, precise shape measurements of sperm are needed for fertility counseling, genotoxic screening, and occupational monitoring schemes. Information pertaining to sperm head morphology is available from flow cytometric analyses. Flow cytometry, another major tool of analytical cytology provides high analytical rate, precision, and sensitivity. In flow cytometry, including fluorescence-activated flow sorting, sperm DNA is stained typically with a fluorophore, the sperm are passed rapidly in single file through one or more illuminating beams, and fluorescence is measured (FIGURE 1). Separation, through use of flow cell-sorting technology, of large numbers of normal and malformed sperm would provide material for biochemical analyses and might provide insight into mechanisms of sperm shaping and the consequences of morphologic abnormalities. Computational confirmation of the potential of flow cytometric analysis of sperm shape has been provided[13] but thus far experimental testing has been undertaken on only a limited scale.[1,8,10,24]

Slit-scan Flow Analysis of Sperm Head Shape

We applied slit-scan flow cytometry (SSFCM) to classification of mammalian sperm according to head shape.[1] When analyzed for shape by SSFCM, fluorescently stained sperm are moved lengthwise at approximately 8 m/sec through an intense blue (1 W, 488 nm) beam from an argon-ion laser that is shaped optically into a ribbon 2.5 × 40 μm in cross-section. The SSFCM measures the distribution of fluorescence in 50 to 100 narrow strips across each sperm head. When these intensities are time-ordered the composite fluorescence profile is a measure of sperm head morphology. Measurements are made on about 100 sperm/sec and, thus, objective results with high statistical precision are obtained quickly.

Mouse, hamster, rabbit, and bull sperm were fixed with formalin and stained with an acriflavine-Feulgen procedure.[9] An average fluorescence profile was generated for each species. Individual sperm were classified as morphologically normal or abnormal by comparison of their profiles to the average profiles by test of sum of squared differences.

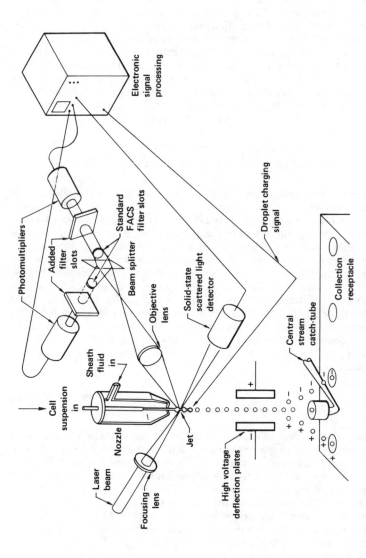

FIGURE 1. Schematic of a fluorescence-activated flow sorter showing orthogonal axes of sample flow, laser beam illumination, and fluorescent light detection. Fluorescently stained particles to be sorted are carried in a fast-moving jet of fluid past an optical detection system that responds to fluorescent light. The jet carrying the particles subsequently breaks up into individual droplets. Those droplets that contain a desired particle can be electronically charged and deflected into a separate receptacle.

Interspecies Comparisons

The profile for each species has a characteristic shape (FIGURE 2). Sperm heads of roughly similar outline produce comparable fluorescence profiles. Mouse and hamster sperm have hooked heads and SSFCM of their sperm yields skew profiles; the paddle-shaped sperm of the bull and the rabbit produce more symmetric profiles. When the average Swiss Webster mouse sperm profile was used as a control and a threshold of fit was set to include 95% of mouse sperm profiles, then only 5% of hamster and 0% of rabbit and bull sperm profiles fit within this threshold. Bull and rabbit sperm, which are difficult to differentiate visually are distinguished by this method. With the average rabbit sperm profile as the control, only 15% of bull sperm were within a threshold that included 95% of rabbit sperm.

Effects of X-irradiation on Mouse Sperm

Caudal epididymal sperm were collected from $AKD2F_1$ mice that had received a single dose of x-irradiation to their testicles 35 days earlier. Doses were 0,100, 300, 450, 600, or 900 rads. The SSFCM profiles were analyzed to determine the frequency of atypical sperm for each dose; the sperm also were scored visually for morphological abnormalities by trained, independent observers. The frequency of atypical sperm estimated by SSFCM correlated remarkably ($r = 0.99$) with frequencies of abnormally shaped sperm estimated by microscopic analysis.[1] The sensitivity of the SSFCM assay was slightly lower than that of visual scoring, but in this study only 100 sperm were assayed by SSFCM per dose. In recent studies[10] between 500 and 1000 sperm per dose were analyzed with SSFCM and sensitivity of the SSFCM assay was equal to or better than the visual assay of sperm shape.

High Resolution DNA Content Measurements

As mammalian sperm are haploid and incapable of DNA synthesis, they should have a narrow distribution of DNA content. However, early flow cytometric analyses[9] revealed a peak of fluorescence with a shoulder (FIGURE 3), a pattern often seen with cycling somatic cells. Sperm with fluorescence intensities from either the peak or the shoulder gave the same skew distribution when subsequently analyzed by flow sorting. The skew distribution has been ascribed to an artifact of measurement[7,24,32] secondary to the extremely compacted, flat sperm nuclei. The dense nucleus has a high refractive index and necessitates special staining protocols[27] for quantitation of sperm DNA. The problems of measuring flattened nuclei, i.e., cellular orientation, are overcome (FIGURE 4) by a commercial flow cytometer, the ICP22 (Ortho Instruments, Westwood, MA), that is largely insensitive to cell orientation or by a specially built orienting flow cytometer (OFCM) that orients the sperm during measurement.[4,27,32]

The difficulty of measuring sperm DNA content with a flow cytometer with orthogonal geometry complicated the studies of Sarkar *et al.*[29,30] in their investigations of population heterogeneity in human sperm DNA content. They obtained broad asymmetric peaks with coefficients of variation (CV) for normal men ranging from 9 to 20%. The asymmetry of the peaks was attributed to subpopulations of sperm bearing either X or Y chromosomes and the variability to diminished

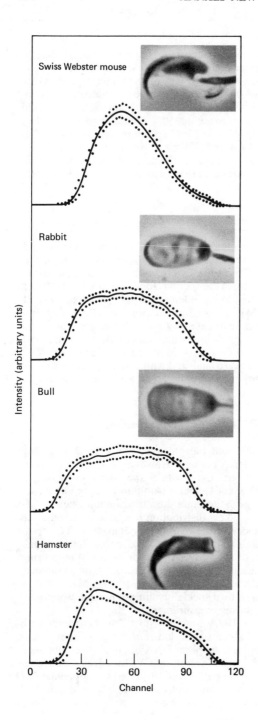

FIGURE 2. Average slit-scan flow cytometric profiles for sperm from four mammals. The flow cytometer used in these studies is not constructed as shown in Figure 1. The solid line is a sample average; the dotted lines represent 1 SD from the average. Sperm from each animal yield an average profile with a distinct length and shape.[1]

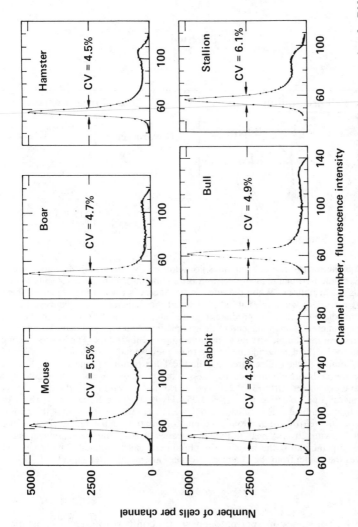

FIGURE 3. Fluorescence distributions of flat sperm heads from six mammals stained by the acriflavine-Feulgen procedure for DNA content show similar asymmetric shapes with skew to the right. Flow cytometer had orthogonal geometry as in FIGURE 1. Modal channel numbers are not indicative of the relative DNA content of the sperm.[9]

(a)

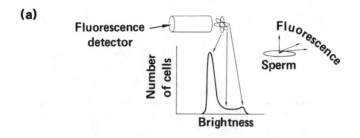

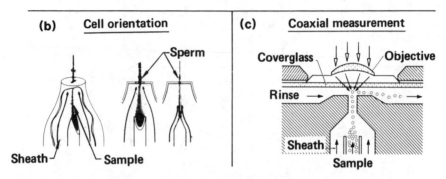

FIGURE 4. Special measurement techniques are required for sperm. (a) Measuring DNA content of flat, condensed mammalian sperm in orthogonal flow cytometers results in distorted frequency distributions. When the edge of the sperm is toward the detector a high fluorescence is recorded; when the flat side is toward the detector, a low fluorescence is recorded; intermediate orientations produce intermediate values. (b) Flow chamber of the orienting flow cytometer: shaping the end of the sample injection tube and using a rectangular flow orifice cause the sample stream to be drawn into a thin ribbon. The hydrodynamic forces encountered by the flat sperm cause them to be preferentially oriented in the plane of the ribbon. The output of the orifice enters a cylindrical quartz tube of quiescent liquid (not shown) where the cells are illuminated by a laser beam. (c) Flow chamber of the epi-illumination flow cytometer (Ortho ICP 22): The sperm flow upward along the optical axis towards the microscope objective (N. A. = 1.25). Hydrodynamic forces cause them to orient with their longitudinal axis parallel to the flow. The emitted light reaching the photomultiplier is not affected by the random rotational orientation of the nuclei because the optics are radially symmetric. A peak in the fluorescence signal occurs as the nuclei move through the focal plane and is the basis of the photometric measurement. The wash fluid rapidly removes the nuclei from the chamber after measurement. After Pinkel.[23]

control of DNA constancy in spermatogenesis (in contrast to greater constancy during the replication of somatic cells). They also found that carriers of balanced translocations were oligospermic and showed a wide dispersion of modal sperm DNA content. These are unexplained findings. Reciprocal events in the alternate form of segregation, which occurs predominantly in male carriers of balanced translocations, should not alter the modal DNA value nor should they be associated with oligospermia. It is more likely that the Sarker observations[29,30] are attributable to poor resolution caused by the artifact just described as well as staining and instrument variability.

The cytotoxicity of ionizing radiation has been studied[11] with murine spermatogenesis as an *in vivo* biologic dosimeter. Changes of the frequency distribution of cellular DNA content of whole testis preparations were analyzed by flow cytometry. A linear increase of the CV of DNA content of cells irradiated as spermatocytes, a dose-dependent arrest of differentiated spermatogonia, and an induction of diploid sperm were observed. However, a shoulder on the dose-effect curve of the irradiated spermatocytes limited the value of the method in the low-dose (< 100 rad) range. Evenson *et al.*[5] found that the DNA of misshapen sperm nuclei from unexposed bulls, mice, and humans has decreased resistance to thermal denaturation. Many morphologically normal nuclei derived from subfertile donors were also abnormally sensitive to thermal denaturation of their DNA. Sperm DNA is readily denatured following exposure to chemical mutagens and carcinogens (D. P. Evenson, personal communication 19 July 1983). Thus, flow cytometry of sperm DNA content might provide a measure of damage in the genetic material of male germ cells following exposure of an individual to a mutagen, carcinogen, or teratogen. We have used several flow cytometric techniques to measure the relative DNA content of sperm.[27]

Mutagen-induced DNA Content Variability

Accuracy of our measurements was established[27] by resolution of X- and Y-chromosome–bearing sperm in normal mice (FIGURE 5a) and those with the Cattanach 7 to X translocation[3] (FIGURE 5b) by two protocols. Additional details are given in the following sections on measuring and separating X and Y sperm. Staining sperm with 4-6-diamidino-2-phenylindole (DAPI) and measuring fluores-

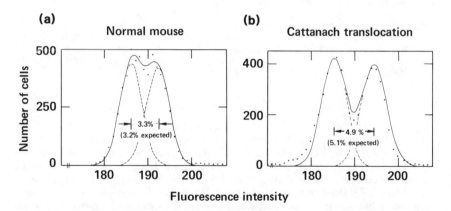

FIGURE 5. The DNA content of Y sperm is measured accurately. Fluorescence distributions of EBMI-stained sperm from normal mice (a) and those with the Cattanach 7 to X translocation (b). The separation of the peaks is determined by fitting a pair of normal distributions to the data. The separations agree with the differences expected from measurements of the individual chromosomes.[27]

cence in an ICPC22 flow cytometer is one protocol we used; the other is measuring ethidium bromide mithramycin (EBMI)-stained cells in the OFCM. Quantitative agreement of the response among these two protocols and another that uses acriflavine-Feulgen stain measured with the OFCM reduces the probability that the response is a staining artifact.

Caudal epididymal mouse sperm collected 35 days after acute localized exposure of testes to X rays show dose-dependent increases of the CV of fluorescence distributions of DNA content (FIGURE 6). Comparison of dose response curves obtained with protocols that overcome optical and cytochemical difficulties in different ways leads to the conclusion that the response is due to X-ray–induced DNA content variability.[26]

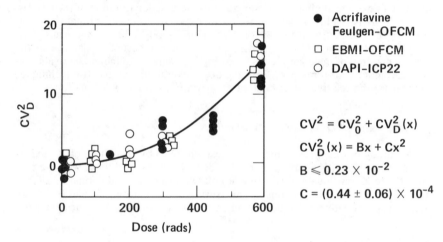

FIGURE 6. The observed X-ray dose response is the same for three measurement techniques. The square of the coefficient of variation of the fluorescence distribution, CV_D^2, increases with radiation for the three protocols. Each symbol represents an independent determination. The solid line is the least squares fit of a second-order polynomial (second equation) to the data.[23]

In the range between 0 and 600 rads the dose dependence of the square of CV of the DNA content variability, CV_D^2, is described by $CV_D^2 = Bx + Cx^2$, with $0 \leq B \leq 0.23 \times 10^{-2}$ and $C = (0.44 \pm 0.06) \times 10^{-4}$. The dose x is measured in rads and CV_D is expressed in percent.[26] Computer modeling of the shapes of the fluorescence distributions shows that at 600 rads 30 to 40% of the sperm have abnormal DNA stain content. Some have deviations as large as two whole chromosomes, but it is not clear whether they are due to whole chromosome nondisjunction, a finer fragmentation of the genome, or an effect of the irradiation on DNA-stain stoichiometry.

Aged mice, 27 to 30 months old, show no increased response relative to 3-month-old controls, and the CV for unexposed animals is independent of age. Benzo(a)pyrene (B(a)P) and mitomycin C (MMC) cause abnormalities of sperm shape but no measurable variability of DNA content. This can be interpreted as a control for morphologic effects on the flow measurement of DNA content. Because the X-ray dose response has a small slope at low doses and B(a)P and MMC cause no detectable response in DNA content, the sensitivity of this technique is low and its utility for detecting mutagen exposure will be limited to agents that produce aneuploidy in sperm. Using another species with fewer chromosomes than the mouse might help optimize detection of exposure-induced errors in DNA content.

X- and Y-Chromosome–Bearing Sperm

The DNA content of spermatids from chromosomally normal mice[18] and from mice carrying Cattanach's translocation[17] has been measured by flow cytometry. These studies, which report two peaks essentially analogous to those in our study (FIGURE 5), help substantiate our belief that the two peaks in our study[27] represent X- and Y-chromosome–bearing sperm. The ability to obtain excellent resolution of the two peaks is useful for other biological applications. For example, using sperm selection methods to influence the sex ratio of agriculturally important animals would have profound genetic importance and marked economic impact. Garner et al.[6] have quantified X- and Y-chromosome–bearing sperm from ram, rabbit, boar, and bull semen using a slight modification of the method in the mouse studies. Although we have yet to resolve the X and Y subpopulations of human sperm, Otto et al.[22] have demonstrated such subpopulations and found a DNA difference between them of 3.4%. Our measurements of cockerel sperm predictably produced one narrow peak as the cockerel is the homogametic sex.

Flow cytometry, when used for X-Y sperm discrimination, exploits the only established difference between X- and Y-sperm; i.e., the quantity of DNA in the sex chromosome. The small differences of X-Y peak separations seem to represent the actual DNA content difference of the chromosomes but could be caused by more subtle effects, e.g., differences of base composition of the DNA. Even small differences of base composition of the sex chromosomes could be magnified by the preference of DAPI for adenine-thymine base pairs.[31] Nonetheless, although the observed fluorescence would not be proportional to the total DNA content of the sperm, the two peaks still would represent X and Y sperm.

Analyses of bimodal frequency distributions by fitting two Gaussian distributions to the data showed that fluorescence intensity of the peaks differed by 3.9, 3.7, 4.1, and 3.9% for bulls, boars, rams, and rabbits.[6] In four replicate analyses of semen from 25 bulls representing five breeds, the average area for the Y peaks was $50 \pm 0.5\%$, as typified in FIGURE 7. The X-Y peak differences did not vary within breeds but varied among breeds. Sperm from Jersey bulls had larger X-Y peak differences ($p < 0.001$) than sperm from Holstein, Hereford, and Angus bulls; sperm from Brahman bulls had smaller X-Y differences ($p < 0.004$). In this context it is interesting to note that the Y chromosome in Brahman cattle is a small acrocentric while that in the other breeds is a small metacentric, said by some[14] to arise as a pericentric inversion of the acrocentric Y.

The work of Garner et al.[6] shows that flow cytometry can assess the relative DNA content of sperm from domestic animals (data not presented here) and determine the natural ratio of X- to Y-chromosome–bearing sperm in fresh semen of at least five species and cryopreserved bull and boar semen. Moreover, it suggests that the ability to determine relative populations of X- and Y-chromo-

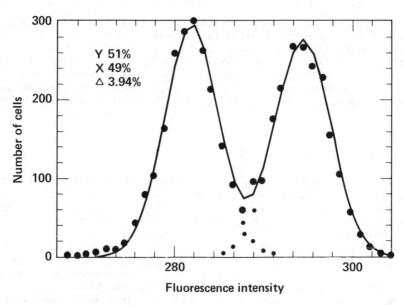

FIGURE 7. Resolution of bull X- and Y-sperm populations. For computer analysis the distribution obtained from flow cytometric measurement was truncated to the channels of fluorescence intensity shown and fitted with a pair of Gaussian distributions. Each of the two distributions is represented by small dots (···) and their sum by the solid line (——). The actual number of sperm per channel are shown as large dots (•). The only restriction placed on the computer fit was that the coefficients of variation be identical. There were 51% of the sperm in the Y peak (lower intensity) and 49% in the X peak. The difference in modal fluorescence intensity of the two peaks was 3.94%.[23]

some–bearing sperm in a semen sample would provide a quick, accurate method to determine the success of a purported sperm selection technique. The practical ability to influence the sex ratio of progeny would have profound impact on the livestock industry. Not only is flow cytometry useful for assessment of enrichment but it also may be used to develop new methods of separating X and Y sperm and to provide quality control for enrichment techniques that reach commercial application.

Separation of Heterogametic Sperm

Development of semen-based sex selection techniques has been impeded by the difficulty of identifying differences that might serve as a basis for enrichment or preferential inactivation of X or Y sperm. Appropriately adapted flow sorting instrumentation can be used to separate sperm based on DNA content. These sperm could be used to search for phenotypic differences that might be exploited for bulk separation of viable cells. However, current staining techniques[27] adequate to resolve a 3 to 4% difference in mean DNA content require decondensation of the highly compact sperm nucleus with proteolytic enzymes, substantially altering many biochemical components and generally disrupting sperm structure. The larger the difference in DNA content between the sex-determining sperm populations, the more biochemically conservative a staining protocol can be and still resolve the populations. For the vole, *Microtus oregoni,* this difference is about 9%, more than double that of most mammals.[20]

M. oregoni is unusual in that it is a gonosomic mosaic;[21] the gonadal and somatic cells have different chromosomal constitutions. Male somatic cells are XY, but spermatogonia are OY. Thus, one of the sperm populations contains the Y chromosome and the other, called "O," contains no sex chromosome. In this animal only Y-linked genes are candidates for coding for markers that differentiate the two sperm classes. This may not be different from other mammals as there is evidence that the X chromosome normally is inactivated during spermatogenesis.[15]

In what we believe to be the first verified sperm separation in a mammal,[25] caudal epididymidal sperm from trapped *M. oregoni* were dispersed for flow sorting, stained with DAPI, and sorted after preparation according to three protocols. (1) Papain and dithioerythritol treatment to decondense the chromatin.[27] Sperm tails and other cytoplasmic structures also are removed. This procedure yields good DNA content resolution (FIGURE 8). (2) Sonication followed by fixation in 80% ethanol. This also removes tails, but staining precision is considerably reduced. (3) Fixation of intact cells in 10% phosphate-buffered formalin. Sperm tails are not removed and resolution is reduced further. Sorting rates in these experiments were on the order of 30 cells/sec for each fraction.

Purity of the sorted fractions was determined by restaining the sperm according to protocol 1, measuring the sperm of each fraction in the ICP22, and computer fitting a pair of normal distributions to the resulting data. The relative areas

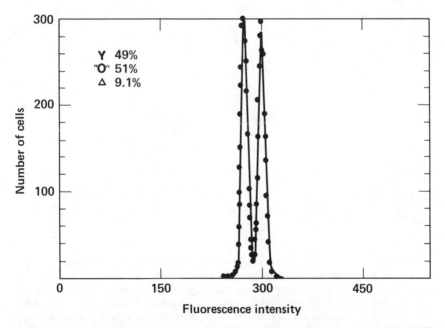

FIGURE 8. The O- and Y-sperm populations are clearly resolved in *M. oregoni* and the 9.1% difference in modal fluorescence intensity of the two peaks[23] corresponds closely to the 8.8% expected based on length of chromosome measurements made by Moruzzi.[20]

of the two fitted curves give the relative Y and O populations in each fraction. FIGURE 9a shows measurement of the O fraction sorted from the sonicated ethanol-fixed cells; the Y fraction is shown in FIGURE 9b. Their photographic superposition, which should be compared to FIGURE 8, is shown in FIGURE 9c. Analysis shows 95, 87, and 82% purity of O fractions for protocols 1, 2, and 3. Purities of Y fractions were 72, 83, and 80%.

Two problems currently prevent insemination of sorted sperm: low sorting rates and lytic staining techniques. Even if vital staining techniques are developed and the sorting rate is increased to about 10^3 sperm/sec use of sorted sperm for artificial insemination will not be widespread because several million cells per insemination are required. Application to *in vitro* fertilization, where the required number of sperm is significantly lower, is more probable.

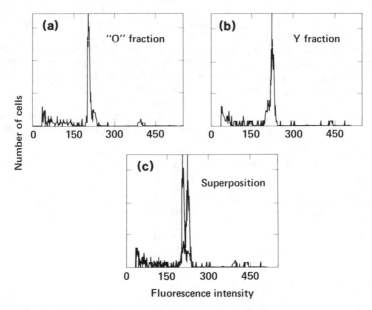

FIGURE 9. Verification of sorting purity of *M. oregoni* sperm. Sperm prepared with protocol 2 were sorted into two fractions. After sorting, the putatively enriched fractions were restained using protocol 1 and analyzed in the ICP22. Analysis of the O and Y fractions are shown in (a) and (b) respectively. The photographic superposition (c) of the peaks should be compared to FIGURE 8.[23]

For the immediate future, flow sorting of *M. oregoni* sperm offers the possibility of directly addressing the question of haploid expression of sex chromosome genes. A genetic marker might permit bulk separation of viable sperm, perhaps with an antibody to bind one population to a column while allowing the other to pass through. If there is a Y-specific *M. oregoni* marker that is conserved across species, it would have general application to mammalian sex selection. In the absence of a common Y-specific marker, extension to other species will require sorting of biochemically preserved sperm differing in DNA content by 3 to 4%.

CONCLUDING REMARKS

Male germ cells respond dramatically to a variety of insults and are important reproductive dosimeters. Semen analyses are very useful in studies on the effects of drugs, chemicals, and environmental hazards on testicular function, male fertility, and heritable germinal mutations. The accessability of male cells makes them well suited for analytical cytology. We might automate the process of determining sperm morphology but should not do so solely for increased speed. Rather, richer tangible benefits will derive from cytometric evaluation through increased sensitivity, reduced subjectivity, standardization between investigators and laboratories, enhanced archival systems, and the benefits of easily exchanged standardized data. Inroads on the standardization of assays for motility and functional integrity are being made. Flow cytometric analysis of total DNA content of individual sperm is an insensitive means to detect exposure to reproductive toxins because of the small size and low frequency of the DNA content errors. Flow cytometry can be used to determine the proportions of X- and Y-chromosome–bearing sperm in semen samples.

ACKNOWLEDGMENT

Many colleagues contributed to the studies reviewed. Special recognition of contributions made is due D. Pinkel, D. L. Garner, S. Lake, D. Stephenson, M. A. Van Dilla, M. L. Mendelsohn, J. W. Gray, A. J. Wyrobek, and L. A. Johnson.

REFERENCES

1. BENARON, D. A., J. W. GRAY, B. L. GLEDHILL, S. LAKE, A. J. WYROBEK & I. T. YOUNG. 1982. Quantification of mammalian sperm morphology by slit-scan flow cytometry. Cytometry 2: 344.
2. CASPERSSON, T. 1936. Uber den Chemischen Aufbau der Strukturen des Zellkernes. Scand. Arch. Physiol. 73 (Suppl. 8):1.
3. CATTANACH, B. M. 1961. A chemically induced variegated-type position effect in the mouse. Z. Vererbungsl 92: 165.
4. DEAN, P. N., D. PINKEL & M. L. MENDELSOHN. 1978. Hydrodynamic orientation of sperm heads for flow cytometry. Biophys. J. 23: 7.
5. EVENSON, D. P., Z. DARZYNKIEWICZ & M. R. MELAMED. 1980. Relation of mammalian sperm chromatin heterogeneity to fertility. Science 210: 1131.
6. GARNER, D. L., B. L. GLEDHILL, D. PINKEL, S. LAKE, D. STEPHENSON, M. A. VAN DILLA & L. A. JOHNSON. 1983. Quantification of the X- and Y-chromosome-bearing spermatozoa of domestic animals. Biol. Reprod. 28:
7. GLEDHILL, B. L., S. LAKE & P. N. DEAN. 1979. Flow cytometry and sorting of sperm and other male germ cells. In Flow Cytometry and Sorting. M. M. Melamed, P. Mullaney, & M. L. Mendelsohn, Eds.:471. John Wiley & Sons. New York.
8. GLEDHILL, B. L., S. LAKE, J. W. GRAY, D. E. BENNETT & A. J. WYROBEK. 1977. Two parameter flow cytometry to detect abnormally shaped sperm. J. Cell Biol. 75: 166a.
9. GLEDHILL, B. L., S. LAKE, L. L. STEINMETZ, J. W. GRAY, J. R. CRAWFORD, P. N. DEAN & M. A. VAN DILLA. 1976. Flow microfluorometric analysis of sperm DNA content: effect of cell shape on the fluorescence distribution. J. Cell Physiol. 87: 367.
10. HALAMKA, J., J. W. GRAY, B. L. GLEDHILL, S. LAKE & A. J. WYROBEK. 1984. Estimation of the frequency of malformed sperm by slit-scan flow cytometry. Cytometry 5: 333.

11. HACKER, U., J. SCHUMANN, W. GÖHDE & K. MÜLLER. 1981. Mammalian spermatogenesis as a biologic dosimeter for radiation. Acta Radiol. Oncology **20:** 279.
12. INGRAM, M. & K. PRESTON. 1970. Automatic analysis of blood cells. Sci. Am. **223:** 78.
13. KERKER, M., D. -S. WANG & H. W. CHEW. 1980. An optical model for flourescence of mammalian sperm in flow cytometry. Cytometry **1:** 161.
14. KIEFFER, N. M. & T. C. CARTWRIGHT. 1968. Sex chromosome polymorphism in domestic cattle. J. Hered. **59:** 35.
15. LIFSCHYTZ, E. 1972. X-chromosome inactivation: an essential feature of normal spermiogenesis in male heterogametic organisms. *In* Edinburgh Symposium on the Genetics of the Spermatozoon. R. A. Beatty & S. Glueckshohn-Waelsch, Eds.: 223. University of Edinburgh Press. Edinburgh, Scotland.
16. MAYALL, B. 1969. Deoxyribonucleic acid cytomorphometry of stained human leukocytes: I. Differences among cell types. J. Histochem. Cytochem. **17:** 249.
17. MEISTRICH, M. L., W. GÖHDE, R. A. WHITE & J. L. LONGTIN. 1979. "Cytogenetic" studies of mice carrying Cattanach's translocation by flow cytometry. Chromosoma **74:** 141.
18. MEISTRICH, M. L., W. GÖHDE, R. A. WHITE & J. SCHUMANN. 1978. Resolution of X and Y spermatids by pulse cytophotometry. Nature (London) **274:** 821.
19. MOORE, II, D. H., D. E. BENNETT, D. KRANZLER & A. J. WYROBEK. 1982. Quantitative methods of measuring the sensitivity of the mouse sperm morphology assay. Anal. Quant. Cytol. **4:** 199.
20. MORUZZI, J. F. 1979. Selecting a mammalian species for the separation of X- and Y-chromosome-bearing spermatozoa. J. Reprod. Fertil. **57:** 319.
21. OHNO, S., J. JAINCHILL & C. STENIUS. 1963. The creeping vole as a gonosomic mosaic. The OY/XY constitution in the vole. Cytogenetics **2:** 232.
22. OTTO, F. J., U. HACKER, J. ZANTE, J. SCHUMANN, W. GÖHDE & M. L. MEISTRICH. 1979. Flow cytometry of human spermatozoa. Histochemistry **61:** 249.
23. PINKEL, D. 1984. Cytometric analysis of mammalian sperm for induced morphologic and DNA content errors. *In* Biological Dosimetry: Cytometric Approaches to Mammalian Systems. W. G. Eisert & M. L. Mendelsohn, Eds.:111. Springer-Verlag. Berlin.
24. PINKEL, D., P. N. DEAN, S. LAKE, D. PETERS, M. L. MENDELSOHN, J. W. GRAY, M. A. VAN DILLA & B. L. GLEDHILL. 1979. Flow cytometry of mammalian sperm: progress in DNA and morphology measurement. J. Histochem. Cytochem. **27:** 353.
25. PINKEL, D., B. L. GLEDHILL, S. LAKE, D. STEPHENSON & M. A. VAN DILLA. 1982. Sex preselection in mammals? Separation of sperm bearing Y and "O" chromosomes in the vole *Microtus oregoni*. Science **218:** 904.
26. PINKEL, D., B. L. GLEDHILL, M. A. VAN DILLA, S. LAKE & A. J. WYROBEK. 1983. Radiation induced DNA content variability in mouse sperm. Radiat. Res. **95:** 550.
27. PINKEL, D., S. LAKE, B. L. GLEDHILL, M. A. VAN DILLA, D. STEPHENSON & G. WATCHMAKER. 1982. High resolution DNA content measurements of mammalian sperm. Cytometry **3:** 1.
28. PREWITT, J. & M. L. MENDELSOHN. 1966. The analysis of cell images. Ann. N.Y. Acad. Sci. **128:** 1035.
29. SARKER, S., O. W. JONES, W. CENTERWALL, E. T. TYLER & N. SHIOURA. 1978. Population heterogeneity in human sperm DNA content. J. Med. Genet. **15:** 271.
30. SARKAR, S., O. W. JONES & N. SHIOURA. 1974. Constancy in human sperm DNA content. Proc. Natl. Acad. Sci. USA **71:** 3512.
31. SUMNER, A. T., J. A. ROBINSON & H. J. EVANS. 1971. Distinguishing between X, Y, and YY-bearing spermatozoa by fluorescence and DNA content. Nature (New Biol.) **229:** 231.
32. VAN DILLA, M. A., B. L. GLEDHILL, S. LAKE, P. N. DEAN, J. W. GRAY, V. KACHEL, B. BARLOGIE & W. GÖHDE. 1977. Measurement of mammalian sperm deoxyribonucleic acid by flow cytometry. Problems and Approaches. J. Histochem. Cytochem. **25:** 763.
33. WYROBEK, A. J., J. A. HEDDLE & W. R. BRUCE. 1975. Chromosomal abnormalities and morphology of mouse sperm heads. Can. J. Genet. Cytol. **17:** 675.

34. WYROBEK, A. J., L. A. GORDON, J. G. BURKHART, M. C. FRANCIS, R. W. KAPP, JR., G. LETZ, H. V. MALLING, J. C. TOPHAM & M. D. WHORTON. 1983. An evaluation of the mouse sperm morphology test and other sperm tests in nonhuman mammals: A report for the GENE-TOX Program. Mutat. Res., Rev. Genet. Toxicol. 115: 10.

35. WYROBEK, A. J., L. A. GORDON, J. G. BURKHART, M. C. FRANCIS, R. W. KAPP, JR., G. LETZ, H. V. MALLING, J. V. TOPHAM & M. D. WHORTON. 1983. An evaluation of human sperm as indicators of chemically induced alterations of spermatogenic function: A report for the GENE-TOX Program. Mutat. Res., Rev. Genet. Toxicol. 115: 73.

36. YOUNG, I. T. 1972. The classification of white blood cells. IEEE Trans. Biomed. Eng. BME-19: 291.

37. YOUNG, I. T., B. L. GLEDHILL, S. LAKE & A. J. WYROBEK. 1982. Quantitative analysis of radiation-induced changes in sperm morphology. Anal. Quant. Cytol. 4: 207.

Genetic Analysis of Mammalian Spermatogenesis:

Use of the t Complex in the Mouse in Studies of Spermatogenesis and Sperm Function[a]

PATRICIA OLDS-CLARKE

Department of Anatomy
Temple University School of Medicine
Philadelphia, Pennsylvania 19140

INTRODUCTION

The use of defective genes to explore the mechanism of action of normal genes is a classic technique that has often uncovered new information or confirmed hypotheses suggested by data gathered through use of other techniques. Two well-known examples are the contribution of the study of testicular feminization syndrome to an understanding of normal androgen receptor function[1] and the use of Kartagener's syndrome, characterized by immotile sperm, chronic sinusitis, bronchiectasis, and situs inversus, to confirm the identity of dynein arms in cilia and flagella.[2] Although the t complex in the mouse is also well-known for its striking effect on sperm carrying it, thus far its study has contributed little to a better understanding of normal spermatogenesis and sperm function. Recent information from our laboratory and others now suggests that the t complex may be useful in studying control of spermiogenesis, capacitation, and hyperactivation of sperm.

THE t COMPLEX CONTAINS SEVERAL FACTORS THAT AFFECT SPERM

The t complex is a group of tightly linked abnormal genes; in a t/+ mouse, sperm carrying the t complex (t sperm) have an advantage over the sperm carrying the normal homolog (+ sperm), since t sperm fertilize most or all of the eggs available,[3] a phenomenon called transmission distortion (TD). TD is dependent on at least two factors (genes or groups of genes) at different sites within the t complex: one is in the region proximal to the centromere, the other more distal.[4] A complete t complex also carries one or more non-allelic lethal factors and several unique H-2 specificities.[5] The constellation of different factors carried by any single t complex is called its haplotype, a term borrowed from immunogenetics. While the phenomenon of TD suggests that sperm carrying a t haplotype may be "super sperm," this is not true when such sperm are produced by a mouse

---

[a] Supported by the National Institutes of Health (grant no. HD15045).

carrying two different t haplotypes. These males are sterile; their sperm are transported abnormally in the female[6] and are incapable of penetrating the egg even after investments have been removed.[7]

Recently, the primary gene product of one of the genes in the t complex has been identified. Tcp-1[a] is a gene carried by all t haplotypes and codes for a cell-surface protein, p63/6.9, found in greatest abundance on round spermatids (Silver and Hecht, personal communication). Normal germ cells have another allele at this locus, Tcp-1[b], that codes for a more basic form of this protein.[8] The function of either protein is as yet unknown; and it is not known whether they remain on sperm as the cells mature and move through the male and female genital tracts. Because of its proximal location within the t complex, Tcp-1[a] could be the proximal factor necessary for TD.[9]

POSSIBLE MECHANISMS OF TRANSMISSION DISTORTION

The abnormally high transmission of the t complex via t/+ males could be caused by either of two mechanisms: the degeneration or removal of + sperm, as occurs in Drosophila carrying a gene complex called segregation distorter[10]; or a physiological advantage of t sperm over + sperm during fertilization. The first possibility is unlikely because t/+ males produce t and + spermatids in equivalent numbers[11] and recent evidence demonstrates that both types of sperm are present in equal proportions in the cauda epididymis and in the uterus 90 minutes after coitus.[12] The second possibility appears more likely: t sperm have a physiological advantage over + sperm in the same population, either because they have normal function while + sperm are dysfunctional, or because t sperm (from a t/+ male) are better or faster at fertilization than normal sperm.

In either case, in t/+ mice the sperm genotype has modified its own phenotype, i.e., haploid gene expression has occurred in the t complex. While there is no direct evidence that the t complex is active post-meiotically, recent studies suggest that other genes are transcribed and translated in round spermatids of mice.[13-15] In the past it has always been assumed that since spermatids are connected by cytoplasmic bridges, any translation product in one spermatid would be shared by all. Advances in our understanding of intracellular traffic and cytoplasmic compartmentalization in other cell types make it clear that few if any proteins are free to diffuse randomly within a cell.[16,17] If t sperm are indeed physiologically different than + sperm in the same population, then the spermatids may not be a functional syncytium.

Identifying physiological differences between t and + sperm in a single population is difficult, since few techniques are sensitive enough to be used on single sperm, and it is not possible to separate the sperm by genotype. As a first step toward determining such differences, we have compared +/+ and t/+ populations. In doing so, we encounter another difficulty: since the sperm characteristics to be studied are usually the result of expression of many genes, effects of the t complex must be distinguished from effects of other genes on spermatogenesis. Although many differences have been found between t/+ and +/+ sperm populations, few of these differences have been shown to be the result of expression of the t complex itself. We have overcome this problem by using congenic strains of mice that differ genetically only in the t complex and closely linked genes. Thus, in these animals, any differences between +/+ and t/+ sperm populations must be due to expression of the t complex.[18]

EPIDIDYMAL SPERM FROM t/+ MICE HAVE ABNORMAL MOTILITY

In vivo, sperm from $t^{w32}/+$ mice (t^{w32} is the particular t haplotype we have chosen for study) begin to penetrate eggs sooner than do sperm from congenic +/+ mice.[19] This could be the result of faster transport to the site of fertilization, faster penetration of the eggs and their investments, or both. A study of sperm transport through the oviduct showed that $t^{w32}/+$ sperm populations began to arrive at the site of fertilization slightly sooner than did congenic sperm populations.[20] Since sperm motility probably plays an important role in passage of sperm through the uterotubal and isthmo-ampullary junctions, as well as through the egg investments,[21] we have also begun to examine the motility of $t^{w32}/+$ sperm populations

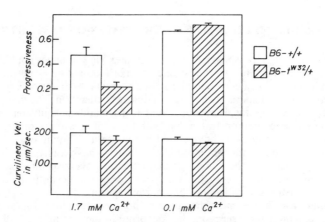

FIGURE 1. Progressiveness (*P*) and curvilinear velocities (V_c) of cauda epididymal sperm from C57BL/6-$t^{w32}/+$ and C57BL/6-+/+ mice, after 1–2 hr incubation in IVF medium containing 2% bovine serum albumin and 1.7 mM Ca^{2+} (4 males) or 0.1 mM Ca^{2+} (3 males). Three samples of 10 sperm each were analyzed from each male, and the mean values for each sample determined. The mean of the 3 sample means was taken as the value for that male. Bars indicate the mean ± SEM. There were significant differences in *P* between $t^{w32}/+$ and +/+ sperm populations incubated in 1.7 mM Ca^{2+}, between +/+ sperm populations incubated in 1.7 mM and 0.1 mM Ca^{2+}, and between $t^{w32}/+$ sperm populations incubated in 1.7 mM and 0.1 mM Ca^{2+} (Mann-Whitney *U* test, *p* = 0.05).

in detail. When sperm from the caudae epididymides of a $t^{w32}/+$ male are first released into a complete culture medium capable of supporting fertilization *in vitro* (IVF), their motility is indistinguishable from that of sperm populations taken from congenic +/+ males. After several hours *in vitro,* however, their net velocity, as determined by the method of Ojakian and Katz,[22] drops sharply. The net velocity of congenic +/+ sperm populations does not change significantly.[23]

Net velocity is a measure of progressive swimming speed, and thus has two components: curvilinear or actual sperm velocity and the progressiveness of the sperm path or trajectory, that is, how closely it resembles a straight line. The method of Ojakian and Katz[22] does not quantitatively evaluate either component. Subjective evaluation of $t^{w32}/+$ sperm populations suggested that there was a change from progressive swimming to a particular type of nonprogressive movement that we called "dancing"; we suggested that this was the cause of the decrease in net velocity.[24] Dancing after incubation *in vitro* is characteristic of sperm from mice carrying t^{w32} on each of three different genetic backgrounds, and of sperm from mice carrying any other complete t haplotype.[25]

Recently, we have begun to analyze sperm motility by videomicrography, a method that can measure net and curvilinear velocities and progressiveness, and objectively describe sperm movement patterns or trajectories.[26] Sperm samples were placed on a hemocytometer on a microscope stage warmed to 37°C and videotaped for up to two minutes. Tapes were played back at $1/10$ normal speed, and a tracing made of the movement of the junction between head and neck of individual sperm, usually for about one second. Net and curvilinear velocities of individual sperm were calculated from the elapsed real time displayed on the monitor simultaneously with the sperm images. Three samples containing 10 sperm each were analyzed from each male, and the mean of the three samples' means was taken as indicative of the sperm populations of that mouse. Net velocity divided by the curvilinear velocity gives a value, P, which is a measure of the progressiveness of the sperm's motility. A P value close to zero indicates very little progressiveness, while a straight line would have a P value of 1.0. The mean $\pm$ SEM curvilinear velocities (V_c) and progressiveness (P) values for sperm populations from C57BL/6 (B6) mice with and without the t^{w32} haplotype are shown on the left in FIGURE 1. (Net velocities are not shown, since they are the result of V_c and P.) The P value of the $t^{w32}/+$ sperm populations is significantly lower than that of the congenic $+/+$ populations. Curvilinear velocities of the two types of populations, however, are similar. These findings confirm our subjective observations, which suggested that after incubation in IVF medium $t^{w32}/+$ cauda epididymal sperm populations appear much less progressive than $+/+$ populations, while retaining vigorous motility.

IS DANCING HYPERACTIVATION?

What is the relevance of dancing to normal sperm motility and function in fertilization? We had noticed a similarity in the shape of the dancing trajectory and that of normal sperm undergoing hypeactivation, which is the change in motility concomitant with the end of capacitation. During hyperactivation, the beat of the sperm's flagellum decreases in frequency and increases in amplitude; the hyperactivated type of motion is usually referred to as "whiplash." As a result of this change in the beat of the sperm's flagellum, the sperm's trajectory becomes nonprogressive[27] and resembles dancing (compare FIGURE 2b in Fraser[28] with FIGURE 4a in this paper). Trajectories of normal sperm occasionally appeared hyperactivated, but the majority remained progressive (e.g., FIGURE 4b). To determine the relationship between dancing and hyperactivation, we have used videomicrography to compare some of the characteristics of normal hyperactivated sperm to dancing sperm from $t^{w32}/+$ mice. Our results suggest a close similarity between the two. Thus, dancing may be an indication that $t^{w32}/+$ epididymal sperm populations are capable of undergoing hyperactivation sooner and to a greater extent than are $+/+$ populations.

We first determined whether dancing is dependent on exogenous calcium, since calcium ions are required for capacitation and hyperactivation.[29,30] The right half of FIGURE 1 shows the V_c and P values for $t^{w32}/+$ and $+/+$ sperm populations incubated in IVF medium with 0.1 mM Ca^{2+}. For both genetic types of sperm populations, V_c is similar to that of sperm incubated in normal IVF medium. P values, however, are significantly higher than the P values for sperm from the same populations in medium with 1.7 mM Ca^{2+}. Moreover, the shapes of the sperm trajectories of normal and mutant populations in low calcium medium are indistinguishable from each other (FIGURE 4c and d). These results suggest that the degree of progressiveness of both $+/+$ and $t^{w32}/+$ sperm populations depends on exogenous calcium, a requirement for hyperactivation.

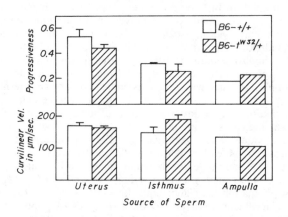

FIGURE 2. P and V_c of sperm from various parts of the genital tracts of B6D2F$_1$/J-$+/+$ females mated to B6-$t^{w32}/+$ or B6-$+/+$ males. Uterine sperm were recovered between 15 min and 2 hr after coitus and oviductal sperm at 2 hr postcoitus. Videotapes were made within 30 min of isolation of the sperm (in IVF medium with 2% bovine serum albumin and 1.7 mM Ca^{2+}) from the female. For each female, 3 samples of 10 uterine sperm each were analyzed, and the mean of the 3 sample means determined. $N = 4$ for B6-$+/+$ sperm populations and $N = 3$ for B6-$t^{w32}/+$ sperm populations. To collect oviductal sperm the ampullae were opened, fluid containing eggs were allowed to flow out onto a slide, and the fluid examined for motile sperm. The remainder of the oviduct was removed to a clean slide, the isthmus teased apart in 20 μl of medium, and the entire suspension examined for motile sperm. One sample was collected from each female, and sample sizes varied. For $+/+$ populations from the isthmus, $N = 3(7, 11,$ and 24 sperm); one sample was analyzed from the ampulla (5 sperm). For $t^{w32}/+$ populations from the isthmus, $N = 2$ (14 and 29 sperm); one sample was analyzed from the ampulla (15 sperm). Bars represent the mean $\pm$ SEM. There were no significant differences in P of either uterine or oviductal sperm between B6-$+/+$ and B6-$t^{w32}/+$ males. Consequently, data from B6-$+/+$ and B6-$t^{w32}/+$ males were pooled; there was a significant difference in P between uterine and oviductal sperm (Mann-Whitney U test, $p < 0.001$). Considering only $t^{w32}/+$ sperm populations, there was a significant difference in P between uterine and epididymal sperm (Mann-Whitney U test, $p = 0.05$).

We also examined the motility of sperm from the female genital tract, since it has been shown for other species that sperm from the oviduct are capacitated and exhibit whiplash motility.[31] FIGURE 2 summarizes the V_c and P values of sperm populations after removal from the uterus, isthmus, or ampullae of B6D2F$_1$-$+/+$ females mated to $t^{w32}/+$ or congenic $+/+$ males. The V_c and P vales of normal uterine sperm were similar to those of normal epididymal sperm. However, unlike $t^{w32}/+$ epididymal sperm, $t^{w32}/+$ uterine sperm populations were as progressive as normal uterine sperm. The shapes of the trajectories resembled those of normal epididymal sperm (FIGURE 4e and f). This suggests that some factor present in the seminal fluid or the uterus but not in the culture medium prevents $t^{w32}/+$ sperm populations from dancing after their deposition in the uterus.

Motile sperm from the oviducts of females mated to either $+/+$ or $t^{w32}/+$ males have very little progressiveness, as indicated by the low P values (FIGURE 2), which are similar to those of $t^{w32}/+$ epididymal populations. The shape of their trajectories is also similar (compare FIGURE 4g and h to a). These data are consistent with the hypothesis that in the oviduct most sperm in both $+/+$ and $t^{w32}/+$ populations are hyperactivated. That there appears to be no difference between the motility of $+/+$ and $t^{w32}/+$ sperm populations in the female genital tract may indicate that our method of measuring progressiveness is not sensitive enough to detect subtle differences in trajectories or that the onset of hyperactivation may occur at a different time in the two types of populations. Determining P values at different times after ejaculation, or measuring other characteristics of the trajectories may uncover differences between normal and mutant populations in the female genital tract. Although the large decrease in progressiveness that occurs in epididymal $t^{w32}/+$ sperm populations may not occur *in vivo,* this decrease in progressiveness does show that these sperm have the potential for abnormal motility, which may be manifested in a different form in the female tract.

EPIDIDYMAL SPERM FROM t/+ MICE HAVE HIGH GALACTOSYLTRANSFERASE LEVELS

Recent evidence suggests that sperm surface galactosyltransferase plays a role in fertilization by binding to substrates in the zona pellucida.[32] Capacitation, as assayed by the ability of sperm to bind to the zona pellucida, was associated with the release of specific galactosyltransferase substrates bound to the sperm, thereby exposing the surface galactosyltransferase for binding to the zona. It was suggested that these substrates were glycoconjugates from epididymal fluid.[33] Cauda epididymal sperm populations from $t^{w32}/+$ mice have four times the galactosyltransferase activity of normal sperm.[34] This is further support for the hypothesis that the t complex increases the ability of the sperm to become capacitated. We have begun to study the effect of galactosyltransferase activity on sperm motility by treating the sperm with alpha-lactalbumin, a protein that changes the substrate specificity of galactosyltransferase so that this enzyme now accepts other sugars, such as glucose or myoinositol, as substrates.[35] An alpha-lactalbumin-like molecule has been found in the epididymis, and it was suggested that this molecule may be adsorbed onto the sperm surface in the epididymis and removed during capacitation.[36]

A representative experiment, in which sperm from a $t^{w32}/+$ male were incubated in either 2% bovine serum albumin (BSA) or in 2% alpha-lactalbumin, is summarized in FIGURE 3. V_c is apparently not affected by alpha-lactalbumin, but progressiveness is increased to a level similar to that of normal epididymal and uterine sperm. That this effect is due to the presence of alpha-lactalbumin, and not to the absence of BSA, was shown by an additional experiment in which sperm of the same genotype were incubated in IVF medium with no protein (FIGURE 3). In protein-free medium, the large majority of sperm adhere to the glass slide. The small number of sperm not stuck to the slide all had very low P values, indicative of nonprogressive motility. The shape of the trajectory of sperm

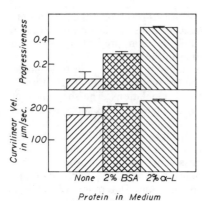

Figure 3. P and V_c of sperm from the cauda epididymides of (B6 × C3H)F_1-T/t^{w32} males, incubated for 20–60 min in IVF medium with no protein, 2% bovine serum albumin (BSA), or 2% alpha-lactalbumin (α-L). The bar for the group without protein represents the mean ± SEM of 6 sample means of 10 sperm each (total of 60 sperm). Sperm incubated in BSA and α-L were taken from the same male and SDs of these group means were not overlapping.

incubated in BSA or in protein-free medium was similar to that of mutant epididymal and oviductal sperm (FIGURE 4i and j), while the shape of the trajectory of sperm incubated in alpha-lactalbumin (FIGURE 4k) was similar to that of normal epididymal and uterine sperm. This preliminary result suggests that alpha-lactalbumin interferes with dancing and is consistent with the hypothesis that dancing is a form of hyperactivation.

IS DANCING IMPORTANT IN TRANSMISSION DISTORTION?

If dancing represents hyperactivation, is this the mechanism by which t sperm gain their advantage over + sperm in the same population? To ask this question, it will be necessary to first answer four others.

(1) Are dancing sperm acrosome-reacted? Under normal circumstances, hyperactivation and the acrosome reaction are coupled. However, in special environments hyperactivation may occur independently.[37] There are also situations in which whiplash motility is not indicative of fertility.[38] If dancing sperm have lost their acrosomes, they should be unable to penetrate the zona pellucida, since acrosome-reacted mouse sperm are unable to bind to the zona.[40] We have already shown that B6-t^{w32}/+ sperm populations have the same fertility *in vitro* as do B6-+/+ sperm populations, but the motility of the sperm was not examined.[41] In future experiments, we will determine whether the acrosome reaction has occurred in dancing populations and whether the degree of progressiveness of a population is correlated with the ability to penetrate eggs *in vitro*.

(2) Are there differences between the motility of t^{w32}/+ and congenic +/+ sperm populations within the female genital tract? Although studies of epididymal sperm demonstrate that the potential for a different motility exists, no differences were apparent in our preliminary study of sperm from the female genital tract. There may be subtle, as yet undetected, differences in the shape of the trajectories or differences in the timing or location of the onset of nonprogressive motility. Since we have already observed differences between the transport of +/+ and t^{w32}/+ sperm populations through the oviduct,[20] these studies are worth pursuing in greater detail.

(3) Are there differences between the motility of t sperm and + sperm in t/+ populations? The motility differences observed between t^{w32}/+ and +/+ sperm

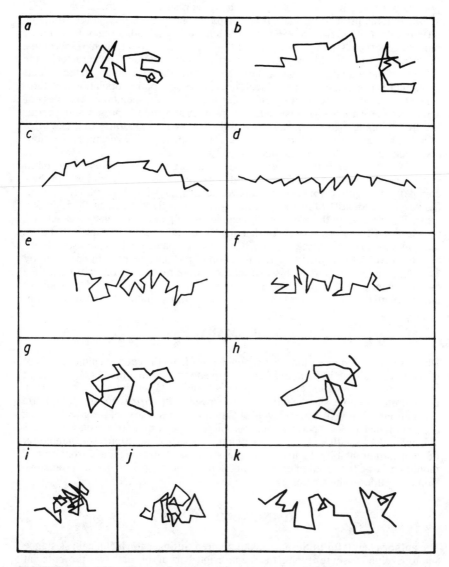

FIGURE 4. Typical tracings of the movement of the junction of head and neck of individual sperm for 1.0 sec. (a–d) B6 epididymal sperm in IVF medium with different levels of Ca^{2+} (refer to FIGURE 1). (a) $t^{w32}/+$ sperm in 1.7 mM Ca^{2+}; (b) $+/+$ sperm in 1.7 mM Ca^{2+}; (c) $t^{w32}/+$ sperm in 0.1 mM Ca^{2+}; (d) $+/+$ sperm in 0.1 mM Ca^{2+}. Magnification $=1,080\times$. (e–h) B6 sperm from the female genital tract (refer to FIGURE 2). (e) $t^{w32}/+$ uterine sperm; (f) $+/+$ uterine sperm; (g) $t^{w32}/+$ sperm from the isthmus; (h) $+/+$ sperm from the isthmus. Magnification $= 1,080\times$. (i–k) $(B6\times C3H)F_1$-T/t^{w32} cauda epididymal sperm in IVF medium (refer to FIGURE 3). (i) no protein; (j) 2% BSA; (k) 2% alpha-lactalbumin. Magnification $= 862\times$. Figure reduction is 70%.

populations could be a diploid effect, that is, the result of the expression of t^{w32} in spermatogonia prior to meiosis. If so, then all sperm in the population would be different than sperm from a $+/+$ male, but similar to each other regardless of their haploid genotype. On the other hand, if this is a haploid effect, then $+$ sperm in a $t^{w32}/+$ population should resemble sperm in a $+/+$ population. To characterize the motility of individual sperm and determine whether they are similar to individuals in another sperm population is difficult because every sperm population is heterogeneous with respect to motility characteristics. In any population, regardless of genotype, there are always fast and slow, progressive and nonprogressive sperm. We are beginning to look for ways to identify the "typical" features of trajectories of individual sperm that characterize them as belonging to a certain population, and to describe those features quantitatively.

(4) Are there other factors within the t complex that are expressed in sperm and are necessary for transmission distortion? Since several factors within the t complex are required for TD, the answer to this question must be affirmative. However, the identity of these other factors and how they influence TD is not yet clear. The possibility that abnormally high levels of galactosyltransferase activity on sperm surfaces are related to dancing needs to be further explored: Is the mechanism causing dancing directly dependent on galactosyltransferase activity or is it a result of capacitation? The function of p63/6.9, the protein produced by Tcp-1[a], is unknown, but if this cell surface protein remains on sperm as they mature, it may have a role in sperm motility and/or capacitation. Other as yet undocumented gene products of the t complex may also influence sperm function.

SUMMARY

Our observations suggest that sperm populations from the caudae epididymides of $t^{w32}/+$ mice undergo hyperactivation *in vitro* sooner and to a much greater extent than do sperm populations from congenic $+/+$ mice: (1) epididymal $t^{w32}/+$ sperm populations become significantly less progressive *in vitro* than do $+/+$ sperm populations; (2) low (0.1 mM) levels of Ca^{2+} prevent this loss of progressiveness; (3) epididymal $t^{w32}/+$ sperm populations have trajectories and progressiveness values similar to both $+/+$ and $t^{w32}/+$ oviductal sperm populations; (4) an inhibitor of capacitation inhibits the loss of progressiveness. This divergence from normal motility may be the result of expression of one of the factors involved in transmission distortion of the t complex.

ACKNOWLEDGMENTS

The author is grateful to Susan Day and Karen Sittinger for technical assistance and to Evelyn Dissin for typing the manuscript. Part of this data was presented at the annual meeting of the Society for the Study of Reproduction and the American Society for Cell Biology in 1982.

REFERENCES

1. ATTARDI, B. 1976. Genetic analysis of steroid hormone action. Trends Biochem. Sci. **1:** 241–244.
2. AFZELIUS, B. A. 1976. A human syndrome caused by immotile cilia. Science **193:** 317–319.

3. BENNETT, D. 1976. The T-locus of the mouse. Cell **6:** 441–454.
4. STYRNA, J. & J. KLEIN. 1981. Evidence for two regions in the mouse t complex controlling transmission ratios. Genet. Res. **38:** 315–325.
5. LYON, M. F. 1981. The t-complex and the genetical control of development. Symp. Zool. Soc. Lond. **47:** 455–477.
6. OLDS, P. 1970. Effect of the T locus on sperm distribution in the house mouse. Biol. Reprod. **2:** 91–97.
7. McGRATH, J. & N. HILLMAN. 1980. Sterility in mutant (t^{Lx}/t^{Ly}) male mice. III. In vitro fertilization. J. Embryol. Exp. Morph. **59:** 49–58.
8. SILVER, L. M. & M. WHITE. 1982. A gene product of the mouse t complex with chemical properties of a cell surface-associated component of the extracellular matrix. Dev. Biol. **91:** 423–430.
9. SILVER, L. 1981. A structural gene (Tcp-1) within the mouse t complex is separable from effects on tail length and lethality but may be associated with effects on spermatogenesis. Genet. Res. **38:** 115–123.
10. KETTANEH, N. & D. HARTL. 1980. Ultrastructural analysis of spermiogenesis in segregation distorter males of *Drosophila melanogaster*: the homozygotes. Genetics **96:** 665–683.
11. HAMMERBERG, C. & J. KLEIN. 1975. Evidence for post-meiotic effect of t factors causing segregation distortion in the mouse. Nature **253:** 137–138.
12. SILVER, L. & P. OLDS-CLARKE. 1984. Transmission ratio distortion of mouse t haplotypes is not a consequence of wild-type sperm degeneration. Dev. Biol. **105:** in press.
13. ERICKSON, R. P., J. M. ERICKSON, C. J. BETLACH & M. L. MEISTRICH. 1980. Further evidence for haploid gene expression during spermatogenesis: heterogeneous, poly(A)-containing RNA is synthesized post-meiotically. J. Exp. Zool. **214:** 13–19.
14. WIEBEN, E. D. 1981. Regulation of the synthesis of lactate dehydrogenase-X during spermatogenesis in the mouse. J. Cell Biol. **88:** 492–498.
15. GOLD, B., L. STERN, F. M. BRADLEY & N. B. HECHT. 1983. Gene expression during mammalian spermatogenesis. II. Evidence for stage-specific differences in mRNA populations. J. Exp. Zool. **225:** 123–134.
16. CLARKE, F. M. & C. J. MASTERS. 1976. Interactions between muscle proteins and glycolytic enzymes. Int. J. Biochem. **7:** 359–365.
17. SABATINI, D.D., G. KREIBICH, T. MORIMOTO & M. ADESNIK. 1982. Mechanisms for the incorporation of proteins in membranes and organelles. J. Cell Biol. **92:** 1–22.
18. OLDS-CLARKE, P. & S. McCABE. 1982. Genetic background affects expression of t haplotype in mouse sperm. Genet. Res. **40:** 249–254.
19. OLDS-CLARKE, P. & A. BECKER. 1978. The effect of the T/t locus on sperm penetration *in vivo* in the house mouse. Biol. Reprod. **18:** 132–140.
20. TESSLER, S. & P. OLDS-CLARKE. 1981. Male genotype influences sperm transport in female mice. Biol. Reprod. **24:** 806–813.
21. OVERSTREET, J. W. & D. F. KATZ. 1977. Sperm transport and selection in the female genital tract. *In* Development in Mammals. M. Johnson, Ed. **2:** 31–65. North-Holland Publishing Co. New York.
22. OJAKIAN, G. & D. KATZ. 1973. A simple technique for the measurement of swimming speed of *Chlamydomonas*. Exp. Cell Res. **81:** 487–491.
23. TESSLER, S., J. E. CAREY & P. OLDS-CLARKE. 1981. Mouse sperm motility affected by factors in the T/t complex. J. Exp. Zool. **217:** 277–285.
24. OLDS-CLARKE, P. 1983. The nonprogressive motility of sperm populations from mice with a t^{w32} haplotype. J. Androl. **4:** 136–143.
25. OLDS-CLARKE, P. 1983. Nonprogressive sperm motility is characteristic of most complete t haplotypes in the mouse. Genet. Res. **42:** 151–157.
26. KATZ, D. F. & J. W. OVERSTREET. 1981. Sperm motility assessment by videomicrography. Fert. Steril. **35:** 188–193.
27. KATZ, D. F., R. YANAGIMACHI & R. D. DRESDNER. 1978. Movement characteristics and power output of guinea-pig and hamster spermatozoa in relation to activation. J. Reprod. Fert. **52:** 167–172.
28. FRASER, L. 1977. Motility patterns in mouse spermatozoa before and after capacitation. J. Exp. Zool. **202:** 439–445.

29. YANAGIMACHI, R. & N. USUI. 1974. Calcium dependence of the acrosome reaction and activation of guinea pig spermatozoa. Exp. Cell. Res. **89:** 161–174.
30. FRASER, L. R. 1982. Ca^{2+} is required for mouse sperm capacitation and fertilization in vitro. J. Androl. **3:** 412–419.
31. KATZ, D. F. & R. YANAGIMACHI. 1980. Movement characteristics of hamster sperm within the oviduct. Biol. Reprod. **22:** 759–764.
32. SHUR, B. D. & N. G. HALL. 1982. A role for mouse sperm surface galactosyltransferase in sperm binding to the egg zona pellucida. J. Cell Biol. **95:** 574–579.
33. SHUR, B. D. & N. G. HALL. 1982. Sperm surface galactosyltransferase activities during in vitro capacitation. J. Cell Biol. **95:** 567–573.
34. SHUR, B. D. 1981. Galactosyltransferase activities on mouse sperm bearing multiple t^{lethal} and t^{viable} haplotypes of the T/t complex. Genet. Res. **38:** 225–236.
35. HILL, R. L. & K. BREW. 1975. Lactose synthetase. Adv. Enzymol. **43:** 411–490.
36. BYERS, S. W., P. K. QASBA, H. L. PAULSON & M. DYM. 1984. Immunocytochemical localization of alpha lactalbumin in the male reproductive tract. Biol. Reprod. **30:** 171–178.
37. BARROS, C. & M. BERRIOS. 1977. Is the activated sperm really capacitated? J. Exp. Zool. **201:** 65–72.
38. FRASER, L. R. 1981. Dibutyryrl cyclic AMP decrease capacitation time *in vitro* in mouse spermatozoa. J. Reprod. Fert. **62:** 63–72.
39. SALING, P. M. & B. T. STOREY. 1979. Mouse gamete interactions during fertilization in vitro. J. Cell Biol. **83:** 544–555.
40. FLORMAN, H. M. & B. T. STOREY. 1982. Mouse gamete interactions: the zona pellucida is the site of the acrosome reaction leading to fertilization in vitro. Dev. Biol. **91:** 121–130.
41. OLDS-CLARKE, P. & J. E. CAREY. 1978. Rate of egg penetration in vitro accelerated by T/t locus in the mouse. J. Exp. Zool. **206:** 323–332.

Scanning Transmission Electron Microscopy of Dynein Arms

KENNETH A. JOHNSON

Department of Biochemistry, Microbiology,
Molecular and Cell Biology,
The Pennsylvania State University
University Park, Pennsylvania 16802

Of the numerous techniques used to study the structure of dynein, none has revealed so much information in such a short period of time as the analysis by scanning transmission electron microscopy (STEM). Recent advances in hardware and in sample preparation techniques at the Brookhaven National Laboratory have enabled the simultaneous observation of structure and accurate measurement of mass of individual protein molecules.[1-4] Such analysis was heretofore unattainable by any other single technique. In this report, I will summarize the unique features provided by STEM and describe the results of our analysis of dyneins isolated from *Tetrahymena* cilia and *Chlamydomonas* flagella.

THE SCANNING TRANSMISSION ELECTRON MICROSCOPE

STEM differs from conventional transmission electron microscopy (TEM) principally in that the signal resulting from scattered electrons is analyzed rather than an image obtained by refocusing the unscattered electrons.[1] Like darkfield light microscopy, one gains a tremendous increase in contrast of the observable sample over background by looking only at the scattered electrons. Unlike darkfield light microscopy, because of the inefficiency of refocusing scattered electrons, an image is generated by scanning the sample with a small beam of electrons and recording the intensity of electron scattering as a function of position over the sample. Since the electron scattering intensities can be measured with quantum yield efficiency, one can directly observe *unstained* protein molecules. By "looking" at the protein rather than heavy metals deposited on or around the protein, the technique is free of some of the potential artefacts of sample preparation. More importantly, the electron scattering intensity is directly proportional to the mass of the protein and therefore provides a measurement of the molecular weight of each particle observed. The ability to determine molecular weight while simultaneously observing the structure of isolated protein molecules is of obvious importance since the mass of a particle serves to define the protein being examined. In addition, one can literally dissect the protein by analyzing the distribution of mass within the particle.

The data obtained in the STEM are recorded digitally as the intensity of electron scattering versus position over the sample and can be replayed to a monitor for photography or for selection of particles for mass analysis. The mass analysis involves integrating the electron scattering intensities over an area of the sample bounded by a given particle and then subtracting the background scattering due to the thin carbon film. The major sources for random error in the method, beyond the limits of the biochemical purity of the sample, are counting statistics and variations in thickness of the supporting film. These two factors tend to limit the method to the examination of larger macromolecules. The smallest biological macromolecule thus far examined is tRNA,[5] where STEM analysis gave a mass of 25 kilodaltons with a standard deviation of 12%; the predicted error due to counting statistics in this case was 9.4%.

Loss of mass due to beam damage can easily be kept to less than 1% by using a low electron density (1–2 electrons per square angstrom) and even this loss of mass is compensated by including an internal standard of tobacco mosaic virus particles.[1] The only significant limitation is in the biochemical quality of the specimen. For example, small amounts of denatured protein become visible as sheets of material shrouding the sample; however, this should be considered as a strength of the method since it provides an extra control for the quality of the preparation.

STEM ANALYSIS OF DYNEIN

An image of unstained *Tetrahymena* dynein, applied to a thin carbon film, freeze dried, and examined in the Brookhaven STEM is shown in FIGURE 1. The image

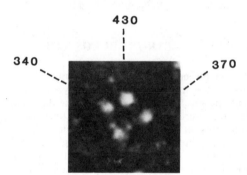

FIGURE 1. STEM analysis of unstained dynein. *Tetrahymena* 30S dynein was applied to a carbon film, freeze-dried, and examined as described.[6] This figure shows one dynein molecule. The entire particle exhibited a mass of 1.85 million daltons. The masses of the individual heads are given in the figure in kilodaltons. The strands connecting the heads to the base can be more easily seen in negatively stained samples.[6] 260,000×.

displays the intensity of electron scattering as a function of position over the sample. The mass of the entire particle and its subdomains were determined by integration of electron scattering intensities. The entire particle had a mass of 1.85 million daltons while the masses of the three heads were 340, 370, and 430 kilodaltons as indicated in the figure. This figure illustrates the analysis as it is applied to a single particle. Examination of a large number of particles in unstained and in negatively stained samples demonstrated that the 30S dynein molecule isolated from *Tetrahymena* cilia consists of three globular domains connected by three slender threads to a somewhat extended base.[6] Averages for the particles analyzed gave a mass of 1.95 million ($\pm$12%) for the entire particle. The average mass of the heads was 416 $\pm$ 76 kilodaltons; however, analogy to the *Chlamydomonas* dyneins as described below suggests that the three heads are not identical.

It is quite remarkable that analysis of dynein by STEM could provide such a wealth of new information to so completely alter our view of the dynein molecule. It is difficult to estimate what would have been required to obtain the same information by any combination of other techniques; although, it is not likely that any other data would be so compelling. For example, one criticism of the work might have been that the three-headed particle was an aggregate or a breakdown product of dynein. However, the mass analysis served to identify the isolated particle and relate it to a dynein molecule bound to the microtubule. Several investigators have established that dynein binds to microtubules with a 24 nm repeat[7-9] and Mary Porter had established conditions required to saturate a microtubule such that there were seven dynein microtubules surrounding a 14-protofilament microtubule.[10] This then provided an independent definition of the dynein molecule, as the unit seen to decorate microtubules with a 24 nm repeat. Mass per unit length measurements performed on the microtubule-dynein complex established that the 24 nm repeating unit had a mass of two million daltons, identical with that observed for the isolated particles.[6] Thus, the mass of the protein as measured by STEM also provides a quantity that can be used to define a particle or to relate one structure to another.

Mass analysis of individual particles also established that the apparently different conformations of the dynein molecule represented particles of the same mass, providing support for the notion that the threads connecting the heads of the dynein to the base are rather flexible and allow various conformations as the molecule adsorbs to the carbon film. Thus, again the mass analysis provided a means to resolve what might have been an insurmountable problem in the interpretation of images obtained by conventional transmission electron microscopy employing shadowing of the specimen to make the particles visible.

A final and perhaps most important advantage provided by STEM analysis is in the small amount of sample (0.5 μg) and the relatively short time required to perform the analysis. Thus it is relatively easy to examine dyneins isolated from different sources. We have successfully analyzed dyneins isolated from *Chlamydomonas* flagella in collaboration with George Witman[11] and are in the process of examining dyneins isolated from sea urchin and bull sperm.

Chlamydomonas outer arm dynein spontaneously breaks down upon extraction from the flagella to yield two particles, a 12S and an 18S ATPase. Analysis of mutants of *Chlamydomonas* lacking the outer dynein arm[12,13] and reconstitution experiments[14] have established that both ATPases are components of the outer arm. FIGURE 2 schematically summarizes the results obtained on the two *Chlamydomonas* dyneins in comparison to the *Tetrahymena* dynein. STEM analysis of the 18S dynein revealed a two-headed particle with a net mass of 1.25 million daltons and each head gave a mass of 370 kilodaltons.[11] The 12S dynein was a single globular unit with a mass of 460 kilodaltons. Thus, the structures as well as the masses of the two *Chlamydomonas* dyneins added together nearly equal the structure and mass, respectively, of the *Tetrahymena* 30S dynein.

Preliminary analysis of sea urchin 21S dynein in collaboration with Ian Gibbons has indicated a structure and mass essentially identical to the *Chlamydomonas* 18S dynein.[15] Although we do not know why sea urchin 21S dynein is a two-headed particle while the outer arm dyneins from both *Chlamydomonas* and *Tetrahymena* are composed of three heads, the results may be taken to indicate that the third head is required for generation of the ciliary waveform seen in *Chlamydomonas* and *Tetrahymena,* but not in sea urchin. Alternatively, the different particles obtained may be due to differences in the way in which the outer/inner arm complex dissociates from the doublet microtubule during extraction. In any event, these studies have led to a unified view of the dynein molecule consisting of two or three globular heads connected to a base by slender threads. Significantly, the analysis has removed what might have been a conflict in the literature concerning disparate results obtained using the three sources of dynein.

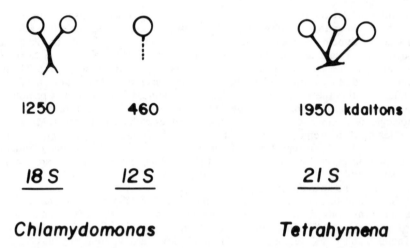

FIGURE 2. Comparison of *Tetrahymena* and *Chlamydomonas* dyneins. The results of STEM analysis of *Tetrahymena* 30S dynein[6] and *Chlamydomonas* 18S and 12S dyneins[11] are summarized (*see text*). Note that the actual sedimentation coefficient of *Tetrahymena* "30S" dynein is 22S[16] although we have continued to use the name 30S dynein for historical reasons.

SUPPORTING EVIDENCE FOR THE BOUQUET MODEL

Electron microscopy provides the only method, short of X-ray crystallography, for determining the subunit arrangement of a multimeric protein. However, the images obtained are necessarily a function of the substrate that the sample is adsorbed to and, whether that substrate is a carbon film or a doublet microtubule, one must consider the effects due to collapse of the sample onto the substrate. Hydrodynamic studies compliment electron microscopy by providing information relating to the structure of the molecule in solution. Recent hydrodynamic analysis of *Tetrahymena* 30S dynein has confirmed the three-headed bouquet model.[16] Independent measurements of the sedimentation and diffusion coefficients of the dynein has given a molecular weight of 1.8–1.9 million. Analysis by light-scattering techniques gave a molecular weight of 1.85 million and provided an estimate of the radius of hydration of the molecule in solution. Combining the information obtained by electron microscopy and light scattering with mathematical modeling of the sedimentation behavior has indicated that the molecule must be rather extended in solution, with the heads far apart from one another. Any model predicting close contact between the heads gave a sedimentation coefficient that was much greater than that actually observed. Thus, the hydrodynamic analysis established that the extended bouquet image seen by electron microscopy is not an artefact of adsorption to the carbon film; moreover, the data support the conclusion that the apparently different morphologies seen in the electron microscope are due to the flexibility of the connections from the heads to the base. In addition, the data suggest that the base of the molecule is extended in solution.

THE MECHANISM OF FORCE GENERATION

Several types of evidence indicate that each of the three globular heads of *Tetrahymena* dynein interacts with the microtubule in an ATP-dependent reaction to produce the force for movement. Kinetic analysis of the ATP-induced dissociation of the microtubule-dynein complex has established that three moles of ATP per mole of dynein are required to dissociate the complex.[17,18] In addition, analysis of the radial distribution of mass about the microtubule in the STEM indicated that the heads were located in close proximity to the microtubule wall.[6] The most reasonable interpretation of these data, and of other views of the dynein attached to the outer doublet as observed by conventional TEM, is that the roots of the bouquet form a structural attachment site on the A-subfiber of the outer doublet and that the heads interact with the adjacent B-subfiber in a reaction to produce the force for movement. A similar model can best account for the sea urchin dynein, but involving only two heads; titration of the ATPase sites by measuring the amplitude of the ATP hydrolysis presteady-state transient has indicated two ATP binding sites per 1.25 million dalton particle.[19]

Kinetic analysis of the ATPase cycle has established that the pathway by which ATP hydrolysis is coupled to the interaction of dynein with the microtubule is essentially identical to that which has been described for actomyosin.[20] Namely, ATP binding induces a very rapid dissociation of the dynein from the microtubule and ATP hydrolysis occurs in a slower step following hydrolysis. In fact, in spite of rather great differences in structure and polypeptide composition, the kinetic constants that govern ATP binding and hydrolysis are quite similar for myosin and dynein.[20] Thus, it would seem that the same principals govern the conversion of chemical energy to mechanical force production in the two systems. Although the structures are greatly different in detail as summarized in FIGURE 3, the two

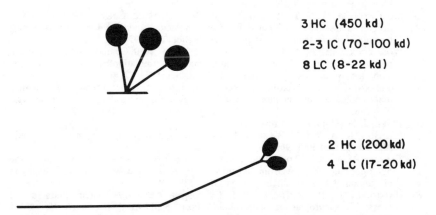

3 HC (450 kd)
2-3 IC (70-100 kd)
8 LC (8-22 kd)

2 HC (200 kd)
4 LC (17-20 kd)

FIGURE 3. Comparison of dynein and myosin structures. The structures of *Tetrahymena* dynein (upper) and skeletal myosin (lower) are drawn to the same scale for comparison. The numbers at the right refer the number and approximate molecular weights of the polypeptides in each molecule, where HC represents heavy chain, IC, intermediate chain, and LC, light chain.

structures appear to be similar in principle. In each case, globular heads containing the ATP and filament (actin or microtubule) binding sites are connected via somewhat flexible strands. Very little is known about the conformational changes responsible for net movement in either system; although, the most favored model for the action of actomyosin suggests that there is a rotation of the head on the actin filament to produce the force for sliding.[21] This would seem to be the most attractive model for understanding the interaction of the dynein heads with the B-subfiber. More complex models have been proposed for dynein,[22,23] but none of them quantitatively account for our current understanding of the dynein molecule in solution and the nature of the ATP-sensitive interaction of the dynein heads with the microtubule.

In summary, STEM analysis has revolutionized our view of the dynein molecule and we have only begun to exploit the wealth of information provided by the STEM. Previous data pertaining to dynein mechanochemistry and interpreted in terms of a single rather bulky arm must now be re-analyzed in terms of a flexible bouquet consisting of two (in the case of sea urchin) or three globular heads connected by independent strands. Current work is aimed at localizing the dozen polypeptides, the microtubule binding sites, and the ATP binding sites within the domains of the bouquet. Of particular interest is the demonstration that a heavy atom cluster compound can be readily visualized in the STEM providing a potential label for specific sites within the molecule.[24] Further STEM analysis of dynein and its subfragments will do much to resolve many of the interesting questions raised by the current study.

REFERENCES

1. WALL, J. S. 1979. Biological scanning transmission electron microscopy. *In* Introduction to Electron Microscopy, J. J. Hren, J. I. Goldstein & D. C. Joy, Eds.: 333–342. Plenum Publishing Co. New York.
2. MOSESSON, M. W., J. HAINFELD, J. WALL & R. H. HASCHEMEYER. 1981. Identification and mass analysis of human fibrinogen molecules and their domains by scanning transmission electron microscopy. J. Mol. Biol. **153:** 695–718.
3. WOODCOCK, C. L. F., L.-L. Y. FRADO & J. S. WALL. 1980. Composition of native and reconstituted chromatin particles: direct mass determination by scanning transmission electron microscopy. Proc. Natl. Acad. Sci. USA **77:** 4818–4820.
4. FREEMAN, R. & K. R. LEONARD. 1981. Comparative mass measurement of biological macromolecules by scanning transmission electron microscopy. J. Microsc. **122:** 275–286.
5. WALL, J. S. (Unpublished results.)
6. JOHNSON, K. A. & J. S. WALL. 1983. Structure and molecular weight of the dynein ATPase. J. Cell Biol. **96:** 669–678.
7. TAKAHASHI, M. & Y. TONOMURA. 1978. Binding of 30S dynein to the B-tubule of the outer doublet axonemes from *Tetrahymena pyriformis* and ATP induced dissociation of the complex. J. Biochem. (Tokyo) **84:** 1339–1355.
8. HAIMO, L. T., B. R. TELZER & J. L. ROSENBAUM. 1979. Dynein binds to and crossbridges cytoplasmic microtubules. Proc. Natl. Acad. Sci. USA **76:** 5759–5763.
9. MITCHELL, D. R. & F. D. WARNER. 1981. Binding of dynein 21S ATPase to microtubules. Effects of ionic conditions and substrate analogs. J. Biol. Chem. **23:** 12535–12544.
10. PORTER, M. E. & K. A. JOHNSON. 1983. Characterization of the ATP-sensitive binding of *Tetrahymena* dynein to bovine brain microtubules. J. Biol. Chem. **258:** 6575–6581.

11. WITMAN, G. B., K. A. JOHNSON, K. K. PFISTER & J. S. WALL. 1983. Fine structure and molecular weight of the outer arm dyneins of *Chlamydomonas*. J. Submicrosc. Cytol. **15:** 193–197.

12. PIPERNO, G. & D. J. L. LUCK. 1979. Axonemal adenosine triphosphatase from flagella of *Chlamydomonas reinhardtii*. J. Biol. Chem. **254:** 3084–3090.

13. HUANG, B., G. PIPERNO & D. J. L. LUCK. 1979. Paralysed flagella mutants of *Chlamydomonas reinhardtii* defective for axonemal doublet microtubule arms. J. Biol. Chem. **254:** 3091–3099.

14. FAY, R. B. & G. B. WITMAN. 1977. The localization of flagellar ATPases in *Chlamydomonas reinhardtii*. J. Cell Biol. **75:** 286a

15. GIBBONS, I. R., K. A. JOHNSON & J. S. WALL. (Unpublished results).

16. CLUTTER, D. B., D. STIMPSON, V. BLOOMFIELD & K. A. JOHNSON. (Manuscript in preparation.)

17. PORTER, M. E. & K. A. JOHNSON. 1983. Transient state kinetic analysis of the ATP-induced dissociation of the dynein-microtubule complex. J. Biol. Chem. **258:** 6582–6587.

18. SHIMIZU, T. & K. A. JOHNSON. 1983. Kinetic evidence for multiple dynein ATPase sites. J. Biol. Chem. **258:** 13841–13846.

19. EVANS, J. A. 1982. A kinetic study of latent and triton potentiated dynein-1 ATPase. Ph.D. thesis. University of Hawaii.

20. JOHNSON, K. A. 1983. The pathway of ATP hydrolysis by dynein: kinetics of a pre-steady state phosphate burst. J. Biol. Chem. **258:** 13825–13832.

21. EISENBERG, E. & T. L. HILL. 1978. A cross-bridge model of muscle contraction. Prog. Biophys. Molec. Biol. **33:** 55–82.

22. WITMAN, G. B. & N. M. MINERVINI. 1982. Dynein arm conformation and mechano-chemical transduction in the eukaryotic flagella. Symposium of the Association of Experimental Biology. *In* Prokaryotic and Eukaryotic Flagella. W. B. Amos & J. G. Ducket, Eds.: 203–223. Cambridge University Press.

23. GOODENOUGH, U. W. & J. E. HEUSER. 1982. Substructure of the outer dynein arm. J. Cell Biol. **95:** 798–815.

24. SAFER, D., J. HAINFELD, J. S. WALL & J. E. RIORDAN. 1982. Biospecific labeling with undecagold: visualization of the biotin binding site on avidin. Science **218:** 290–291.

Incorporation of Radiolabeled Amino Acids into Protein Subunits of the Rat Leydig Cell Gonadotropin Receptor:

Application to the Study of Receptor Structure and Turnover[a]

PHILIPPE CRINE and MURIEL AUBRY

Département de Biochimie
Université de Montréal
Montréal, Canada H3C 3J7

MICHEL POTIER

Section de Génétique Médicale
Hôpital Sainte-Justine
Université de Montréal
Montréal, Canada H3T 1C5

The initial step in the action of many hormones and neurotransmitters is their binding to specific receptors localized in the plasma membrane of target cells.[1-3] Plasma membrane receptors for gonadotropins in Leydig cells of the testis were initially recognized more than a decade ago.[4-7] The initial response of testicular Leydig cells to gonadotropins is an increase in cyclic AMP formation, which stimulates testosterone secretion.[8] Administration of luteinizing hormone (LH) or human chorionic gonadotropin (hCG) to rats is followed by a dose- and time-dependent refractory period where desensitization of Leydig cell has been shown to depend on several factors, including gonadotropin receptor loss from the plasma membrane.[9,10] The mechanisms involved in this receptor loss have not yet been fully defined. Recent reports suggest that receptor-hormone complexes are internalized by hormone-induced endocytosis and are then degraded in lysosomes.[12-14] This period of net receptor loss is followed by restoration of the receptor number to normal over the next 6 to 10 days.[9]

In order to approach the questions of receptor down-regulation and replenishment it would be very useful to follow the biosynthesis of receptor components as well as the fate of newly synthesized receptor subunits at the cell surface. Unfortunately, a detailed description of the structural components of the gonadotropin receptor is still lacking mainly because of the low concentration of the receptor in target cells and difficulties encountered in purifying highly active forms of the protein.

The purpose of this study was to determine whether biosynthesis of gonadotropin receptor components could be observed in rat Leydig cells. Obtaining radiolabeled receptor components could pave the way for more detailed structural studies and lead to a better understanding of the molecular mechanisms involved in receptor turnover.

[a] Supported by the Medical Research Council of Canada (MA8064).

In order to purify Leydig cells, collagenase-dispersed cells were first prepared from testes of 250–300 g Sprague-Dawley male rats (Charles River Laboratories, St. Constant, Qúebec) essentially as described by Dufau *et al.*[15] and then fractionated on discontinuous Percoll gradients. For making isoosmotic Percoll gradients, a stock solution was first prepared by mixing nine parts of Percoll (Pharmacia) with one part of a tenfold concentrated solution of Earle's salts (Gibco) containing 7% bovine serum albumin (BSA) and buffered with 250 mM HEPES pH 7.4.[16] Discontinuous Percoll gradients were prepared by successively layering appropriate dilutions of this stock solution in a 50 ml polyethylene centrifuge tube (FIGURE 1). The bottom layer (5 ml) had a density of 1.123 g/ml (as measured by refractive index). The upper layers (8 ml each) had densities of 1.050 g/ml and 1.033 g/ml,

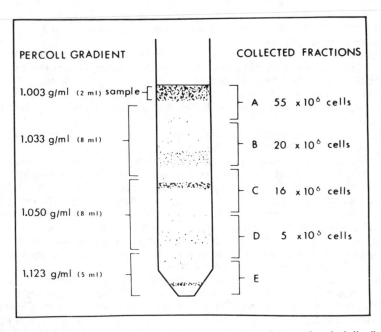

FIGURE 1. Characteristics of the discontinuous Percoll gradients and typical distribution of the testicular collagenase-dispersed cells after centrifugation.

respectively. In a typical experiment, 10^8 collagenase-dispersed cells obtained from two testes were resuspended in 2 ml of a mixture of Ham's F12 and Dulbecco's modified Eagle medium (F12/DME) (1 : 1) (Gibco) containing 0.1% BSA and layered on top of the gradient. Centrifugation was performed at 800 *g* for 15 min at 4°C, in the swinging bucket rotor of a IEC centrifuge. Four visible bands were observed after the centrifugation. Approximately 55×10^6 cells were recovered in band A (FIGURE 1). Band B was the broadest in width and contained approximately 20×10^6 cells, most of which appeared to be germ cells. Band C was sharply delineated; it migrated at a density of 1.053 g/ml and was largely composed of cells that had a morphology very similar to those of band D, when observed with a light microscope. Band D was found at an average density of 1.075 g/ml. It was composed of a 90% homogeneous preparation of cells and more than 95% of these were viable as judged by trypan blue dye exclusion. The very sharp band E migrating at the bottom of the tube consisted almost exclusively of red blood cells.

In order to determine hCG binding as a function of cell location in the gradient, we next incubated about 30×10^6 crude interstitial cells for 1 hr at 36°C in 2 ml of medium containing 1.5×10^6 cpm of $[^{125}I]$hCG prepared as described by Dufau et al.[15] (specific activity 11.8 μCi/μg; 13,500 IU/mg; Boehringer Mannheim Canada). The nonspecific binding was evaluated in parallel on an identical sample after the addition of an excess of unlabeled hCG (500 IU). The cells were then washed twice with 10 ml of medium and applied to Percoll gradients. After centrifugation, the bottom of the tube was punctured and the gradient fractionated. The number of cells and $[^{125}I]$hCG binding was determined for each fraction. Nonspecific binding was substracted from the total amount of $[^{125}I]$hCG bound and the results expressed as cpm/10^6 cells.

The ability of cells from each fraction to respond to hCG stimulation by increased testosterone production was also determined during *in vitro* incubations. The cells were washed, resuspended at a density of 5×10^5 cells/ml, and incubated in the presence or in the absence of 100 mIU hCG (APL-Ayerst) for 3 hr at 34°C. Testosterone levels in the incubation medium were measured by radioimmunoassay.[18]

As seen in TABLE 1 and in FIGURE 2, only cells from band D exhibited high basal and hCG-stimulated testosterone production as well as high $[^{125}I]$hCG binding activity. Band C (found at a density of 1.053 g/ml) corresponded to a small hCG binding activity but did not respond to hCG by increased testosterone production. This fraction is thought to contain Leydig cells, possibly from a second population as already reported by others.[19-23] Band A, remaining at the top of the gradient, was composed of damaged cells and viable large cells with a morphology completely different from that of the Leydig cells of band D. The small hCG binding activity recovered at this position is probably due to the presence of Leydig cell membrane fragments. Band B showed virtually no hCG binding and only small basal level testosterone production.

Only purified Leydig cells from band D were used for metabolic labeling. They were washed and resuspended at a density of 4×10^6 cells/ml in methionine-free RPMI 1640 medium containing $[^{35}S]$methionine (0.2–0.4 mCi/ml, 1200 Ci/mmol, Amersham) and 10% dialyzed fetal calf serum. The cells were then plated in Petri dishes and incubated for 17 hr at 37°C under an atmosphere of 5% CO_2 and 95% air. At different times during the incubation, the cells were washed to remove free $[^{35}S]$methionine and the amount of radioactivity incorporated into cell proteins in

TABLE 1. Basal and hCG-stimulated Testosterone Production of Rat Testis Cells Fractionated on Percoll Gradients

	Testosterone Production (ng/10^6 cells/3 hr)	
Cell Fraction	Basal	hCG-stimulated
A	0.55 ± 0.01	0.61 ± 0.00
B	0.51 ± 0.01	0.53 ± 0.01
C	0.70 ± 0.01	0.94 ± 0.04
D	6.36 ± 0.86	19.98 ± 0.14

Values are means ± S.D.

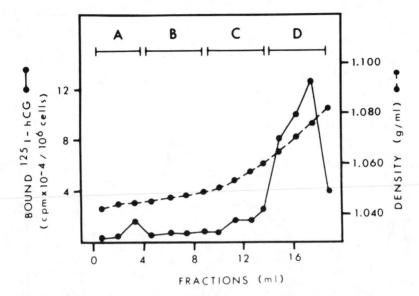

FIGURE 2. Typical [^{125}I]hCG profile obtained for testicular collagenase-dispersed cells fractionated on discontinuous Percoll gradient. The bars at the top of the figure delineate the different bands of cells used for measuring testosterone production.

each culture was determined by the procedure of Mans and Novelli.[24] FIGURE 3 shows that incorporation of [^{35}S]methionine into trichloroacetic acid–precipitable material was linear for at least 18 hr. These results demonstrate that discontinuous Percoll gradients can be used for the isolation of a highly purified, viable rat Leydig cell population. These gradients can very easily be prepared in large numbers and under sterile conditions. These features make them amenable to routine laboratory use, particularly when cell culture is anticipated.

In order to identify eventual labeled receptor components in crude extracts of Leydig cells, we have attempted to purify the proteins by affinity chromatography on an agarose-hCG resin. Previous studies by Dufau *et al.*[25] had shown that gonadotropin receptors could be purified 15,000-fold by this procedure. An affinity resin was therefore prepared by covalently linking partially purified hCG (Ayerst Canada) to Affigel-10 (BioRad) according to the manufacturer's instructions (2,500–3,000 IU of hCG coupled/ml of packed gel).

In a pilot experiment, we verified first that this affinity resin was capable of removing all hCG binding components from a Triton X-100–solubilized receptor preparation. For this purpose 1 ml of packed agarose–hCG derivative was shaken for 16 hr at 4°C with solubilized testicular particules (from 20 testes) in 50 mM phosphate-buffered saline (pH 7.4) (PBS) containing 0.2% Triton X-100 (BDH) as described by Dufau *et al.*[26] The gel suspension was then allowed to settle and the supernatant was incubated overnight at 4°C with [^{125}I]hCG. No binding activity was detected in the supernatant as evaluated by precipitation with polyethylene glycol.[27] By contrast, 38% of the original binding activity of the crude soluble receptor preparation was recovered when the agarose derivative was covalently coupled to ethanolamine. Taking into account that approximately 66% degradation of the original binding capacity was observed when the detergent-solubilized

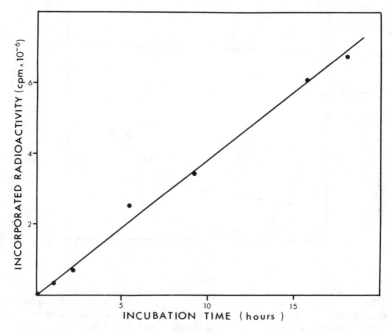

FIGURE 3. Incorporation of [³⁵S]methionine into proteins of purified Leydig cells.

receptor preparation was stored at 4°C, these results allow us to conclude that, under our experimental conditions, the affinity resin was capable of binding completely and selectively gonadotropin receptor components. Unlike Dufau et al.,[25] we were unable to recover active binding components by acid elution from the affinity resin. Similar problems have also been encountered by others[28] and were assumed to be due to very tight binding of receptor components to the affinity resin. In our hands, proteins bound to the resin could be eluted only under highly denaturing conditions such as those provided by the sample buffers used for one- or two-dimensional gel electrophoresis.[29,30] Under those conditions however, receptor components lost all binding activity. Therefore, in order to distinguish between specific binding of receptor components and eventual non-specific trapping of radioactive proteins by the resin, we performed control experiments where binding of the solubilized Leydig cell proteins to the resin was done in the presence of a 100-fold excess of soluble hCG (Ayerst).

In order to prepare ³⁵S-labeled receptor components, Leydig cells that had been incubated for 17 hr in the presence of [³⁵S]methionine as described above were washed twice with ice-cold 50 mM phosphate-buffered saline at pH 7.4 (PBS) and proteins from washed cells were then solubilized for 60 min at 4°C in 400 μl of PBS containing 1% Triton X-100 and 1 mM phenylmethylsulfonyl fluoride (PMSF) (Sigma). This preparation was diluted five fold with PBS, centrifuged at 100,000 × g for 90 min at 4°C and the pellet was discarded. The supernatant was mixed with 50 μl of the affinity resin. The mixture was rotated at 4°C for 16 hr and the resin was washed extensively by centrifugation in 1.5 ml Eppendorf microcentrifuge tubes with PBS solutions containing decreasing concentrations of Triton X-100 (0.2%, 0.1%, and 0.05%) and finally with PBS alone. All washing solutions contained 2 mM methionine to help removal of trapped [³⁵S]methionine.

After washing, the resin was boiled for 3 min in Laemmli's sample buffer[29] also containing 2 mM PMSF and 2 mM methionine. Labeled proteins were submitted to electrophoresis under reducing conditions in a 7.5% polyacrylamide gel containing 0.1% sodium dodecyl sulfate under reducing conditions exactly as described by Laemmli.[29] The labeled protein bands were revealed by autoradiography and the pattern compared to the ones obtained from an experiment where identical aliquots of the solubilized extract had been mixed with an excess of hCG (compared to the amount of hCG bound to the gel) prior to the affinity purification step. FIGURE 4 shows that in the absence of hCG (lane 1), the affinity resin had

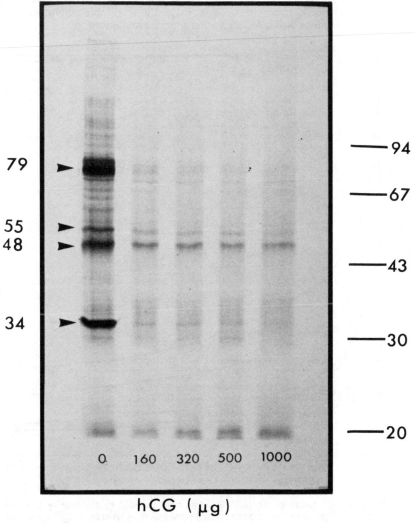

FIGURE 4. Autoradiography of one-dimensional gel electrophoresis of [^{35}S]methionine proteins bound to the hCG affinity resin in the absence (lane 1) or in the presence of excess of soluble hCG (lanes 2 to 5).

retained four major protein species migrating with apparent molecular weights of 79,000, 55,000, 48,000 and 34,000, respectively. However, in the presence of an amount of hCG varying from a 17-fold to 111-fold excess (lanes 2 to 5), most of the radioactivity associated with these bands disappeared. Microdensitometric scanning of each lane allowed an estimation of the amount of radioactivity associated with each protein species. The results, when plotted as a function of the amount of competing hCG (FIGURE 5), clearly show that the 79,000 dalton and the 39,000 dalton proteins behaved quite similarly during the competition experiment. They were readily displaced from the affinity matrix by low concentrations of competing hCG. On the contrary, displacement of the 55,000 and 48,000 dalton proteins required larger amounts of competing hCG. The 48,000 and 55,000 proteins seemed to bind more strongly to the resin, suggesting a preferential binding to the immobilized hormone and a reduced affinity for the natural ligand.

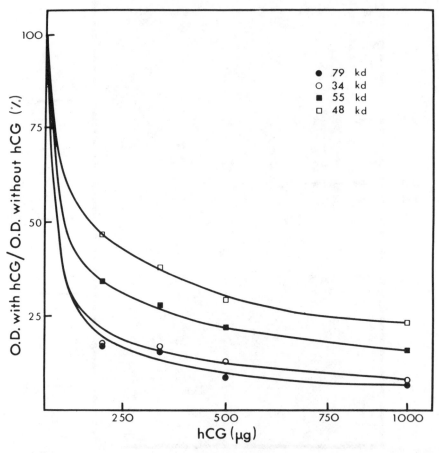

FIGURE 5. Displacement of the four major proteins retained by the affinity resin with increasing concentrations of soluble hCG. Each point was calculated by using the microdensity scanning of each lane of FIGURE 4 and was expressed as a percentage of the control without hCG.

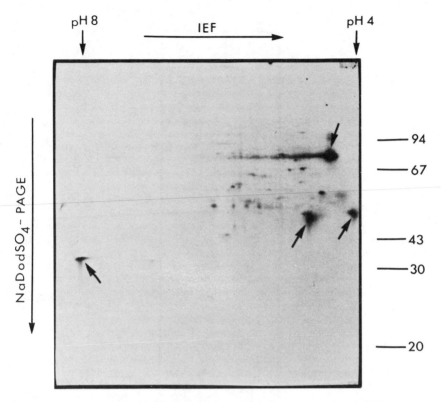

FIGURE 6. Autoradiography of a two-dimensional gel electrophoresis of [^{35}S]methionine proteins bound to the hCG affinity resin.

These [^{35}S]methionine-labeled proteins were next analyzed on two-dimensional gels according to the method of O'Farrell.[30] As can be seen on FIGURE 6, the 79,000 dalton protein was quite acidic and migrated in the electrofocusing dimension of the gel with an isoelectric point of 4.5. The 55,000 and 48,000 dalton proteins also focused in the acidic region of the gel. By contrast, the 34,000 dalton protein was found to be very basic and focused at a pH of 8.0.

In order to test the possibility that the 34,000, 48,000, and 55,000 dalton proteins could represent degradation products of a 79,000 dalton true binding component, we repeated the isolation of these proteins in the absence of protease inhibitors. As shown in FIGURE 7, the 34,000 and 79,000 dalton proteins were recovered with the same yield whether protease inhibitors were omitted or present throughout the whole experiment. Unless the proteases responsible for protein degradation in the testis are insensitive to aprotinin and PMSF fluoride, it seems therefore unlikely that the smaller molecular weight species could represent artifacts of extraction. Moreover, if smaller fragments had appeared through the degradation of a true receptor component of 79,000 daltons, it is most probable that they would have grossly altered binding properties.

By contrast, FIGURES 4 and 5 show that the affinity of the 34,000 and 79,000 dalton proteins for the ligand was quite similar. It is also highly improbable that a

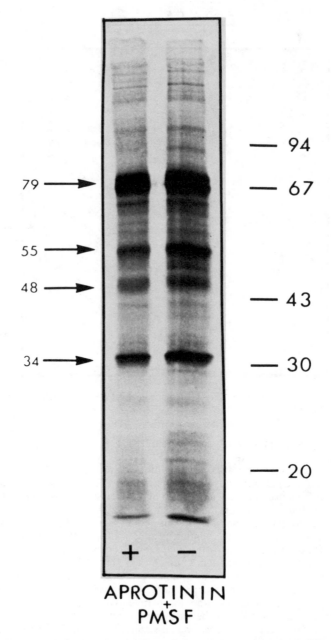

FIGURE 7. Autoradiography of a one-dimensional gel electrophoresis of [^{35}S]methionine proteins bound to the hCG affinity resin in the absence (*right lane*) or the presence (*left lane*) of phenylmethylsulfonyl fluoride and aprotinin.

79,000 dalton protein with an isoelectric point of 4.5 could contain within its sequence a 34,000 dalton fragment focusing at the basic end of the pH scale.

Taken together, these results suggest that the 34,000 and 79,000 dalton proteins could represent true receptor subunits. However, we are still at a loss to assign a precise function for the 48,000 and 55,000 dalton proteins. We cannot rule out completely the possibility that degradation by a protease insensitive to aprotinin and PMSF occurs during the solubilization step in our procedure.

Although direct proof of the true receptor nature of the 34,000 and 79,000 dalton radiolabeled proteins isolated by affinity chromatography is still lacking, several lines of evidence support the idea that they represent specific subunits of the gonadotropin receptor. First, when solubilized material from purified rat Leydig cells was mixed with a 100-fold excess of partially purified hCG, a significant decrease in the binding of the labeled protein was observed. This effect was due to the gonadotropin itself and not to contaminants of the preparation since it was observed with purified hCG (as prepared by concavalin A affinity chromatography) and not with the other proteins of the preparation unrelated to hCG or with ovalbumin (results not shown). Moreover, these proteins were not observed when a bovine serum albumin-affigel resin was used. Second, the electrophoretic characteristics of this protein are in good agreement with previously published reports. Using the same procedure for solubilizing and purifying rat testis receptors, Dufau *et al.*[25] have proposed a molecular weight of 90,000 for the main receptor subunit, after correcting for the hydrophobicity of the protein. In good agreement with our data, Saxena[31] has also reported the presence of an 80,000 dalton receptor component with a pI of 4.5 in bovine corpora lutea membranes. More recently Dattatreyamurty *et al.*[32] have found an additional component of $M_r = 38,000$ from the same source.

From several other studies it would appear however that the molecular weight of the testicular and ovarian LH-hCG receptor may range from 194,000 to 280,000.[32,33] It should be emphasized that these molecular weights have been obtained mostly by gel permeation chromatography in which detergent molecules bound to the receptor could substantially affect the conformation and thereby the Stokes radius of the molecules. In order to avoid the drawbacks of these methods, we have sought to determine the molecular weight of the gonadotropin receptor in Leydig cells by radiation inactivation. With this method, the receptors do not need to be solubilized and can be studied *in situ* in crude lyophilized preparations. Kempner *et al.*[34] suggested that the radiation inactivation method takes into account the functional unit (i.e. the minimal structural assembly necessary for a given biological activity) and the degree of coupling between subunits that would allow energy transfer rather than the structural size of the molecule. Relatively large dose rates (1–2 Mrad/min) are usually employed. For our studies, we used a ^{60}Co bomb that delivers about 10^4 rad/min. Beauregard and Potier[35] indicate that such a relatively low dose-rate apparatus can be used, providing an appropriate calibration curve with enzymes of known radiation sensitivities is constructed.

Testicular homogenates were prepared in PBS buffer as described by Tsuruhara,[36] lyophilized in 1.5 ml Eppendorf microcentrifuge tubes and flushed with nitrogen. Such receptor preparations were stable for at least two weeks at room temperature. No difference in binding activities of lyophilized samples were found when compared to identical non-lyophilized samples.

The tubes were exposed to the 5,000 Ci ^{60}Co source (Gamma-cell model 220, Atomic Energy of Canada, Ottawa) at room temperature (26 ± 2°C). Appropriate controls of nonirradiated preparations were run concurrently. At least three tubes were exposed for each radiation dose. Hormone binding assays were done

essentially as described by Tsuruhara.[36] The radiation inactivation curve of go-
nadotropin receptor is shown in FIGURE 8. It can be seen that specific binding of
[^{125}I]hCG to testicular homogenates decreases as the irradiation dose increases.
Irradiation had no significant effect on the value of the dissociation constant
($K_d = 8.8 \pm 4.3 \times 10^{-11}$ M). The observed decreases in binding therefore re-
sulted from loss of functional binding sites.

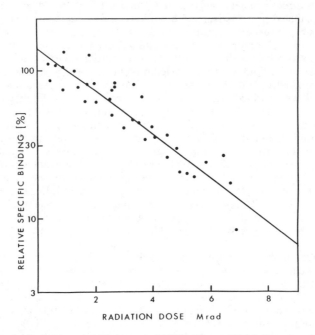

FIGURE 8. Radiation inactivation curve of [^{125}I]hCG-specific binding sites in testicular
homogenates. Each value recorded is the mean of triplicate determinations and the figure is
representative of four separate irradiation experiments.

The empirical equation of Kepner and Macey[37] relates the radiation dose (in
megarads) necessary to inactivate a given protein activity (enzyme or receptor) to
37% of its initial value (D_{37}) to the molecular mass,

$$M_r = (6.4 \times 10^5)/D_{37}.$$

Using this relation we determined a molecular weight of 170,000 $\pm$ 20,000 (mean
$\pm$ SD, $N = 5$) for the testicular gonadotropin receptor.

In spite of the limits inherent in the radiation inactivation technique for the
determination of molecular weight, two conclusions can be reached from all these
data. (1) The M_r found here for the hCG binding component from rat testis ($M_r =$
170,000) agrees reasonably well with those of previously reported results. A molecular weight of 194,000 was determined by sucrose density gradient ultracentrifugation and by gel filtration by Dufau et al.[27] In a recent study on the
gonadotropin receptor of the luteinized rat ovary, Wimalasena and Dufau[38] also

found a hormone binding component of 165,000 by gel chromatography and by nonreducing polyacrylamide gel electrophoresis. Dattatreyamurty *et al.*[32] recently reported on the isolation of a high molecular mass aggregate ($M_r = 5.9 \times 10^6$) that could be dissociated further into $M_r = 280,000$ and $M_r = 140,000$ species. The smaller molecular weight species reported here by us and elsewhere by others[25,31,32,38-40] must certainly be part of a larger receptor complex with a molecular weight in the range of 140,000–200,000. As indicated by our radiation inactivation studies, this complex could represent the minimal binding species present in the membrane.

In conclusion, our studies agree well with many other reports suggesting an oligomeric nature of the LH-hCG receptor. In addition, the present study demonstrates that rat Leydig cells prepared by Percoll gradient centrifugation can incorporate radioactive amino acids into proteins that are specifically retained by a hCG affinity matrix and are for this reason thought to represent gonadotropin receptor subunits. This new strategy could provide a convenient alternative for studying receptor structure, using only a limited amount of starting material. The ability to biosynthetically label the gonadotropin receptor could also open new avenues for the study of receptor regulation in various cell types and under various physiologic conditions.

ACKNOWLEDGMENTS

We are grateful to Ayerst Laboratories for a generous gift of hCG. We thank Dr. R. Collu and J.-R. Ducharme for performing the testosterone radioimmunoassays, for providing space in their laboratory and for stimulating discussions during the early part of this work. The dedicated help of Rose-Mai Roy for the preparation of this manuscript is also acknowledged.

REFERENCES

1. KAHN, C.R. 1976. J. Cell Biol. **70:** 261–286.
2. CATT, K. J., J. P. HARWOOD, G. AGUILERA & M. L. DUFAU. 1979. Nature **280:** 109–116.
3. TELL, G. P., F. HAOUR & J. M. SAEZ. 1978. Metabolism **27:** 1566–1592.
4. LEIDENBERGER, F. & L. E. JR. REICHERT. 1972. Endocrinology **91:** 901–909.
5. MENDELSON, C., M. L. DUFAU & K. J. CATT. 1975. J. Biol. Chem. **250:** 8818–8823.
6. BELLISARIO, R. & D. P. BAHL. 1975. J. Biol. Chem. **250:** 3837–3844.
7. ASCOLI, M. & D. PUETT. 1978. Proc. Natl. Acad. Sci. USA **75:** 99–102.
8. DUFAU, M. L. & K. J. CATT. 1978. Vitam. Horm. **36:** 461–592.
9. TSURAHARA, T., M.L. DUFAU, S. CIGORRAGA & K. J. CATT. 1977. J. Biol. Chem. **252:** 9002–9009.
10. CIGORRAGA, S. B., M. L. DUFAU & K. J. CATT. 1978. J. Biol. Chem. **253:** 4294–4304.
11. HAOUR, J. & J. M. SAEZ. 1977. Mol. Cell Endocrinol. **1:** 17–24.
12. CONN, P. M., M. CONTI, J. P. HARWOOD, M. L. DUFAU & K.J. CATT. 1978. Nature **274:** 598–600.
13. ASCOLI, M. & D. PUETT. 1978. J. Biol. Chem. **253:** 4892–4899.
14. RAJANIEMI, H. J., M. MANNINEN & I. T. HUHTANIEMI. 1979. Endocrinology **105:** 1208–1214.
15. DUFAU, M. L., C. R. MENDELSON & K. J. CATT. 1974. J. Clin. Endocrinol. Metab. **36:** 1132–1142.
16. SCHUMACHER, M., G. SCHÄFER, A. F. HOLSTEIN & H. HILZ. 1978. FEBS Lett. **91:** 333–338.

17. DUFAU, M. L., E. J. PODESTA & K. J. CATT. 1975. Proc. Natl. Acad. Sci. USA **72:** 1272–1275.
18. FOREST, M. G., A. M. CATHIARD & J. A. BERTRAND. 1973. J. Clin. Endocrinol. Metab. **36:** 1132–1142.
19. JANSZEN, F. H. A., B. A. COOKE, M. J. A. VAN DRIED & H. J. VAN DER MOLEN. 1976. J. Endocrinol. **70:** 345–359.
20. PAYNE, A. H., J. R. DOWNING & K. L. WONG. 1980. Endocrinology **106:** 1424–1429.
21. COOKE, B. A., R. MAGEE-BROWN, M. GOLDING & C. J. CIX. 1981. Int. J. Androl. **4:** 355–366.
22. DEHEJIA, A., K. NOZU, K. J. CATT & M. L. DUFAU. 1982. Ann. N.Y. Acad. Sci. **383:** 204–211.
23. LEFEBVRE, A., J. M. SAEZ & C. FINAZ. 1983. Hormone Res. **17:** 114–120.
24. MANS, R. J. & G. D. NOVELLI. 1961. Arch. Biochem. Biophys. **94:** 48–53.
25. DUFAU, M. L., D. W. RYAN, A. J. BAUKAL & K. J. CATT. 1975. J. Biol. Chem. **250:** 4822–4824.
26. DUFAU, M. L. & K. J. CATT. 1974. FEBS Lett. **52:** 273–277.
27. DUFAU, M. L., E. H. CHARREAU & K. J. CATT. 1973. J. Biol. Chem. **248:** 6973–6982.
28. METSIKKO, K. & H. RAJANIEMI. 1979. FEBS Lett. **106:** 193–196.
29. LAEMMLI, U. K. 1970. Nature **227:** 680–685.
30. O'FARRELL, P. H. 1975. J. Biol. Chem. **250:** 4007–4021.
31. SAXENA, B. B. *In* Methods in Receptor Research. M. Blecher, Ed. **1:** 251–295. Marcel Dekker. New York.
32. DATTATREYAMURTY, B., P. RATHNAM & B. B. SAXENA. 1983. J. Biol. Chem. **258:** 3140–3158.
33. DUFAU, M. L., E. H. CHARREAU & K. J. CATT. 1973. J. Biol. Chem. **248:** 6973–6982.
34. KEMPNER, E. S. & W. SCHLEGEL. 1979. Anal. Biochem. **92:** 2–10.
35. BEAUREGARD, G. & M. POTIER. 1982. Anal. Biochem. **122:** 379–384.
36. TSURUHARA, T., M. L. DUFAU, S. CIGORRAGA & K. J. CATT. 1977. J. Biol. Chem. **252:** 9002–9009.
37. KEPNER, G. R. & R. I. MACEY. 1968. Biochim. Biophys. Acta **163:** 188–203.
38. WIMALASENA, J. & M. L. DUFAU. 1981. Endocrinology **110:** 1004–1012.
39. METSIKKO, K. & H. RAJANIEMI. 1980. Biochem. Biophys. Res. Commun. **95:** 1730–1736.
40. REBOIS, R. V., F. OMEDEO-SALE, R. D. BRADY & P. H. FISHMAN. 1981. Proc. Natl. Acad. Sci. USA **78:** 2086–2089.

Studies on Leydig Cell Purification

DANIEL R. AQUILANO and MARIA L. DUFAU

Section of Molecular Endocrinology
Endocrinology and Reproduction Research Branch
National Institute of Child Health and Human Development
National Institutes of Health
Bethesda, Maryland 20205

Studies on purified Leydig cells have been of considerable value in the analysis of hormonal regulation of gonadotropin receptors and the control of androgen biosynthesis.[1,2] Also, Leydig cell purification has been useful for studies on specific aspects of gonadotropin action and cyclic AMP–mediated events, including occupancy of protein kinase regulatory subunits[3] and phosphorylation of endogenous protein substrates.[4] Leydig cell purification has been performed in a number of laboratories by using density gradient centrifugation (TABLE 1). Most methods have employed continuous or discontinuous Percoll gradients and continuous Metrizamide gradients. The recovery and degree of purity of the final Leydig cell preparation, as well as the number of cell bands obtained, depended on the range of concentrations used in the gradients. However, since less than 100 million cells can be resolved on each gradient, and testicular interstitial cell suspensions obtained by collagenase digestion contain only 15–25% Leydig cells, a considerable number of gradients must be performed to prepare large quantities of pure Leydig cells. This limitation of the density gradient method led us to evaluate the efficacy of centrifugal elutriation, which has a higher capacity and is more rapid than most other methods for preparing homogeneous cell fractions. This technique has been used for separating a variety of cell types including mast cells,[11] spermatogenic cells,[12] liver cells,[13] solid tumor cells,[14] and more recently, pituitary cells.[15] Centrifugal elutriation combines centrifugal and hydrodynamic forces for separating cells or other particles of different sedimentation velocities.[16,17] The system consists of a separation chamber located in a specially designed centrifuge rotor (JE-6E, Beckman, Palo Alto, CA) through which buffer and sample can be injected and further collected from outside, while the rotor is spinning (FIGURE 1). The flow rate is controlled by a pump (Masterflex 7014, Cole Parmer, Chicago, IL) that must be calibrated before each run to ensure reproducibility of the separation. The chamber is made of transparent plastic so that with the illumination provided by a strobe light mounted in the centrifuge well, the movements of the cell boundary can be observed through a window located in the centrifuge lid. Cells are subjected to two opposing forces within the separation chamber: the centrifugal field generated by the spinning rotor and the counterflow of fluid in the opposite direction (FIGURE 2). Each cell tends to migrate to a zone where its sedimentation velocity is exactly balanced by the flow rate of the fluid through the separation chamber. By increasing the flow rate in steps, or decreasing the rotor speed, successive populations of relatively homogeneous cell sizes can be washed from the chamber.

TABLE 1. Comparison of Various Rat Leydig Cell Purification Procedures

Authors	Year	Method	Degree of Purity of the Final Preparation (%)	Leydig Cell Recovery (%)
Janszen et al.[5]	1976	Ficoll gradient	42–76	29
Conn et al.[1]	1977	Metrizamide gradient	94	25
Schumacher et al.[6]	1978	Percoll gradient	90–95	<36
Payne et al.[7]	1980	Metrizamide gradient	90–95	30–35
Browning et al.[8]	1981	Percoll gradient	90–95	5–10
Dehejia et al.[9]	1982	Metrizamide gradient	90–95	50–60
Gale et al.[10]	1982	Percoll gradient	71–79	51

CENTRIFUGAL ELUTRIATION OF TESTICULAR INTERSTITIAL CELLS

To determine the resolution of testicular interstitial cells in terms of their sedimentation velocities, the crude preparation obtained by collagenase digestion of decapsulated testes from adult Sprague-Dawley rats[18] was applied to the elutriator. Approximately one billion nucleated cells suspended in 50 ml of elutriation buffer (medium 199 containing 1.4 g/l $NaHCO_3$, 0.5% BSA, 1 mM EDTA, 50

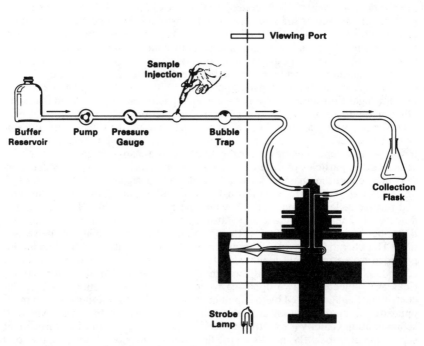

FIGURE 1. The centrifugal elutriation system. See explanation in the text. (Reproduced with permission from the elutriator manual. Beckman, Palo Alto, CA).

U/ml heparin, 12.5 μg/ml DNase I, and 50 μg/ml gentamycin) were injected into the chamber at a flow rate of 3.5 ml/min while the rotor speed was kept constant at 2,000 rpm. The flow rate was then increased to 7 ml/min, collecting 150 ml of elutriation buffer to allow the cells of a given sedimentation velocity to exit (Fraction 1, TABLE 2). This procedure was repeated until the maximal speed of the pump was reached (Fraction 11). Then, the rotor was stopped and cells

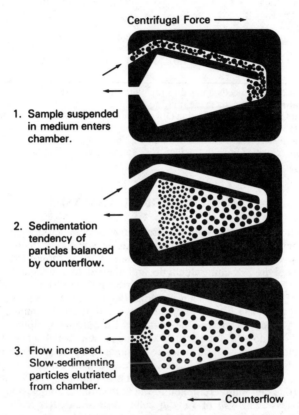

Centrifugal Force ⟶

1. Sample suspended
   in medium enters
   chamber.

2. Sedimentation
   tendency of
   particles balanced
   by counterflow.

3. Flow increased.
   Slow-sedimenting
   particles elutriated
   from chamber.

⟵ Counterflow

FIGURE 2. The separation chamber. See explanation in the text. (Reproduced with permission from publication DS-534. Beckman, Palo Alto, CA).

remaining in the chamber were collected in fraction 12 (wash out). Sedimentation velocities of the cells were calculated using the equation:

$$s = 1.93 \times f/R^2,$$

where s is the sedimentation velocity (mm/h $\cdot$ g), f is the volumetric flow rate (ml/min), R the rotor speed expressed in units of 10^3 rpm, and 1.93 is a constant factor involving chamber and rotor characteristics and conversions from minutes to hours and centimeters to millimeters.[12] Cells from each fraction were pelleted at 400 $\times$ g and were further subjected to morphological and functional analyses.

TABLE 2. Centrifugal Elutriation of Collagenase-dispersed Rat Testicular Interstitial Cells

Fraction Number	1	2	3	4	5	6	7	8	9	10	11	12
Flow rate (ml/min)	7	10	13	15	17.5	20	25	30	35	40	45.5	wash out
Sedimentation velocity (mm/h · g)	3.3	4.8	6.2	7.2	8.4	9.6	12	14.4	16.8	19.3	22	>22
Recovered cells (%)[a]	56	2.1	11	4.2	3.5	3.4	4.0	3.4	3.0	3.5	2.8	3.1
Leydig cells (%)[b]	0	0	0.9	1.0	2.5	7	12	93	95	94	92	93

[a] From total nucleated cells applied to the elutriation chamber.

[b] From total nucleated cells present in the fraction.

The crude interstitial cell preparation (10^9 nucleated cells) was separated into 12 fractions. Fractions 1–11 were obtained by collecting 100–150 ml of elutriation buffer at each indicated flow rate. Fraction 12 was obtained by stopping the rotor and collecting a further 150 ml. Sedimentation velocities of each fraction were calculated as indicated in the text.

MORPHOLOGICAL ANALYSIS

The total number of viable cells per fraction was obtained after methylene blue staining, whereas the Leydig cell number was obtained after histochemical staining for Δ_5-3β-hydroxysteroid dehydrogenase.[19] For microphotography, cell pellets were fixed in 2% glutaraldehyde and then dehydrated and embedded in Epon.[20] Thick sections (1 μm) for light microscopy were stained with methylene blue-azure II (1 : 1 vol/vol). Thin sections (50–60 nm) for electron microscopy were stained with OsO_4[21] and uranyl acetate,[22] and further examined in a Siemens Elmiskop 1A electron microscope. Samples for autoradiography were preincubated with [^{125}I]iodo-hCG for 3 hr at 35°C in the presence or absence of an excess of cold hCG and washed several times to eliminate free tracer. Specimens for microscopy were prepared as indicated above and then exposed to photographic emulsion for one month. As shown in TABLE 2, fractions 1 to 7 contained 80 to 85% of the total cell number applied to the elutriation chamber, and only a minor proportion (less than 4%) of Leydig cells were found. Red cells were mostly concentrated in fractions 1 and 2. Fractions 8 to 12 comprised 15–20% of the original cells, and contained 90–95% positive stained Leydig cells. FIGURE 3A shows a light micrograph of the crude interstitial cell preparation containing approximately 20% Leydig cells (dark cells). Electron microscope analysis of this preparation (FIGURE 3B) indicated the presence of normal Leydig cells, germinal cells, lymphocytes, endothelial cells, macrophages, damaged cells, and cellular debris. After elutriation, light microscopy of fractions 1–7 (FIGURE 4A) showed the absence of dark cells, indicating the absence of Leydig cells. These fractions were shown to be composed of germinal cells, endothelial cells, lymphocytes, red cells, macrophages, cellular debris, and damaged cells (FIGURE 4B). On the other hand, fractions 8 to 12 contained highly purified Leydig cells (FIGURE 5A). Electron micrographs of these fractions (FIGURE 5B) showed the presence of morphologically intact Leydig cells displaying their ultrastructural characteristics such as abundant smooth endoplasmic reticulum, mitochondria with lamellar cristae, lipid droplets, and a nucleus with a rim of heterochromatin.[23,24] Only a small contami-

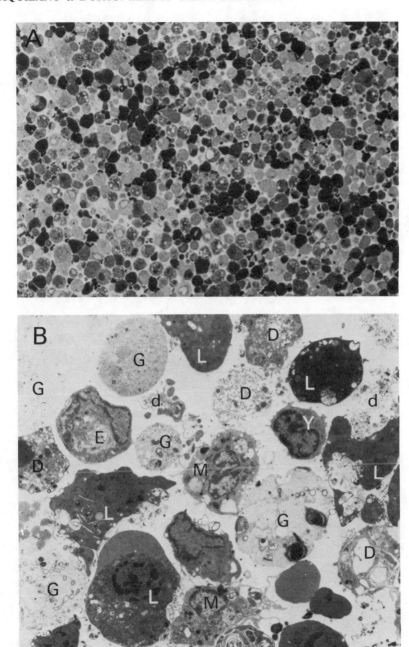

FIGURE 3. (A) Light micrograph (× 300) of the crude interstitial cell preparation from the adult rat testis. Leydig cells (dark cells) represent approximately 20% of the total population. (B) Electron micrograph (× 2,100) of the same preparation showing intact Leydig cells (L), germinal cells (G), endothelial cells (E), lymphocytes (Y), damaged cells (D), macrophages (M), and cellular debris (d).

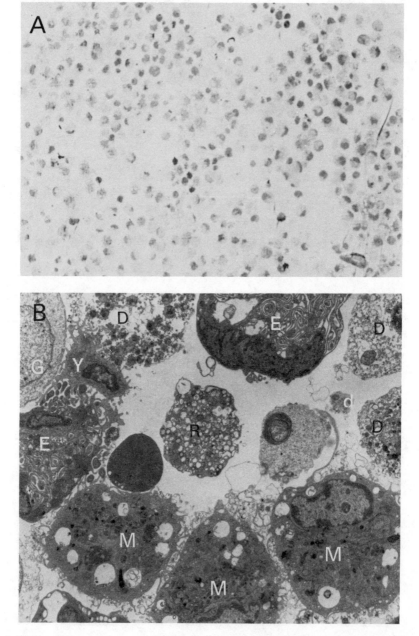

FIGURE 4. (A) Light micrograph (× 300) of a pool of fractions 1–7 from elutriation. (B) Electron micrograph (× 4,000) of the same preparation showing germinal cells (G), endothelial cells (E), lymphocytes (Y), macrophages (M), residual bodies (R), damaged cells (D), and cellular debris (d).

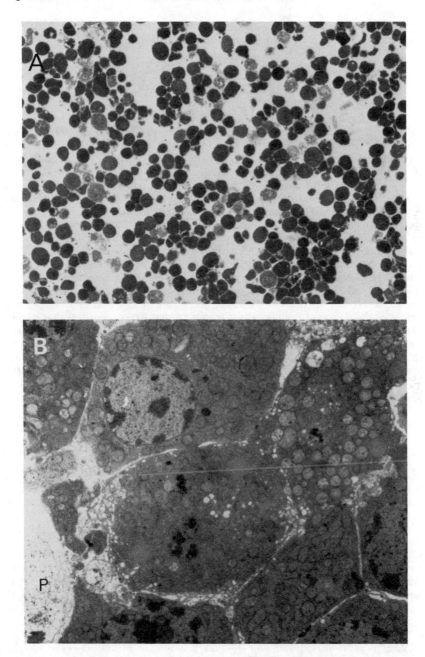

FIGURE 5. (A) Light micrograph (× 300) of a pool of fractions 8–12 from elutriation containing more than 90% Leydig cells. (B) Electron micrograph (× 3,100) of the same preparation showing morphologically intact Leydig cells and a minor contamination with pachytene spermatocytes (P).

nation (6–8%) with pachytene spermatocytes was observed, as judged by their characteristic nucleus containing synaptolema complexes.[25]

FUNCTIONAL ANALYSIS

Studies on the functional activity of the individual fractions obtained by centrifugal elutriation were performed by incubation of the cells in medium 199 and 0.1% BSA for 3 hr under 95% O_2 : 5% CO_2 in the presence or absence of hCG to measure testosterone[26] (FIGURE 6, upper panel) and cyclic AMP production[3] (FIGURE 6, middle panels), and in the presence of [125I]iodo-hCG plus or minus an excess of cold hCG to measure the receptor binding capacity[2] (FIGURE 6, lower panel). This study demonstrated that the heaviest fractions[8–12] showed the highest binding to labeled hCG and gave the largest cAMP and steriodogenic responses to the acute in vitro hCG stimulation. In contrast, fractions 1 and 2, containing cells of low sedimentation velocities, showed no testosterone or cAMP production, and only minor responses were noted in fractions 3–7, which contained a small proportion of morphologically intact Leydig cells. In addition, the binding to labeled hCG was very low in the first five fractions, and somewhat higher in fractions 6 and 7. Electron microscope autoradiograms indicated that the radioactivity observed in fractions 1–7 was due to [125I]iodo-hCG binding to membrane debris and to damaged Leydig cells (FIGURE 7A and B), components that cannot exhibit membrane-coupling events and/or steroidogenic activity. In contrast, the radioactivity found in fractions 8–12 was entirely due to binding of the tracer to intact Leydig cells (FIGURE 8A and B). The specificity of the binding was confirmed by the absence of silver grains associated with other cell types and by the absence of silver grains when cells were incubated in the presence of an excess of cold hCG.

GnRH BINDING TO ELUTRIATION-PURIFIED LEYDIG CELLS

The existence of specific gonadotropin releasing hormone (GnRH) receptor sites in the rat testis is now recognized.[27–32] Although the physiological significance of the presence of these receptors is still unclear, GnRH and its agonistic analogs have been shown to have stimulatory effects within 16 hr of treatment,[32,33] but inhibitory effects after prolonged exposure.[34,35] However most of the information available on the binding properties of these receptors has been derived from studies using whole testis homogenates,[27] crude Leydig cells,[28,29] and crude Leydig cell membranes,[30,31] which demonstrated that testicular GnRH receptors are located on the Leydig cell surface. In order to extend our study on the functional characterization and integrity of Leydig cells obtained by centrifugal elutriation, a pool of fractions 8–12 containing more than 90% Leydig cells was incubated with increasing concentrations of the 125I-labeled form of the agonistic GnRH analog (D-Ala[6] desGly-10-GnRH-N-ethylamide, specific activity 2000 $\mu Ci/\mu g$) as previously described.[27] FIGURE 9 shows the saturation curve and the Scatchard plot (inset) of the GnRH-analog binding to Leydig cells, indicating the presence of a single class of GnRH binding sites. The association constants (K_a) derived from Scatchard analyses, as well as the concentration of receptors expressed per Leydig cell or per testis were in the order of magnitude of those

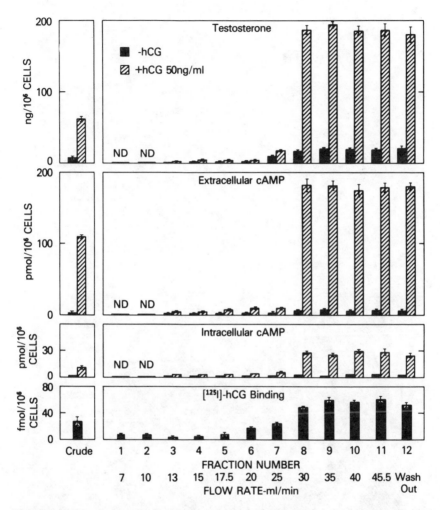

FIGURE 6. Functional analysis of fractions obtained by centrifugal elutriation of collagenase-dispersed interstitial cells from the rat testis. Fractions were collected as indicated in the legend to TABLE 2. Cells from the crude and elutriated fractions were then individually pelleted, resuspended, and counted. Approximately 10^6 nucleated cells/ml were incubated in a shaking water bath at 35°C for 3 hr under atmosphere of 95% O_2/5% CO_2, with or without 50 ng/ml pure hCG (for testosterone and cAMP production) or with 200,000 cpm [^{125}I]iodo-hCG (5–10 ng) plus or minus 10 μg of cold hCG (for the [^{125}I]iodo-hCG binding assay). Results are the mean±SD of triplicate incubations.

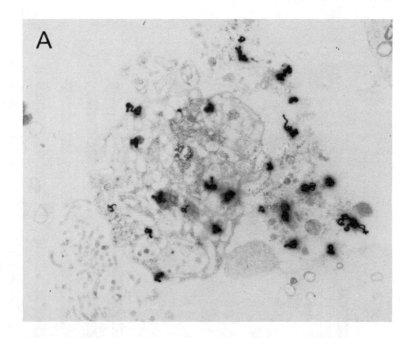

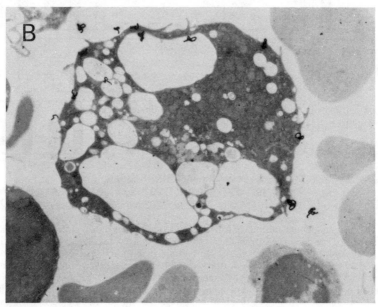

FIGURE 7. Electron microscope autoradiographs (× 5,675) of a pool of fractions 1–7 showing binding of radiolabeled hCG to membrane debris (A) and to damaged Leydig cells (B).

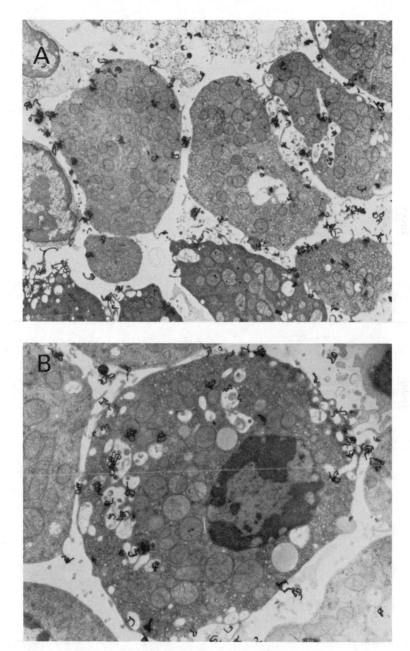

FIGURE 8. Electron microscope autoradiographs of a pool of fractions 8–12 showing binding of radiolabeled hCG to intact Leydig cells. (A) × 4,250; (B) × 5,675. The hormone molecules bound to the plasma membrane are associated with microvilli, whereas those internalized are associated with endocytic vesicles.

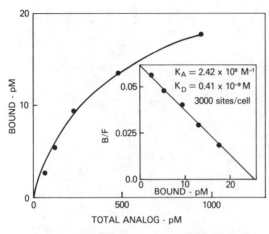

FIGURE 9. Saturation curve and Scatchard analysis (*inset*) of GnRH analog binding to Leydig cells purified by centrifugal elutriation. Cells (1.5×10^6) from a pool of fractions 8–12 were incubated at 4°C for 80 min with increasing concentrations of [^{125}I]GnRH analog, as previously described.[27] Results are the mean of three closely agreeing experiments.

previously obtained from a variety of testicular preparations (TABLE 3). These experiments confirmed previous findings on the localization of testicular GnRH receptors and indicated that the process of Leydig cell purification does not affect the binding properties of this receptor.

RESOLUTION OF FRACTIONS FROM CENTRIFUGAL ELUTRIATION IN GRADIENTS OF METRIZAMIDE

In further studies, fractions obtained by elutriation were analyzed in gradients of Metrizamide. For these experiments fractions 1 to 7 were pooled into a fraction

TABLE 3. [^{125}I]GnRH Binding to the Adult Rat Testis

Authors	Preparation	$K_a(nM^{-1})$	Sites/Cell	fmol/10^6 cells	fmol/testis
Clayton et al.[27]	27000 × g pellet from teased testes	4.0	–	–	93 ± 3
Lefebvre et al.[28]	Crude Leydig cells	8.3	2500	–	–
Sharpe et al.[29]	Crude Leydig cells	1.2	–	–	–
Perrin et al.[30]	Membranes from crude Leydig cells	3.84	–	–	–
Bourne et al.[31]	Membranes from crude Leydig cells	7.0	–	–	–
Hunter et al.[32]	Percoll-purified Leydig cells	–	–	3.8 ± 0.7	–
This study	Elutriation-purified Leydig cells	2.42 ± 0.19	3000 ± 400	5.0 ± 0.5	100 ± 10[a]

[a] This value was figured assuming the adult rat testis to have approximately 20×10^6 Leydig cells.

named H (heterogeneous) and fractions 8 to 12 were pooled into another fraction named L (Leydig cell-rich). These two fractions were separately fractionated on gradients of 16–24% Metrizamide.[36] Both the heterogeneous and the Leydig cell–rich fractions separated into five bands. (FIGURE 10). Red cells from fraction H

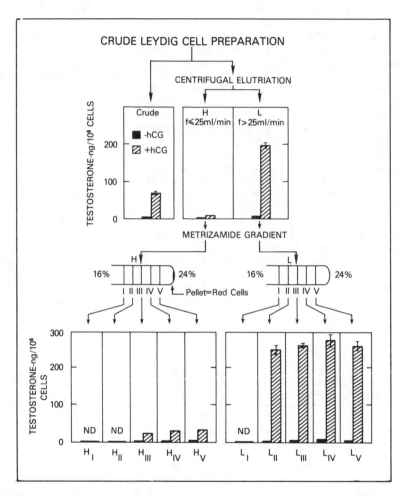

FIGURE 10. Subfractionation in Metrizamide gradients of interstitial cell fractions H and L obtained by centrifugal elutriation. Fractions H and L were obtained, as indicated in the legend to TABLE 4, and then subfractionated in 16–24% Metrizamide gradients. Cell bands were collected, washed, and then incubated for testosterone production as indicated in the legend to FIGURE 6.

were pelleted in the gradient tube. The cell bands were aspirated, washed with medium 199 and 0.1% BSA, and pelleted at $200 \times g$ for 10 min. Functional analysis indicated that Leydig cells were present in bands II–V from resolution of the fraction L (L_{II-V}, FIGURE 10). Band L_I contained the only contaminating cell type of the preparation—pachytene spermatocytes. On the other hand, the steroido-genic activity seen in the heterogeneous bands H_{III-V} was due to the presence of Leydig cells normally present in the fraction H from elutriation in a small propor-tion lower than 4%. Quantitative analysis on the composition of those bands indicated that most of the cells from the heterogeneous fraction H migrated to lower density positions (Bands H_{I-II}, TABLE 4), whereas the Leydig cells of frac-tion H and those of the enriched fraction L separated at higher densities (Bands H_{III-V} and L_{II-V}, respectively). Electron microscope analysis of the Leydig cell–rich bands demonstrated that none of the procedures (centrifugal elutriation or Metrizamide fractionation) affected the morphology of the Leydig cell (FIGURE 11). The functional study (FIGURE 10) correlated well with the morphological analysis (TABLE 4 and FIGURE 11) indicating that only morphologically intact Leydig cells showed functional activity. Less responsive or inactive cells dis-played some degree of structural damage and therefore were not considered as normal cells. The cell damage should not be attributed to the purification proce-dure or to Metrizamide exposure since it was already observed in the crude preparation (FIGURE 3B). This experiment also demonstrated that a complete Leydig cell purification can be achieved by using a combination of centrifugal elutriation and Metrizamide fractionation (Bands L_{III-V}, TABLE 4), an outcome that is not readily achieved by other separation techniques. In fact, centrifugal elutriation separates cells by taking advantage of their different sedimentation velocities, whereas centrifugation on density gradients does so according to their differences in density. Therefore, the overlapping of sedimentation velocities or densities for cells of different types yields partially rather than totally purified cells. However, when a combination of both methods is used, the results are significantly improved since cells with similar sedimentation velocities may have different densities and can further be easily separated by density gradient centrifu-gation. In our preparations, this was the case for pachytene spermatocytes and Leydig cells. The purity of the final Leydig cell preparation obtained by centrifu-gal elutriation followed by centrifugation on gradients of Metrizamide was the

TABLE 4. Separation in 16–24% Metrizamide Gradients of Fractions Obtained by Centrifugal Elutriation of Rat Interstitial Cells

	H_I	H_{II}	H_{III}	H_{IV}	H_V
Density (g/ml)	1.048	1.069	1.090	1.099	1.108
Recovered cells (%)[a]	47	39	5.2	6.4	2.4
Leydig cells (%)[b]	0	0	3	9	12

	L_I	L_{II}	L_{III}	L_{IV}	L_V
Density (g/ml)	1.048	1.075	1.088	1.098	1.110
Recovered cells (%)[a]	12.8	11.6	14	31	30.6
Leydig cells (%)[b]	0	95	100	100	100

[a] From total nucleated cells applied to the gradient.
[b] From total nucleated cells present in the band.

The crude interstitial cell preparation was separated by elutriation into 12 fractions, as indicated in the legend to TABLE 2. Fractions 1–7 containing heterogeneous cells, were pooled into one fraction (H), whereas fractions 8–12 containing highly purified Leydig cells, were pooled into another fraction (L). Both fractions were then separately centrifuged on 16–24% Metrizamide gradients. Densities of the bands were obtained from their refractive indexes. Cell bands were aspirated and counted as indicated in the text.

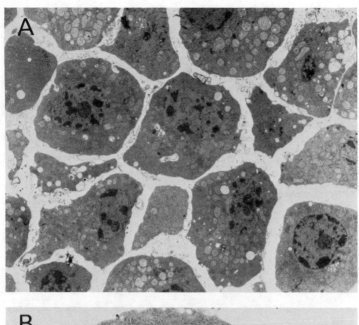

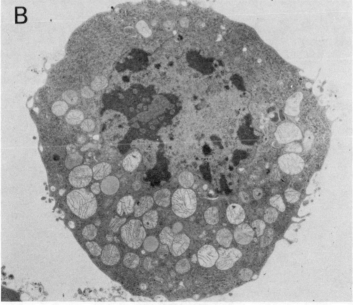

FIGURE 11. Electron micrograph of Leydig cells purified by centrifugal elutriation followed by centrifugation on gradients of Metrizamide (Bands L_{II-V}, TABLE 4). (A) × 2,100; (B) × 5,700. Cells show their characteristic cytoplasm containing abundant smooth endoplasmic reticulum, mitochondria with lamellar cristae, lipid droplets, and a nucleus with a rim of heterochromatin.

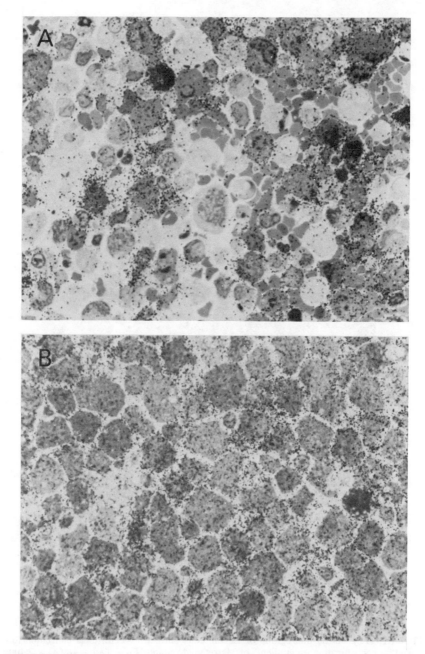

FIGURE 12. Light microscope autoradiographs (× 800) of rat interstitial cell before (A) and after (B) the purification by a combination of centrifugal elutriation and centrifugation on gradients of Metrizamide.

TABLE 5. Comparison between Centrifugal Elutriation Alone and Centrifugal Elutriation Followed by Centrifugation on Gradients of Metrizamide for Purifying Leydig Cells

Method	Degree of Purity of the Final Preparation (%)	Leydig Cell Recovery (%)
Centrifugal elutriation	90–95	60–70
Centrifugal elutriation + Metrizamide fractionation	98–100	45–55

highest, with a minor loss in recovery (TABLE 5). Autoradiographs of the double purified Leydig cells also demonstrated the ability of this procedure to achieve a complete purification (FIGURE 12). The Leydig cell size taken as the cross-sectional area from the micrographs (120 ± 38 μm^2) was not significantly different among the elutriation fractions or Metrizamide bands, and was similar to that reported by Risbridger et al.[37] and Mori et al.[38] by in situ fixation.

CENTRIFUGAL ELUTRIATION OF DESENSITIZED LEYDIG CELLS AND FURTHER SUBFRACTIONATION IN METRIZAMIDE GRADIENTS

Desensitization of Leydig cells in adult rats can be evoked by the acute action of gonadotropin upon the testis, which induces a loss of LH receptors and a decreased in vitro maximum pregnenolone and testosterone response to hCG in isolated Leydig cells.[3,39,40] An "early" steroidogenic defect prior to pregnenolone formation is induced by high doses of gonadotropin (above 40 μg/kg BW, s.c.) and was shown to be caused by a mitochondrial protein factor able to inhibit the cleavage of the cholesterol side chain leading to pregnenolone synthesis.[41] On the other hand, treatment with lower doses of gonadotropin induces a "late" steroidogenic lesion with reduction of the activities of the microsomal enzymes 17α-hydroxylase and 17-20 desmolase,[34] which appear to be mediated by estradiol.[42–45] In order to investigate whether desensitization induced selective changes in the different cell bands of the gradient, Leydig cells from control rats and animals treated 48 hr earlier with 5 or 10 μg hCG were purified by elutriation and further applied to gradients of Metrizamide (FIGURE 13). Analysis of the elutriated Leydig cells indicated that treatment with 5 μg hCG induced a 75% depletion in the binding to labeled hCG, with significant reduction of testosterone response to hCG in vitro. However there was no difference as compared to control cells, in the maximum response of pregnenolone to the stimulus in vitro. This indicated the presence of a steroidogenic lesion, which must have occurred after pregnenolone formation. The increased basal levels of testosterone and pregnenolone arise from the initial trophic effect of hCG. Further subfractionation on 16–24% Metrizamide gradients indicated that all the Leydig cell bands were desensitized to the same extent. On the other hand, in vivo treatment with 10 μg hCG caused a more marked decrease in the [^{125}I]iodo-hCG binding to the Leydig cell, with reduction of both testosterone and pregnenolone maximum responses to hCG in vitro. This indicated the presence of an additional "early" steroidogenic lesion that occurred before pregnenolone formation. The in vivo hormonal treatment induced the same degree of desensitization in each Leydig cell band. This experiment demonstrated that the different Leydig cell bands were functionally identical.

It has been suggested by Payne et al.[7] that rat testes contain two populations of Leydig cells with similar LH receptor number, but with different in vitro testoster-

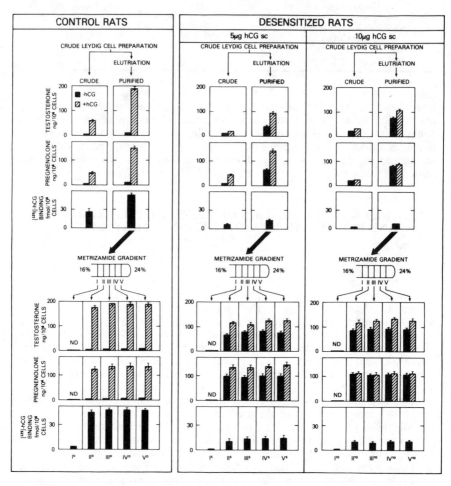

FIGURE 13. Subfractionation in 16–24% Matrizamide gradients of elutriation-purified Leydig cells after in vivo desensitization with hCG. (*Upper panels*) In vitro [125I]iodo-hCG binding and testosterone and pregnenolone responses to hCG of crude and elutriation-purified Leydig cells from adult rats treated 48 hr earlier with 5 or 10 μg of hCG in PBS. Control rats received vehicle alone. (*Lower panels*) The same evaluation performed in the individual bands obtained after separation of the elutriation-purified Leydig cells in 16–24% Metrizamide gradients. Cell incubations were performed as indicated in the legend to Figure 6. For pregnenolone measurement,[46] inhibitors of 3β-hydroxysteroid dehydrogenase (1 μM cyanoketone) and 17α-hydroxylase (10 μM spironolactone) were added to cell incubations 20 min before the addition of stimulus. Results are the mean±SD of triplicate incubations.

TABLE 6. Relative Distribution of Control and Desensitized Leydig Cells in 16–24% Metrizamide Gradients

| | Density | Leydig Cells/Band (%) | |
Band	(g/ml)	Control	Desensitized
I	1.048	0	0
II	1.072	12	48
III	1.089	32	22
IV	1.098	30	17
V	1.110	26	13

Rats were treated with 10 μg hCG (desensitized) or PBS (control) 48 hr before the cells were isolated. Centrifugal elutriation-purified Leydig cells from each group were then applied to the gradient.

one responses to hCG (Leydig cell responsiveness is markedly greater in population II than I). These authors claimed that a single subcutaneous administration of a desensitizing dose of gonadotropin (150 μg LH) decreased the *in vitro* testosterone response to hCG in population II but had no effect on responsiveness in population I.[47] The present study, in which same strain and age of rats were employed, has indicated that population I corresponds to the densities of the gradient with a major proportion of Leydig cells displaying atypical ultrastructure but maintaining the capacity to bind the labeled gonadotropin (FIGURE 7). This could explain the absence of differences in the LH receptor number between both populations observed by Payne *et al.*[7] In contrast to their findings, in our experiments using pure and intact Leydig cells no functional differences were observed between these cells when separated either according to their sedimentation velocities or their densities.

A redistribution of the Leydig cells was observed after treatment with desensitizing doses of hCG (TABLE 6). As shown in comparison to the control cells, the concentration of desensitized Leydig cells in bands III, IV, and V (densities 1.089, 1098, and 1.110 g/ml, respectively) was decreased, whereas that of band II (density 1.072 g/ml) was increased. The shifting of a significant proportion of desensitized Leydig cells to lower density positions in the gradient could arise from changes in the lipid content following stimulation with gonadotropins, since the cell size was not significantly affected ($p > 0.5$).

CONCLUSIONS

In summary, we have demonstrated that (1) centrifugal elutriation is a rapid and convenient method for purifying large quantities of functionally intact Leydig cells since up to 1 billion interstitial cells can be processed in less than 1 hr; (2) the combination of centrifugal elutriation and centrifugation on gradients of Metrizamide yields 100% pure Leydig cell preparations; (3) unresponsive Leydig cells displayed various degrees of structural damage and therefore should not be considered a separate population of physiological significance; (4) the active Leydig cell population of the testicular interstitial tissue is composed of cells with different densities and sedimentation velocities, showing similar morphology and biological activity. This suggests that functionally there is only one population of Leydig cells with comparable LH receptor number, steroidogenic activity, and susceptibility to desensitization by gonadotropins; and (5) desensitized Leydig cells undergo a significant reduction of their flotation densities, which is possible related to changes in their lipid content.

ACKNOWLEDGMENTS

We thank Dr. Kenneth Tung for his helpful advice on morphological aspects of this study.

REFERENCES

1. CONN, P. M., T. TSURUHARA, M. L. DUFAU & K. J. CATT. 1977. Isolation of highly purified Leydig cells by density gradient centrifugation. Endocrinology **101:** 639–642.

2. DUFAU, M. L. & K. J. CATT. 1978. Gonadotropin receptors and regulation of steroidogenesis in the testis and ovary. Vitam. Horm. **36:** 461–592.

3. DUFAU, M. L., T. TSURUHARA, K. A. HORNER, E. PODESTA & K. J. CATT. 1977. Intermediate role of adenosine 3′ : 5′-cyclic monophosphate and protein kinase during gonadotropin-induced steroidogenesis in testicular interstitial cells. Proc. Natl. Acad. Sci. USA **74:** 3419–3423.

4. DUFAU, M. L., S. SORREL & K. J. CATT. 1981. Gonadotropin-induced phosphorylation of endogenous proteins in the Leydig cell. FEBS Lett. **131:** 229–234.

5. JANSZEN, F. H. A., E. A. COOKE, M. J. VON DRIEL & H. J. VAN DER MOLEN. 1976. Purification and characterization of Leydig cells from rat testes. J. Endocrinol. **70:** 345–359.

6. SCHUMACHER, M., G. SCHAFER, A. F. HOLSTEIN & H. HILTZ. 1978. Rapid isolation of mouse Leydig cells by centrifugation in Percoll gradients with complete retention of morphological and biochemical integrity. FEBS Lett. **91:** 333–338.

7. PAYNE, A. H., J. R. DOWNING & K. L. WONG. 1980. Luteinizing hormone receptors and testosterone synthesis in two distinct populations of Leydig cells. Endocrinology **106:** 1424–1429.

8. BROWNING, J. Y., R. D'AGATA & H. E. GROTJAN, JR. 1981. Isolation of purified Leydig cells using continuous Percoll gradients. Endocrinology **109:** 667–669.

9. DEHEJIA, A., K. NOZU, K. J. CATT & M. L. DUFAU. 1982. Luteinizing hormone receptors and gonadotropic activation of purified rat Leydig cells. J. Biol. Chem. **257:** 13781–13786.

10. GALE, J. S., J. ST J. WAKEFIELD & H. C. FORD. 1982. Isolation of rat Leydig cells by density gradient centrifugation. J. Endocr. **92:** 293–302.

11. GLICK, D., D. VON REDLICK, E. T. JUHOS & C. R. MCEWEN. 1971. Separation of mast cells by centrifugal elutriation. Exp. Cell Res. **65:** 23–26.

12. GRABBSKE, R. J., S. LAKE, B. L. GLEDHILL & M. L. MEISTRICH. 1975. Centrifugal elutriation: Separation of spermatogenic cells on the basis of sedimentation velocity. J. Cell Physiol. **86:** 177–190.

13. KNOOK, D. L. & E. C. SLEYSTER. 1976. Separation of Kupffer and endothelial cells of the rat liver by centrifugal elutriation. Exp. Cell Res. **99:** 444–449.

14. MEISTRICH, M. L., D. J. GRDINA, R. E. MEYN & B. BARLOGIE. 1977. Separation of cells from mouse solid tumors by centrifugal elutriation. Cancer Res. **37:** 4291–4296.

15. HYDE, C., G. CHILDS (MORIARTY), L. M. WAHL, Z. NAOR & K. J. CATT. 1982. Preparation of gonadotropin-enriched cell populations from adult rat anterior pituitary cells by centrifugal elutriation. Endocrinology **111:** 1421–1423.

16. SANDERSON, R. J. & K. E. BIRD. 1977. Cell separations by counterflow centrifugation. In Methods in Cell Biology. D. M. Prescott, Ed. **15:** 1–14. Academic Press. New York.

17. GRABBSKE, R. J. 1978. Separating cell populations by elutriation. Fractions 1:1. Beckman Instruments, Inc. Palo Alto, CA.
18. DUFAU, M. L., C. MENDELSON & K. J. CATT. 1974. A highly sensitive in vitro bioassay for luteinizing hormone and chorionic gonadotropin: Testosterone production by dispersed Leydig cells. J. Clin. Endocrinol. Metab. **39:** 610–613.
19. MENDELSON, C., M. L. DUFAU & K. J. CATT. 1975. Gonadotropin binding and stimulation of ciclic adenosine 3':5'-monophosphate and testosterone production in isolated Leydig cells. J. Biol. Chem. **250:** 8818–8823.
20. LUFT, J. H. 1961. Improvements in epoxy resin embedding methods. J. Biophys. Biochem. Cytol. **9:** 409–414.
21. MILLONING, G. 1962. Further observations on a phosphate buffer for osmium solutions. *In* 5th International Congress for Electron Microscopy. S. S. Breese, Jr., Ed. **2:** 8. Academic Press. New York.
22. WATSON, M. L. 1958. Staining of tissue sections for electron microscopy with heavy metals. J. Biophys. Biochem. Cytol. **4:** 475–478.
23. CHRISTENSEN, A. K. 1975. Leydig cells. Handb. Physiol. **5:** 57–94.
24. CONNELL, C. J. & G. M. CONNELL. 1977. The interstitial tissue of the testis. *In* The Testis. A. D. Johnson & W. R. Gomes, Eds. **4:** 333–369. Academic Press. New York.
25. SOLARI, A. J. & L. L. TRES. 1970. Ultrastructure and histochemistry of the nucleus during male meiotic prophase. *In* Advances in Experimental Medicine and Biology. E. Rosemberg & C. A. Paulsen, Eds. **10:** 127–138. Plenum Press. New York.
26. CIGORRAGA, S. B., M. L. DUFAU & K. J. CATT. 1978. Regulation of luteinizing hormone receptors and steroidogenesis in gonadotropin-desensitized Leydig cells. J. Biol. Chem. **253:** 4297–4304.
27. CLAYTON, R. N., M. KATIKINENI, V. CHAN, M. L. DUFAU & K. J. CATT. 1980. Direct inhibition of testicular function by gonadotropin-releasing hormone: Mediation by specific gonadotropin-releasing hormone receptors in intersitital cells. Proc. Natl. Acad. Sci. USA **8:** 4459–4463.
28. LEFEBVRE, F. A., J. J. REEVES, J. SEGUIN, J. MASSICOTTE & F. LABRIE. 1980. Specific binding of a potent LHRH agonist in rat testis. Mol. Cell. Endocrinol. **20:** 127–134.
29. SHARPE, R. M. & H. M. FRASER. 1980. Leydig cell receptors for luteinizing hormone releasing hormone and its agonists and their modulation by administration or deprivation of the releasing hormone. Biochem. Biophys. Res. Commun. **95:** 256–262.
30. PERRIN, M. H., J. M. VAUGHAN, J. E. RIVIER & W. W. VALE. 1980. High affinity GnRH binding to testicular membrane homogenates. Life Sci. **26:** 2251–2255.
31. BOURNE, G. A., S. REGIANI, A. B. PAYNE & J. C. MARSHALL. 1980. Testicular GnRH receptors: Characterization and localization on interstitial tissue. J. Clin. Endocrinol. Metab. **51:** 407–409.
32. HUNTER, M. G., M. H. F. SULLIVAN, C. J. DIX, F. ALDRED & B. A. COOKE. 1982. Stimulation and inhibition by LHRH analogues of cultured rat Leydig cell function and lack of effect on mouse Leydig cells. Mol. Cell. Endocrinol. **27:** 31–44.
33. SHARPE, R. M. & I. COOPER. 1982. Stimulatory effect of LHRH and its agonists on Leydig cell steroidogenesis *in vitro*. Mol. Cell. Endocrinol. **26:** 141–150.
34. HSUEH, A. J. W. & G. F. ERICKSON. 1979. Extra-pituitary inhibition of testicular function by luteinizing hormone releasing hormone. Nature **281:** 66–67.
35. HSUEH, A. J. W., J. R. SCHRIEBER & G. F. ERICKSON. 1981. Inhibitory effect of gonadotropin releasing hormone upon cultured testicular cells. Mol. Cell. Endocrinol. **21:** 43–49.
36. AQUILANO, D. R. & M. L. DUFAU. 1984. Functional and morphological studies on isolated Leydig cells: Purification by centrifugal elutriation and Metrizamide fractionation. Endocrinology. (In press.)
37. RISBRIDGER, G. P., J. B. KERR, R. A. PEAKE & D. M. DE KRETSER. 1981. An assessment of Leydig cell function after bilateral or unilateral efferent duct ligation: Further evidence for local control of Leydig cell function. Endocrinology **109:** 1234–1241
38. MORI, H. & A. K. CHRISTENSEN. 1980. Morphometric analysis of Leydig cells in the normal rat testis. J. Cell Biol. **84:** 340–354.

39. TSURUHARA, T., M. L. DUFAU, S. B. CIGORRAGA & K. J. CATT. 1977. Hormonal regulation of testicular luteinizing hormone receptors J. Biol. Chem. **252:** 9002–9009.
40. HSUEH, A. J. W., M. L. DUFAU & K. J. CATT. 1977. Gonadotropin-induced regulation of luteinizing hormone receptors and desensitization of testicular 3′ : 5′-cyclic AMP and testosterone responses. Proc. Natl. Acad. Sci. USA **74:** 592–595.
41. HATTORI, M. 1982. Gonadotropins modulate the affinity of cholesterol side-chain cleavage enzyme for NADPH in rat Leydig cell mitochondria. Endocrinology **110:** 41 (Abstract).
42. NOZU, K., S. MATSUURA, K. J. CATT & M. L. DUFAU. 1981. Modulation of Leydig cell androgen biosynthesis and human chorionic gonadotropin-induced desensitization. J. Biol. Chem. **256:** 10012–10017.
43. CIGORRAGA, S. B., S. SORRELL, J. BATOR, K. J. CATT & M. L. DUFAU. 1980. Estrogen dependence of a gonadotropin-induced steroidogenic lesion in rat testicular Leydig cells. J. Clin. Invest. **64:** 699–705.
44. NOZU, K., A. DEHEJIA, L. ZAWISTOWICH, K. J. CATT & M. L. DUFAU. 1981. Gonadotropin-induced receptor regulation and steroidogenic lesions in cultured Leydig cells. J. Biol. Chem. **256:** 12875–11882.
45. AQUILANO, D. R. & M. L. DUFAU. 1983. Changes in RNA polymerase activities in gonadotropin-treated Leydig cells: An estradiol-mediated process. Endocrinology **113:** 94–103.
46. DIPIETRO, D. L., R. D. BROWN & C. A. STROTT. 1972. A pregnenolone radioimmuno assay utilizing a new fractionation technique for sheep antiserum. J. Clin. Endocrinol. Metab. **35:** 729–735.
47. PAYNE, A. H., K. L. WONG & M. M. VEGA. 1980. Differential effects of a single and repeated administration of gonadotropins on luteinizing hormone receptors and testosterone synthesis in two populations of Leydig cells. J. Biol. Chem. **225:** 7118–7122

Regulation of the Synthesis of Cholesterol Side-chain Cleavage Cytochrome P-450 and Adrenodoxin in Rat Leydig Cells in Culture[a]

CHRISTEN M. ANDERSON and CAROLE R. MENDELSON[b]

The Departments of Biochemistry and Obstetrics-Gynecology
The Cecil H. and Ida Green Center
for Reproductive Biology Sciences
The University of Texas Health Science Center
Dallas, Texas 75235

INTRODUCTION

Luteinizing hormone (LH) and human chorionic gonadotropin (hCG) stimulate testosterone production both in freshly dispersed rat Leydig cells[1] and in such cells in primary culture.[2] This increase in androgen synthesis is mediated by the binding of LH and hCG to specific receptors, activation of adenylate cyclase, and increased cyclic AMP (cAMP) formation.[3] The subsequent cAMP-mediated events presumably result in an increase in the activity of one or more steroidogenic enzymes. The finding that stimulation of testosterone synthesis by hCG in freshly dispersed Leydig cells is dependent upon both RNA and protein synthesis[4,5] is suggestive that acute stimulation of testosterone synthesis may be mediated by a rapid increase in the synthesis of a protein(s) that modulates the activity of one or more steroidogenic enzymes. Recently, Pedersen and Brownie[6] reported that treatment of rats with adrenocorticotropin (ACTH) resulted in a rapid increase in the amount of a cytosolic peptide ($M_r \simeq 2200$) in adrenal cortex that increased the rate of association of cholesterol with cholesterol side-chain cleavage cytochrome P-450 (cytochrome P-450$_{scc}$).

On the other hand, chronic treatment with LH and hCG may increase testosterone production by stimulating the synthesis of one or more steroidogenic enzymes in the testis. In primary cultures of bovine adrenocortical cells, treatment with ACTH for 24–48 hr increased the rates of synthesis of cytochrome P-450$_{scc}$,[7] adrenodoxin,[8,9] 11β-hydroxylase cytochrome P-450,[9] and steroid 21-hydroxylase cytochrome P-450.[10] The increased synthesis of these steroidogenic enzymes was mediated by an increase in the translatability of mRNA coding for these proteins. Such effects are assumed to account, at least in part, for the increased cytochrome P-450$_{scc}$ activity and corticosteroid synthesis observed with chronic

[a] This research was supported, in part, by National Institutes of Health (grant 1-RO1-AM31206-01A1). C.M.A. is supported by Training Grant 1-T32-HD07190.

[b] Address correspondence to Carole R. Mendelson, Ph.D., Department of Biochemistry, University of Texas Southwestern Medical School, 5323 Harry Hines Boulevard, Dallas, Texas 75235.

ACTH treatment *in vitro*. While it is known that the activity of testicular cytochrome P-450$_{scc}$ is increased by LH or hCG in rat Leydig cells,[11-13] the long term effects of gonadotropins on the synthesis of cytochrome P-450$_{scc}$ or other steroidogenic enzymes in the testis have not been reported previously.

Cytochrome P-450$_{scc}$, which catalyzes the removal of the cholesterol side-chain to form pregnenolone, is localized in the inner mitochondrial membrane. This enzyme functions as the terminal oxidase in an electron transport chain that also includes adrenodoxin (an iron-sulfur protein) and adrenodoxin reductase (a flavoprotein). The scission of the cholesterol side-chain is the first committed step in the steroidogenic pathway, and is generally considered to be the rate-limiting step in steroid synthesis;[14,15] the regulation of synthesis of cytochrome P-450$_{scc}$ is, therefore, crucial to the regulation of testicular androgen synthesis. It was our objective, in the present study, to investigate the effects of hCG and dibutyryl cAMP (Bu$_2$cAMP) on the synthesis of testicular cytochrome P-450$_{scc}$ and adrenodoxin in rat Leydig cells in primary culture. We found that both hCG and Bu$_2$cAMP increased the rate of synthesis of cytochrome P-450$_{scc}$ and adrenodoxin in these cells, suggesting that the stimulatory effect of gonadotropins and cyclic AMP on testosterone synthesis *in vitro* is mediated, at least in part, by an increase in the rate of synthesis of these proteins.

MATERIALS AND METHODS

Tissue Culture

A crude Leydig cell suspension, containing 40–50% Leydig cells as determined by histochemical staining for 3β-hydroxysteroid dehydrogenase activity[16,17] was prepared by incubation of decapsulated testes from adult Sprague-Dawley rats with collagenase as described previously.[18,19] The cells were washed in Dulbecco's modified Eagle's medium : F12 nutrient mixture (1 : 1) that contained HEPES (15 mM), antibiotic/antimycotic (10 μg/ml), glucose (4.5 mg/ml), insulin (5 μg/ml), transferrin (5 μg/ml), selenium (5 ng/ml), and glutathione (0.5 μg/ml) (hereafter referred to as DMEM : F12 medium). The cells were plated at a density of 5.0×10^5 cells/35 mm dish in the same culture medium. After eight days of culture with daily medium changes, treatment with hCG or Bu$_2$cAMP was begun. Testosterone concentrations in the culture media were measured by a specific radioimmunoassay.[20]

Cell Labeling and Immunoisolation

After eight days of incubation in the absence of serum or stimulatory factors, hCG (10 mIU/ml) or Bu$_2$cAMP (1 mM) was added to some of the cultures and the incubations were continued for an additional 72 hr. After the addition of stimulatory factors, media were collected at 24 hr intervals for testosterone determination. After various intervals of culture, the DMEM : F12 medium was replaced with methionine-free F12 nutrient mixture for a 2 hr incubation period, followed by the addition of [^{35}S]methionine (75 μCi/ml) for an additional 2 hr. The cells were harvested by scraping in Gey's balanced salt solution and washed twice in fresh balanced salt solution. The cells were lysed and the proteins were solubilized by the addition of cholate (1%, w/vol) and SDS (0.1%, w/vol), followed by two freeze-thaw cycles. Cytochrome P-450$_{scc}$ and adrenodoxin were immunoisolated from equivalent amounts of trichloroacetic acid (TCA)-precipitable radioactivity in lysates from control and treated cells by the method of Dubois *et al.*[7] using specific antibodies directed against bovine adrenal cytochrome P-450$_{scc}$ and bovine adrenal adrenodoxin. The immunoisolates were subjected to electrophoresis on 7–15% linear gradient polyacrylamide gels by the method of Laemmli.[21] Immunoisolated cytochrome P-450$_{scc}$ and adrenodoxin were visualized by autoradiography.

Protein Immunoblotting

Cultured Leydig cells were harvested and lysed as described above. Protein concentrations of cell lysates were determined by the method of Bradford.[22] The solubilized proteins were separated by SDS-polyacrylamide gel electrophoresis on 7–15% linear gradient gels. The resolved proteins were then electrophoretically transferred to nitrocellulose paper,[23] which was subsequently incubated with rabbit-anti-bovine-P-450$_{scc}$ IgG. Bound antibody was localized by a second incubation with [^{125}I]goat-anti-rabbit IgG, followed by autoradiography of the immunoblot.

Hormone Source

Human chorionic gonadotropin (CR-121, 13,450 IU/mg) was generously provided by Dr. R. E. Canfield, Center for Population Research of the National Institute of Child Health and Human Development, National Institutes of Health.

Purified Proteins and Antibodies

Purified bovine adrenal cytochrome P-450$_{scc}$ and bovine adrenal adrenodoxin were kindly provided by Dr. J. D. Lambeth, Emory University. Specific antibodies raised in rabbits against these proteins[24] were a generous gift from Dr. M. R. Waterman, University of Texas Health Science Center at Dallas.)

RESULTS

Effect of hCG and Bu$_2$cAMP on Testosterone Production by Cultured Leydig Cells

Testosterone concentrations were measured in media collected every 24 hr from Leydig cells cultured in the absence or presence of stimulatory factors. Testosterone production by cells incubated in the absence of stimulatory factors was 5–10 pg/24 hr/5 × 10^5 cells. Inclusion of hCG (10 mIU/ml) in the culture medium caused 10- and 30-fold increases in testosterone formation after incubation for 24 and 48 hr, respectively (FIGURE 1). Testosterone synthesis by cultured cells was also increased markedly by Bu$_2$cAMP (1 mM); maximal stimulation was observed after 24 hr of incubation (200 × control). After 48 hr of incubation the stimulatory effect of Bu$_2$cAMP was reduced (50 × control).

Effect of hCG and Bu₂cAMP on the Synthesis of Cytochrome P-450_scc and Adrenodoxin

The effects of hCG and Bu$_2$cAMP on the synthesis of cytochrome P-450$_{scc}$ and adrenodoxin were studied by immunoisolation of the newly synthesized proteins from cells that were radiolabeled with [^{35}S]methionine during the last 2 hr of culture. Changes in the rates of synthesis of each of these proteins after incubation of cells for various periods in the absence or presence of stimulatory factors were determined by measuring the densities of autoradiographic bands that co-migrated with purified bovine cytochrome P-450$_{scc}$ or adrenodoxin on polyacrylamide gels. In FIGURES 2 and 3 are shown representative autoradiograms of immunoisolates from cells incubated in the presence or absence of stimulatory factors for periods of 24 or 48 hr. Both hCG and Bu$_2$cAMP increased the rate of synthesis of cytochrome P-450$_{scc}$, as indicated by the greater radiographic densities of the bands corresponding to cytochrome P-450$_{scc}$ in hormone-treated samples with respect to controls. The apparent rate of synthesis of cytochrome P-450$_{scc}$ in hCG-treated cells was increased 5.1- and 2.5-fold over the corresponding controls after 24 and 48 hr, respectively. In cells incubated with Bu$_2$cAMP for 24 and 48 hr, the rate of cytochrome P-450$_{scc}$ synthesis was increased sevenfold and fivefold, respectively (FIGURE 2B). In parallel immunoisolations conducted in the presence of an excess of nonradiolabeled purified cytochrome P-450$_{scc}$, no radiographic band corresponding to the bovine cytochrome P-450$_{scc}$ standard was present (data not shown).

The rate of synthesis of adrenodoxin was also increased by hCG and Bu$_2$cAMP treatment. Adrenodoxin synthesis in hCG-treated cells was increased twofold over that of controls after 24 hr of incubation; after 48 hr, only a small stimulatory effect of hCG was observed. In contrast, in cells incubated with Bu$_2$cAMP for 24 and 48 hr, adrenodoxin synthesis was increased 15- and 11-fold, respectively. In each case, the greatest stimulation was observed in cells that had been incubated with the appropriate stimulatory factor for 24 hr.

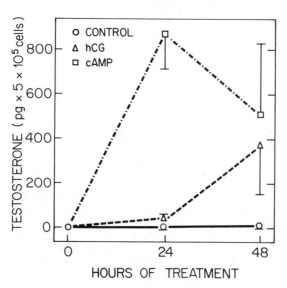

FIGURE 1. Effects of hCG and Bu$_2$cAMP on testosterone secretion by cultured Leydig cells. Leydig cells were maintained in culture for 8 days in the absence of serum or stimulatory factors; hCG (10 mIU/ ml) or Bu$_2$cAMP (1 mM) were then added to the cultures (time = 0). Testosterone concentrations were measured by radioimmunoassay of the media collected at 24 hr intervals. Data are expressed as the mean ± SEM of results from four experiments.

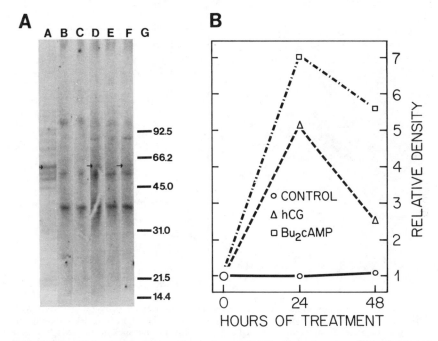

FIGURE 2. (A) Immunoisolation of cytochrome P-450$_{scc}$ from Leydig cells radiolabeled with [^{35}S]methionine. Leydig cells that were maintained in culture for 8 days were incubated with or without hCG (10 mIU/ml) for 24 or 48 hr. The cell proteins were radiolabeled and newly synthesized cytochrome P-450$_{scc}$ was immunoisolated as described in METHODS. Lane A: purified cytochrome P-450$_{scc}$ stained with Coomassie blue. Lanes B–F are autoradiograms. Lane B: control, time = 0. Lane C: control, 24 hr. Lane D: hCG-treated, 24 hr. Lane E: control, 48 hr. Lane F: hCG-treated, 48 hr. Lane G: molecular weight standards (MW × 10^{-3}). (B) Relative densities of radiographic bands corresponding to cytochrome P-450$_{scc}$. Densities were determined by calculating the areas under the appropriate peaks of densitometric scans from two experiments. Relative density = sample density/density of control, time = 0.

The Effect of hCG and Bu$_2$cAMP on the Content of Cytochrome P-450$_{scc}$ in Cultured Leydig Cells

To determine the effects of hCG and Bu$_2$cAMP on the content of cytochrome P-450$_{scc}$ in cultured Leydig cells, cells were incubated in the presence or absence of hCG (10 mIU/ml) or Bu$_2$cAMP (1 mM) for 24, 48, or 72 hr; the cells were harvested, and equivalent amounts of cell protein separated by SDS polyacrylamide gel electrophoresis. The relative amounts of cytochrome P-450$_{scc}$ were estimated by the immunoblotting technique described in MATERIALS AND METHODS. In FIGURE 4A is shown a representative autoradiogram of a cytochrome P-450$_{scc}$ immunoblot from lysates of cultured cells; relative densities of the bands that co-migrated with purified cytochrome P-450$_{scc}$ are shown in FIGURE 4B. Both hCG and Bu$_2$cAMP increased the concentration of immunoreactive cytochrome P-450$_{scc}$ in cultured Leydig cells. In hCG-treated cells, the relative concentrations of immunoreactive cytochrome P-450$_{scc}$ were 1.5, 1.8, and 1.3

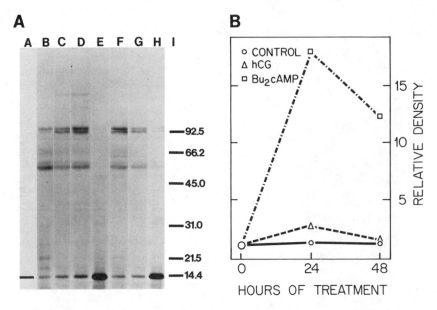

FIGURE 3. (A) Immunoisolation of adrenodoxin from Leydig cells radiolabeled with [^{35}S]methionine. Cultured Leydig cells were treated as described in FIGURE 2A; adrenodoxin was immunoisolated from the radiolabeled cell lysates by use of a specific antibody. Lane A: Position of purified adrenodoxin. Lanes B–H are autoradiograms. Lane B: Control, time = 0. Lane C: Control, 24 hr. Lane D: hCG-treated, 24 hr. Lane E: Bu$_2$cAMP-treated, 24 hr. Lane F: Control, 48 hr. Lane G: hCG-treated, 48 hr. Lane H: Bu$_2$cAMP-treated, 48 hr. Lane I: Molecular weight standards (MW × 10^{-3}). (B) Relative densities of radiographic bands corresponding to adrenodoxin. Band densities from a representative experiment were determined as described in FIGURE 2B.

times that of the corresponding controls at 24, 48, and 72 hr, respectively. In Leydig cells incubated with Bu$_2$cAMP the concentration of cytochrome P-450$_{scc}$ was increased to 3.2, 5.8, and 6.9 times that of control at 24, 48, and 72 hr, respectively.

DISCUSSION

The results of this study are indicative that the stimulatory effects of chronic treatment with hCG and Bu$_2$cAMP on testosterone synthesis by rat Leydig cells in culture are mediated, in part, by an increase in the synthesis of cytochrome P-450$_{scc}$ and adrenodoxin. These findings are suggestive that the capacity of LH to maintain testicular steroidogenesis and cytochrome P-450$_{scc}$ activity may be mediated by regulation of the synthesis of steroidogenic enzymes. Administration of LH or hCG to hypophysectomized rats was found to restore cytochrome P-450$_{scc}$ activity,[13] 3β-hydroxysteroid dehydrogenase activity,[25] and testosterone synthesis[17,26] to normal levels after a period of hours to days. In previous studies, the rate of synthesis of cytochrome P-450$_{scc}$ was found to be increased in bovine adrenocortical cells in culture by

ACTH[7-9] and in bovine granulosa cells in culture by follicle-stimulating hormone (FSH).[27] In both of these systems the rate of synthesis of cytochrome P-450$_{scc}$ was also increased by cyclic AMP analogs, suggesting that the stimulatory effects of ACTH and FSH in their respective target tissues are mediated by an increase in cyclic AMP formation. ACTH and Bu$_2$cAMP also increased the rate of synthesis of adrenodoxin in bovine adrenocortical cells in vitro.[8,9]

In the present study, we found that the rates of synthesis of cytochrome P-450$_{scc}$ and adrenodoxin were stimulated maximally by hCG and Bu$_2$cAMP after 24 hr of incubation; the cellular concentrations of these proteins were maximally increased after somewhat longer periods of culture. The finding that the rates of synthesis of cytochrome P-450$_{scc}$ and adrenodoxin were maximally stimulated by hCG and by Bu$_2$cAMP after 24 hr of incubation and declined, thereafter, is suggestive of a form of desensitization. Nozu et al.[28] reported that in acute preparations of Leydig cells incubated for 24 hr with hCG (100–1000 mIU/ml) there was a decrease in the concentration of receptors for hCG, as well as a decrease in responsiveness of the cells to hCG. Although incubation of cells for 24 hr with hCG at a concentration comparable to that used in the present study (10 mIU/ml)

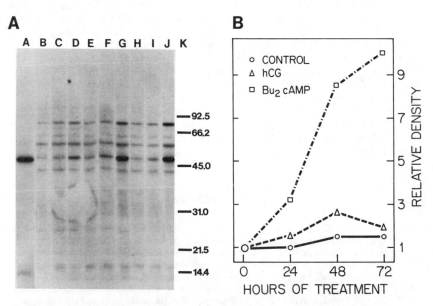

FIGURE 4. (A) Protein immunoblot of cytochrome P-450$_{scc}$ from cultured Leydig cells. Rat Leydig cells in culture were incubated with or without hCG or Bu$_2$cAMP as described in FIGURE 2A. After 24 or 48 hr, the cell lysates were analyzed for cytochrome p-450$_{scc}$ content by immunoblotting as described in METHODS. Lanes A–J are autoradiograms. Lane A: purified cytochrome P-450$_{scc}$. Lane B: control, 24 hr. Lane C: hCG-treated, 24 hr. Lane D: Bu$_2$cAMP-treated, 24 hr. Lane E: control, 48 hr. Lane F: hCG-treated, 48 hr. Lane G: Bu$_2$cAMP-treated, 48 hr. Lane H: control, 72 hr. Lane I: hCG-treated, 72 hr. Lane J: Bu$_2$cAMP-treated, 72 hr. Lane K: molecular weight standards (MW $\times$ 10^{-3}). (B) Relative densities of radiographic bands corresponding to cytochrome P-450$_{scc}$. Band densities were determined in a representative experiment as described in FIGURE 2B.

resulted in an increase in hCG receptor concentration and an increase in testosterone synthesis in response to acute hCG stimulation, the finding of an accumulation of progesterone and 17α-hydroxyprogesterone was indicative of a decrease in the activity of 17α-hydroxylase and 17,20-lyase. This so-called late steroidogenic lesion is thought to be caused by the accumulation of locally produced steroid intermediates, especially estrogens.[29] This phenomenon could account for the decline in Bu_2cAMP-stimulated testosterone formation that we observed in Leydig cells after 48 hr of incubation.

The decreased stimulatory effect of hCG on the rates of synthesis of cytochrome $P-450_{scc}$ and adrenodoxin that we observed after 48 hr is also suggestive of a decrease in hCG receptor number and/or coupling to adenylate cyclase. Alternative mechanisms must be considered, however, since the magnitude of the stimulatory effect of Bu_2cAMP on the rates of synthesis of cytochrome $P-450_{scc}$ and adrenodoxin also was decreased at 48 hr. It is possible that chronic treatment of Leydig cells with relatively low concentrations of hCG or Bu_2cAMP results in an accumulation of steroid intermediates or other regulatory factors that, in turn, inhibits the synthesis of cytochrome $P-450_{scc}$ and adrenodoxin. A similar biphasic effect of ACTH on the synthesis of cytochrome $P-450_{scc}$,[7] adrenodoxin,[8,9] and other steroidogenic enzymes[9,10] was observed in bovine adrenocortical cells in culture.

In the present study, the finding that both hCG and Bu_2cAMP increased the rates of synthesis of cytochrome $P-450_{scc}$ and adrenodoxin is suggestive that this inductive effect of hCG is mediated by an increase in cyclic AMP formation. The increase in cyclic AMP may act to increase cytochrome $P-450_{scc}$ and adrenodoxin synthesis by one or more of the following mechanisms. (1) Increased cyclic AMP levels may cause an increase in the transcriptional activity of the genes that code for these steroidogenic enzymes. (2) The translatability of existing or newly synthesized mRNAs may be increased. (3) The stability of mRNAs coding for cytochrome $P-450_{scc}$ and adrenodoxin may be increased by a cyclic AMP–mediated mechanism. Studies to clarify the molecular mechanisms by which hCG and Bu_2cAMP induce the synthesis of cytochrome $P-450_{scc}$ and adrenodoxin are currently in progress.

REFERENCES

1. MENDELSON, C. R., M. L. DUFAU & K. J. CATT. 1975. Gonadotropin binding and stimulation of cyclic adenosine $3':5'$-monophosphate and testosterone production in isolated Leydig cells. J. Biol. Chem. 250: 8818–8823.
2. HSUEH, A. J. W. 1980. Gonadotropin stimulation of testosterone production in primary culture of adult rat testis cells. Biochem. Biophys. Res. Commun. 97: 506–512.
3. CATT, K. J. & M. L. DUFAU. 1978. Gonadotropin receptors and regulation of interstitial cell function in the testis. In Receptors and Hormone Action. L. Birnbaumer & B. O'Malley, Eds. 3: 291–339. Academic Press. New York.
4. MENDELSON, C. R., M. L. DUFAU & K. J. CATT. 1975. Dependence of gonadotropin-induced steroidogenesis upon RNA and protein synthesis in the interstitial cells of the rat testis. Biochim. Biophys. Acta 41: 222–230.
5. COOKE, B. A., F. H. JANSZEN, W. F. CLOTSCHER & H. J. VAN DER MOLEN. 1975. Effect of protein-synthesis inhibitors on testosterone production in rat testis interstitial tissue and Leydig-cell preparations. Biochem. J. 150: 413–418.
6. PEDERSEN, R. C. & A. C. BROWNIE. 1983. Cholesterol side-chain cleavage in the rat adrenal cortex: Isolation of a cycloheximide-sensitive activator peptide. Proc. Natl. Acad. Sci. USA 80: 1882–1886.

7. DuBois, R. N., E. R. Simpson, R. E. Kramer & M. R. Waterman. 1981. Induction of synthesis of cholesterol side chain cleavage cytochrome P-450 by adrenocorticotropin in cultured bovine adrenocortical cells. J. Biol. Chem. **256:** 7000–7005.
8. Kramer, R. E., C. M. Anderson, J. A. Peterson, E. R. Simpson & M. R. Waterman. 1982. Adrenodoxin biosynthesis by bovine adrenal cells in monolayer culture. J. Biol. Chem. **257:** 14921–14925.
9. Kramer, R. E., C. M. Anderson, J. L. McCarthy, E. R. Simpson & M. R. Waterman. 1982. Coordinate induction of synthesis of adrenal mitochondrial steroid hydroxylases by ACTH. Fed. Proc. **41:** 1928 (abstr.).
10. Funkenstein, B., J. McCarthy, K. M. Dus, E. R. Simpson & M. R. Waterman. 1983. Effect of adrenocorticotropin on steroid 21-hydroxylase synthesis and activity in cultured bovine adrenocortical cells. J. Biol. Chem. **258:** 9398–9405.
11. Menon, K. M. J., M. Drosdowsky, R. I. Dorfman & E. Forchielli. 1975. Side-chain cleavage of cholesterol-26-^{14}C and 20α-hydroxycholesterol-22-^{14}C by rat testis mitochondrial preparations and the effects of gonadotropin administration and hypophysectomy. Steroids Suppl. **1:** 95–111.
12. Purvis, J. L., J. A. Canick, S. A. Latif, J. H. Rosenbaum, J. Hologgitas & R. H. Menard. 1973. Lifetime of microsomal cytochrome P-450 and steroidogenic enzymes in rat testis as influenced by human chorionic gonadotrophin. Arch. Biochem. Biophys. **159:** 39–49.
13. Menon, K. M., R. I. Dorfman & E. Forchielli. 1967. Influence of gonadotrophins on the cholesterol-side-chain cleavage reaction by rat-testis mitochondrial preparations. Biochim. Biophys. Acta **148:** 486–494.
14. Jefcoate, C. R. 1975. Cytochrome P-450 of adrenal mitrochondria. J. Biol. Chem. **250:** 4663–4670.
15. Simpson, E. R. 1979. Cholesterol side-chain cleavage, cytochrome P-450 and the control of steroidogenesis. Mol. Cell. Endocrinol. **13:** 213–227.
16. Bilinska, B. 1979. Histochemical demonstration of Δ^5-3β-hydroxysteroid dehydrogenase activity in cultured Leydig cells under the influence of gonadotropic hormone and testosterone. Int. J. Androl. **2:** 385–394.
17. Fisher, T. V. & R. H. Kahn. 1972. Histochemical studies of rat ovarian follicular cells *in vitro*. In Vitro **7:** 201–205.
18. Catt, K. J. & M. L. Dufau. 1973. Interactions of LH and hCG with testicular gonadotropin receptors. Adv. Exp. Med. Biol. **36:** 379–418.
19. Dufau, M. L., C. R. Mendelson & K. J. Catt. 1974. A highly sensitive *in vitro* bioassay for luteinizing hormone and chorionic gonadotropin: testosterone production by dispersed Leydig cells. J. Clin. Endocrinol. Metab. **39:** 610–613.
20. Dufau, M. L., K. J. Catt & T. Tsuruhara. 1972. A sensitive gonadotropin responsive system: radioimmunoassay of testosterone production by the rat testis *in vitro*. Endocrinology **90:** 1032–1040.
21. Laemmli, U. K. 1970. Cleavage of structural proteins during the assembly of the head of bacteriophage T4. Nature **227:** 680–685.
22. Bradford, M. M. 1976. A rapid and sensitive method for the quantitation of microgram quantities of protein utilizing the principle of protein-dye binding. Anal. Biochem. **72:** 248–254.
23. Towbin, H., T. Staehelin & J. Gordon. 1979. Electrophoretic transfer of proteins from polyacrylamide gels to nitrocellulose sheets: procedure and some applications. Proc. Natl. Acad. Sci. USA **9:** 4350–4354.
24. DuBois, R. N., E. R. Simpson, J. Tuckey, J. D. Lambeth & M. R. Waterman. 1981. Evidence for a higher molecular weight precursor of cholesterol side-chain-cleavage cytochrome P-450 and induction of mitochondrial and cytosolic proteins by corticotropin in adult bovine adrenal cells. Proc. Natl. Acad. Sci. USA **78:** 1028–1032.
25. Samuels, L. T. & M. L. H. Helmreich. 1956. The influence of chorionic gonadotropin on the 3β-ol-dehydrogenase activity of the testes and adrenals. Endocrinology **58:** 435–442.
26. Purvis, K., L. Cusan & V. Hansson. 1981. Regulation of steroidogenesis and steroid action in Leydig cells. J. Steroid Biochem. **15:** 77–86.

27. FUNKENSTEIN, B., M. R. WATERMAN, B. S. S. MASTERS & E. R. SIMPSON. 1983. Evidence for the presence of cholesterol side chain cleavage cytochrome P-450 and adrenodoxin in fresh granulosa cells. J. Biol. Chem. **258:** 10187–10191.
28. NOZU, K., A. DEHEJIA, L. ZAWISTOWICH, K. J. CATT & M. L. DUFAU. 1981. Gonadotropin-induced receptor regulation and steroidogenic lesions in cultured Leydig cells. J. Biol. Chem. **256:** 12875–12882.
29. NOZU, K., M. L. DUFAU & K. J. CATT. 1981. Estradiol receptor-mediated regulation of steroidogenesis in gonadotropin-desensitized Leydig cells. J. Biol. Chem. **256:** 1915–1922.

Control of Steroidogenesis in Leydig Cells: Roles of Ca^{2+} and Lipoxygenase Products in LH and LHRH Agonist Action

B. A. COOKE, C. J. DIX, A. D. HABBERFIELD, and
M. H. F. SULLIVAN

Department of Biochemistry and Chemistry
Royal Free Hospital School of Medicine
University of London
London NW3 2PF, England

INTRODUCTION

Previous studies from this laboratory[1] demonstrated that LHRH agonists bind specifically to purified rat but not mouse Leydig cells. During short term (less than 24 hr) these agonists stimulate steroidogenesis in the rat Leydig cells[1-3] but long term (in excess of 24 hr) effects are inhibitory on LH-stimulated steroidogenesis.[1,4] Further studies have now been carried out[5-7] to determine the effects and roles of cyclic AMP and Ca^{2+} in LHRH agonist action during stimulation of steroidogenesis and to determine the effects of LHRH agonist on cholesterol side-chain cleavage enzyme activity.[5] The effects of inhibitors of the cyclooxygenase and lipoxygenase pathways of arachidonic acid metabolism on LH and LHRH agonist–stimulated steroidogenesis have also been investigated.[8] These more recent studies will now be reviewed.

METHODS AND MATERIALS

Rat Leydig cells were prepared and purified as described previously.[1,9] All preparative procedures were carried out in media containing 2.0–2.5 mM Ca^{2+}. Media depleted in Ca^{2+} were prepared by adding 2.8 mM EGTA to complex the calcium.

Purified rat Leydig cells were plated out in Costar culture wells (10^5 cells/well unless otherwise stated) and the media (Dulbecco's Modified Eagles Medium) added. LHRH agonist (ICI 118630) (dissolved in medium) and LH (LH-NIH-S 20; 2.3 IU NIH-SI/mg) (dissolved in medium) were added as stated in the text. The calcium ionophore A23187 was dissolved in dimethylsulfoxide at 100 times the final concentration and 10 μl/ml medium was added. The same amount of dimethylsulfoxide was added to the controls. 1-Methylisobutylxanthine (MIX) was dissolved in medium at the final concentration stated in the text. Hydroxycholesterol or pregnenolone (in ethanol, 10 μl/ml) medium were added as appropriate after two hours in culture, unless stated otherwise in the text. The cells were then incubated at 32°C. After four hours, incubations were stopped with $HClO_4$ (final concentration 0.5 M) and frozen at −20°C until neutralized with K_3PO_4 (final

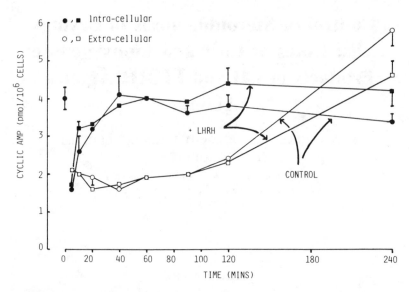

FIGURE 1. LHRH agonist effect on cyclic AMP production in rat Leydig cells. Intracellular (●,■) and extracellular cyclic AMP (○,□) were measured in the presence (□,■) and absence (○,●) of LHRH agonist (10^{-7} M) over the time period shown in freshly cultured Leydig cells. Results are means ± S.E.M. (N = 3). (Data from Sullivan & Cooke.[7])

concentration 0.23 M) and assayed for testosterone[10] and cyclic AMP[11] as modified by Harper and Brooker.[12] ICI 118530 (<Glu-His-Trp-Ser-Tyr-D-Ser(Bu^t)-Leu-Arg-Pro-*Aza*Gly-NH$_2$) was a gift from ICI plc. All data are total (intracellular plus extracellular) levels of testosterone and cyclic AMP, unless stated otherwise. Initial levels were not subtracted.

To measure intra- and extracellular cyclic AMP and testosterone levels, the medium was removed from the cells, acidified with HClO$_4$ as above, and frozen. 150 μl of HClO$_4$ was added to the cells, and this was followed by freezing. Before assay, the cellular extract was neutralized with 300 μl K$_3$PO$_4$; the medium was treated as above.

[^{14}C]Arachidonic Acid Metabolism

This was carried out with purified tumor Leydig cells for 30 min at 32°C. The products were separated by thin layer chromatography in an ether:hexane:glacial acetic acid system (60:40:1) at 4°C. The chromatography was autoradiographed then cut into fractions as indicated and the radioactivity estimated. The inhibitors used were indomethacin, aspirin, nordihydroguaiaretic acid (NDGA), BW 755C (3-amino-1-[3(trifluoromethyl)-phenyl]-2-pyrazoline hydrochloride), and benoxaprofen (Opren®, 2-[4-chloropophenyl]-methyl-5-benzoxazole acetic acid).

RESULTS

Effects of LHRH Agonist

Cyclic AMP Production

An investigation of the initial two hours of incubation of rat testis Leydig cells showed (FIGURE 1) that intracellular and extracellular cyclic AMP levels are unaffected by LHRH agonist in the presence of the phosphodiesterase inhibitor, MIX. A significant increase in extracellular testosterone production was detected after 40 minutes incubation and the major increase occurred in the period from 120 minutes to 240 minutes incubation (FIGURE 2).

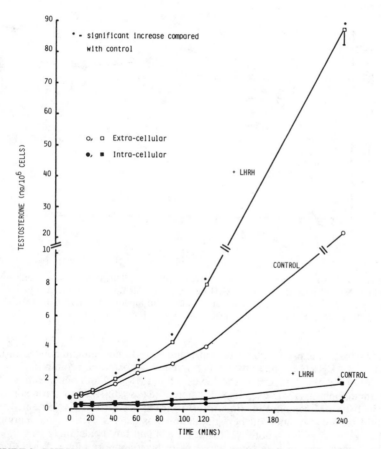

FIGURE 2. LHRH agonist effect on testosterone production in rat Leydig cells. Intracellular ($\bullet$,$\blacksquare$) and extracellular testosterone ($\bigcirc$,$\square$) were measured in the presence ($\square$,$\blacksquare$) and absence ($\bigcirc$,$\bullet$) of LHRH agonist (10^{-7} M) over the time period shown in freshly cultured Leydig cells. Results are means $\pm$ S.E.M. ($N = 3$). (Data from Sullivan & Cooke.[7])

Calcium

To determine the effect of the calcium ionophore A23187 on LHRH agonist–stimulated testosterone production, cells were incubated with different concentrations of the ionophore in the presence and absence of the agonist (10^{-7} M) for four hours (in 2.5 mM calcium). The results obtained (FIGURE 3) show that the ionophore itself stimulated testosterone production and that this occurred in a concentration-dependent manner. LHRH agonist had little or no additional effect in the presence of 0.2–1.0 μM A23187. The effect of changing the calcium concentration in the incubation medium in the presence and absence of the ionophore and LHRH agonist was investigated (FIGURE 4). LHRH agonist and ionophore A23187 were added as before at the beginning of the four-hour incubation period.

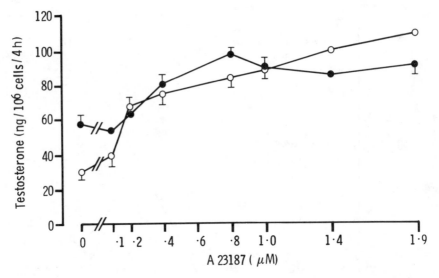

FIGURE 3. Response curves to ionophore A23187 (0–1.9 μM) for testosterone in the presence (●) and absence (○) of LHRH agonist (10^{-7} M) during 4 hours incubation. All values are means ± S.E.M. of triplicate cultures. Ionophore was added in DMSO (dimethylsulfoxide) at 10 μl/ml media. (Data from Sullivan & Cooke.[7])

Basal testosterone production was unaffected by different calcium concentrations (FIGURE 4). LHRH agonist (10^{-7} M) stimulated testosterone production two- to threefold ($p < 0.05$) except at the lowest (1.1 μM) calcium concentration. The calcium ionophore A23187 significantly increased ($p < 0.01$) testosterone production in 1–10 mM calcium; maximum testosterone production was obtained with 2.5 mM calcium. A small further stimulation was caused by the combination of LHRH agonist and ionophore A23187 at 1.1 μM and 1 mM calcium ($p < 0.05$) but not at higher calcium levels compared with the ionophore alone. With 10 mM calcium, the ionophore effect (in the presence or absence of LHRH agonist) was the same as the effect of LHRH agonist alone. In the presence of low calcium levels (1.1 μM and 1.0 mM) LH-stimulated testosterone production was less than 50% of the production with 2.5 mM calcium (FIGURE 5). Concentrations of cal-

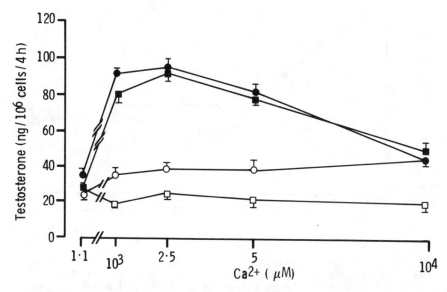

FIGURE 4. Response curves to calcium (1.1 μM–10 mM) for testosterone during a 4 hour incubation period. (□): Basal. (○): LHRH agonist (10⁻⁷ M) present. (■): A23187 (1.9 μM) present. (●): A23187 and LHRH agonist present. All points are means ± S.E.M. of triplicate cultures. (Data from Sullivan & Cooke.[7])

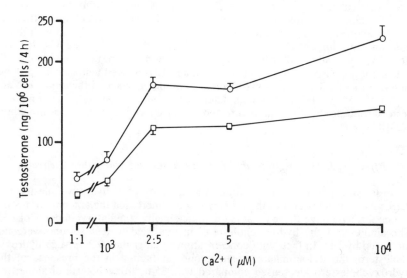

FIGURE 5. Response curve to calcium (1.1 μM–10 mM) for testosterone production in the presence of LHRH agonist (10⁻⁷ M) (○), or control (□). LH (100 ng/ml) was present for the final 2 hours of incubation of the total incubation period of 4 hours. All points are means ± S.E.M. of triplicate incubations. (Data from Sullivan & Cooke.[6])

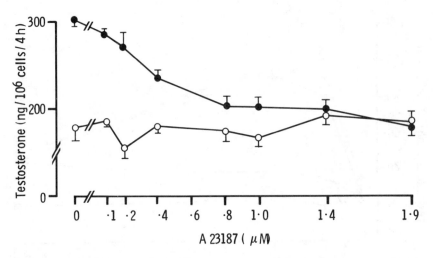

FIGURE 6. Response curves to ionophore A23187 (0–1.9 μM) for testosterone and cyclic AMP production in the presence (●) and absence (○) of LHRH agonist (10^{-7} M). LH (100 ng/ml) was added for the final 2 hours of the 4 hour incubation period. All values are means ± S.E.M. of triplicate cultures.

cium higher than 2.5 mM had little further effect. The LHRH agonist potentiated LH-stimulated testosterone production at all calcium concentrations, and was highest at the highest calcium concentration used (10 mM) ($p < 0.05$, with 1.1 μM and 1 mM calcium; $p < 0.01$, with 2.5–10 mM calcium) (FIGURE 5).

To examine the effect of the ionophore A23187 on the potentiating effects of LHRH agonist on LH-induced steroidogenesis, cells were incubated with different concentrations of the ionophore with and without LHRH agonist for four hours; LH was added after two hours of incubation. Again, in the absence of the calcium ionophore, LHRH agonist potentiated LH-induced testosterone production (FIGURE 6). This effects was decreased in the presence of the ionophore and with 0.8 μM A23187 it was completely inhibited. In contrast, LH-stimulated testosterone production was unaffected by all concentrations of the ionophore A23187 used.

Effects of LHRH Agonist and LH on Cholesterol Side-chain Cleavage

In initial experiments it was found that addition of 25-hydroxycholesterol or 22(R)hydroxycholesterol to the rat Leydig cells increased the amounts of testosterone formed above those obtained with maximally stimulatory amounts of LH. The amounts of the hydroxycholesterol metabolized to testosterone were not increased by LH. In fact, with concentrations greater than 0.37 μM 25-hydroxycholesterol the LH-stimulated testosterone production in the presence of the hydroxycholesterol decreased compared with 25-hydroxycholesterol alone; the LH-induced stimulation of testosterone production above basal decreased from 69.5 ± 3.8 ng/10^6 cells/4 hr over a range 0–0.37 μM 25-hydroxycholesterol to 38.4 ± 6.2 ng with 3.7 μM hydroxycholesterol and to 13.2 ± 5.4 ng with 37 μM hydroxycholesterol. In contrast, LHRH agonist markedly stimulated more 25-

hydroxycholesterol metabolism to testosterone with concentrations of the former greater than 0.37 μM; the increase due to LHRH agonist was 16.6 ± 1.2 ng testosterone/10^6 cells/4 hr with no hydroxycholesterol present, and increased to 83.5 ± 7.9 testosterone/10^6 cells/4 hr in the presence of 37 μM 25-hydroxycholesterol.

Because more testosterone is formed from 22(R)-hydroxycholesterol than the 25-hydroxy compound the metabolism of the former was also investigated. In the above experiments the Leydig cells were incubated with the LHRH agonist for a total of 4 hr and the hydroxycholesterol and LH were present during the last 2 hr of incubation. An additional experiment was carried out in which LH and/or LHRH agonist was present for 4 hr. The 22(R)-hydroxycholesterol (0.1, 1.0 and 10.0 μM) was added after 1 hr. LHRH agonist increased the production of testosterone as the concentration of 22(R)-hydroxycholesterol was increased (from 23.4 ng testosterone/10^6 cells/4 hr with no hydroxysteroid to 101.2 ng testosterone/10^6 cells/4 hr with 10 μM hydroxysteroid) ($p < 0.05$) (FIGURE 7). In contrast, the stimulation by LH compared with the hydroxysteroid alone remained constant (61.9 ± 5.2 ng/10^6 cells/4 hr over the whole concentration range). LH plus LHRH agonist potentiated steroidogenesis further ($p < 0.05$) compared with the effects of LH and LHRH agonist when present separately, e.g., with 10 μM 22(R)-hydroxycholesterol the testosterone production due to LH + LHRH agonist was 326.4 compared with 101.2 and 52.5 ng/10^6 cells/4 hr for LHRH agonist and LH, respectively (FIGURE 7).

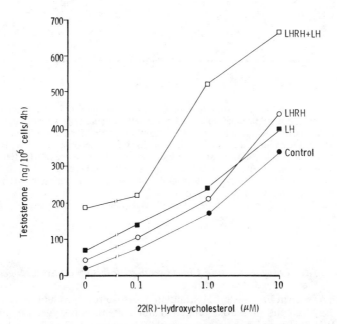

FIGURE 7. Testosterone production in the presence of LHRH agonist, LH, LH plus LHRH agonist, and various concentrations of 22(R)-hydroxycholesterol. The cells were incubated with LHRH agonist (10^{-7} M) and LH (100 ng/ml) for 4 hr. 22(R)-hydroxycholesterol was present for the final 2 hr of incubation. (Data from Sullivan and Cooke.[5])

Substitution of 1.6 μM pregnenolone (added in 10 μl ethanol) for 22(R)-hydroxysteroid in the incubations with the Leydig cells also resulted in high testosterone production (562 $\pm$ 24 ng/10^6 cells/4 hr), but the addition of LHRH agonist had no additional effect on testosterone production (pregnenolone + LHRH agonist: 558 $\pm$ 16 ng/10^6 cells/4 hr).

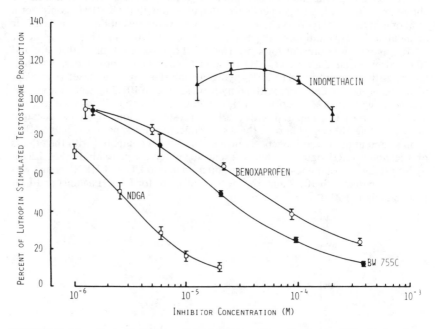

FIGURE 8. The effect of inhibitors of arachidonic acid metabolism on LH-stimulated testosterone and cyclic AMP production in rat Leydig cells. Leydig cells were preincubated for 2 hr in DMEM + 0.1% BSA and isobutylmethylxanthine (0.5 mM) and then incubated in the presence of various concentrations of (▲) indomethacin, (○) benoxaprofen, (●) BW 755C, and (□) NDGA for 15 min followed by a 2 hr incubation in the presence of LH (100 ng/ml) at 32°C in an atmosphere of 90% air, 10% CO_2. Values represent percent $\pm$ S.D. of duplicate determinations carried out on triplicate samples. In a typical experiment LH increased testosterone production from 1.6 $\pm$ 1.3 to 103 $\pm$ 2.9 ng/10^6 cells/2 hr and cyclic AMP production from 13.7 $\pm$ 2.3 to 225.1 $\pm$ 8.4 pmol/10^6 cells/2 hr (means $\pm$ S.D., $N = 3$). (Data from Dix *et al.*[8])

Effects of Cyclooxygenase and Lipoxygenase Inhibitors on Steroidogenesis

As can be seen in FIGURE 8, LH-stimulated testosterone production is inhibited in testis Leydig cells in a dose-related manner by the lipoxygenase inhibitors NDGA, BW 755C, and benoxaprofen with ID_{50} values of 2.5, 25, and 30 μM, respectively. However, indomethacin or cyclooxygenase inhibitors, at all concentrations tested (10–200 μM), had no inhibitory effect on LH-stimulated testosterone production. Indomethacin also had no significant effect on LH-stimulated cyclic AMP production and BW 755C and benoxaprofen only inhibited at the highest concentrations tested (330 and 380 μM, respectively). NDGA inhibited LH-stimulated cyclic AMP production over the same concentration range that inhibited testosterone production. However, if steroidogenesis was stimulated with dibutyryl cyclic AMP, it was found that NDGA still inhibited testosterone production with similar potency to that seen with LH-stimulated steroidogenesis.[8]

In order to investigate further the site of action of these inhibitors, experiments were performed in which the conversion of pregnenolone to testosterone by the Leydig cells was inhibited with SU 10603 (an inhibitor of 17β-hydroxylase, E.C.1.14.1.7) and cyanoketone (an inhibitor of 3β hydroxysteroid dehydrogenase E.C.1.1.1.51) and the dibutyryl cyclic AMP–stimulated production of pregnenolone was measured. Again NDGA produced a dose-related inhibition of pregnenolone production with a similar ID_{50} as seen for testosterone production (2–3 μM). BW 755C (75 μM) and benoxaprofen (70 μM) also inhibited pregnenolone production to 27% $\pm$ 4.7% and 30% $\pm$ 4.7%, respectively of the LH-stimulated pregnenolone production (190 $\pm$ 24 ng/10^6 cells/2 hr). When pregnenolone was added to the Leydig cells its conversion to testosterone was not inhibited by NDGA using concentrations up to 10 μM; with 1.25 μM NDGA a significant increase ($p < 0.001$) in the conversion of pregnenolone to testosterone was found. Indomethacin again had no significant effect on this conversion at concentrations up to 100 μM. When 22(R)-hydroxylcholesterol was used instead of pregnenolone the results were essentially the same, again with the only significant effect being an increased conversion of 22R(OH)-cholesterol to testosterone with 1.25 μM NDGA ($p < 0.05$).

In order to study the possible production of lipoxygenase products by Leydig cells, the Leydig tumor was used since a large number of pure tumor cells can be obtained, which is essential for the detection of these metabolites of arachidonic acid. It was found that the effects of aspirin, indomethacin, BW 755C, benoxaprofen, and NDGA on pregnenolone production in the purified rat tumor Leydig cells were essentially the same as those for the rat testes Leydig cells. Both aspirin and indomethacin at concentrations up to 80 μM had no significant effect on LH-stimulated pregnenolone production whereas both BW 755C and benoxaprofen produced a dose-dependent inhibition over the same range of concentrations as that seen for the rat testes Leydig cells. NDGA again inhibited LH-stimulated cyclic AMP production in the tumor Leydig cell to the same extent as in the testis Leydig cell but still inhibited dibutyryl cyclic AMP–stimulated pregnenolone production with the same order of potency as seen for the rat testis Leydig cell.

Metabolism of [^{14}C]Arachidonic Acid by Leydig Tumor Cells

When tumor Leydig cells were incubated with [^{14}C]arachidonic acid and the extracts subjected to thin layer chromatography followed by autoradiography, a number of products were evident. FIGURE 9 shows a typical autoradiograph of these products and indicates the mobilities of arachidonic acid, leukotriene B_4, 5-HETE (hydroxyeicosatetraenoic acid), and 12-HETE. Compared with the control product pattern seen in lane 1, LH had variable and inconsistent effects on the products in fractions 2, 3, and 4 (FIGURE 9, lane 2). However in all experiments there was an increased conversion of arachidonic acid to products found in fractions 1 and 6 (results not shown). In contrast the calcium ionophore, A23187, increased the metabolism of arachidonic acid to products found in fractions 2, 3, and 4 (FIGURE 9, lane 3); these fractions contain products that have similar mobili-

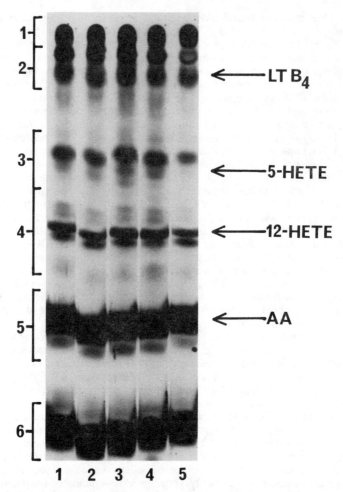

FIGURE 9. Autoradiograph of ^{14}C metabolites of arachidonic acid produced by rat tumor Leydig cells. Rat tumor Leydig cells were incubated with either [^{14}C]arachidonic acid (0.5 × 10[6] dpm, lane 1) or [^{14}C]arachidonic acid plus LH (1.0 μg/ml, lane 2), plus A23187 (1.9 μM, lane 3), plus A23187 and indomethacin (50 μM, lane 4), or A23187 and NDGA (10 μM, lane 5), under conditions described in the legend of TABLE 1, and the subsequent thin layer chromatograph of the products was autoradiographed as described in the MATERIALS AND METHODS, the arrows represent the positions of radiolabeled markers run in separate lanes on the thin layer chromatogram. Fractions 1–6 are the areas of each lane for this and subsequent experiments in which the radioactivity was determined, summed, and represented as a percentage of the total radioactivity as seen in TABLE 1. (Data from Dix *et al.*[8])

ties to leukotriene B$_4$, 5-HETE, and 12-HETE, respectively. The results seen for the calcium ionophore are typical of those seen in several experiments. In contrast, although indomethacin caused an increase in the formation of products in fractions 2, 3, and 4, this effect was inconsistent and never reached levels of significance (TABLE 1). NDGA reduced the amount of radioactive products in fractions 2, 3, and 4 (FIGURE 9, lane 5) and in three comparable experiments the percentage reduction of these products was statistically significant (TABLE 1). BW755C and benoxaprofen also produce a similar pattern of inhibition of the arachidonic acid metabolites in these fractions while aspirin had similar inconsistent effects to indomethacin (TABLE 1).

DISCUSSION

The results show that the LHRH agonist requires at least 1 mM Ca^{2+} to exert its effects on steroidogenesis, and has no detectable effect on cyclic AMP levels at any Ca^{2+} concentration. Detailed kinetic studies using a sensitive radioimmunoassay for cyclic AMP also showed that the LHRH agonist had no detectable effect on cyclic AMP levels. This stimulatory effect on LHRH agonist on steroidogenesis is apparently, therefore, dependent on Ca^{2+} rather than cyclic AMP. That the stimulatory effect of LHRH agonist was mimicked by A23187 also supports a role of Ca^{2+} in LHRH agonist action.

The role of Ca^{2+} in the potentiation of LH stimulation of steroidogenesis by LHRH agonist is less certain, especially in view of the negating effect of low concentrations of Ca^{2+} ionophore A23187. This requires further investigation.

It was demonstrated that the LHRH agonist increases 22(R)- and 25-hydroxycholesterol metabolism to testosterone. At high concentrations of 22(R)-hydroxycholesterol, LHRH agonist plus LH also increased testosterone production more than that obtained with the hydroxysterol alone. In contrast, LH did not increase metabolism of the hydroxysterols; this is in agreement with the results of Taoff *et al.*,[13] who found that the metabolism of 25-hydroxycholesterol by dispersed rat luteal cells was not influenced by addition of LH. The present results, therefore,

TABLE 1. Effect of Various Inhibitors of Arachidonic Acid Metabolism on the Metabolism of [^{14}C]Arachidonic Acid by Rat Tumor Leydig Cells

| | Percent of Control [^{14}C]Arachidonic Acid Metabolism | | | | |
| | A | | B | | |
Fraction Number	Indomethacin (50μM)	NDGA (10μM)	BW755C (50μM)	Benoxaprofen (50μM)	Aspirin (50μM)
1	74.9 ± 11.69	61.0 ± 38.62	46.7 ± 3.60	67.3 ± 1.65	48.0 ± 4.3
2	108.5 ± 6.05	36.2 ± 17.65[a]	68.0 ± 6.20	35.2 ± 14.7	97.4 ± 12.79
3	105.8 ± 32.2	36.8 ± 2.86[b]	27.0 ± 4.45	61.3 ± 4.8	89.5 ± 13.65
4	93.1 ± 15.61	45.1 ± 16.19[b]	53.5 ± 7.45	59.0 ± 23.1	113.6 ± 0.10
5	122.7 ± 15.05	109.4 ± 14.67	169.6 ± 22.20	146.4 ± 18.05	123.7 ± 3.46
6	105.0 ± 6.97	103.4 ± 30.67	49.8 ± 3.15	228.3 ± 68.9	192.4 ± 57.4

Rat tumor Leydig cells were incubated in DMEM for 30 min at 32°C in the presence of various inhibitors of arachidonic acid metabolism. At the end of the incubation period products were extracted and run on thin layer chromatograms as described in the MATERIALS AND METHODS section, after which each lane of the chromatogram was cut into 0.5 cm sections and counted for radioactivity. The radioactivity of six main regions of each lane as indicated in FIGURE 9 was summed and represented as a percentage of the control lane containing no inhibitors. The results represent means ± S.D. from 3 separate experiments for indomethacin and NDGA (A) and means ± range for 2 separate experiments for BW755C, benoxaprofen, and aspirin (B). (Data from Dix *et al.*[8])

A: [a] $p < 0.05$, [b] $p < 0.001$.
B: Values represent means ± range of means, $N=2$.

indicate a specific action of the LHRH agonist on steroidogenesis, which is different from that of LH.

The hydroxysteroids were used in this study because it was previously shown that they could increase steroidogenesis both in the ovary and testis in dispersed cells and isolated mitochondria and that more steroid was formed than from added cholesterol.[13,14] Also in agreement with these studies, it was found that the amount of steroid formed in the presence of the hydroxysteroids is higher than could be achieved with LH alone. As Taoff et al.[13] pointed out these results suggest that not enough endogenous substrate is available and/or cannot be mobilized to achieve the highest rates of steroidogenesis possible. Taoff et al.[13] found that there was a direct relationship between cytochrome P_{450} content and 25-hydroxycholesterol-supported steroid production in the ovary. The evidence obtained by Bakker et al.,[14] using tritiated hydroxycholesterol, suggests that added hydroxycholesterols are directly metabolized by testis mitochondria rather than these compounds increasing metabolism of endogenous cholesterol. The metabolism of the hydroxysteroids with saturating levels of substrate in the present study is, therefore, probably a reflection of the amounts of the cytochrome P_{450} cholesterol side-chain cleavage enzyme present in the Leydig cell mitochondria and the results indicate that LHRH analogs increase the synthesis of the cytochrome P_{450} enzyme. Further evidence for the specific effect of LHRH agonist on the cholesterol side-chain cleavage enzyme in the present study was obtained by the finding that LHRH agonist had no effect on the conversion of exogenous pregnenolone to testosterone. The results of the present study, therefore, indicate that the LHRH agonist, in contrast to LH, increases the metabolism of 22(R)- and 25-hydroxycholesterol in rat testis Leydig cells to testosterone. This may well result from an increased synthesis of the mitochondrial cytochrome P_{450} enzyme.

It is apparent that inhibitors of lipoxygenase but not cyclooxygenase activity inhibit LH- and dibutyryl cyclic AMP–stimulated steroidogenesis in purified testis and tumor Leydig cells. The potency of inhibition of LH-stimulated steroidogenesis by NDGA, BW 755C, and benoxaprofen is very similar to the known potencies of these compounds for inhibition of lipoxygenase activity in other cell systems.[15,16] These findings, together with the observation that [^{14}C]arachidonic acid is metabolized to products whose formation are inhibited by NDGA, BW 755C, and benoxaprofen but not by aspirin or indomethacin and that the degree of metabolism of arachidonic acid to these products is further increased by the calcium ionophore A23187, strongly suggest that lipoxygenase products are involved in the stimulation of steroidogenesis.

It has been known for some time that calcium is required for hormone-stimulated steroidogenesis[17,18] and that the requirement for calcium is primarily at a step before the conversion of cholesterol to pregnenolone.[19] The metabolism of arachidonic acid, particularly the release of arachidonic acid from membrane phospholipids by phospholipase A_2 is considered to be a calcium-dependent mechanism.[20] Results from the present study indicate a potentiation of arachidonic acid metabolism by the calcium ionophore A23187 and A23187 was shown to have stimulatory activity on steroidogenesis. Phosphatidyl inositol metabolism/turnover has been implicated in steroidogenesis[21] and this turnover is the possible mechanism of calcium entry into the cell.[22] It is interesting to speculate that the activation of arachidonic acid metabolism and the production of lipoxygenase products may be the link between phosphatidyl inositol metabolism, calcium, and steroidogenesis and evidence from the present study would suggest that a lipoxygenase product of arachidonic acid metabolism stimulates the transport of cholesterol or cholesterol ester to the mitochondria (FIGURE 10).

A role for lipoxygenase products in stimulus secretion coupling has also been implicated in the pancreatic beta cell for the stimulation of insulin release by glucose and other agents[23] and in the release of LH by LHRH in pituitary gonadotrophs.[24] Preliminary results carried out in the present study with LHRH instead of LH agonist indicate that LHRH agonist–stimulated steroidogenesis is also inhibited to the same extent by the lipoxygenase inhibitors as LH; again the cyclooxygenase inhibitors had no effect.[25] Lipoxygenase products may play, therefore, a pivotal role in many stimulus secretion coupling events in endocrine cells. An interesting result is the potentiation of the conversion of both pregnenolone and 22R(OH)-cholesterol to testosterone by low concentrations of NDGA. The reason for this is unclear. It is possible that NDGA increases the activity of one of the enzymes in the steroid pathway between pregnenolone and testosterone in a biphasic manner. However, until a more detailed study of a range of doses and compounds is carried out any conclusions can only be speculative.

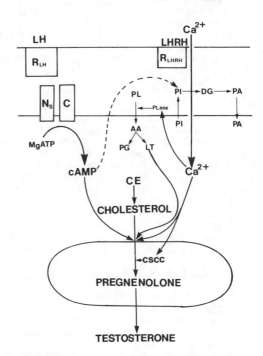

FIGURE 10. A scheme for the control of steroidogenesis in Leydig cells.

In conclusion, we have demonstrated for the first time that inhibitors of lipoxygenase activity but not cyclooxygenase activity cause a potent inhibition of LH- and dibutyryl cyclic AMP–stimulated steroidogenesis in rat Leydig cells. Preliminary evidence indicates that these inhibitors also inhibit products of arachidonic acid metabolism that have similar relative mobilities to those of reported lipoxygenase products of other systems. Our results indicate that lipoxygenase products may be essential for one of the steps before the conversion of cholesterol or cholesterol esters to pregnenolone. Since these steps are common to all steroidogenic pathways such findings may be important in the control of steroidogenesis not only in the testis but also in the ovary and the adrenal gland.

ACKNOWLEDGMENTS

We are grateful to ICI plc and the Science and Engineering Research Council and the Medical Research Council for financial support and Miss B. E. Macey for typing the manuscript. M.H.F.S. is a S.E.R.C. Case Student.

REFERENCES

1. HUNTER, M. G., M. H. F. SULLIVAN, C. J. DIX, L. F. ALDRED & B. A. COOKE. 1982. Mol. Cell. Endocrinol. **27:** 31–44.
2. SHARPE, R. M. & I. COOPER. 1982. Mol. Cell. Endocrinol. **26:** 141–150.
3. SHARPE, R. M., D. G. DOOGAN & I. COOPER. 1982. Biochem. Biophys. Res. Commun. **106:** 1210–1217.
4. MASSICOTTE, J., R. VEILLEUX, M. LAVOIE & F. LABRIE. 1980. Biochem. Biophys. Res. Commun. **94:** 1362–1366.
5. SULLIVAN, M. H. F. & B. A. COOKE. 1983. Biochem. J. **216:** 747–752.
6. SULLIVAN, M. H. F. & B. A. COOKE. 1983. Molec. Cell. Endocr. **34:** 17–22.
7. SULLIVAN, M. H. F. & B. A. COOKE. 1984. Biochem. J. **218:** 621–624.
8. DIX, C. J., A. D. HABBERFIELD, M. H. F. SULLIVAN & B. A. COOKE. 1984. Biochem. J. **219:** 529–537.
9. ALDRED, L. F. & B. A. COOKE. 1982. Int. J. Androl. **5:** 191–195.
10. VERJANS, M. L., B. A. COOKE, F. H. DE JONG, C. M. M. DE JONG & H. J. VAN DER MOLEN. 1973. J. Steroid Biochem. **4:** 665–676.
11. STEINER, A. L., C. W. PARKER & D. M. KIPNIS. 1972. J. Biol. Chem. **247:** 1106–1113.
12. HARPER, T. F. & G. BROOKER. 1975. J. Cycl. Nucl. Res. **1:** 207–218.
13. TAOFF, M. E., H. SCHLEGER & J. F. STRAUSS. 1982. Endocrinology **111:** 1785–1790.
14. BAKKER, C. P., M. VAN DER PLANK, M. P. I. VAN WINSEN & H. J. VAN DER MOLEN. 1979. Biochim. Biophys. Acta **584:** 94–103.
15. WALKER, J. R. & W. DAWSON. 1979. J. Pharm. Pharmacol. **31:** 778–780.
16. HIGGS, G. A., R. J. FLOWER & J. R. VANE. 1979. Biochem. Pharmacol. **28:** 1959–1961.
17. BIRMINGHAM, M. K., F. H. ELLIOT & P. H. VALERE. 1953. Endocrinology **53:** 687–689.
18. JANSZEN, F. H. A., B. A. COOKE, M. J. A. VAN DRIEL & H. J. VAN DER MOLEN. 1976. Biochem. J. **160:** 433–437.
19. HALL, P. F., S. OSAWA & J. MROTEK. 1981. Endocrinology **109:** 1677–1682.
20. CRAVEN, P. A., R. K. STRUDER & F. R. DERUBERTIS. 1981. J. Clin. Invest. **68:** 722–732.
21. FARESE, R. V., A. M. SABIR, S. L. VANDOR & R. E. LARSON. 1980. J. Biol. Chem. **255:** 5728–5734.
22. MICHELL, R. H. 1975. Biochim. Biophys. Acta **415:** 81–147.
23. METZ, S. A., W. Y. FUJIMOTO & R. P. ROBERTSON. 1982. Endocrinology **111:** 2141–2143.
24. NAOR, Z. & K. J. CATT. 1981. J. Biol. Chem. **256:** 2226–2229.
25. SULLIVAN, M. H. F., C. J. DIX & B. A. COOKE. (Unpublished results.)

Functional Maturation of Rat Testis Leydig Cells

ILPO T. HUHTANIEMI[a]

*Departments of Clinical Chemistry and Immunology and
Bacteriology
University of Helsinki
SF-00290 Helsinki 29, Finland*

DWIGHT W. WARREN and KEVIN J. CATT

*Endocrinology and Reproduction Research Branch
National Institute of Child Health and Human Development
National Institutes of Health
Bethesda, Maryland 20205*

INTRODUCTION

Testicular steroidogenesis has two active phases during life. The first one starts in fetal life, when the androgens produced by the testis are responsible for differentiation of the male genitalia.[1,2] Depending on species, the peak of this fetal activity is in early to mid pregnancy (human and other primates)[3-7] or in later gestation (rodents).[8-12] The testicular steroidogenic activity continues (rodents) or becomes reactivated (human and primates) during the immediate postnatal life, but thereafter it stays quiescent until puberty. The second phase of testicular steroidogenic activity starts at puberty and lasts for the rest of life.

A parallel developmental variation with steroidogenesis is seen in the testicular steroidogenic cells, Leydig cells, which are known to appear in two growth phases, one in fetal-neonatal life and the other during sexual maturation.[13-15] These two cell generations have been generally termed the fetal and adult Leydig cell populations. Because the two cell populations differentiate and function in vastly different hormonal environments (*in utero* versus in adult life), it is reasonable to assume that there are differences in their functional and regulatory characteristics. Besides some morphological differences in their arrangement in the interstitial space, and their ultrastructure,[13,14,16-19] very little is known about these possible functional differences. The present review describes some of our recent results from studies on the characterization of the regulatory and functional differences between the fetal and adult Leydig cell generations of the rat testis.

[a] Correspondence: Dr. Ilpo T. Huhtaniemi, Department of Clinical Chemistry, University of Helsinki, Meilahti Hospital, SF-00290 Helsinki 29, Finland.

LEYDIG CELL NUMBER, LH RECEPTORS, AND ENDOGENOUS STEROIDS IN THE RAT TESTIS FROM FETAL PERIOD UNTIL SEXUAL MATURITY

Morphological differentiation of Leydig cells begins at fetal age of 15.5 to 16.5 days.[13] The volume density of these cells reaches the peak on intrauterine day 19.5 (68×10^6 cells/g tissue), and starts a gradual decrease thereafter, attaining a nadir on day 14 post partum (5×10^6 cells/g tissue).[15] On the basis of morphological criteria it seems that a transition from a predominately fetal Leydig cell population to one of adult Leydig cells takes place at the same age.[13,14,17] After 2 weeks of age, the Leydig cell density increases again and reaches the adult level (about 20×10^6 cells/g) by about 30 days of age.[15]

Several pieces of evidence indicate that the number of LH receptors per Leydig cell is lower in the fetal than adult population. Quantitation of LH binding in both fetal Leydig cell suspensions and whole testis homogenates (related to Leydig cell density) has yielded this result.[20–22] Furthermore, we found in a quantitative autoradiographic study (Huhtaniemi *et al.,* unpublished) that the number of [^{125}I]hCG grains per Leydig cell in the neonatal testis was only about 50% of that counted in the adult (FIGURE 1). Likewise, the mean diameter of the grain-positive cells in the neonatal testis was about half of that of the adult.

The appearance of Leydig cells in the fetal testis is accompanied by the activation of the testicular steroidogenesis, as depicted by the endogenous steroid content of the rat fetal testes (FIGURE 2). At the same time as the maximum endogenous steroid content,[15,20] the LH receptor level of the fetal testis reaches a maximum,[20] and fetal testicular testosterone shows a maximum response to gonadotropin stimulation *in vitro.*[23–25] When either endogenous steroid content or *in vitro* steroidogenesis in rat testes of different ages (ranging from fetal period until sexual maturity) were compared, it was evident that the steroidogenic capacity of the fetal Leydig cells is higher than that of the adult cells.[15,17,20,22]

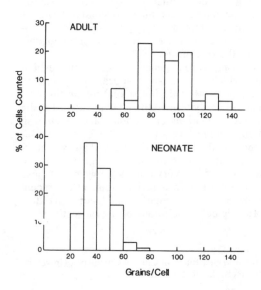

FIGURE 1. Grain distribution in autoradiography of [^{125}I]hCG binding to Leydig cell suspensions prepared from adult and 5-day-old rat testes. 100 grain-positive cells were counted in each case, and the %-distribution of the number of grains per cell (by the nearest 10) is presented.

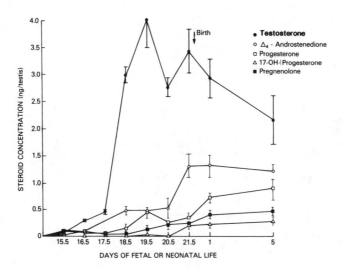

FIGURE 2. Content of various steroids in the androgenic pathway in the fetal rat testis.[20] Each point is the mean ± SE of 6 replicate determinations.

DIFFERENCES IN THE REGULATION OF LEYDIG CELL LH AND PROLACTIN RECEPTORS BETWEEN THE NEONATAL AND ADULT TESTIS

Gonadotropin-induced negative regulation, or down-regulation, of testicular and ovarian LH receptors is now well-established.[26,27] In the adult rat, a high dose of hCG or LH completely eliminates free LH receptors from the testis in 1–2 days and the recovery takes as long as 12–14 days.[22,26,72] We first wanted to see whether the negative LH receptor autoregulation would also take place in the fetal-neonatal testis.[21] The 5-day-old male rat was chosen as the experimental model of fetal Leydig cell function. Animals of this age are technically easier to handle than fetuses, while their Leydig cells are still exclusively derived from the fetal growth phase.

The neonatal and adult (60-day-old)rats were injected with increasing doses of hCG, and their testicular free LH receptors were measured 24 hr (neonates) and 48 hr (adults) after the injections, which were the times known to represent maximal loss of free receptors in these ages. As shown before, there was a dose-dependent loss of LH receptors in the adult testis (FIGURE 3). In the neonatal testis, the loss of binding was preceded by a transient increase in binding with lower hCG doses that has not been detected in the adult testis. A short-lived increase in LH and prolactin (Prl) receptors of the adult testis has been shown a few hours after gonadotropin stimulation[28-31] but this response is clearly distinct from the present findings and is probably due to rearrangement in plasma membrane conformation and exposure of cryptic binding sites, apparently related to the steroidogenic response of the testis.[31] It seems, therefore, that the neonatal testis LH receptors are regulated both positively and negatively by acute gonadotropin exposure, but those of the adult exhibit predominately negative regulation.

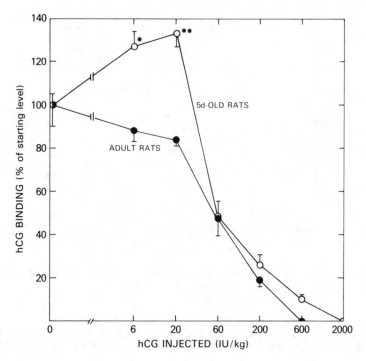

FIGURE 3. Effect of 0–2000 IU/kg subcutaneous injections of hCG on *in vitro* [125I]hCG binding (percent of controls) to 5-day-old and adult rat testis homogenates.[21] Binding of the 5-day-old rat testes was measured at 24 hr and that of the adult testis 48 hr after the injections, since these were in each case the times of maximal receptor loss. Each point depicts the mean ± SE of measurements from 5–7 animals. The asterisks indicate statistically significantly higher binding than the control (0 IU hCG): **, $p<0.01$; *, $p<0.05$.

The positive effect of hCG in the neonate is analogous to that observed in hypophysectomized adult animals,[32] which in the absence of pituitary LH show an increase in LH receptors after gonadotropin treatment. This effect does not occur in the intact adult animal, and after hypophysectomy it is most clearly seen during concomitant treatment with LH and prolactin.[32] Although the neonatal animal has a relatively high level of immunoreactive LH in the circulation,[33-35] the serum level of bioactive LH may be insufficient to maintain function of the regressing fetal Leydig cell population. This may be the reason why exogenous gonadotropin is able to induce trophic effects in the neonatal testis, as seen in the Leydig cell number, LH receptors, and steroidogenic capacity (see below).

The absence of a positive effect of gonadotropin stimulation on adult testis LH receptors is corroborated by our recent studies with a GnRH antagonist, in which short-term deprivation from gonadotropin support had no effect on testicular LH receptors.[36] In contrast, the GnRH antagonist reduced LH binding in the immature testis.[37] Therefore, maintenance of the existing LH receptor population in the adult testis may not need continuous gonadotropic stimulation, but the induction of new receptors in the growing gonads of immature animals is critically dependent on gonadotropin support. This could also be relevant to the ability of low-dose hCG treatment to increase testicular LH receptors in the neonatal rat but not in the adult.

The time-course of LH receptor down-regulation in the neonatal and adult rat testis was studied using a similarly effective dose of hCG (600 IU/kg) at both ages (FIGURE 3). Free receptors were lost in the adult testis in 24–48 hr, and the slow recovery of binding took about two weeks (FIGURE 4). There was also a fast loss of free receptors in the neonatal testis but the recovery of binding followed a completely different time-course, being completed in less than three days. When the receptor occupancy of the neonatal testis was assessed by low pH elution and assay of hCG released from the tissue,[21] there was no clear evidence for the net loss of binding sites (decreased sum of free and occupied receptors) that is a characteristic feature of receptor down-regulation in the adult.

The above conclusion is somewhat complicated by the fact that the number of Leydig cells in the neonatal testis increases during the days following gonadotropin stimulation.[21] There is a possibility that the new cells, 30–50% of the total Leydig cell mass on day 3 after hCG injection, have higher number of receptors per cell, which would thus mask the down-regulation receptor loss in the pre-existing cells. To investigate this possibility we performed a quantitative autoradiographic study on the amount of LH receptors per cell in neonatal control testes and in testes of animals injected three days earlier with the high hCG dose (Huhtaniemi *et al.*, unpublished observation). The number of grains per cell was distributed in a Gaussian manner in each case, and was 40.9 ± 1.1 in the control testes and 41.0 ± 1.2 in the testes three days after hCG injection. These data imply that the apparent lack of down-regulation is not explained by the presence of "old" cells with decreased receptors and "new" cells with a compensatory increase in receptor number.

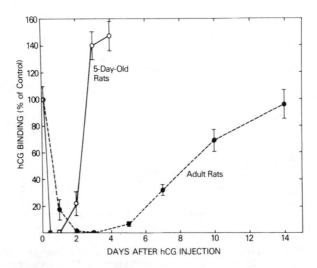

FIGURE 4. Comparison of the effects of a 600 IU/kg injection of hCG on free LH-receptors in 5-day-old (O——O) and adult (●-----●) rat testes.[21] Each point is the mean ± SE of measurements from 5–7 individual testes.

These results have shown that LH receptor down-regulation does not occur in the neonatal testis. High gonadotropic stimulation results in free receptor loss through occupancy but as soon as the bound hormone dissociates, the binding sites are replenished by new functional LH receptors. Whether the "old" receptor sites regain their binding capacity or whether they are replaced by new molecules, remains to be studied.

Specific receptors for another pituitary hormone, Prl, are also located in the Leydig cells.[38,39] Adult testis Prl receptors are known to disappear transiently during the phase of gonadotropin-induced LH receptor down-regulation, a phenomenon termed "heterologous down-regulation."[40] The duration of the heterologous Prl receptor loss is shorter than that of the LH receptors. As this phenomenon represents some form of functional coupling of LH and Prl receptors during their negative regulation, we found it of interest to see whether it would occur in a situation where the homologous down-regulation could not be demonstrated.[41] The 600 IU/kg dose of hCG was again administered to 5-day- and 60-day-old rats, and the time-course of changes in Prl receptors was followed. Interestingly, no loss of Prl binding could be seen in the neonate. In contrast, there was gradual increase of these binding sites that reached statistical significance in two days (FIGURE 5). Thus, heterologous down-regulation does not occur in the fetal growth phase of Leydig cells, consistent with the absence of true LH receptor loss during hCG stimulation.

Since LH and Prl receptors are concomitantly lost in the adult testis, this may be a consequence of the same regulatory mechanism, which possibly involves internalization and intracellular degradation of both receptor sites.[26,27,42,43] These processes may be both qualitatively and quantitatively different in the fetal Leydig cells. For instance, the bound hormone in the neonatal testis could be released from the cell surface receptors by mechanisms other than internalization, and the receptor could resume its function after hormone release. This could

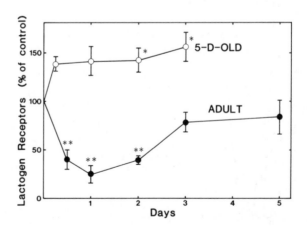

FIGURE 5. Effects of a 600 IU/kg injection of hCG on testicular lactogen receptors in the neonatal (○) and adult (●) testis.[41] Each point is the mean ± SE of measurements from 6 pools of 6 testes (5 days) or from 6 individual testes (60 days). Statistically significant differences from controls: **, $p < 0.01$; *, $p < 0.05$.

FIGURE 6. Effects of bromo-criptine(BR)-induced hypoprolactinemia on the recovery of LH receptors of 5-day-old rat testes after a 600 IU/kg injection of hCG. LH receptors were measured 2 days and 3 days after the hCG injection. Control = saline-injected animals; hCG = 600 IU/kg hCG on day 0; BR = 1 mg/kg BR each 12 hr between day 0 and sacrifice; hCG + BR = combined treatment. Each bar shows the mean ± SE of measurements from five testes.

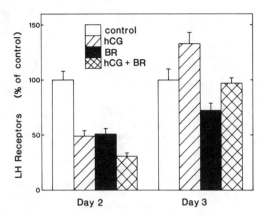

explain the lack of the negative functional coupling between the LH and Prl receptors. In fact, we have evidence (Huhtaniemi *et al.*, unpublished) that the association and dissociation rates of LH binding in the neonatal testis are faster than in the adult, and that the progression from 'loose' to 'tight' binding, which is possibly the initial step in LH receptor internalization,[44,45] does not progress in the same way in the neonatal testis as in the adult testis.

There is further evidence suggesting that the receptor recovery in the neonatal testis is different from the replenishment taking place in down-regulated adult Leydig cells. Bromocriptine-induced hypoprolactinemia significantly delays the increase in LH receptors in pubertal animals and during the recovery phase after hCG-induced down-regulation,[47] consistent with earlier findings on the permissive role of Prl in induction and maintenance of LH receptors.[32] Neonatal animals rendered hypoprolactinemic by bromocriptine also show a decrease of LH receptors, indicating their dependence on Prl (FIGURE 6). However, when these hypoprolactinemic animals are treated with hCG, their LH receptor recovery is as fast as in the normoprolactinemic animals, indicating that the receptor recovery in the neonate is a phenomenon distinct from the Prl-dependent LH receptor replenishment of the adult testis after down-regulation, and that synthesis of new receptors is probably not involved in this recovery of binding.

DIFFERENCES IN THE REGULATION OF STEROIDOGENESIS BETWEEN THE NEONATAL AND ADULT TESTIS

The steroidogenic response of the neonatal and adult testis to gonadotropic stimulation was compared in the next experiments. It was of particular interest to see whether the same kind of refractoriness in androgen production as in the adult after gonadotropin stimulation could be demonstrated in the neonate. Gonadotropin stimulation of the adult induces desensitization of cytochrome P-450–dependent enzymes of the androgen biosynthetic pathway in about 24 hr, which is seen as a decrease of testosterone formation and compensatory accumulation of the C_{21} form androgen precursors, progesterone and 17-hydroxyprogesterone, due to a defect in the C_{21} steroid side-chain cleavage activity.[47-50] The time-course of serum

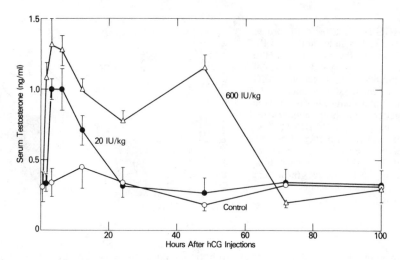

FIGURE 7. Serum testosterone levels in 5-day-old rats up to 100 hr after subcutaneous injections of 20 (●———●) or 600 (△———△) IU/kg hCG.[21] The controls (○———○) received saline injections. Each point gives the mean ± SE of measurements from 5–8 animals.

testosterone response to a low (20 IU/kg) and high (600 IU/kg) dose of hCG is seen in FIGURE 7. As in the adult, an acute increase in testosterone was seen with both doses between 1–2 hr. Thereafter, testosterone returned to control level in 24 hr with the lower dose, evidently because hCG had decreased in the circulation below the stimulating level. There was also a decrease at 24 hr after the high dose, but a secondary rise was seen at 48 hr. The decrease at 24 hr suggests a similar steroidogenic lesion as known to occur in the adult testis (see above). On the other hand, the free LH receptors were unmeasurable at this time (FIGURE 4), and therefore gonadotropin stimulation, in spite of normally functioning steroidogenesis, would be impossible. At 48 hr the receptors already had recovered to some extent, which explains the second testosterone peak.

To find out whether the testosterone synthetic capacity was really impaired at 24 hr, we incubated the control and hCG-stimulated testes of neonatal and adult rats in the presence and absence of a maximally stimulating dose of hCG (FIGURE 8), and measured the production of cAMP, testosterone, and pregesterone.[51] Progesterone was chosen as indicator of the blockade of C_{21} steroid side-chain cleavage. The hCG injection induced down-regulation of the cAMP response at both ages. In the neonate this was probably at least partly due to loss of free LH receptors capable of stimulating adenylate cyclase. The hCG-stimulated part of the testosterone response was lost in the adult, and in keeping with the well-characterized blockade of C_{21} steroid side-chain cleavage, progesterone production was increased. No decrease in the *in vitro* rate of testosterone production was seen in the neonate, since the basal and hCG-stimulated testosterone production rates were the same as the stimulated rates in the controls. Progesterone production was increased about twofold, but this was minimal in comparison with the 20-fold increase in the adult testis. Thus, there was no clear evidence that steroidogenic desensitization occurred in the neonatal tests after gonadotropic stimulation.

The same lack of the C_{21} steroid response was also seen in serum steroids after hCG stimulation (FIGURE 9). Only marginal changes occurred in the neonatal testis in the levels of progesterone and 17-hydroxyprogesterone in response to gonadotropic stimulation, whereas in the adult the levels of progesterone and 17-hydroxyprogesterone were at a maximum (on day 1), 15- and 35-fold elevated, respectively.

Taken together, these results indicate that steroidogenesis in the 5-day-old rat testis does not respond to gonadotropic stimulation with decreased responses in androgen production and a reduction in C_{21} steroid side-chain cleavage activity. In contrast to the adult, the active androgen production of the neonatal testis persists for as long as the gonadotropin stimulation is maintained.

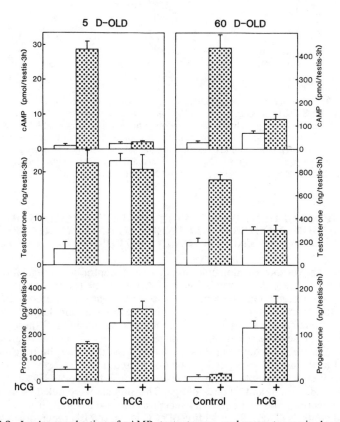

FIGURE 8. *In vitro* production of cAMP, testosterone, and progesterone in decapsulated testes of 5- and 60-day-old rats.[51] Testes of either control animals or those injected with hCG (600 IU/kg) 24 hr prior to sacrifice were used. The incubations were performed either in the absence (−) or presence (+) of maximally stimulating concentration of hCG (Pregnyl, 3 IU/ml).

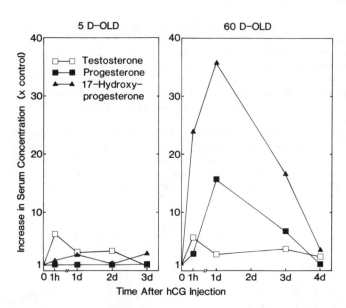

FIGURE 9. Response of serum testosterone (□), progesterone (■), and 17-hydroxyproges-
terone (▲) to 600 IU/kg hCG in 5-day-old (*left panel*) and 60-day-old (*right panel*) male rats.[51]
The levels are presented as relative increased in comparison to the basal levels. Each point
is the mean of five individual measurements. The standard errors of the observations are
from 2–14% on the means, and are omitted for the sake of clarity. Also pregnenolone and
androstenedione were measured. The former steroid did not change after stimulation, and
the levels of androstenedione were similar to testosterone at both ages.

DEVELOPMENT OF LH RECEPTOR DOWN-REGULATION, FUNCTIONAL COUPLING BETWEEN LH AND PRL RECEPTORS, AND STEROIDOGENIC LESION IN THE POSTNATAL RAT TESTIS

As shown above, the gonadotropin-induced LH-receptor down-regulation, heterologous Prl receptor down-regulation, and steroidogenic lesion are not functional
in the neonatal testis. Our working hypothesis was that these differences indicate
specific functional features of fetal and adult Leydig cell populations. We therefore did a time-course study to find out the ages of transition of these fetal-type
features to those observed in the adult testis. It was of special interest to see
whether a correlation between these functional features and the transition from
the fetal to the adult Leydig cell population would occur.

In the first experiment,[22] rats were given two injections of 10 IU/kg hCG, 24 hr
apart, at 3, 8, 13, 23, and 50 days of age. The animals were killed 24 hr after the
second injection, and testicular LH receptors were measured in these and age-
matched controls (TABLE 1). Injection of hCG increased LH receptors in the three
youngest age groups (5, 10, 15 days) but not in 25- and 52-day-old animals. The
trophic effect of hCG on LH receptors thus gradually disappears with age, and the
transition from positive to negative regulation occurs around day 15, which is the
same age at which the fetal Leydig cells are replaced by those of the adult population.

TABLE 1. Effect of Two Daily Injections of hCG (10 IU/kg) on Testicular LH Receptors Measured on the Third Day[22]

Age of Animals (days)[a]	Binding in Controls (fmol/testis)	Binding in Treated Animals (fmol/testis)	Increase in Binding (%)
5	0.57 ± 0.06	1.10 ± 0.13	91[b]
10	1.10 ± 0.05	1.50 ± 0.11	35[b]
15	1.70 ± 0.10	2.60 ± 0.24	52[b]
25	61 ± 1.40	64 ± 0.85	5
52	2000 ± 110	1700 ± 110	−16

Values are the mean ± SE for pairs of testes from five to seven rats. Control animals were injected with saline.

[a] At the time of death.

[b] Different from age-matched control, $p < 0.01$.

The effect of a single high dose of hCG (600 IU/kg) on unoccupied LH receptors was studied next at different ages ranging from 5 to 60 days (FIGURE 10). At all ages, the available LH receptors were almost completely lost in 12–24 hr. When the hCG injection was given at 5 days of age, the binding recovered completely in 72 hr, exceeding the age-matched controls at this time. In the 10-day-old group, binding recovered almost as rapidly as on day 5, but in 20-day-old animals, only 20% of the binding sites had been recovered on day 3. The length of time required for the recovery of binding became gradually longer, and 14 days were needed for complete receptor recovery in 60-day-old rats. As with the positive

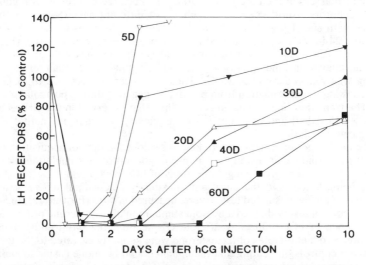

FIGURE 10. Effects of a single subcutaneous injection of hCG (600 IU/kg) on free LH receptors of rat testes.[22] The ages of the animals were 5, 10, 20, 30, 40, or 60 days at the time of injection. Testicular Lh receptor binding was measured for up to 10 days after hCG injection. At 60 days of age, the binding was 100% of control binding 14 days after the hCG injection (not shown). Each point represents the mean of measurements from five testes, and results are expressed as percentage of binding measured in age-matched animals. The individual values were 6–13% of the means.

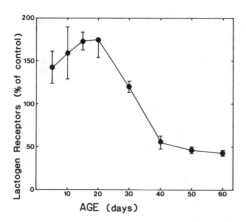

FIGURE 11. Effects of 600 IU/kg hCG on lactogen receptors of 5–60-day-old rats.[41] The receptors were measured 24 hr after injection of hormone or saline (controls). Each point is the mean ± SE of measurements of 6 testis pools (6 testes per pool at day 5, 4 at day 10) or 6 individual testes (15 days and older). The binding is expressed as percentage of the mean binding of controls. Statistically significant differences from controls: **, $p < 0.01$; *, $p < 0.05$.

hCG effect on LH receptors, a transition from the fetal-type receptor response to the long adult-type response seems to occur between 10 and 20 days, again suggesting that the fast and slow rates of recovery are features of the fetal and adult Leydig cell populations, respectively. The fetal cells are gradually involuted and replaced by adult cells, which explains the gradual transition from fetal to adult-type responses. The long time needed for development of the full adult-type response indicates that this is a slow process associated with pubertal maturation.

We also assessed the time of appearance of negative heterologous regulation of Prl receptors. Another group of animals at different ages (5–60 days) were injected with 600 IU/kg hCG, and the lactogen receptor sites in the testes were measured 24 hr later, and compared to those of saline-injected controls (FIGURE 11). Up to 20 days of age, there was an increase of Prl binding by about 50%. At 30 days, no change in binding was found, and in animals older than 40 days, the binding was reduced by about 50%. Thus, Prl receptor response to hCG also undergoes a gradual transition from positive to negative during postnatal maturation. The transition time (30 days) is later than that observed in the LH receptor response (15 days), and does not follow as closely the changing nature of the Leydig cell population.

The next experiment was undertaken to explore the time of acquisition of the adult-type steroidogenic lesion in response to gonadotropic stimulation. Rats (2–55 days of age) were given single injections of hCG (600 IU/kg), 1, 2, or 3 days before being killed, and the basal and maximally hCG-stimulated testosterone synthesis of the decapsulated testes were measured *in vitro* (FIGURE 12). In 5-day-old rats, control testes showed a fivefold stimulation of testosterone production in the presence of hCG. One day after hCG injection, the basal and maximally stimulated production rates of testosterone were similarly elevated to the level of stimulated controls, indicating that the *in vivo* bound hormone is able to maintain maximal steroidogenic response and that no steroidogenic lesion is present. At 2 and 3 days, basal testosterone production was decreased as the injected hCG disappeared from the circulation. In contrast, the hCG-stimulated steroidogenesis increased (2.5-fold on day 3) in comparison to the control.

In 10-day-old animals, a similar response was seen although the testosterone production rate and rate of stimulation by hCG were less marked. A further decrease in testosterone production per testis was seen on day 17, being only

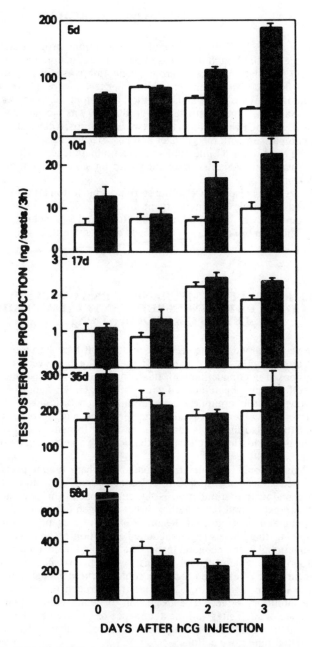

FIGURE 12. Effects of single injections of 600 IU/kg hCG on *in vitro* testosterone production by testes of 5-, 10-, 17-, 35-, and 58-day-old rats.[22] Each panel represents measurements from one age group, as indicated in the upper left corner of the panels. A single hCG injection was given on 1 of 3 consecutive days; each animal received only one injection. All the animals were killed on day 4. (○), uninjected controls. The ages refer to the age on the day of death. (□), testosterone production in the absence of hCG; (■), testosterone production in the presence of maximally stimulating concentration of hCG. Each bar is the mean ± SE of results from five incubations.

1.5% of that on day 5. hCG did not stimulate testosterone production in control testes of this age, and although it increased basal T production about twofold on day 3, the hCG stimulation of testosterone production was still only marginal.

The rate of *in vitro* testosterone production per testis increased over 100-fold between 17 and 35 days of age, and a further 1.5–2-fold increase occurred between 35 and 58 days. When testosterone production was measured 1, 2, and 3 days after the *in vivo* hCG injection in these two age groups, a clear difference was observed in comparison with the younger animals. Basal testosterone production was unchanged after the hCG injection and the stimulation seen with hCG in the control testes was lost, which is in keeping with the gonadotropin-induced steroidogenic lesion.[47–50]

These observations also show that the steroidogenic lesion after hCG stimulation is acquired by the developing testis at around 15–20 days of age, which is again in agreement with the hypothesis that this feature is lacking in the fetal Leydig cell population but appears in the newly differentiating Leydig cells of the adult growth phase.

POSSIBLE REGULATORY MECHANISMS RESPONSIBLE FOR THE FUNCTIONAL DIFFERENCES BETWEEN FETAL AND ADULT LEYDIG CELL POPULATIONS

No evidence was obtained for the presence of the adult-type steroidogenic lesion after hCG treatment in the neonatal testis. In the adult testis, several mechanisms have been proposed in connection with this gonadotropin-induced phenomenon, since similar effects have been induced with estrogen, GnRH-agonists, prolactin, epidermal growth factor, arginine vasotocin, and glucocorticoids.[47–50,52–56] Most evidence exists for involvement of intratesticular estrogen in this process. Gonadotropin stimulation also increases testicular estrogen formation and it has been shown that the desensitizing effects can be duplicated with estrogen treatment and prevented with antiestrogen.[47–50]

This mechanism could form an intratesticular feed-back loop to prevent excessive or sustained androgen response after gonadotropin stimulation. Since this response to gonadotropin stimulation is not functional in the neonatal testis it would be of interest to find out whether direct estrogen effects on the neonatal testis could induce the steroidogenic lesion. We have at present several pieces of evidence implying that the estrogen-mediated inhibition of androgen synthesis may not be functional in the neonatal testis. The fetal and neonatal circulation are rich in α-fetoprotein, which binds avidly estrogens in this species.[57,58] Furthermore, the occurrence of estrogen receptor could not be demonstrated in the rat testis before 6 days of age (TABLE 2). Since the estrogen receptor presumably mediates the inhibitory effects of estrogen on testicular steroidogenesis,[49] the apparent absence of such sites and the abundance of estrogen-binding α-fetoprotein in the circulation could account for the resistance of the neonatal rat testis to estrogen-mediated inhibitory actions.

Although the details of the molecular mechanisms involved in gonadotropin-induced down-regulation are still unknown, there is some evidence that estrogen could also be involved in LH receptor regulation.[59,60] Since estrogen-mediated inhibitory actions on steroidogenesis seem to be inoperative in the neonate, it is therefore possible that lack of LH receptor down-regulation is also related to the insensitivity of neonatal Leydig cells to estrogen.

Direct effects of gonadotropin-releasing hormone (GnRH) and its agonist analogues on the rat testis have been revealed recently.[52,61] The testis tissue has GnRH receptors,[62,63] and these peptides have been shown to decrease testicular LH binding and induce a steroidogenic lesion similar to that caused by hCG in C_{21} steroid side-chain cleavage.[52] There is no conclusive evidence about the physiological mediator for these actions, although there exist several reports about extraction of GnRH-like activity from the testis.[65,66] Despite the lack of gonadotropin effect, it is possible that the alternative GnRH-mediated induction of the steroidogenic lesion is functional in the fetal Leydig cells. To investigate this possibility, we injected neonatal rats with hCG, a GnRH-agonist analogue (GnRH-A) (Buserelin, Hoechst), and their combination, and compared their effects on LH receptor levels and steroidogenesis.[66] GnRH-A induced only a transient and minor decrease of LH receptors at 24 hr (FIGURE 13), in contrast with the clear down-regulation seen in the adult testis with this peptide,[46] again indicating absence of true LH receptor down-regulation in the neonatal testis.

TABLE 2. Estradiol Binding in 4- to 60-day-old Rat Testicular Cytosol, Measured by Density Gradient Centrifugation Analysis[22]

Age (days)	8S Binding		5S Binding	
	fmol/mg protein	fmol/testis	fmol/mg protein	fmol/testis
4	ND	ND	538	85
6	5.6	1.4	500	42
11	6.6	3.8	240	140
18	15.0	15	164	170
60	6.3	280	ND	ND

ND, not detectable. A single pool of testicular tissue (1–2 g) was measured at each age; 100 testes were pooled at 4–6 days of age, 50 testes were pooled at 11–18 days of age, and 100–200 mg aliquots of 10 testes were pooled at 60 days of age.

The steroidogenic responses of the testes to the hCG and GnRH agonist treatments were studied 24 hr after the injections by incubating the decapsulated testes in the presence and absence of a maximally stimulating dose of hCG (FIGURE 13).[66] As before, the hCG injection resulted in high testosterone production in the absence and presence of hCG, due to maximal effect of the *in vivo* injected hormone. GnRH-A did not influence the *in vitro* production of testosterone at this time when compared to the control. When the hormone treatments were combined, slightly decreased levels of basal and maximal testosterone production were seen, suggesting minor inhibition of the hCG-stimulated testosterone production by the peptide.

When *in vitro* progesterone production was measured (FIGURE 14), only a marginal increase was observed with hCG, which is in striking contrast to the adult testis (FIGURE 8). However, GnRH-A induced a clear increase in hCG-stimulated progesterone production (FIGURE 14), and when both treatments were combined a similar increase in hCG-stimulated progesterone production was seen. This finding indicates a relative steroidogenic lesion of C_{21} steroid side-chain cleavage activity, with compensatory accumulation of progesterone. This effect was only induced by GnRH-A, or when hCG and GnRH-A treatments were combined. A

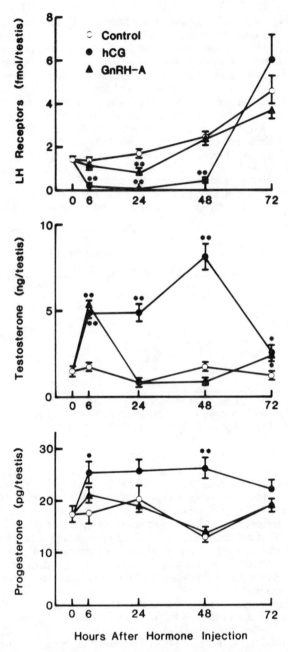

FIGURE 13. Testicular LH receptors (*upper panel*), testosterone (*middle panel*), and progesterone (*lower panel*) at times 0, 6, 24, 48, and 72 hr in relation to injection of hCG (●) and GnRH-A (▲).[66] Control animals (○) were injected with saline. Each point is the mean ± SE of measurements from 5–6 animals. The asterisks indicate statistically significant differences of the treatment groups from the time-matched controls (**, $p<0.01$; *, $p<0.05$).

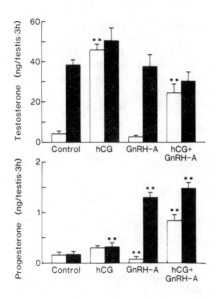

FIGURE 14. Testosterone and progesterone production *in vitro* of decapsulated testes from 5-day-old rats 24 hr after injection of hCG (600 IU/kg), GnRH-A (4 μg/kg), or their combination.[66] Each testis was incubated for 3 hr in the absence (left one of the pairs of bars) or presence of 8 nM hCG, and the steroids accumulated in the medium were analyzed. Each bar is the mean ± SE of 6 incubations. Asterisks indicate statistically significant differences from respective incubations with the control tissue (*, $p<0.05$; **, $p<0.01$). Furthermore, the differences between testosterone production of the hCG and hCG + GnRH-A groups, both basal and hCG-stimulated, were found statistically significant ($p<0.05$).

direct gonadal action of GnRH-A is the most likely explanation for this finding since the high hCG dose injected in combined treatment would totally mask the effects of increased levels of LH. Further evidence for the possibility of direct gonadal action of GnRH-A at this age was provided by our finding of GnRH receptors in the neonatal testis.[66]

This result demonstrates that the hCG- and GnRH-induced steroidogenic lesions must have two distinct mechanisms functioning through separate routes, since absence of the hCG-mediated lesion does not exclude the GnRH-mediated response. It also indicates that the GnRH-receptor–mediated functions are not involved in the gonadotropin actions on the testis.

CONCLUSIONS

We have identified several functional differences between the fetal and adult populations of Leydig cells in the rat testis. The nature of these differences, and the several mechanisms involved in them, indicate that we are dealing with a complex network of regulatory functions, all of which differ between the fetal and adult Leydig cell populations in a fashion to ensure persistent androgen production of the fetal-neonatal testis.

In evaluating the significance of these findings it is clearly important to question their relevance to the physiological regulation of the immature testis. Is there a reason why the fetal-neonatal testis is selectively immune to the inhibitory effects on gonadotropin stimulation that are prominently expressed in the adult testis? From a functional point of view it is obvious that the fetal testis maintains active steroidogenesis in conditions that would be inhibitory in the adult. This is especially clear in the human fetus, which is exposed to high levels of placental hCG and estrogens. It is well established that testosterone production is essential for differentiation of the genitalia and certain areas of the brain in the male fetus.[1,2,67] Castration of the newborn male rat prevents the masculinization of hypo-thalamic-pituitary function that is brought about by androgen secretion during the first few days of life.[68] The masculinization of hypothalamus in newborn rats takes place during the first day of life[69] and may be initiated during the LH-related testosterone surge of the first hours.[35] The immunity of the fetus and neonate to the gonadotropin- and estrogen-induced inhibitory functions could be a means to maintain the constant production of testosterone during these critical events in androgen-dependent differentiation.

REFERENCES

1. Jost, A. 1953 Problems of fetal endocrinology: The gonads and hypophyseal hormones. Rec. Prog. Horm. Res. **8:** 379–418.
2. Jost, A., B. Vigier, J. Prepin & J. P. Perchellet. 1973. Studies on sex differentiation in mammals. Rec. Prog. Horm. Res. **29:** 1–34.
3. Reyes, F. I., J. S. D. Winter & C. Faiman. 1973. Studies on human sexual development. I. Fetal gonadal and adrenal sex steroids. J. Clin. Endocrinol. Metab. **37:** 74–78.
4. Siiteri, P. K. & J. D. Wilson. 1974. Testosterone formation and metabolism during male sexual differentiation in the human embryo. J. Clin. Endocrinol. Metab. **38:** 113–125.
5. Tapanainen, J., P. Kellokumpu-Lehtinen, L. J. Pelliniemi & I. Huhtaniemi. 1981. Age-related changes in endogenous steroids of human fetal testes during early and midpregnancy. J. Clin. Endocrinol. Metab. **52:** 98–102.
6. Dang, D. C. & N. Meusy-Dessolle. 1979. Testosterone levels in umbilical cord blood, maternal peripheral plasma and amniotic fluid of the crab-eating monkey (*Macaca fascicularis*). Ann. Biol. Anim. Biochim. Biophys. **19:** 1307–1316.
7. Ellinwood, W. E., R. M. Brenner, D. L. Hess & J. A. Resko. 1980. Testosterone synthesis in rhesus fetal testes: Comparison between middle and late gestation. Biol. Reprod. **22:** 955–963.
8. Warren, D. W., G. Haltmeyer & K. B. Eik-Nes. 1973. Testosterone in the fetal rat testis. Biol. Reprod. **8:** 560–565.
9. Brinkmann, A. O. 1977. Testosterone synthesis *in vitro* by the fetal testis of the guinea pig. Steroids **29:** 861–873.
10. Buhl A. E., L. M. Pasztor & J. A. Resko. 1979. Steroids in guinea pig fetuses after sexual differentiation of the gonads. Biol. Reprod. **21:** 905–908.
11. Pointis, G. & J. A. Mahoudeau. 1976. Demonstration of a pituitary gonadotropic activity in the male foetal mouse. Acta Endocrinol. **83:** 158–165.
12. George, F. W., K. J. Catt, W. B. Neaves & J. D. Wilson. 1978. Studies on the regulation of testosterone synthesis in the fetal rabbit testis. Endocrinology **102:** 665–673.
13. Roosen-Runge, E. C. & D. Anderson. 1959. The development of the interstitial cells in the testis of the albino rat. Acta Anat. **37:** 125–137.
14. Lording, D. W. & D. M. De Kretser. 1972. Comparative ultrastructural and histochemical studies of the interstitial cells of the rat testis during fetal and postnatal development. J. Reprod. Fert. **29:** 261–269.
15. Tapanainen, J., T. Kuopio, L. J. Pelliniemi & I. Huhtaniemi. 1984. Developmental changes in the rat testicular endogenous steroids and Leydig cell density between the fetal period and sexual maturity. Biol. Reprod. (In press.)
16. Niemi, M. & M. Ikonen. 1963. Histochemistry of the Leydig cells in the postnatal prepubertal testis of the rat. Endocrinology **72:** 443–448.
17. Kuopio, T., J. Tapanainen, I. Huhtaniemi & L. J. Pelliniemi. 1982. Morphological and steroidogenic characteristics of fetal and adult type Leydig cells in the rat testis. Abstracts of The IInd European Workshop on Molecular and Cellular Endocrinology of the Testis, No. D7. Rotterdam.

18. CHRISTENSEN, A. K. & G. B. CHAPMAN. 1959. Cup-shaped mitochondria in interstitial cells of the albino rat. Exp. Cell Res. **18:** 576–579.

19. NARBAITZ, R. & R. ADLER. 1967. Submicroscopical aspects in the differentiation on rat testis Leydig cells. Acta Physiol. Lat. Am. **17:** 286–291.

20. WARREN, D. W., I. T. HUHTANIEMI, J. TAPANAINEN, M. L. DUFAU & K. J. CATT. 1984. Ontogeny of gonadotropin receptors in the fetal and neonatal rat testis. Endocrinology **114:** 470–476.

21. HUHTANIEMI, I. T., M. KATIKINENI & K. J. CATT. 1981. Regulation of luteinizing-hormone-receptors and steroidogenesis in the neonatal rat testis. Endocrinology **109:** 588–595.

22. HUHTANIEMI, I. T., K. NOZU, D. W. WARREN, M. L. DUFAU & K. J. CATT. 1982. Acquisition of regulatory mechanisms for gonadotropin receptors and steroidogenesis in the maturing rat testis. Endocrinology **111:** 1711–1720.

23. WARREN, D. W., G. HALTMEYER & K. B. EIK-NES. 1975. The effect of gonadotrophins on fetal and neonatal rat testis. Endocrinology **96:** 1226–1229.

24. PICON, R. & A. KTORZA. 1976. Effect of LH on testosterone production by foetal rat testis *in vitro*. FEBS Lett. **68:** 19–22.

25. FELDMAN, S. C. & E. BLOCH. 1978. Developmental pattern of testosterone synthesis by fetal rat testes to luteinizing hormone. Endocrinology **102:** 999–1007.

26. CATT, K. J., J. P. HARWOOD, G. AGUILERA & M. L. DUFAU. 1979. Hormonal regulation of peptide receptors and target cell responses. Nature **97:** 176–180.

27. CATT, K. J., J. P. HARWOOD, R. N. CLAYTON, T. F. DAVIES, V. CHAN, M. KATIKINENI, K. NOZU & M. L. DUFAU. Regulation of peptide hormone receptors and gonadal steroidogenesis. Rec. Prog. Horm. Res. **36:** 557–622.

28. HSUEH, A. J. W., M. L. DUFAU & K. J. CATT. 1977. Gonadotropin-induced regulation of luteinizing hormone receptors and desensitization of testicular 3′ : 5′-cyclic AMP and testosterone responses. Proc. Natl. Acad. Sci. USA **74:** 592–595.

29. HUHTANIEMI, I., H. MARTIKAINEN & L. TIKKALA. 1979. hCG-induced changes in the number of rat testis LH/hCG receptors. Mol. Cell. Endocr. **11:** 43–50.

30. SUTER, D. E., P. W. FLETCHER, P. M. SLUSS, L. E. REICHERT, JR. & G. D. NISWENDER. 1980. Alterations in the number of ovine luteal receptors for LH and progesterone secretion induced by homologous hormone. Biol. Reprod. **22:** 205–210.

31. HUHTANIEMI, I. T., M. KATIKINENI, V. CHAN & K. J. CATT. 1981. Gonadotropin-induced regulation of testicular luteinizing hormone receptors. Endocrinology **108:** 58–65.

32. ZIPF, W. B., A. H. PAYNE & R. P. KELCH. 1978. Prolactin, growth hormone and luteinizing hormone in the maintenance of testicular luteinizing hormone receptors. Endocrinology **103:** 995–600.

33. DÖHLER, K. D. & W. WUTTKE. 1975. Changes with age in levels of serum gonadotropins, prolactin and gonadal steroids, in prepubertal male and female rats. Endocrinology **97:** 898–907.

34. KETELSLEGERS, J.-M., W. D. HETZEL, R. J. SHERINS & K. J. CATT. 1978. Developmental changes in testicular gonadotropin receptors: Plasma gonadotropins and plasma testosterone in rats. Endocrinology **103:** 212–222.

35. CORBIER, P., B. KERDELHUE, R. PICON & J. ROFFI. 1978. Changes in testicular weight and serum gonadotropin and testosterone level before, during and after birth in the prenatal rat. Endocrinology **103:** 1985–1991.

36. HUHTANIEMI, I. T., J. M. STEWART, K. CHANNABASAVAIAH, H. M. FRASER & R. N. CLAYTON. 1984. Effect of treatment with GnRH antagonist, GnRH antiserum and bromocriptine on pituitary-testicular function of adult rats. Molec. Cell. Endocr. **34:** 127–135.

37. HUHTANIEMI, I. T., J. M. STEWART, K. CHANNABASAVAIAH, H. M. FRASER & R. N. CLAYTON. 1984. Pituitary-testicular function in immature rats after treatment with GnRH antagonist, GnRH antiserum and bromocriptine. Molec. Cell. Endocr. **34:** 137–143.

38. ARAGONA, C., H. G. BOHNET & H. G. FRIESEN. 1977. Localization of prolactin binding in prostate and testis. The role of serum prolactin concentration on the testicular LH receptors. Acta Endocrinol. (Copenh.) **84:** 403–409.

39. CHARREAU, E. H., A. ATTRAMADAL, P. A. TORJESEN, K. PURVIS, R. CALANDRA & V. HANSSON. 1977. Prolactin binding in rat testis: Specific receptors in interstitial cells. Mol. Cell. Endocr. **6:** 303–307.
40. DAVIES, T. F., M. KATIKINENI, V. CHAN, J. P. HARWOOD, M. L. DUFAU & K. J. CATT. 1979. Lactogenic receptor regulation in hormone-stimulated steroidogenic cells. Nature **283:** 863–865.
41. HUHTANIEMI, I. T., D. W. WARREN & K. J. CATT. 1983. Development of heterologous down-regulation of lactogen receptors in the rat testis. Mol. Cell. Endocr. **29:** 287–294.
42. AMSTERDAM, A., A. NIMROD, A. LAMPRECHT, Y. BURSTEIN & H. R. LINDNER. 1979. Internalization and degradation of receptor-bound hCG in granulosa cell cultures. Am. J. Physiol.: Endocrinol. Metab. Gastrointest. Physiol. **5:** E129–E138.
43. POSNER, B. I., J. J. M. BERGERON, Z. JOSEFSBERG, N. M. KHAN, B. A. PATEL, R. A. SIKSTROM & A. K. VERMA. 1981. Polypeptide hormones: Intracellular receptors and internalization. Rec. Prog. Horm. Res. **37:** 539–582.
44. KATIKINENI, M., T. F. DAVIES, I. T. HUHTANIEMI & K. J. CATT. 1980. Luteinizing hormone-receptor interaction in the testis: Progressive decrease in reversibility of the hormone-receptor complexes. Endocrinology **108:** 1980–1988.
45. VAN DER GUGTEN, A. A., M. J. WATERS, G. S. MURTHY & H. G. FRIESEN. 1980. Studies on the irreversible nature of prolactin binding to receptors. Endocrinology **106:** 402–411.
46. HUHTANIEMI, I. T. & K. J. CATT. 1981. Induction and maintenance of gonadotropin and lactogen receptors in hypoprolactinemic rats. Endocrinology **109:** 483–490.
47. CIGORRAGA, S. B., M. L. DUFAU & K. J. CATT. 1978. Regulation of luteinizing hormone receptors and steroidogenesis in gonadotropin-desensitized Leydig cells. J. Biol. Chem. **253:** 4297–4304.
48. CIGORRAGA, S. B., S. SORRELL, J. BATOR, K. J. CATT & M. L. DUFAU. 1980. Estrogen dependence of a gonadotropin-induced steroidogenic lesion in rat testicular Leydig cells. J. Clin. Invest. **65:** 699–705.
49. NOZU, K., M. L. DUFAU & K. J. CATT. 1981. Estradiol receptor-mediated regulation of steroidogenesis in gonadotropin-desensitized Leydig cells. J. Biol. Chem. **256:** 1915–1922.
50. NOZU, K., S. MATSUURA, K. J. CATT & M. L. DUFAU. 1981. Modulation of Leydig cell androgen biosynthesis and cytochrome P-450 levels during estrogen treatment and human chorionic gonadotropin-induced desensitization. J. Biol. Chem. **256:** 10012–10017.
51. HUHTANIEMI, I. T., D. W. WARREN, D. APTER & K. J. CATT. 1983. Absence of gonadotropin-induced desensitization of testosterone production in the neonatal rat testis. Mol. Cell. Endocr. **32:** 81–90.
52. HSUEH, A. J. W. 1982. Direct effects of gonadotropin releasing hormone on testicular Leydig cell functions. Ann. N.Y. Acad. Sci. **383:** 249–271.
53. WELSH, T. H. & A. J. W. HSUEH. 1983. Prolactin regulation of gonadotropin-stimulated androgen biosynthesis in cultured testicular cells. The Endocrine Society Annu. Mtg. Abstract No. 376.
54. WELSH, T. H., JR. & A. J. W. HSUEH. 1982. Mechanism of the inhibitory action of epidermal growth factor on testicular androgen biosynthesis in vitro. Endocrinology **110:** 1498–1506.
55. WELSH, T. H., JR., T. H. BAMBINO & A. J. W. HSUEH. 1982. Mechanism of glucocorticoid-induced supression of testicular androgen biosynthesis in vitro. Biol. Reprod. **27:** 1138–1146.
56. ADASHI, E. Y. & A. J. W. HSUEH. 1982. Direct inhibition of rat testicular androgen biosynthesis by arginine vasotocin. J. Biol. Chem. **257:** 1301–1308.
57. URIEL, J., B. DE NECHAUD & S. M. DUPIER. 1972. Estrogen-binding properties of rat, mouse and man fetospecific serum proteins, demonstration by immuno-autoradiographic methods. Biochem. Biophys. Res. Commun. **46:** 1175–1180.
58. RAYNAUD, J.-P., C. MERCIER-BODARD & E.-E. BAULIEU. 1977. Rat estradiol binding plasma protein (EBP). Steroids **18:** 767–788.

59. HSUEH, A. J. W., M. L. DUFAU & K. J. CATT. 1978. Direct inhibitory effects of estrogen on Leydig cell function of hypophysectomized rats. Endocrinology **103:** 1096–1102.

60. HUHTANIEMI, I. T., P. LEINONEN, G. L. HAMMOND & R. VIHKO. 1980. Effect of oestrogen treatment on testicular LH/hCG receptors and endogenous steroids in prostatic cancer patients. Clin. Endocr. **13:** 561–568.

61. HSUEH, A. J. W. & P. B. C. JONES. 1981. Extrapituitary action of gonadotropin-releasing hormone. Endocr. Rev. **2:** 437–461.

62. CLAYTON, R. N., M. KATIKINENI, V. CHAN, M. L. DUFAU & K. J. CATT. 1980. Direct inhibition of testicular function by gonadotropin-releasing hormone: mediation by specific gonadotropin-releasing hormone receptor in interstitial cells. Proc. Natl. Acad. Sci. USA **77:** 4459–4463.

63. BAMBINO, T. H., J. R. SCHREIBER & A. J. W. HSUEH. 1980. Gonadotropin-releasing hormone and its agonist inhibit testicular luteinizing hormone receptor and steroidogenesis in immature and adult hypophysectomized rats. Endocrinology **107:** 908–917.

64. SHARPE, R. M., H. M. FRASER & I. COOPER. 1982. The secretion, measurement, and function of a testicular LHRH-like factor. Ann. N.Y. Acad. Sci. **383:** 272–294.

65. BHASIN, S., D. HEBER, M. PETERSON & R. SWERDLOFF. 1983. Partial isolation and characterization of testicular GnRH-like factors. Endocrinology **112:** 1144–1146.

66. HUHTANIEMI, I. T., R. N. CLAYTON & K. J. CATT. 1984. GnRH agonist-analogue induced steroidogenic lesion in the neonatal rat testis—evidence for direct gonadal action. Endocrinology **115:** 233–238.

67. DONOVAN, B. T. 1980. Role of hormones in prenatal brain differentiation. *In* The Endocrine Functions of The Brain. M. Motta, Ed.: 117–141. Raven Press. New York.

68. PFEIFFER, C. A. 1936. Sexual differences of the hypophyses and their determination by the gonads. Am. J. Anat. **58:** 195–225.

69. HARRIS, G. W. & H. J. CAMPBELL. 1966. The regulation of the secretion of luteinizing hormone and ovulation. *In* The Pituitary Gland. G. W. Harris & B. T. Donovan, Eds. **2:** 99–165. University of California Press. Berkeley, Calif.

Maturation of the Human Testicular Response to hCG[a]

MAGUELONE G. FOREST

Unité de Recherches Endocriniennes et
Métaboliques chez l'Enfant
INSERM-U.34
Hôpital Debrousse
69322 Lyon Cedex 05 France

INTRODUCTION

Although testosterone was isolated from testicular tissues almost 50 years ago[1] it was 20 years later that the Leydig cell was definitely established as the major site of testosterone synthesis and secretion.[2] It is now well established that testosterone is the major secretory product of the interstitial tissue.[3] *In vitro* and *in vivo* studies have shown that other biosynthetic precursors of testosterone in the Δ^4 pathway, such as progesterone, 17α-hydroxyprogesterone (OHP), Δ^4-androstenedione, (Δ^4), and 17β-estradiol (E$_2$), are secreted by the adult testis.[3–10] Measurement of plasma hormone levels under varying conditions may reflect their testicular production, despite the fact that blood concentrations are also influenced by peripheral or hepatic metabolism, excretion, and/or by another site of production. In adult men, testosterone precursors in the Δ^5 pathway have either a mixed testicular and adrenal origin (17α-hydroxypregnenolone) or a predominant adrenal origin (pregnenolone and dehydroepiandrosterone.[3,11] In the human, there is a marked postnatal testicular steroidogenic activity (reflected in testosterone, OHP and Δ^4 blood levels) that, decreasing by about the seventh month of life onward,[12,13] is not apparent until a few years after the pubertal rise in gonadotropins. There is limited information concerning the secretory activity of the prepubertal testis. Despite the fact that plasma levels of testosterone and gonadotropins are similar in prepubertal boys and girls of comparable age,[14,15] maintenance of some testicular secretion during childhood has been suggested by the increased gonadotropins levels observed in agonadal boys.[16] Only recently has the secretory activity of the pubertal testis been documented *in vivo*.[17,18] These studies, together with previous *in vitro* experiments,[19] provided evidence that the secretory pattern of the prepubertal testis is quite different from that of the adult. Although both testosterone and progesterone testicular secretion is present at all ages, that of OHP and Δ^4 appears to be negligible in prepubertal boys. A pubertal change in testicular secretions has for long been suspected to occur in animals as well as in humans. The exact mechanism of this phenomenon is still unknown, although it is probably attributable to different physiological gonadotropin stimulation. Indeed, it is well established that testicular secretions are dependent on normal luteinizing hormone (LH) secretion.[20] Human chorionic gonadotropin (hCG) has been widely used for evaluating Leydig cell function in males of all ages.[21,22,24] Those studies of hCG stimulation testis were purely empirical and at first based on the sole mea-

[a] This work supported by INSERM (grant PRC 129047).

surement of urinary or plasma testosterone. Although it has been known for many years that besides testosterone, other testicular steroids (progesterone, OHP, Δ^4, E_2) respond to hCG/LH stimulation by increasing their secretion or excretion,[5,6,8,21,25] the great variability in the protocols of hCG stimulation used have resulted in confusing or conflicting data on the steroidogenic capacity of the maturing testis. It is only during recent years that it has been progressively understood that hCG and LH have selective effects on the intermediate enzymes of the testosterone biosynthetic pathways and that in adult men the dynamic of response of testosterone, its precursors, or E_2 is not uniform with respect to the dose or the duration of hCG stimulation.

Part of the problem is that in the last few years it has become apparent that the actions of LH and hCG have proved more complicated[26–28] than originally thought.[29] Indeed, experimental studies in rodents have shown that in addition to acutely stimulating testosterone production, hCG induces a temporary state of steroidogenic refractoriness to further gonadotropin stimulation. This phenomenon, hCG-induced testicular desensitization, is dose dependent and complex including receptor losses[28,30–34] or modification of the coupling system between the binding sites and the adenylate cyclase[35–37] and lesions beyond cAMP formation. The latter process is related to a partial blockade of the 17α-hydroxylase and 17,20-desmolase enzyme activities[34,38–40] and to a decreased conversion of cholesterol to pregnenolone when high dosages of hCG are used.[34,35,40] These enzymatic alterations are reflected by a biphasic response of plasma or testicular testosterone, with transient accumulation of C21 steroids after acute hCG stimulation.[28,35,41] Previous studies have shown that the normal adult testis exposed to pharmacological doses of hCG may be similar to the desensitized Leydig cells in the rodent.[23,42–46] Likewise a single injection of LH induces a state of testicular steroidogenic desensitization[47] indicating that the testicular response to hCG is comparable to that of native hormone. This report will summarize our experience with respect to the steroidogenic testicular response following various protocols of hCG administration, according to age and physiopathological conditions. These studies have been designed to provide a better understanding of the endocrine function of the maturing testis and to delineate some rational basis for the establishment of protocols for optimal use of hCG testing. Despite the limitation of interpreting testicular responses by estimating plasma steroid levels, certain working concepts emerge from such clinical studies, which in the main correspond to the information derived from *in vivo* and *in vitro* animal studies.

MATERIAL AND METHODS

Patients and Protocols

Three categories of subjects have been studied after prior informed consent. The first group consisted of adults or children with normal pituitary-gonadal function, who were subjects for, respectively, three and four different protocols. The adults were eugonadal volunteer men aged 29 ± 7 yr (ranges 23–43 yr). The children received the hCG stimulation tests at the request of their physicians for various reasons,[22] including retractile or undescended testis. They were in good health and normal by clinical and biological parameters. Among the cryptorchid boys, only those who showed a normal testicular capacity in response to a standard hCG stimulation test, previously established in normal boys,[48] were included in the results.

Protocol I consisted of a single i.m. hCG injection (Pregnyl®, Organon), administered at 9.00 hr to 7 adults and at 08.00 hr to 6 prepubertal (stage P_1 of Tanner) boys ($4/12$ to $13^2/12$ yr) with undescended testis. Blood was obtained before and 2, 4, 8, and 12 hr after the hCG injection, then every 24 hr for 7 and 6 days, respectively. The adults received a standard dose of 6,000 IU of hCG, corresponding to 95 ± 8 IU/kg BW or to a mean of 3,430 IU/m² of body surface area (the range was 3,060 to 3,700), while the children were given a constant dose for a body size (100 IU/kg BW). However, the dosages of hCG were quite comparable in both.

Protocol II consisted of two injections of hCG at 24-hr intervals administered i.v. at 09.00 hr to 6 adults (4 of whom participated in protocol 1, at random 1 to 6 months earlier or later) and at 08.00 hr to 2 prepubertal boys (P_1, $1^1/12$ and $11^7/12$ yr). In the last subject, a pubertal (stage P_2 of Tanner) boy aged $12^6/12$ yr, hCG was given i.m. at 08.00 hr. The dose of hCG used was 6,000 IU in the adults (or a mean of 3420 IU/m²) and 1,050, 2,000, and 1,500 IU in the 3 boys, respectively (83.5 ± 33 IU/kg). Blood was obtained before hCG injection, 2, 4, 8, 12, and 24 hr after the first injection, 2, 4, and 8 hr after the second, and then every 24 hr after the second injection for 1 week.

In protocol III, 4 adults and 4 prepubertal boys (P_1, 1 to $5^6/12$ yr) received 4 hCG injections every 5 days. A standard dose of hCG was used: 6,000 IU in adults (97 ± 3 IU/kg BW or 3225 to 3465 IU/m²) and 1,500 IU in children (99 ± 51 IU/kg BW or 2850 ± 370 IU/m²). Blood was sampled before, 2, 4, and 8 hr after each injection.

The protocol IV, utilized in children only, consisted of 7 i.m. injections, each of 1,500 IU hCG (82 ± 22 IU/kg BW) at 48 hr intervals. Blood was obtained before the first injection and the morning (09.00–12.00 hr) following the last injection. A large number (120) of children have been so studied and classified according to age and prepubertal stage (P_1 or P_2). The dynamic of response has been followed in only 6 boys, 5 at stage P_1 ($3^8/12$ to $9^{10}/12$ yr) and one at stage P_2 ($11^{10}/12$ yr) in whom blood was drawn before the test and 4 hr following each hCG injection.

The second group of subjects presented with congenital abnormal testicular function due to either 17,20-desmolase (17,20-D) or 17-ketosteroid reductase (17-KSR) deficiency. The 17,20-D patients were two adults (17 and 35 yr) and one prepubertal boy ($9^3/12$ yr, whose clinical and biological characteristics have been reported in part.[49–51] Because of the adrenal involvement in the enzyme defect all three, as well a control prepubertal boy matched for age ($9^6/12$ yr), were studied during adrenal supression (2 mg/day of dexamethasone from the day before until the end of the test). In addition the 17,20-D boy was restudied several months later ($9^{10}/12$ yr) without adrenal suppression. The 17-KSD–deficient patients were one adult (25 yr) and one child ($3^3/12$ yr). All these patients received a single i.m. hCG injection of 100 IU/kg BW between 08.00–09.00 hr (Protocol I as detailed above).

The third group consisted of adults with congenitally impaired gonadotrophic function, i.e. hypogonadic hypogonadotrophic (HH) subjects. Seven adult males affected with either Kallman's syndrome (4 subjects, 23 to 28 years old, 2 were siblings) or isolated hypogonadotropic hypogonadism (3 subjects, 18 to 30 yr). All subjects had eunuchoid habitus, prepubertal testicular volume, no cryptorchidism, and testosterone blood levels in the prepubertal range. None of them had received any form of hormonal therapy (neither androgens nor gonadotropins) prior to the study. They first received a single i.m. injection of 100 IU/kg BW of hCG at 09.00 hr (Protocol I). Blood samples were obtained 30 min and just prior hCG injection and then at various times detailed above for a week. The subjects were then put on hCG treatment consisting of a weekly i.m. hCG injection of 100 IU/kg for 3 months. The kinetics of the steroidogenic responses to hCG was restudied (daily for a week) after the 13th hCG injection in six of the subjects.

Steroid Analysis

Heparinized blood samples were centrifuged immediately and plasma stored at $-20°C$ until analyzed. After addition of tritiated tracers to monitor procedural losses, plasma was extracted with 10 volumes of ethyl ether and the dried extracts submitted to Celite column chromatographies as reported elsewhere.[14,52] An equivalent of 0.2 to 3 ml of plasma (according to age and or steroid) was used to measure testosterone, Δ^4, OHP, 17α-hydroxypregnenolone, progesterone, dihydrotestosterone (DHT), or E_2 in progressive triplicates by specific radioimmunoassays, the details of which have been reported earlier.[12-14,22,42,52] All samples from the same subjects (in one or two protocols when realized) were run in the same assay. Intra- and inter-assay coefficients of variations were $\leq 7\%$ and $\leq 12\%$, respectively. Unless stated, the results are expressed as mean $\pm$ SE. In addition, the results obtained in HH patients have been computed as the net area under the curve starting with the mean of the two samples (-30 min and 0) before hCG injection and using the samples obtained every day for the ensuing week. Steroid responses to hCG were expressed in area units equivalent to ng/dl/hr for testosterone, Δ^4, OHP and to pg/ml/hr for E_2. The data were analyzed by analysis of variance, paired or unpaired student's t test, as appropriate. A p value of <0.05 was selected as the limit of statistical significance.

RESULTS AND DISCUSSION

Developmental Changes in the Dynamic of the Steroidogenic Responses to hCG in Eugonadal Subjects

Testosterone Response

In adult men. A single injection of hCG (Protocol I) induced a biphasic response of plasma testosterone. A rapid and transient increase was followed by a plateau intermediate between the peak and the basal levels at about 24 hr. Plasma testosterone levels started to rise again at 24–48 hr, reaching a secondary peak maximum at 3–4 days, (FIGURE 1).[23] A similar pattern of response is observed in monkeys[53] and rodents[30,42] after a single high dose of hCG. However, species differences are observed in the respective amplitude of the early or late responses to hCG. In humans, the rapid response is much less (1.5- to 2-fold) than in rodents (10–20-fold)[30,42] and its significance has been questioned. We have studied this early response in 12 eugonadal men by determining plasma testosterone levels hourly for 8 hours after an i.v. or i.m. injection of 6,000 IU hCG. A significant rise in circulating testosterone levels was observed in all subjects, but individual maximal values were observed at any time between 1 and 6 hours and were independent of the mode of administration (data not shown). During this period, circulating hCG levels remain very high.[23] These data and other studies[44,54] emphasize the need for multiple blood sampling to establish the significance of the acute testosterone response to hCG, or to 3 hr LH infusion.[55] The former has also been documented by direct measurement of spermatic testosterone levels.[56] The early response to hCG is however different in the morning (short-lived) than during the evening (plateauing through 6 hr).[57,58] In contrast, the magnitude (2–3-fold) and the average time of the secondary testosterone response to hCG are similar in humans and rodents and the amplitude of response is clearly hCG dose-dependent in both species.[35,36,44]

A state of temporary refractoriness to further hCG stimulation is observed at least 24–36 hr following an initial hCG injection, since during this period a second injection of hCG is ineffective in significantly increasing plasma testosterone levels (FIGURE 2). Another study has shown that the acute testosterone release is the same before and 72 hr after a single hCG injection, despite the persistence of high serum levels of hCG,[54] suggesting that by that time the testis has become resensitized to gonadotropin stimulation. The desensitization period also lasts 2 days in the rodents given high doses of hCG.[59]

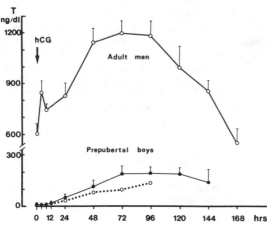

FIGURE 1. Responses of plasma testosterone (T) to a single dose of hCG (given at time 0) in adult men (open circle) and prepubertal boys (closed circles) (Protocol I). The testosterone response observed in a boy during dexamethasone suppression (*see* MATERIAL AND METHODS) is illustrated by the dotted curve.

The only apparent effect of repeating hCG stimulation at 24-hr intervals was to delay the secondary rise by about 24 hr without increasing its maximal value (FIGURE 2 versus FIGURE 1). Similar conclusions can be drawn from the study of adult men with our third protocol, one hCG injection every 5 days (FIGURE 3). Despite the fact that plasma testosterone levels had not returned to basal values 120 hr after each hCG injection, the rapid testosterone responses to hCG (maximal at 2–4 hr) were comparable before and 120 hr after any of the three subsequent injections. There was no cumulative effect (FIGURE 3) of repeating testicular stimulation. Plasma testosterone values achieved at 48–120 hr after one,[23,43–46,57,58] two at 2–3-day intervals,[23,43,54,61] three daily,[43,60] or four injections at 5-day intervals reported in the literature are strikingly comparable whatever the dosages used (1,500–10,000 IU), inducing supraphysiological circulating levels of hCG. This suggests that delayed maximal testicular testosterone production is already obtained after a single hCG injection. Indirect evidence is also given by the study of patients with choriocarcinomas in whom plasma testosterone levels remain in the upper normal range despite high levels of tumor hCG.[62]

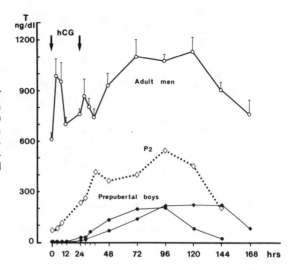

FIGURE 2. Responses of plasma testosterone (T) to two hCG injections, one at time 0 and the second 24 hr later, in adult men (○), one early pubertal boy (◇), and two prepubertal (●, ◆) boys (Protocol II).

In Prepubertal Children. Whatever the protocol used (I to IV), we noted a distinctly different pattern of response in prepubertal boys compared to that in adult men (FIGURES 1–4). Following a single hCG injection, plasma testosterone levels increased steadily in all boys, reaching peaks levels (237 ± 33 ng/dl) at about 96 hr (range 72–120 hr).[63] There was no rapid testosterone response, the first significant ($p < 0.01$) rise being observed at 24 hr (FIGURE 1). Results similar to ours just appeared in the literature,[64,65] in respect to the pattern of response and peaks values observed at 96 hr, i.e. 213 ± 57 and 296 ± 69 ng/dl in, respectively, 9 and

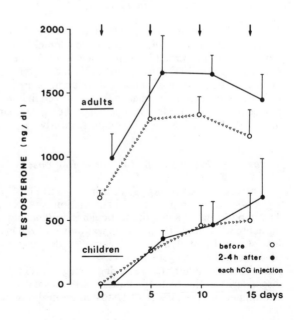

FIGURE 3. Effect of four successive hCG injections administered at five-day intervals on the plasma levels of testosterone in adult men or prepubertal boys. The dotted lines join the values observed before and 120 hr after each hCG injection; the solid lines those observed 4 hr after each hCG injection. The rapid response to each injection is the gradient between open and closed circles on days 0, 5, 10, and 15 in both groups (Protocol III).

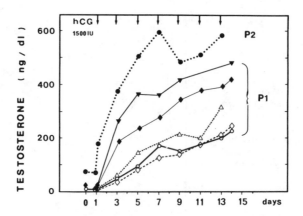

FIGURE 4. Dynamic of the plasma testosterone response to seven hCG injections given at 48-hr intervals in one early pubertal and five prepubertal boys (Protocol I).

12 prepubertal boys of similar ages. Although the absolute increases in plasma testosterone were small in prepubertal boys, probably reflecting a limited potential of Leydig cells, the relative late testosterone response was higher (18–36-fold) than in adult men (2–3-fold).

A second hCG injection administered 24 hr after the first (Protocol II) neither modified the profile of the response (FIGURE 2), nor increased peak values of plasma testosterone levels (218 ± 9 ng/dl).[24-63] Repeated hCG stimulation, either four at five-day intervals (Protocol III) or seven every 48 hr (Protocol IV), resulted in higher end-test testosterone levels (in the range of adult values), but did not induce a significant rapid testosterone response (FIGURE 3 and data not shown).

Early Pubertal Boys. Obviously due to ethical limitations, only very scarce results are currently available at this developmental stage: three subjects studied with Protocol I reported by Tapanainen et al.,[64] one with Protocol II (FIGURE 2), one with Protocol IV (FIGURE 4). From these preliminary data it appears that in boys at an early stage of pubertal development (P_2), the pattern of plasma testosterone response is still similar to that observed in immature boys (lack of an early response at 2–4 hr). Maximal increases, being comparable in the three protocols used (519 ± 231, 548, and 595 ng/dl, respectively), are greater.

Testosterone Precursors and Estrogen Responses

The dissociated responses of urinary excretions[25] or plasma testosterone and E_2[60,66] to single or repeated hCG stimulation have been observed for many years. That modifications along the testicular steroidogenic pathway also occur following acute hCG and LH stimulation was only realized in the last few years. This was first shown by studying the dynamic of the responses of plasma testosterone precursors and estrogens to hCG.[42]

Adult Men. In adult men receiving a single hCG injection, there was a striking dissimilarity in this temporal pattern. After a small (about 1.5-fold) initial rise, the two immediate precursors of testosterone in the Δ^4 pathway showed a different behavior. OHP continued to rise to peak levels at 24–48 hr whereas Δ^4 showed a biphasic profile with a maximal delayed response (2.5-fold) at the same time (72–96 hr) as did plasma testosterone (FIGURE 4). The response of plasma estrone (E_1) was similar to that of Δ^4 although more modest.[42] In contrast, E_2 rose abruptly (3- to 7-fold) from the eighth hour and reached surprisingly high levels, maximal at 24 hr in all subjects (FIGURE 4). Studies by others have confirmed[43,55] and extended our findings.[45,47,54] Measurement of practically all steroids in the testosterone biosynthetic pathways, in multiple peripheral bloods samples obtained every 10 or 30 min,[47,54,55] or in spermatic vein blood,[45] have provided direct or indirect evidence that there is an initial, transient, and non-selective release of all testicular steroids 2–3 hr following acute hCG (IV, i.m.) or LH (four i.v. injections at 90-min intervals or 1 hr and 6 hr infusions) administration, regardless the protocol used. Also, the initial rises in plasma progesterone, OHP, 17α-hydroxypregnenolone, E_1 are not affected by dexamethasone suppression.[47] Thereafter a different behavior is observed among C21, C19, or C18 steroids. Progesterone, OHP, 17α-hydroxypregnenolone responses are maximal at about 24 hr decreasing at the time when testosterone starts to rise again. E_2 displays a very similar temporal pattern. The profiles of response of plasma Δ^4, E_1, and 5α-dihydrotestosterone (DHT) are rather similar to that of testosterone, but their absolute and relative increases are smaller. In contrast, plasma pregnenolone and dehydroepiandrosterone (DHA) remain unaffected. Repetition of the same hCG injection, 24 hr after the first one, did not modify in the main the temporal patterns described above.[42] The amplitude of the maximal rise in E_2 (24 ± 2 to 140 ± 10 pg/ml) was greater than after a single hCG injection (22.5 ± 3 to 106 ± 12 pg/ml), whereas those of OHP were similar with both protocols (118 ± 15 to 292 ± 26 versus 121 ± 16 to 298 ± 37 ng/dl). For both hormones the peak response was observed 24 hr after the first hCG injection. The patterns of Δ^4 and E_1 followed again that of testosterone, their late and maximal rises being delayed by about 24 hr, but not significantly greater than those observed after a single hCG injection. However, the decline in plasma E_1,

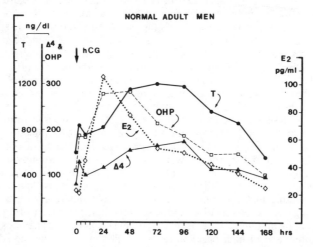

FIGURE 5. Kinetics of response of plasma testosterone (T), Δ^4-androstenedione (Δ^4), 17α-hydroxyprogesterone (OHP), and 17β-estradiol (E_2) to a single dose (94 ± 7 IU/kg BW) of hCG in adult men. Mean profiles observed in seven subjects (Protocol I).

Δ^4, and E_2 was slower and none of them had returned to basal levels seven days after the beginning of the test, in contrast to OHP the levels of which had returned to control values within five days. This "residual" effect on Δ^4, E_1, and E_2 was even more pronounced when the hCG injections were repeated every five days (Protocol III). Baseline levels observed before each of the four injections tend to rise further for Δ^4 and E_1, or to plateau at twice basal values for E_2. Early (2–4 hr) responses were no longer observed after the third or fourth injection. In contrast, OHP levels were not different from basal values before each of the four injections and any of the four injections induced an early rise (1.5- to 2-fold) similar to that observed after a single hCG injection.[42] However, as shown by another study in the literature,[54] more frequent repetition of hCG stimulation (daily) at similar dosage (4,000 IU) not only increases baseline levels of OHP and abolishes its acute release (1–4 hr) after the third injection, but seems to induce a shift in the pattern of testosterone biosynthesis from the Δ^4 to the Δ^5 pathway (significant acute release of DHA). Unfortunately the 24 hr response of testosterone precursors or estrogens has not been studied in those protocols using three or more hCG injections at various intervals.

Taken together, these data show the inability of the human adult testis to increase substantially its testosterone production for 4–48 hr after an acute hCG stimulation. Steroidogenic desensitization seems to be related to a temporary block in the conversion of OHP to testosterone, which is reflected by a plateau in circulating testosterone levels and by an accumulation of C21 biosynthetic testosterone precursors (progesterone and OHP). This blockade in 17,20-desmolase enzyme activity appears more pronounced in the Δ^4 than in the Δ^5 pathway and is accompanied by a large increase in plasma E_2. Although direct evidence is lacking in the human studies summarized here, the small and slow peripheral conversion of androgens to estrogen[67,68] is unlikely to account for the marked surge in plasma E_2. It thus appears that high doses of LH and hCG are capable of specifically increasing aromatase activity within the testis and to stimulate considerably its E_2 secretion within 8–24 hr. Recovery from testicular desensitization begins two to three days after one hCG injection, but full resensitization with regard to testosterone production seems to require four to five days and is contemporary to the return of plasma OHP to control values (apparently reflecting the disappearance of the 17,10-desmolase block). The recognition of such hCG-induced temporal changes in testicular steroidogenesis was of importance for realizing that the frequency of repeated hCG injections also influences the pattern of testicular secretions. Daily hCG injections obviously maintain a certain degree of 17,20-desmolase inhibition, as reflected by increased OHP levels and increased ratio of OHP to testosterone. This specific enzymatic inhibition is however less apparent with time (as judged on plasma OHP levels, OHP/testosterone ratio, or acute responses to hCG clearly decreasing after three daily hCG injection).[43,54] It is possible that such changes reflect the progressive occurrence of other relative enzymatic blocks, either early in the biosynthetic pathway as shown in rodents given very high doses of hCG[34,40,42] or in the conversion of Δ^5 to Δ^4 steroids.[54] There is at the moment no direct evidence to support these hypotheses. By contrast, repeating hCG injections at 5-day intervals apparently results in alternate steroidogenic desensitization and resensitization periods. During the latter there seems to be an overall increased activity in steroidogenic enzymes as judged by the maintenance of high baseline levels of all steroids along the Δ^4 pathway (FIGURE 3 and data in Smals et al.[43])

Prepubertal Children. The temporal pattern of response of progesterone, OHP, Δ^4, and E_2 to a single hCG injection observed in prepubertal boys are illustrated in

FIGURE 6. Basal levels of plasma progesterone (8.8 ± 2.3 ng/dl), OHP (40 ± 10.5 ng/dl), Δ^4 (28.5 ± 7 ng/dl), testosterone (11 ± 2 ng/dl), DHT (3.4 ± 2.9 ng/dl), or E_2 (13 ± 3 pg/ml) were all normal for age. Plasma levels of progesterone, OHP, and Δ^4 showed normal diurnal variations the first day following the hCG injection (values observed at 20,000 hr being respectively 47%, 17%, and 37% of morning ones) but did not vary significantly throughout the study (FIGURE 6). The temporal pattern of DHT was quite similar to that of testosterone[63] but the maximal rise was only 3- to 6-fold. Despite individual fluctuations, E_2 levels tend to rise steadily until 96–120 hr by about twofold. Maximal E_2 levels (37 ± 15 pg/ml) were observed at slightly different individual times and were significantly ($p < 0.02$) higher than control values (paired t-test). Except for this small late rise in E_2 levels, probably due to the peripheral conversion of increasing testosterone levels

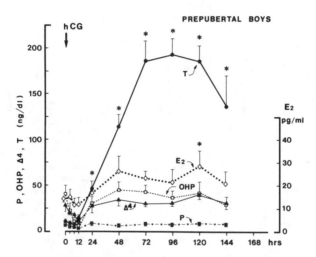

FIGURE 6. Kinetics of response of plasma T, E_2, OHP, Δ^4, and progesterone (P) to a single injection (100 IU/kg BW) of hCG in prepubertal boys (Protocol I). The asterisk indicates responses that are significantly different from basal values for T (analysis of variance) or E_2 (paired Student' t-test).

(FIGURE 6), our results (absolute values and temporal patterns) are strictly comparable to the two studies in the literature.[64,65] Thus, an acute hCG stimulation does not change the steroidogenic pattern of the human infantile testis as it does in the adult. We were also unable to detect any significant changes in the plasma levels of OHP, Δ^4, or E_2 in the prepubertal boys receiving either two injections at 24-hr interval (Protocol II) or four injections at 5-day intervals (Protocol III) (unpublished data). These observations are in accordance with earlier reports of a lack of response of plasma E_2 to three injections of 2,000 IU of hCG administered at 24 hr[69,70] or 48-hr intervals[71–73] in prepubertal boys. However, in an earlier study we found that more prolonged hCG stimulation (seven injections every other day, Protocol IV) induced a significant rise in both OHP and Δ^4 levels[22] in immature boys regardless of their age. The net increments (obtained by subtracting the basal value from the end-test value obtained for each subject) in plasma testosterone,

Δ^4, and OHP that we observed are summarized in FIGURE 7. They were all significant (paired student t-test). The apparent discrepancy between the results of this earlier study and those observed after short-term hCG stimulation by us[63] and others,[69–71] prompted us to reinvestigate the steroidogenic responses in 20 prepubertal boys 3 to $12^{8/12}$ yr old (mean age $8^{5/12}$ yr) submitted to this long term hCG stimulation (Protocol IV). Their testosterone, Δ^4, and OHP responses to hCG fell in the range of those reported earlier. Plasma E_2 levels were significantly ($p <$ 0.01 at paired student's t test) higher 16–24 hr after the seventh injection (24 ± 5 pg/ml) than before the first one (9.5 ± 1.4 pg/ml).

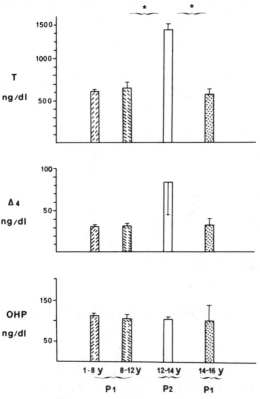

FIGURE 7. Net increase in plasma T, Δ^4, or OHP levels following seven i.m. injections of 1,500 IU hCG at 48-hr intervals (Protocol IV) in a total of 100 prepubertal (P_1) boys divided in two age groups, early pubertal boys (P_2), boys with simple delayed puberty (P_1, 14–16 years). The greater responses of T and Δ^4 with engaged puberty was only significant for T (*).

Pubertal Boys. We did not have the opportunity to study in detail the steroidogenic responses to hCG in pubertal boys, but the scarce information gleaned in the literature indicates that a shift from the prepubertal pattern of both basal testicular secretion and steroidogenic responses to single or repeated hCG stimulation is noticeable in boys who had just entered puberty (stage P_2 of Tanner). The pattern of the steroidogenic response to a single hCG injection in three early pubertal (P_2) boys is already intermediate between the prepubertal and adult response patterns:[64] a small but significant rise in plasma E_2 (from 8.5 ± 2 to 14.2 ± 6.7 pg/ml at 12 hr), followed by a more substantial rise in plasma OHP, maximal at 24 hr. Thus a temporal dissociation in the rises of E_2 and OHP and that of testosterone, similar to that seen in adult, was already observed in boys at stage P_2. It has been known for some years that the hCG-induced response of E_2 gradually increases throughout puberty;[69,72,73] but since only end-test values have been estimated in those studies, it is not known if this increasing response results from a cumulative effect of three consecutive hCG injections or from an increasing capacity of the maturing testis acutely to secrete E_2. Apart from the study showing that the net increment in plasma OHP after two weeks hCG stimulation (Protocol IV) does not vary between stage 1 and 2 of puberty, the pattern of response of OHP has not been investigated in detail throughout pubertal development.

In the early pubertal stage, plasma Δ^4 begins to rise significantly after either one[64] or three daily[69] hCG injections. The amplitude of plasma Δ^4 response to hCG increases throughout pubertal development whatever the protocol used, three daily injections[70] or seven every other day (FIGURE 7.)

Collectively, these data show clearly that significant hCG-induced responses of plasma OHP levels are only observed in parallel with the appearance of E_2 responses. The relative hCG-induced testosterone response (fold rise over basal levels) decreases markedly between childhood (18–70-fold according to the studies) early puberty (6–10-fold), and adulthood (about 2–3-fold). Because of the limitations of extrapolating these figures to an index of testosterone responsiveness to hCG stimulation, it would appear that the sensitivity of the Leydig cell to hCG decreases coincidently with pubertal development and with an increasing capacity of testicular secretion of Δ^4, E_2, and possibly OHP. Finally, the dissociation seen in temporal patterns of testosterone and OHP suggests that the early pubertal testis is already sensitive to hCG-induced steroidogenic desensitization.

Studies in Subjects with Testicular Enzymatic Defects

Inborn errors in testosterone biosynthesis are rare diseases. In the cases reported in the literature, testicular endocrine function has been studied by repeating hCG stimulation daily or every 48 hr for 3 to 14 days. These hCG tests, emphasizing the biological feature of a given enzyme defect, have been useful for the diagnosis.[74] However, the effects of an acute hCG stimulation on testicular steroidogenesis have not been documented in such patients. The results of our earlier studies demonstrating that the patterns of hCG-induced steroid responses were radically different between immature boys and adult men (see above) prompted us to analyze, in relation to age, the steroidogenic responses to a single hCG stimulation in patients with a pre-existing block in one of the two enzymes in Δ^4-androgen biosynthesis (17,20-D and 17-KSR). A total of seven patients is reported. The first two children with 17,20-D have been described in detail.[76] With the kind clinical collaboration of Drs. M. David, J. Rollet, J. Touniaire in Lyon, Dr. C. Sainmont in Besançon, and Dr. D. Bosson in Brussels, we had the rare opportunity to study five additional patients (three adults and two children) with either defect. The 17,20-D patients have been studied during adrenal suppression (2 to 3 mg of dexamethasone daily). All subjects received a single i.m. hCG injection at 08.00–09.00 a.m. at similar dosages. The protocol used was designed to examine whether acute hCG stimulation caused steroidogenic desensitization and to investigate further the site of the hCG-induced enzymatic block.

Adult Patients

The dynamics of the hCG responses of plasma testosterone, Δ^4, OHP, and E_2 observed in the three adult patients are illustrated in FIGURES 8 and 9, in comparison of those observed using the same methodology in normal adult men. The high OHP : T or Δ^4 : T ratio observed in basal conditions in, respectively, 17,20-D or 17-KSR patients were pathognomic of the given enzymatic defects. In basal conditions, plasma testosterone levels (180–266 ng/dl) were two to three times lower than normal, those of E_2 (55–115 pg/ml) were markedly elevated (normal 24 ± 6). Despite relative variations in their amplitude of responses to hCG, the four steroids exhibited temporal changes qualitatively similar to those found in normal men, i.e., biphasic testosterone and Δ^4 responses with a modest initial rise and a delayed peak at 72–96 hr (FIGURE 8) and concomitant rises in plasma OHP and E_2 levels, maximal at 24 hr (FIGURE 9). The relative rises (2.7- to 3.2-fold) in plasma testosterone were the same as in normal men. As expected the amplitude of the responses of the two precursors on the Δ^4 pathway differed between 17,20-D and 17-KSR patients, but their temporal patterns were somewhat similar.

In 17,20-D patients, after an initial twofold rise at 24 hr, plasma OHP levels plateaued for about three days before returning to basal values or lower (FIGURE 9). As expected in this enzyme deficiency, Δ^4 response was very poor (FIGURE 8). This suggests that acute hCG stimulation temporarily aggravated the pre-existing block in 17,20-desmolase activity.

In the patient with 17-KSR defect, plasma OHP was not only elevated in basal state (249 ng/dl) but its absolute and relative (3.8-fold) increase after hCG was noticeably greater than normal. Plasma Δ^4 levels, in basal and stimulated state were in the range of those observed for testosterone in normal subjects. This further documented the 17-KSR enzymatic block (FIGURE 8).

In all three patients, the plasma E_2 responses were surprisingly very large, maximal levels (269 to 320 pg/ml) being about three times higher than those observed in normal men, and returning more slowly to basal values. Because of their incapacity to produce physiological amounts of testosterone, both 17,20-D and 17-KSR patients usually have high endogenous levels of LH, as it was also found in our patients. This, together with the steroidogenic patterns and the profiles of the acute responses to hCG that we observed, suggests that such patients may well be in a chronic state of testicular desensitization induced by high endogenous gonadotropic stimulation.

Prepubertal Patients

In all boys, the response to hCG was strikingly different from that observed in adult patients. Their temporal patterns resembled those of prepubertal boys with normal testicular function.

A boy with undescended testis, matched for age was first studied during adrenal suppression (3 mg of dexamethasone daily). In this control subject, plasma progesterone, OHP, and Δ^4 were suppressed but showed no significant rise, whereas the testosterone response fell in the range of the group of prepubertal boys not receiving dexamethasone (FIGURE 1), suggesting that dexamethasone did not alter the response to hCG in prepubertal age. In the first two 17,20-D boys studied during adrenal suppression, there was a modest progressive rise in plasma testosterone (FIGURE 10). The temporal hCG responses of OHP or 17α-hydroxy-pregnenolone (OHPreg) were parallel to that of testosterone, but absolute and

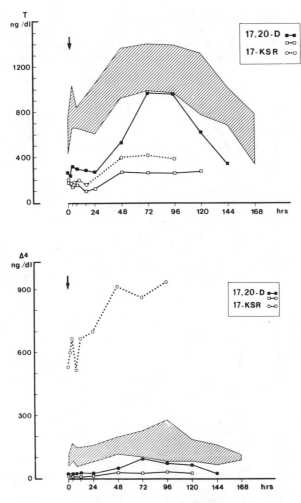

FIGURE 8. Effect of a single hCG injection (100 IU/kg BW) at time 0 (indicated by the arrow) on the plasma levels of T and Δ^4 in three adults patients with either 17,20-desmolase [17 yr (■) and 35 yr (□)] or 17-ketosteroid reductase (17-KSR) (25 yr = ○··○) deficiency. The mean ± SD responses observed in normal adult men are represented by the hatched areas (for detailed protocol see MATERIAL AND METHODS.)

relative rises were greater. The third boy was studied with and without adrenal suppression (FIGURE 11). In basal state, plasma progesterone and OHP showed marked diurnal variations but did not rise further after the single hCG injection. The high basal OHP levels were drastically suppressed by dexamethasone and rose only slightly and progressively when hCG was administered during adrenal suppression (FIGURE 11). There was a modest progressive rise in plasma testosterone in both hCG tests while plasma E_2 levels remained at the limit of detection in the second test (data not shown). The high ratio of OHP to testosterone in the delayed hCG response (72–96 hr) observed in the three patients probably accounts for the pre-existing testicular enzyme defect. But there was apparently not a superimposed block in 17,20-desmolase–induced by hCG administration (accumulation of OHP at 24 hr) as observed in adult patients. The data also indicate that

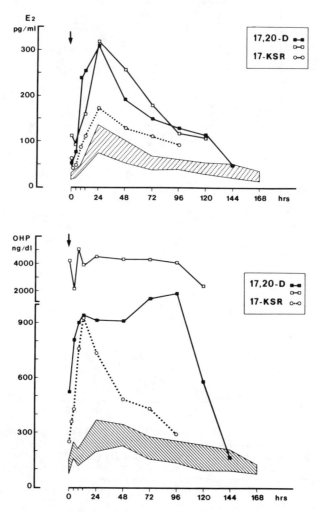

FIGURE 9. Dynamic of the responses of plasma E_2 and OHP levels in three adults with testicular enzyme defects. Symbols as in FIGURE 8.

the inborn 17,20-desmolase defect is mostly expressed in the adrenals in the prepubertal stage.

The profiles of the steroid responses to a single hCG-injection observed in the 17-KSR child are illustrated in FIGURE 12. The testosterone response was modest,

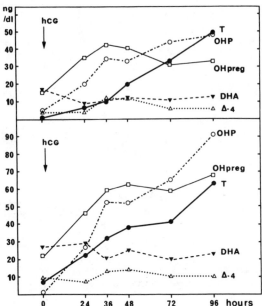

FIGURE 10. Dynamic of the response of plasma T, OHP, 17α-hydroxypregnenolone (OHPreg), DHA, and Δ⁴ to a single i.m. injection of 5,000 IU hCG in two male children with 17,20-desmolase deficiency, aged 6½ yr (*upper panel*) and 9½ year (*lower panel*). The study was made during adrenal suppression (2 mg of dexamethasone daily) (From Forest *et al.*[75] By permission of the *Journal of Clinical Endocrinology and Metabolism*).

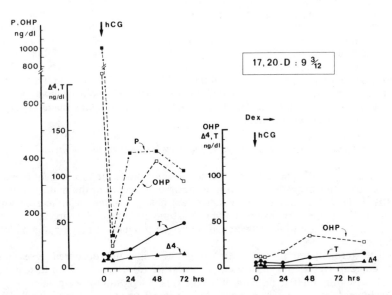

FIGURE 11. Kinetics of the steroidogenic response to a single hCG injection administered without (*left panel*) or during adrenal suppression in a prepubertal boy (*see* MATERIAL AND METHODS).

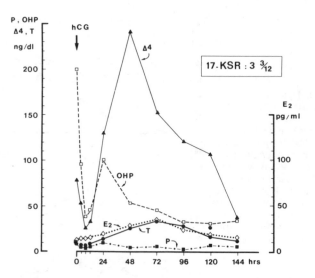

FIGURE 12. Steroidogenic response to a single hCG injection (100 IU/kg BW) in a child with 17-ketosteroid reductase deficiency.

maximal at 72 hr. There was no initial rise, but a diurnal variation in plasma Δ^4. Its further rise was diagnostic of the condition. Plasma progesterone did not change. The high OHP levels for age might be due to stress since a normal diurnal variation was observed. Plasma E_2 levels were surprisingly rather elevated for age, possibly due to peripheral conversion from relatively high Δ^4 levels, but they did not show any significant surge in response to hCG stimulation. It is a pediatric endocrinologist's experience that making the diagnosis of testicular enzymatic defects in prepubertal children requires an hCG stimulation. This is illustrated by the present data and may be accounted for by the low, if not lacking, 17α-hydroxylase activity in the prepubertal testis.[19,77] Finally, despite the limitations in drawing conclusions from a limited number of observations, it would appear that maturing processes in testicular steroidogenesis are also taking place in subjects with testicular enzymatic defects.[75]

Studies in Subjects with Hypogonadotropic Hypogonadism

These studies[78,79] have been designed to investigate the mechanism responsible for the shift in testicular steroidogenesis that occurs in the maturing human testis. Indeed, the cumulative evidence that changes in testicular secretory patterns and/or in the response to acute hCG stimulation take place in early puberty suggests that maturation in testicular androgen production may be a gonadotropin-induced phenomenon.

The steroidogenic responses to a single hCG injection observed in seven untreated adult HH men is illustrated in FIGURE 13 (a). Basal levels of testosterone (18.4 ± 3 ng/dl), OHP (27 ± 5 ng/dl), and E_2 (12 ± 4 pg/ml) were significantly ($p < 0.01$) lower than in normal adult men, but similar to what was observed in 8–12-yr-old prepubertal boys. Mean plasma Δ^4 levels (66 ± 10 ng/dl) were however not significantly lower than in eugonadal adults, in the range of those observed in boys

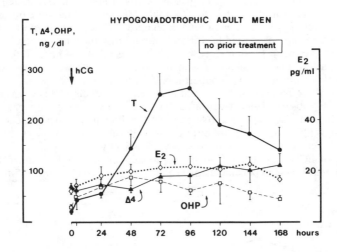

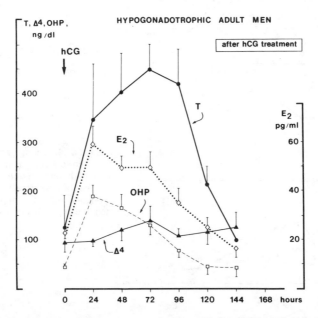

FIGURE 13. Dynamic of the responses of plasma T, E_2, OHP, and Δ^4 in hypogonado-trophic hypogonadic men following a single injection of hCG (100 IU/kg), before any hormonal treatment (*upper panel*), and following three months of a weekly administration of the same dose of hCG (*lower panel*).

with delayed puberty and normal adrenarche. The first hCG injection induced a substantial (mean 17.7-fold) rise in plasma testosterone in all HH patients with marked individual variations (6.7- to 27.4-fold). Maximal values were observed at 72–120 hr, average values at 96 hr (264 ± 56 ng/dl). Plasma OHP and Δ^4 showed large day-to-day and/or individual variations, but no significant temporal changes (analysis of variance). Plasma E_2 rose to 23 ± 3 pg/ml at 144 hr ($p < 0.05$). The temporal pattern and the absolute and relative responses were thus strikingly similar to those observed in prepubertal boys (FIGURE 6).

Despite three months of hCG treatment, plasma levels of testosterone, Δ^4, OHP, and E_2 observed one week after the twelfth hCG injection were strictly comparable to those observed 168 hr after the first injection and, except for testosterone (125 ± 68 ng/dl), not different from basal levels (FIGURE 13 b). However, the kinetics of response to hCG was drastically changed after 13 weekly injections of hCG. The early (2–4 hr) responses could only be studied in two patients: an early rise in plasma testosterone was observed (1.7- and 4–5-fold) but

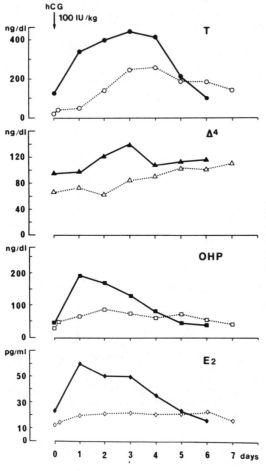

FIGURE 14. Changing pattern of the steroidogenic responses to hCG with three months of hCG treatment in previously untreated hypogonadotrophic hypogonadic men (mean profile in six subjects).

FIGURE 15. Cumulative responses of T, Δ^4, OHP, and E_2 during the week following the first and the 13th weekly injection of 100 IU/kg BW of hCG in previously untreated hypogonadotrophic hypogonadic men. The asterisks indicate significant ($p < 0.05$) changes (Student paired t test).

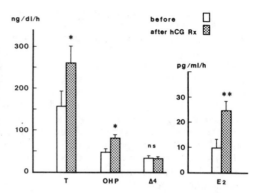

not analyzable statistically. The ensuing temporal patterns now resembled those observed in normal adults: the testosterone response was somewhat more rapid and relatively less (11-fold), peak values (447 ± 141 ng/dl) still being delayed and observed at about 72 hr. The Δ^4 response somewhat paralleled that of testosterone, but was blunted (1.5-fold). Plasma OHP and E_2 both rose significantly (4.4- and 2.2-fold) within 24 hr, declining progressively thereafter. This shifting temporal pattern is illustrated in FIGURE 14. Estimation of testicular production during the week following each hCG stimulation, by comparing (paired Student's t test) the net areas of the response curves before and after three months of hCG treatment, showed a significant increased production for testosterone ($p < 0.02$), OHP ($p < 0.01$), E_2 ($p < 0.005$), but not for Δ^4 (FIGURE 15).

Our results of a constant, although less substantial than in normal men, testosterone response to hCG in untreated HH patients are in accordance with previous reports, considering the fourth-day response to a single high dose (10,000 IU) of hCG,[46] the dynamic of testosterone response to a low dose (1,500 IU),[80] or the testosterone levels achieved after four daily injection of 5,000 IU of hCG.[81] There seems to be no correlation between the stimulated testosterone levels observed and the dose of hCG used in these studies. Two daily[61] or three daily injections[80] do not modify the testosterone response. This is quite similar to what we observed in prepubertal children. The apparent discordance between results of our and three other studies[82–84] with respect to OHP or E_2, probably accounts for the difference in protocols. In the first two,[82,83] all patients were previously treated with hCG and/or testosterone for several years and off treatment for various periods of time at the time of the study. Nevertheless they showed hCG responses not so different from what we observed in untreated HH patients or prepubertal children with, in particular, no clear-cut rise in OHP.[83] In the third study,[84] basal levels only were obtained from previous hCG treatment and the dynamic of testosterone and E_2 responses to hCG examined 48 hr after the last dose of a four-month treatment (three doses weekly). According to the patterns that we observed seven days after repeated weekly hCG injections (FIGURE 13b), testicular steroidogenic desensitization is induced by chronic hCG treatment. Studying the dynamics of the response to hCG starting with the 48th hour of the last of multiple hCG injections obviously results in superimposed temporal responses as we described earlier.[43] This may account for the high basal level and the small rise in E_2 24 hr later observed by these authors.[84] As hypothesized, chronic hCG treatment is thus able to induce testicular steroidogenic desensitization in HH patients. This effect is most likely mainly due to the LH-like activity of the molecule. Indeed, the commercial preparations have extremely low FSH contaminant and/or FSH-like bioactivity.[85] The same desensitization pattern is observed with high doses of LH.[47] Endogenous FSH is suppressed after both acute exogenous[86] or chronic endogenous[87] hCG stimulation, and three-day priming with FSH had no effect on the steroidogenic responses to hCG.[54] However, chronic treatment up to 2 yr[84] (FIGURE 13 b) does not restore normal pubertal testicular secretion. Testosterone production eventually reaches adult levels with frequent hCG injections, but is not sustained between weekly injections, not to mention the various patterns in testosterone precursors observed with varying protocols of hCG stimulation. During puberty the changing pattern in testicular secretion (rise in Δ^4, OHP, and DHT) also observed in monkeys[88] is accompanied by not only increasing "tonic" LH and FSH secretions but also changes in circadian rhythms and in the amplitude and/or frequency of secretory pulses.[89] It is likely that the maturing testis first responds to such a physiological gonadotropic stimulation by recruiting new Leydig cells and increasing steroidogenic enzymatic activities[29] including the 17α-hydroxylase/17,20-desmolase enzymatic complex, which appears to be rate-limiting in the immature testis,[77,90] and aromatizing capacity. The latter appears to respond to synergistic action of LH and FSH.[91] Also, experimental studies in the rat suggest that a different mode of treatment (a single high dose or repeated twice-daily small doses) may have inverse stimulatory or inhibitory effects on Leydig cell steroidogenesis.[90] In contrast, hCG-induced desensitization apparently inhibits the enzyme complex 17α-hydroxylase/17,20-desmolase but no other enzyme of the testosterone biosynthetic pathway. The exact mechanisms of this inhibition are still not understood. It may well be at the level of the common cytochrome P-450,[92] which is affected by estrogens.[93] Indeed, although subject to controversy, the hypothesis that hCG-induced steroidogenic desensitization is estrogen-mediated is strongly supported by experimental evidences in the rat model,[94] by the observation that the anti-estrogen, tamoxifen, prevents the hCG-induced testicular steroidogenic desensitization in the human,[95] and by our results.

The physiological relevance of effects observed with hCG, which has a much longer half-life than LH[23] and is administered at pharmacological doses and unphysiological frequency, is uncertain. However, since the ultimate function of mature Leydig cells is to produce testosterone at optimal amounts for physiological needs, it is conceivable that LH- and hCG-induced desensitization represents a form of defense mechanism against gonadotrophic hyperstimulation, acting as a "short-loop negative feedback" to keep the production of testosterone within optimal limits for physiological needs (for instance, slowing down testosterone secretion during sexual maturation to allow for more prolonged and/or optimal pubertal linear growth). During sexual maturation, the Δ^4: testosterone ratio increases in both basal and hCG-desensitizing conditions. This shift in the testicular secretory pattern might also be estrogen mediated. This hypothesis is supported by earlier in vivo studies,[96] that show that E_2 increases the transfer constant of blood testosterone to Δ^4, and therefore favors the oxidative versus the reductive action of the reversible 17β-hydroxysteroid dehydrogenase.

From a practical viewpoint, our studies provide some rationale basis for hCG-stimulation tests and/or hCG treatments in clinical practice and stress the importance of considering the dose, the number, the rhythm of the hCG injections, and the timing of blood sampling in interpreting results of any hCG stimulation.[97] Standardized protocols appear to be a prerequisite for comparing absolute results in the literature.

CONCLUSION

Testicular secretory patterns change during sexual maturation. A single hCG stimulation neither induces a block in 17,20-desmolase activity nor is capable of acutely stimulating an aromatizing activity in prepubertal or hypogonadotrophic subjects. The steroidogenic desensitization phenomenon is evidenced, in early puberty and after hCG treatment, on the accumulation of both OHP and E_2 24 hr after a single hCG stimulation. This suggests that testicular desensitization is both estrogen mediated and dependent upon previous gonadotrophic exposure. Thus a single hCG-injection test could be proposed as a marker of normal sexual maturation.

ACKNOWLEDGMENT

The author wishes to thank Drs. R. Roulier and M. David for their invaluable collaboration, the many clinicians who referred patients, the staff of the endocrine unit of the Hospital Debrousse for their kind help in the realization of some protocols, and all the adult volunteers for the studies performed. The excellent technical assistance by A. Lecoq and M. P. Monneret and the careful secretarial help by M. Montagnon are also greatly appreciated.

REFERENCES

1. DAVID, K. , E. DINGEMANSE, J. FREUD & E. LAQUEUR. 1935. Z. Physiol Chem. **233:** 281–282.
2. CHRISTENSEN, A. K. & S. W. GILLIN. 1969. In The Gonads. K. W. McKern, Ed.: 415–488. Appleton Century-Crofts. New York.
3. LIPSETT, M. B. 1970. In The Human Testis. E. Rosenberg & C. A. Paulsen, Eds. **10:** 407–418. Plenum Press. New York.
4. EIK-NES, K. B. 1970. In Handbook of Physiology. M. O. Greep & D. W. Hamilton, Eds. **5:** 95–115. Waverly Press. Baltimore.
5. LAATIKAINEN, T., E. A. LAITINEN & R. VIHKO. 1971. J. Clin. Endocrinol. Metab. **32:** 59–64.
6. KELCH, R. P., M. R. JENNER, R. L. WEINSTEIN, S. L. KAPLAN & M. M. GRUMBACH. 1972. J. Clin. Invest. **51:** 824–830.
7. BAIRD, D. T., A. GALBRAITH, I. S. FRASER & J. E. NEWSAM. 1973. J. Endocrinol. **57:** 285–288.
8. WEINSTEIN, R. L., R. P. KELCH, M. R. JENNER, S. L. KAPLAN & M. M. GRUMBACH. 1974. J. Clin. Invest. **53:** 1–6.
9. BELL, J. B. G. & D. LACY. 1974. Proc. R. Soc. London Ser. B **186:** 99–120.
10. HAMMOND, G. L., A. MEROKONEN, M. KONTTURI, E. KOSKELA & R. VIHKO. 1977. J. Clin. Endocrinol. Metab. **45:** 16–24.
11. MARTIKAINEN, H., I. HAHTANIEMI, O. LAKKARINEN & R. VIHKO. 1982. J. Steroid Biochem. **16:** 287–291.
12. FOREST, M. G., P. C. SIZONENKO, A. M. CATHIARD & J. BERTRAND. 1974. J. Clin. Invest. **53:** 819–828.
13. FOREST, M. G. & A. M. CATHIARD. 1978. Pediatr. Res. **12:** 6–11.
14. FOREST, M. G., A. M. CATHIARD & J. A. BERTRAND. 1973. J. Clin. Endocrinol. Metab. **36:** 1132–1142.
15. FAIMAN, C., J. S. D. WINTER & F. I. REYES. 1976. Clin. Obstet. Gynaecol. **3:** 467–483.
16. WINTER, J. S. D. & C. FAIMAN. 1972. J. Clin. Endocrinol. Metab. **35:** 561–564.

17. FORTI, G., S. SANTORO, G. A. GRISOLIA, F. BASSI, R. BONINSEGNI, G. FIORELLI & M. SERIO. 1981. J. Clin. Endocrinol. Metab. **53:** 883–886.
18. FORTI, G., F. FACCHINETTI, S. SARDELLI, G. A. GRISOLIA, S. SANTORO, F. BASSI & M. SERIO. 1983. **56:** 831–834.
19. BERG, A. A., B. KJESSLER & K. LUNDQVIST. 1976. Acta Endocrinol. Suppl. 207 **83:** 23–35.
20. EWING, L. L., J. C. DAVIS & B. R. ZIRKIN. 1980. Int. Rev. Physiol. **22:** 41–115.
21. LIPSETT, M. B., H. WILSON, M. A. KIRSHNER, S. G. KORENMAN, L. M. FISHMAN, G. A. SARFATY & C. W. BARDIN. 1966. Rec. Prog. Hormone Res. **22:** 245–281.
22. FOREST, M. G. 1979. J. Clin. Endocrinol. Metab. **49:** 132–137.
23. SAEZ, J. M. & M. G. FOREST. 1979. J. Clin. Endocrinol. Metab. **49:** 278–283.
24. FOREST, M. G., M. DAVID, A. LECOQ, M. JEUNE & J. BERTRAND. 1980. Pediatr. Res. **14:** 819–824.
25. LEACH, R. B., W. O. MADDOCK, I. TOKUYAMA, C. A. PAULSEN & W. O. NELSON. 1956. Rec. Prog. Hormone Res. **2:** 377–398.
26. PURVIS, K. & V. HANSSON. 1978. Mol. Cell. Endocrinol. **12:** 123–138.
27. DUFAU, M. L. & K. J. CATT. 1978. Vitam. Horm. **36:** 461–592.
28. CATT, K. J., J. P. HARDWOOD, R. N. CLAYTON, T. F. DAVIES, V. CHAN, M. KATIKI-NIEMI, K. NOZU & M. C. DUFAU. 1980. Rec. Prog. Hormone Res. **36:** 557–622.
29. HALL, P. F. 1970. *In* The Androgens of the Testis. K. B. Eik-Nes, Eds.: 73–116. Dekker. New York.
30. HSUEH, R. J. W., M. L. DUFAU & K. J. CATT. 1976. Biochem. Biophys. Res. Commun. **72:** 1145–1152.
31. SHARPE, R. M. 1976. Nature **264:** 644–646.
32. PURVIS, K., P. A. TROJESEN, E. HANG & V. HANSSON. 1977. Mol. Cell. Endocrinol. **8:** 73–80.
33. HAOUR, F. & J. M. SAEZ. 1977. Mol. Cell. Endocrinol. **7:** 17–24.
34. CIGORRAGA, S. B., M. L. DUFAU & K. J. CATT. 1978. J. Biol. Chem. **253:** 4257–4304.
35. SAEZ, J. M., A. M. MORERA & F. HAOUR. 1979. *In* Hormones and Cell Regulation. J. Dumont & J. Nunez, Eds.: 187–217. North Holland. Amsterdam.
36. TSURUHARA, T., M. L. DUFAU, S. CIGORRAGA & K. J. CATT. 1977. J. Biol. Chem. **252:** 9002–9009.
37. DIX, C. J. & B. A. COOKE. 1982. Biochem. J. **204:** 613–616.
38. NOZU, K., A. DEHEJIA, L. ZAWISTOWITCH, K. J. CATT & M. L. DUFAU. 1981. J. Biol. Chem. **256:** 12875–12887.
39. DUFAU, M. L., A. J. HSUEH, S. CIGORRAGA, A. J. BAUKAL & K. J. CATT. 1978. Int. J. Androl. Suppl 2 (part 1):193–239.
40. CHASALOW, F., H. MARR, F. HAOUR & J. M. SAEZ. 1979. J. Biol. Chem. **254:** 5613–5617.
41. MOGER, W. H. 1980. Endocrinology **106:** 496–503.
42. FOREST, M. G., A. LECOQ & J. M. SAEZ. 1979. J. Clin. Endocrinol. Metab. **49:** 284–291.
43. SMALS, A. G. H., G. F. F. M. PIETERS, D. C. LOZEKOOT, T. J. BENRAAD & P. W. C. KLOPPENBORD. 1980. J. Clin. Endocrinol. Metab. **50:** 190–193.
44. PADRON, R. S., J. WISCHUSEN, B. HUDSON, H. G. BURGER & D. M. DE KRETSER. 1980. J. Clin. Endocrinol. Metab. **50:** 1100–1104.
45. MARTIKAINEN, H., I. HUHTANIEMI & R. VIHKO. 1980. Clin. Endocrinol. **13:** 157–166.
46. OKUYAMA, A., M. NAMIKI, T. KOIDE, H. ITATANI, S. MIZUTANI, T. SONODA, T. AONO & K. MATSUMOTO. 1981. Arch. Androl. **6:** 75–81.
47. WANG, C., R. W. REBAR, B. R. HOPPER & S. C. C. YEN. 1980. J. Clin. Endocrinol. Metab. **51:** 201–208.
48. SAEZ, J. M. & J. BERTRAND. 1968. Steroids **12:** 749–761.
49. DAVID, M., M. G. FOREST, M. ZACHMANN & E. DE PERETTI. 1981. Ped. Res. **15:** 83.
50. TOURNIAIRE, J., E. DE PERETTI, B. ESTOUR & M. G. FOREST. 1982. Ann. Endocrinol. (Paris) **43:** 148.
51. FOREST, M. G., E. DE PERETTI & M. DAVID. 1982. Ann. Endocrinol. (Paris) **43:** 148.
52. FOREST, M. G., E. DE PERETTI, A. LECOQ, E. CADILLON, M. T. ZABOT & J. M. THOULON. 1980. J. Clin. Endocrinol. Metab. **51:** 815–823.

53. DAVIES, T., G. HODGEN, M. L. DUFAU & K. J. CATT. 1979. J. Clin. Invest. **64:** 1070–1073.
54. GLASS, A. R. & R. A. VIGERSKY. 1980. J. Clin. Endocrinol. Metab. **51:** 1395–1400.
55. NANKIN, H. R., T. LIN, E. MURONO, J. OSTERMAN & P. TROEN. 1980. Acta Endocrinol. (Copenhagen) **95:** 110–116.
56. MARTIKAINEN, H., I. HUHTANIEMI, O. LUKKARINEN & R. VIHKO. 1982. J. Steroid Biochem. **16:** 287–291.
57. NIESCLAG, E. & H. G. LEIENDECKER. 1981. IRCS Med. Sci. **9:** 143.
58. NANKIN, H. R., E. MURONO, T. LIN & J. OSTERMAN. 1980. Acta Endocrinol. **95:** 560–565.
59. HAOUR, F., P. SANCHEZ, A. M. CATHIARD & J. M. SAEZ. 1978. Biochem. Biophys. Res. Commun. **81:** 547–551.
60. MAHOUDEAU, I. A., I. C. VALCKE & H. BRICAIRE. 1975. J. Clin. Endocrinol. Metab. **41:** 13–20.
61. ANDERSON, D. C., J. C. MARSHALL, J. L. YOUNG & T. R. FRASER. 1972. Clin. Endocrinol. **1:** 127–140.
62. KIRSCHNER, M. A., J. A. WIDER & J. T. ROSS. 1970. J. Clin. Endocrinol. Metab. **30:** 504–511.
63. FOREST, M. G. & J. BERTRAND. 1984. Arch. Franç. Pédiatr. **41:** 103–109.
64. TAPANAINEN, J., H. MARTIKAINEN, L. DUNKEL, J. PERHEENTUPA & R. VIHKO. 1983. Clin. Endocrinol. **18:** 355–362.
65. TOSCANO, V., R. BALDUCI, M. V. ADAMO, M. L. MANCA BITTI, F. SCIARRA & B. BOSCHERINI. 1983. J. Clin. Endocrinol. Metab. **57:** 421–424.
66. JONES, T. M., V. S. FANG, R. L. LANDAU & R. ROSENFIELD. 1978. J. Clin. Endocrinol. Metab. **47:** 1368–1373.
67. LONGCOPE, C., T. KATO & R. HORTON. 1969. J. Clin. Invest. **48:** 2191–2201.
68. MacDONALD, P. C., J. M. GRODIN & P. K. SIITERI. 1971. *In* Gonadal Steroid Secretion. D. T. Baird & J. A. Strong, Eds.: 158–174. Edinburgh University Press. Edinburgh.
69. WINTER, J. S. D., S. TARASKA & C. FAIMAN. 1972. J. Clin. Endocrinol. Metab. **34:** 348–353.
70. HERRERA-JUSTINIANO, E., M. D. GALVEZ, A. M. AZNAR, S. M. M. GOMEZ, P. A. SEUDON, A. R. ZURITA, C. M. MALAGON & R. A. AZNAR. 1979. Acta Endocrinol. **90:** 113–121.
71. CACCIARI, E., A. CICOGNANI & P. TASSONI. 1974. Helvet. Pédiatr. Acta **29:** 27.
72. CANLORBE, P., J. E. TOUBLANC, J. C. JOB, R. SCHOLLER, M. ROGER, M. CASTANIER & P. LEYMARIE. 1974. Ann. Pédiatr. **21:** 13–26.
73. SCHOLLER, R., M. ROGER, P. LEYMARIE & M. CASTANIER. 1975. J. Steroid Biochem. **6:** 95–99.
74. FOREST, M. G. 1981. *In* The Intersex Child. N. Josso, Ed. **8:** 133–155. Karger. Basel.
75. FOREST, M. G., A. LECOQ & M. P. MONNERET. 1983. Ann. Endocrinol. (Paris) **44:** 179.
76. FOREST, M. G., M. LECORNU & E. DE PERETTI. 1980. J. Clin. Endocrinol. Metab. **50:** 826–833.
77. RICHARDS, G. & A. M. NEVILLE. 1974. J. Endocrinol. **61:** XVIII–XIX.
78. ROULIER, R. & M. G. FOREST. 1982. Endocrinology **110** (Suppl.):405.
79. FOREST, M. G. & R. ROULIER. 1982. Second European Workshop on Molecular and Cellular Endocrinology of the Testis. Boekelo, 11–14 May, 1982 Miniposters' book B9. Rotterdam, the Netherlands.
80. SMALS, A. G. H., G. F. M. PIETERS, J. I. M. DRAYER, T. J. BENRAAD & P. W. C. KLOPPENBORG. 1979. J. Clin. Endocrinol. Metab. **49:** 12–14.
81. SANTEN, R. J. & C. A. PAULSEN. 1972. J. Clin. Endocrinol. Metab. **36:** 55–63
82. WANG, C., C. A. PAULSEN, B. R. HOPPER, R. W. REBAR & S. S. C. YEN. 1980. J. Clin. Endocrinol. Metab. **51:** 1269–1273.
83. SMALS, A. G. H., G. F. F. M. PIETERS, P. W. C. KLOPPENBORG, D. C. LOZEKOOT & T. J. BENRAAD. 1980. J. Clin. Endocrinol. Metab. **50:** 879–881.
84. D'AGATA, R., E. VICARI, A. ALIFFI, G. MANGERI, A. MONGIOI & S. GULIZIA. 1982. J. Clin. Endocrinol. Metab. **55:** 76–80.

85. NORTHAITT, R. C. & A. ALBERT. 1970. J. Clin. Endocrinol. Metab. **31:** 91–95.
86. REITER, E. O., H. E. KULIN & D. L. LORIAUX. 1972. J. Clin. Endocrinol. Metab. **34:** 1080–1084.
87. REITER, E. O. & H. E. KULIN. 1971. J. Clin. Endocrinol. Metab. **33:** 957–961.
88. BERCU, B. B., B. C. LEE, J. L. PINEDA, B. E. SPILIOTIS, D. W. DENMAN III, H. J. HOFFMAN, T. J. BROWN & H. C. SACHS. 1983. J. Clin. Endocrinol. Metab. **56:** 1214–1226.
89. KNOBIL, E. 1980. Rec. Prog. Hormone Res. **36:** 53–88.
90. PAYNE, A. P. J. O'SHAUGNHESSY, D. J. CHASE, G. E. K. DIXON & A. K. CHRISTENSEN. 1982. Ann. N.Y. Acad. Sci. **383:** 174–200.
91. POMERANTZ, D. K. 1981. Endocrinology **109:** 2004–2008.
92. PURVIS, J. L., J. A. CANICK, S. A. LATIF, J. H. ROSENBAUM, J. HOLOGGITAS & R. H. MENARD. 1973. Arch. Biochem. Biophys. **159:** 39–49.
93. BRINKMANN, A. O., F. G. LEEMBORG & H. J. VAN DER MOLEN. 1980. Biol. Reprod. **23:** 801–809.
94. NOZU, K., A. DEHEJIA, L. K. J. ZAWISTOWICH, K. J. CATT & M. L. DUFAU. 1982. Ann. N.Y. Acad. Sci. **383:** 212–228.
95. SMALS, A. G. H., G. F. F. M. PIETERS, J. I. M. DRAYER, G. H. J. BOERS, T. J. BENRAAD & P. W. C. KLOPPENBORG. 1980. J. Clin. Endocrinol. Metab. **51:** 1026–1029.
96. MIGEON, C. J., M. A. RIVAROLA & M. G. FOREST. 1969. *In* Transsexualism and Sex Reassignment. R. Green & J. Money, Eds.: 203–211. Johns Hopkins Press. Baltimore, MD.
97. FOREST, M. G. 1983. Int. J. Androl. **6:** 1–4.

Trophic Influences of Luteinizing Hormone on Steroidogenesis by Percoll-separated Rat Leydig Cells in Culture[a]

MICHAEL J. BORDY,[b] JOEL H. SHAPER,[c] and
LARRY L. EWING[b,d]

[b] Division of Reproductive Biology
Department of Population Dynamics
School of Hygiene and Public Health
The Johns Hopkins University
Baltimore, Maryland 21205

[c] The Oncology Center
Department of Pharmacology and Experimental Therapeutics
The Johns Hopkins University School of Medicine
Baltimore, Maryland 21205

INTRODUCTION

Leydig cells of the testicular interstitium primarily synthesize and secrete testosterone.[1] This function is influenced both acutely and chronically by luteinizing hormone (LH). LH acutely regulates Leydig cell metabolism, as evidenced by changes in cyclic $3':5'$ adenosine monophosphate (cAMP) formation,[2] by changes in protein kinase activities,[3,4] by changes in the conversion of cholesterol to testosterone,[5,6] and by increasing the incorporation of radiolabeled precursors into proteins.[7–9]

LH also exerts trophic (chronic) effects on Leydig cell growth and differentiation as evidenced by changes in Leydig cell morphology during breeding season,[10] puberty,[11,12] or aging[13] and by changes in Leydig cell morphology and steroidogenic activity following hypophysectomy,[14] exogenous administration of luteinizing hormone,[15] or subdermal implantation of Silastic capsules filled with testosterone and estradiol.[16–19]

The results of the present study show that LH withdrawal *in vivo* inhibits subsequent testosterone production *in vitro* by Percoll-separated Leydig cells. At least one site of this trophic effect of LH probably involves enzymes sequestered in the smooth endoplasmic reticulum because Percoll-separated Leydig cells obtained from LH-deprived rats lost the capacity to synthesize testosterone from pregnenolone *in vitro*. In initial studies, we have demonstrated that Percoll-separated Leydig cells are capable of *de novo* protein synthesis as analyzed by metabolic labeling and 2D IEF/SDS-PAGE. Percoll-separated Leydig cells therefore

[a] Supported in part by the National Institutes of Health (grant 07204) and the Population Center (grant 06268 for the electron microscope core lab). M. J. B. was a postdoctoral fellow supported by a Mellon foundation grant.
[d] To whom reprint requests should be addressed.

should be amenable to the correlation of structural changes in smooth endoplasmic reticulum with changes in specific polypeptides and the steroidogenic reactions involved in the conversion of pregnenolone to testosterone.

MATERIALS AND METHODS

Experimental Design

Adult, male, Sprague-Dawley–derived rats (Flow Labs, Dublin, VA) were used in the study. The rats were kept in an air-conditioned (20 ± 2°C) and light-controlled (14 hours per 24 hours) room and supplied with rat chow and water *ad libitum*. Experimental rats were implanted with testosterone and estradiol-filled Silastic capsules as described elsewhere.[16] One group of rats (16) was implanted for 1, 2, 4, and 8 days. Another group of rats (19) was implanted for six weeks, and LH was restored endogenously by removing the implants or exogenously by administering ovine LH (NIH LH S21) via ALZET mini-osmotic pumps for 2, 4, 8, 10, or 12 days. Control rats received no Silastic (PDS, Silastic) implants.

Collagenase Dispersion of Rat Testicular Cells

Rats were killed by cranial concussion, and their testes were removed following laparotomy. Rat seminiferous tubules were teased apart and placed into a 50 ml polypropylene centrifuge tube (Corning, Corning, NY) that contained 20 ml of medium 199 (Grand Island Biological Company [GIBCO], Grand Island, NY) supplemented with 0.1% collagenase (134 U/mg, Millipore Corp., Freehold, NJ), 0.1% bovine serum albumin (4× crystalline BSA, ICN Pharmaceuticals, Cleveland, OH), and 25 mM HEPES (GIBCO, Grand Island, NY), pH 7.25. The seminiferous tubules were dispersed in a shaking water bath set at 34°C.[20] After ten minutes, collagenase dispersion was terminated by adding excess medium 199 containing 0.1% BSA, protease inhibitors, leupeptin (50 μg/ml), aprotinin (200 U/ml) (Sigma, St. Louis, MO), and 25 mM HEPES, pH 7.25. The dispersed rat testicular cell suspension was filtered through a 28 μm Nitex cloth mesh to remove cell clumps and seminiferous tubules. Subsequently, dispersed testicular cells were collected by centrifugation at 800 × g for 15 minutes at room temperature and resuspended in medium 199 containing 0.1% BSA and 25 mM HEPES, pH 7.25.

Separation of Dispersed Testicular Cells by Centrifugation in Percoll

Collagenase-dispersed testicular cells were separated on the basis of buoyant density by centrifugation in a density gradient of Percoll (Pharmacia, Piscataway, NJ).[21] Five ml of resuspended, collagenase-dispersed rat testicular cells were combined with 35 ml of 50% Percoll (vol/vol) in a 40 ml capacity centrifuge tube. Multiple centrifuge tubes containing resuspended cells and 50% Percoll were loaded in a fixed angle rotor (International). These tubes were centrifuged at 20,000 × g for one hour at 4°C. Percoll formed a density gradient *in situ* under these conditions.[21]

After one hour of centrifugation, the centrifuge tubes were carefully removed from the rotor. The distances from the top of the gradient to the marker beads were measured. The gradients were fractionated into 20 2-ml fractions. These fractions were washed in excess Hanks' balanced salt solution containing 0.1% BSA and 24 mM HEPES, pH 7.25. The cells from each fraction were collected by centrifugation at 1000 × *g* for 15 minutes at room temperature and resuspended in medium 199.

Cell Cultures of Collagenase-dispersed Rat Testicular Cells and Percoll-separated Leydig Cells

Collagenase-dispersed rat testicular cells (1 × 10^6 cells/ml) or Percoll-separated Leydig cells (1 × 10^6 cells/ml) were incubated in supplemented medium 199 for four hours at 34°C under 95% air : 5% CO_2 atmosphere. The incubation was terminated by collecting the media and removing the cells from the media by centrifugation. Cell-free media were frozen at −20°C subsequent to determination of testosterone content.

Assays for Production of Testosterone

Testosterone production was determined by a radioimmunoassay specific for testosterone.[22] The assay has been completely validated elsewhere.[22]

Light and Electron Microscopic Examination

Dispersed rat testicular cells and Percoll-separated Leydig cells were counted with a hemacytometer and a Nikon phase-contrast microscope. Trypan blue dye exclusion was determined by combining 100 μl cell suspension and 100 μl 1% trypan blue. Stained cells were counted with a hemacytometer and a Nikon phase-contrast microscope.

Samples of cells separated by centrifugation in Percoll were pelleted in glass test tubes and fixed for light and electron microscopy with 2.5% glutaraldehyde buffered with cacodylate, as described elsewhere.[18]

Cytochemical Staining for 3β-Hydroxysteroid Dehydrogenase

Collagenase-dispersed testicular cells and Percoll-separated Leydig cells were stained with nitro blue tetrazolium (NBT) to determine 3β-hydroxysteroid dehydrogenase (3β-HSD) activity. The staining solution contained 0.05 M potassium phosphate buffer, pH 7.4, 10 mg/ml NAD, 1 mg/ml NBT, and 1 mg/ml etiocholan-3-ol-17-one.[23] Cells were stained for 1.5 hours. Following staining, the cells were washed in water and allowed to dry. Subsequently, the cells were fixed with 10% formalin and counterstained with 0.25% eosin. The cells were examined at 400× magnification for the presence of a blue-purple stain indicative of a positive reaction for 3β-HSD.

[³⁵S]Methionine Incorporation into Percoll-separated Rat Leydig Cells

Aliquots of 1.5 × 10^6 Percoll-separated rat Leydig cells were added to 1.0 ml of methionine-free Ham's F12 containing 200 μCi [³⁵S]methionine (New England

Nuclear, Boston, MA). The cultures were incubated at 34°C in 95% air : 5% CO_2 for 2, 4, 8, 16, or 24 hours.

To terminate [^{35}S]methionine incorporation, the media was removed and the cells were washed with Ca^{2+}, Mg^{2+} free phosphate-buffered saline containing aprotinin (200 U/ml) and leupeptin (50 μg/ml). The washed cells were scraped with a rubber policeman into Ca^{2+}, Mg^{2+} free phosphate-buffered saline containing aprotinin and leupeptin. The cells were pelleted by centrifugation, and the cell pellet was solubilized by a 10 mM Tris-HCl buffer, pH 7.5, containing 1% NP-40, aprotinin (200 U/ml), and leupeptin (50 μg/ml) (1 $\times$ 10^7 cells/ml disruption buffer). An aliquot was precipitated with 25% trichloroacetic acid to determine [^{35}S]methionine incorporation into protein. The NP-40–solubilized cell pellet was prepared for isoelectric focusing (IEF) as described by O'Farrell.[24]

Two-dimensional Polyacrylamide Gel Electrophoresis

NP-40–solubilized extracts of non-labeled and [^{35}S]methionine-labeled Percoll-separated rat Leydig cells were analyzed by two-dimensional isoelectric focusing/SDS-electrophoresis as described by O'Farrell.[24]

NP-40–solubilized extracts were subjected to isoelectric focusing in the first dimension in 4% (w/vol) acrylamide gels containing bisacrylamide as a cross-linker, 9 M urea, 2% (vol/vol) NP-40, and 2% (vol/vol) ampholines. Isoelectric focusing gels were prepared for SDS-polyacrylamide gel electrophoresis by equilibration in 0.065 M Tris·HCl buffer, pH 6.8, containing Tris·HCl, 12.5% glycerol, 1% SDS, and 1% β-mecaptoethanol. SDS-polyacrylamide gel electrophoresis was performed according to the procedure described by Laemmli.[25] Equilibrated tube gels were overlaid on 10% (w/vol) acrylamide gel slabs. The slab gels were fixed and stained in Coomassie blue R-250 (Bio-Rad, Richmond, CA).

Analysis of Two-dimensional Polyacrylamide Gels

Slab gels were prepared for fluorography by impregnating with En^{3}Hance (New England Nuclear, Boston, MA), drying on filter paper, and exposing at -70°C to Kodak X-O-Mat X-ray film (Kodak, Rochester, NY) for 1–14 days, using an intensifying screen.

Slab gels were stained with silver as described earlier.[26] Briefly, the gels were fixed in 50% methanol and 12% acetic acid, washed in 10% ethanol and 5% acetic acid, and soaked in 3.4 mM potassium dichromate in 3.2 mM nitric acid. The gels were impregnated with silver nitrate and developed in 0.28 M sodium carbonate containing 0.5 ml formalin per liter.

RESULTS

Testosterone Production in Vitro by Collagenase-dispersed Testicular Cells

Collagenase dispersion of rat testicular cells provided approximately 1.25 $\times$ 10^8 cells per two testes. Approximately 92% of the collagenase-dispersed testicular cells excluded trypan blue, and 20–30% stained positively for 3β-HSD. Collagenase-dispersed testicular cells *in vitro* produced 2.5 and 15 ng of testosterone per million 3β-HSD staining cells per hour in the absence and in the presence of a maximally stimulating dose of LH (0.3 ng NIH LH S21, ovine), respectively. Testosterone production *in vitro* was found to be dependent on cell number, type of media, amount of BSA, and length of incubation. Optimal LH-stimulated testosterone production *in vitro* was achieved by incubating approximately 1.2×10^5 collagenase-dispersed testicular cells for four hours in medium 199 containing 0.1% BSA and 0.3 ng LH in 95% air : 5% CO_2.

Collagenase-dispersed testicular cells *in vitro* produced increasing amounts of testosterone following addition of increasing concentrations of exogenous substrates to supplemented medium 199 (FIGURE 1). Maximal testosterone production *in vitro* was elicited by concentrations of 5 μg/ml pregnenolone, 5.0 μg/ml progesterone, or 87.5 μg/ml androstenedione.

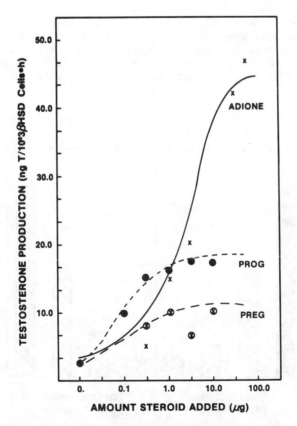

FIGURE 1. Substrate effects (μg/ml) on testosterone production *in vitro* by collagenase-dispersed rat testicular cells. Collagenase-dispersed rat testicular cells were incubated with pregnenolone (PREG), progesterone (PROG), or androstenedione (ADIONE) as described in the text and testosterone production *in vitro* was measured by a radioimmunoassay specific for testosterone. Testosterone production was plotted as a function of the substrate concentration ($N=3$).

The Effect of LH Withdrawal on Testosterone Production by
Collagenase-dispersed Testicular Cells

The results in FIGURE 2 show the effects of LH withdrawal and restoration *in vivo* on testosterone production *in vitro* by collagenase-dispersed testicular cells taken from rats in which LH was withdrawn or from rats in which LH was withdrawn and then restored. The left panel shows the effects of LH withdrawal *in vivo* on testosterone production *in vitro*. Testosterone production by collagenase-dispersed testicular cells from intact rats was 16 ng testosterone per million 3β-HSD staining cells per hour (100% control). By four days after implantation of testosterone- and estradiol-filled Silastic capsules, collagenase-dispersed testicular cells *in vitro* produced only 20% of the testosterone produced by collagenase-dispersed testicular cells from intact rats. The right panel of FIGURE 2 shows the effects of LH restoration *in vivo* on *in vitro* testosterone production by cells from rats in which LH had been withdrawn for six weeks. Collagenase-dispersed testicular cells obtained from rats implanted with testosterone and estradiol-filled Silastic capsules for six weeks after which implants were removed progressively regained the capacity to produce testosterone *in vitro* as a function of time. Collagenase-dispersed testicular cells obtained from rats, which were implanted for six weeks and then had the implants removed for twelve days, produced as much testosterone *in vitro* as collagenase-dispersed testicular cells from intact rats.

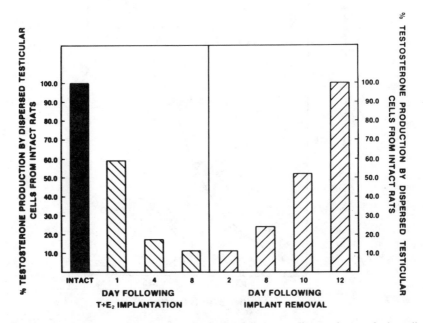

FIGURE 2. Changes in testosterone production by collagenase-dispersed rat testicular cells *in vitro* caused by changes in LH *in vivo*. LH withdrawal *in vivo* was accomplished by subdermal implants of testosterone- and estradiol-filled Silastic capsules. The left panel shows the effects of LH withdrawal for 1, 4, and 8 days on the testosterone production *in vitro* by collagenase-dispersed testicular cells. The right panel shows the effects of LH restoration to rats that previously had LH withdrawn for six weeks by testosterone and estradiol-filled Silastic implants (*N* = 4).

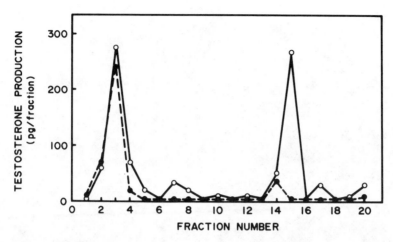

FIGURE 3. Testosterone production *in vitro* by fractions of collagenase-dispersed testicular cells separated on a Percoll density gradient. Collagenase-dispersed testicular cells from intact rats were separated by centrifugation in a Percoll density gradient. The gradients were separated into 2 ml fractions, and the cells from each fraction were collected, washed, and resuspended in medium 199. An aliquot of cells from each fraction was incubated in supplemented medium 199 in absence (-----) or in the presence of a maximally stimulating dose of LH (——). The amount of testosterone produced *in vitro* was plotted as a function of the fraction number. Cultures of cells from the third 2 ml fraction (buoyant density of 1.010 g/ml) produced approximately 300 pg testosterone whether incubated in the absence or presence of LH. Cultures of cells from the fifteenth 2 ml fraction (buoyant density of 1.060 g/ml) produced approximately 300 pg of testosterone only in the presence of LH (The graph represents a typical experiment.)

Percoll Separation of LH-responsive, Testosterone-producing Leydig Cells

The results in FIGURE 3 show testosterone production by collagenase-dispersed testicular cells from intact rats separated by centrifugation in Percoll density gradients. Cells with a buoyant density of 1.010 g/ml (in the third 2 ml fraction) and cells with a buoyant density of 1.060 g/ml (in the fifteenth 2 ml fraction) produced approximately 300 pg testosterone per fraction. Cells with a buoyant density of 1.010 g/ml (in the third 2 ml fraction) produced as much testosterone *in vitro* in the absence as in the presence of LH. In contrast, cells with a buoyant density of 1.060 g/ml (in the fifteenth 2 ml fraction) produced 10–15-fold more testosterone *in vitro* in the presence than in the absence of LH (FIGURE 3).

Morphologically, cells with a buoyant density of 1.010 g/ml (in the third 2 ml fraction) showed discontinuous plasma membranes, swollen mitochondria, vacuoles, and degenerating nuclei (results not shown). Only 65% ($N = 4$) of the cells in fraction three excluded trypan blue. In contrast, cells with a buoyant density of 1.060 g/ml (in the fifteenth 2 ml fraction) contained intact plasma membranes with somewhat expanded mitochondria and relatively normal nuclei (FIGURE 4). The results in TABLE 1 show that 96.5% ($N = 4$) of the cells with a buoyant density of 1.060 g/ml (in fifteenth 2 ml fraction) excluded trypan blue and 83% ($N = 4$) stained positively for 3β-HSD. Most of the other cells (17%) were condensed spermatids (results not shown). Percoll-separated rat Leydig cells with a buoyant

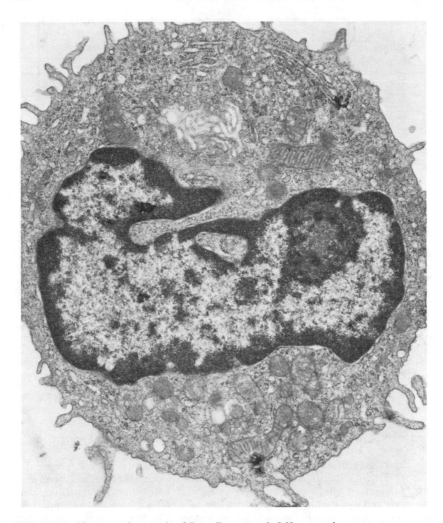

FIGURE 4. Electron micrograph of Percoll-separated, LH-responsive, testosterone-producing cells with a buoyant density of 1.060 g/ml. Collagenase-dispersed rat testicular cells were separated by centrifugation in Percoll density gradients. The gradient was divided into 20 2-ml fractions. LH-responsive, testosterone-producing cells with a buoyant density of 1.060 g/ml (the fifteenth 2 ml fraction) were fixed with 2.5% glutaraldehyde in 0.1 cacodylate buffer and embedded in Epon-Araldite. The micrograph presented is an electron micrograph of a typical Leydig cell. Note the ovoid nucleus, smooth endoplasmic reticulum, Golgi bodies, and slightly swollen mitochondria.

density of 1.060 g/ml produced 16.7 ng testosterone per million 3β-HSD staining cells per hour (TABLE 1), which was identical to the rate of testosterone production by 3β-HSD staining cells in the collagenase-dispersed testicular cell preparation. Taken together, these results suggested that most of the cells from fraction fifteen were intact Leydig cells that produced testosterone in response to LH.

TABLE 1. Characteristics of Percoll-separated Leydig Cells from Intact Rats

Characteristic	N	Mean	±	S.E.M.
Buoyant density (g/ml)	4	1.060	±	0.005
Trypan blue dye exclusion (%)	4	96.5	±	0.65
3β-HSD cytochemistry (%)	4	83.0	±	6.70
Testosterone production				
(ng/10⁶ Leydig cells·hr)				
minus LH	4	3.3	±	1.13
plus LH	4	16.7	±	2.41

Effect of LH Restoration in Vivo *on Testosterone Production* in Vitro *by Percoll-separated Rat Leydig Cells*

Subdermal implants of testosterone- and estradiol-filled Silastic capsules in rats caused LH withdrawal *in vivo*, inhibited testosterone biosynthesis, and after six weeks terminated spermatogenesis.[16] Based on an earlier report,[18] it seemed likely that LH restoration *in vivo* after six weeks of implantation of testosterone- and estradiol-filled Silastic capsules would restore Leydig cell morphology and testosterone biosynthetic capacity prior to the reappearance of condensed spermatids in the testis. Centrifugation of collagenase-dispersed cells from a testis treated in this way in a Percoll gradient should provide a highly enriched preparation of steroidogenically active Leydig cells free of condensed spermatids. That this was achieved is shown by the results in TABLE 2. Ninety-five percent of the cells with a buoyant density of 1.060 g/ml excluded trypan blue. Moreover, these putative Leydig cells constituted 94% of the cell types found in this fraction of the Percoll gradient (TABLE 2). Electron microscopic examination showed that these cells contained an ovoid nucleus, prominent smooth endoplasmic reticulum, and mitochondria characteristic of Leydig cells (FIGURE 5). Virtually no condensed spermatids were present. LH-stimulated testosterone production by these Percoll-separated rat Leydig cells (TABLE 2) was identical to that found in Leydig cells in a collagenase-dispersed testicular cell preparation or Percoll-separated Leydig cells from intact rats (TABLE 1).

The results in FIGURE 6 show the effects of LH withdrawal (left panel) and LH restoration (right panel) *in vivo* on testosterone-producing capacity of Percoll-separated rat Leydig cells *in vitro*. The results in the left panel show that Percoll-separated rat Leydig cells from LH-withdrawn rats progressively lost the capacity to produce testosterone in response to LH *in vitro*. By four days after implanta-

TABLE 2. Characteristics of Percoll-separated Leydig Cells that Were Atrophied by LH Withdrawal and then Restored by LH *in Vivo*

Characteristic	N	Mean	±	S.E.M.
Buoyant density (g/ml)	4	1.060	±	0.005
Trypan blue dye exclusion (%)	4	95.1	±	2.41
3β-HSD cytochemistry (%)	4	94.0	±	1.15
Testosterone production *in vitro*				
(ng/10⁶ Leydig cells·hr)				
minus LH	4	3.1	±	1.83
plus LH	4	16.0	±	3.72

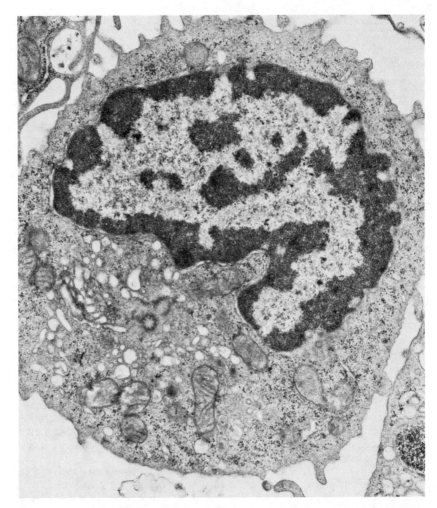

FIGURE 5. Electron micrograph of Percoll-separated Leydig cell from rats implanted for six weeks and then administered LH for twelve days. Percoll-separated Leydig cells from rats implanted for six weeks and then administered LH for twelve days were fixed with 2.5% glutaraldehyde and embedded in Epon-Araldite. The micrograph presented is an electron micrograph of a typical Leydig cell from this preparation. It has the same characteristics as a Percoll-separated Leydig cell from an intact rat.

tion, Percoll-separated 3β-HSD staining cells from rats treated in this fashion produced about a third as much testosterone as Percoll-separated 3β-HSD staining cells from intact rats. In the experiment depicted in the right panel, Percoll-separated Leydig cells from rats implanted for six weeks and then administered LH for 7 to 12 days were cultured *in vitro* to determine testosterone synthesizing capacity. Percoll-separated Leydig cells from rats given LH for twelve days produced as much testosterone *in vitro* as Percoll-separated Leydig cells from intact rats (FIGURE 6).

Loss of testosterone production by *in vitro* perfused rat testes from rats in which LH was withdrawn *in vivo* has been correlated with a diminution in surface areas of smooth endoplasmic reticulum,[18,19] which contains the steroidogenic enzymes that convert pregnenolone to testosterone.[27,28] FIGURE 7 shows the testosterone production *in vitro* by Percoll-separated 3β-HSD staining cells from intact rats (left panel) or rats implanted with testosterone- and estradiol-filled Silastic capsules for five days (right panel) and incubated with a maximally stimulating dose of LH or a saturating concentration of pregnenolone. Percoll-separated 3β-HSD staining cells from intact rats (left panel) produced significantly more testosterone *in vitro* when incubated with a maximally stimulating dose of LH or a saturating concentration of pregnenolone. The right panel shows that the addition of LH failed to stimulate testosterone production *in vitro* by Percoll-separated Leydig cells from implanted rats; nor was it restored by the addition of saturating concentrations of pregnenolone.

Protein Synthesis in Percoll-separated Rat Leydig Cells

As discussed above, one of the most dramatic trophic effects of LH withdrawal *in vivo* is the apparent decrease in the amounts of smooth endoplasmic reticulum of the Leydig cell. Consequently, one would anticipate that LH with-

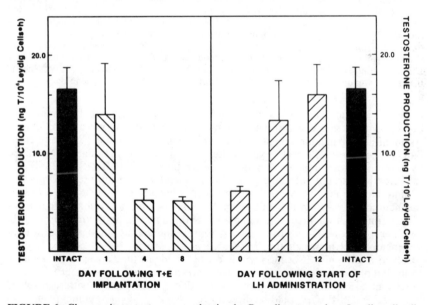

FIGURE 6. Changes in testosterone production by Percoll-separated rat Leydig cells elicited by changes in LH *in vivo*. LH withdrawal *in vivo* was accomplished by subdermal implantation of testosterone and estradiol filled Silastic capsules in rats; LH restoration by exogenous administration of 24 μg ovine LH per day via an ALZET mini-osmotic pump. The left panel shows the effect of testosterone and estradiol filled Silastic implants on testosterone produced *in vitro* by Percoll-separated Leydig cells from intact rats. The right panel shows the effect of seven and twelve days of LH administration in rats implanted for six weeks. The Percoll-separated Leydig cells from rats treated in this manner produce as much testosterone as Percoll-separated Leydig calls from intact rats.

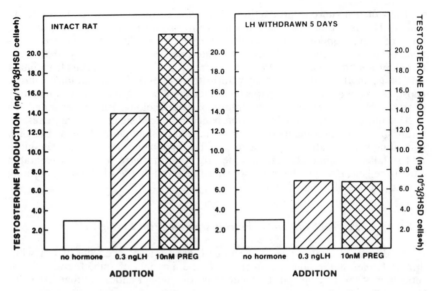

FIGURE 7. Conversion of pregnenolone to testosterone *in vitro* by Percoll-separated Leydig cells from intact and LH-withdrawn rats. The left panel shows *in vitro* testosterone production by Percoll-separated Leydig cells from intact rats incubated in supplemented medium 199 in the absence of hormone, in the presence of maximally stimulating dose of LH (0.3 ng LH/ml), or a saturating concentration of pregnenolone (10 nM). The right panel shows *in vitro* testosterone production by Percoll-separated Leydig cells from rats in which LH was withdrawn for five days incubated in the absence of hormone or in the presence of maximally stimulating dose of LH or a saturating concentration of pregnenolone.

drawal should affect quantitatively (and possibly qualitatively) the amounts of both enzymatic and constitutive proteins of the smooth endoplasmic reticulum. As an initial step in addressing this question, the incorporation of [^{35}S]-methionine into polypeptides in Percoll-separated Leydig cells from intact rats was examined by two-dimensional polyacrylamide gel electrophoresis (2D-IEF/SDS-PAGE).

Percoll-separated rat Leydig cells from intact rats in culture incorporated [^{35}S]methionine into TCA-precipitable material linearly over eight hours. During the incubation less then 10% of the input [^{35}S]methionine was utilized. In a series of experiments, total incorporation of [^{35}S]methionine was approximately 1×10^6 cpm per 10^6 3β-HSD–positive cells. A representative autoradiograph of a two-dimensional gel in which the ^{35}S-labeled proteins from NP-40 cell extract are resolved is shown in FIGURE 8. As is readily evident, the Leydig cells obtained from Percoll gradients have the requisite enzymatic machinery intact for the *de novo* synthesis of a variety of proteins. In addition, the protein pattern resolved by 2D-IEF/SDS-PAGE could be directly visualized by silver staining (results not shown).

DISCUSSION

Purification and Characterization of Rat Leydig Cells

We obtained a purified population of LH-responsive, testosterone-producing Leydig cells as have other investigators.[29–34]

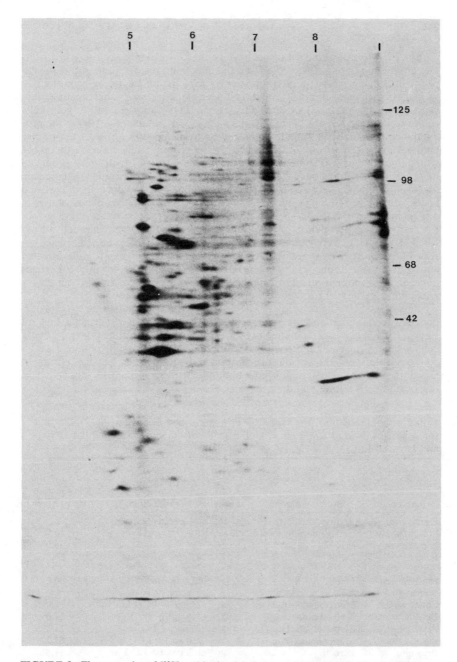

FIGURE 8. Fluorography of [^{35}S]methionine-labeled proteins from NP-40–solubilized extracts of Percoll-separated rat Leydig cell cultures. NP-40–solubilized extracts of [^{35}S]methionine-labeled, Percoll-separated rat Leydig cells were subjected to equilibrium isoelectric focusing followed by SDS-polyacrylamide gel electrophoresis. Slab gels were impregnated with En^{3}Hance, dried, and exposed to X-ray film at −70°C for 4 days. The pI gradient is indicated at the top of the gel and the molecular weight scale is indicated at the right of the gel.

Since *in vitro* perfused rat testes have been shown to mimic closely testosterone production *in vivo*,[35] we compared the maximum testosterone-producing capacity of collagenase-dispersed rat testicular cells and rat Leydig cells purified by us and other investigators[23,29–34] with testosterone secretion by maximally stimulated rat testes perfused *in vitro* (TABLE 3). Purification of rat Leydig cells achieved in these reports ranged from 55–95%. LH-stimulated testosterone production by isolated rat Leydig cells ranged from 3.6–105 ng testosterone per million Leydig cells per hour. The results of the present study compare favorably with all but two previous reports[23,32] in which the purified Leydig cells produced more testosterone than did cells obtained by us or other investigators. The reason for this discrepancy between testosterone production by Leydig cells in perfused testes and purified Leydig cells or in purified Leydig cells between laboratories is not apparent.

Testosterone production rates by collagenase-dispersed testicular cells or purified Leydig cells were not as high as production rates for *in vitro* perfused rat testes (TABLE 3). This suggested that enzymatic dispersion significantly affected subsequent testosterone production *in vitro* by rat Leydig cells in culture. Perhaps collagenase treatment affected cellular architecture or interactions required for maximum Leydig cell testosterone production.

Regardless, Leydig cells lose some capacity to convert substrate to testosterone. A recent summary[36] of published reports on this topic suggested that rat Leydig cells *in vitro* accumulated more 17α-hydroxyprogesterone than rat Leydig cells *in vivo*. Consequently, one must cautiously interpret results obtained with a collagenase-dispersed testicular preparation and with purified Leydig cells given this difference in testosterone production between the purified Leydig cells and the Leydig cells within an intact testis.

TABLE 3. Comparison of the Isolation Procedure and Testosterone Production for *in Vitro* Perfused Rat Testes, Collagenase-dispersed Rat Testicular Cells, and Isolated Rat Leydig Cells

Reference	Isolation Medium	Purity	Reported Testosterone Production	Calculated Testosterone Production (ng/10^6LC·hr)
Ewing *et al.*[19]	Perfused rat testis	3–5	6 μg/testis·hr	200
Present study	Collagenase-dispersed	20–30		16.7
Present study	Percoll	85–95		16.0
Janszen *et al.*[29]	Ficoll	55	42.4 ng/10^6 cells·3 hr	25.8
van Beurden *et al.*[30]	Ficoll	55	55.0 ng/10^6 cells · 2 hr	50.0
Conn *et al.*	Metrizamide	94	78 ng/10^6 LC·3 hr	25.0
Dehejia *et al.*[32]	Metrizamide	95	315 ng/10^6 LC·3 hr	105.0
Payne *et al.*[23]	Metrizamide (Pop I)	95	75 ng/10^6 LC·3hr	25.0
Payne *et al.*[23]	Metrizamide (Pop II)	95	250 ng/10^6 LC·3 hr	83.3
Browning *et al.*[33]	Percoll	70	120 pM/10^6 LC·3 hr	11.5
Gale *et al.*[34]	Percoll	71–79	36 pM/10^6 LC·3hr	3.6

Testosterone production was calculated by us as ng testosterone produced per million Leydig cells (LC) per hour from representative results in each publication. This represents our interpretation of the authors' data. For the *in vitro* perfused rat testis, the testosterone production rate was divided by the average number of Leydig cells per rat testis.[37]

Payne and colleagues have reported the separation of two populations of Leydig cells using Metrizamide gradients.[15,23] In the experiments reported here, we observed a continuum of Leydig cells throughout the Percoll gradient. That is, we observed that almost every fraction contained some 3β-HSD staining cells. However, only the cells with buoyant density of 1.060 g/ml consistently produced testosterone when stimulated by LH *in vitro*.

Trophic Effects of LH on Rat Leydig Cells

LH exerts trophic effects on Leydig cell growth and differentiation.[10–16] The results in FIGURES 2 and 6 confirm that LH withdrawal *in vivo* caused a reversible reduction in subsequent testosterone production *in vitro* both by collagenase-dispersed testicular cells and Percoll-separated rat Leydig cells. One site of the trophic effect of LH on Leydig cell testosterone production involves the conversion of pregnenolone to testosterone because loss in testosterone production by *in vitro* perfused testes from rats in which LH was withdrawn *in vivo* has been correlated with a loss in surface area of the Leydig cell smooth endoplasmic reticulum and because administration of LH *in vivo* restored testosterone secretion by *in vitro* perfused testes.[19]

Percoll-separated rat Leydig cells from intact rats produced as much testosterone when a saturating concentration of pregnenolone was added to the culture medium *in vitro* as when maximally stimulated with LH (left panel, FIGURE 7). Percoll-separated Leydig cells obtained from rats in which LH was withdrawn for five days did not produce as much testosterone as Percoll-separated Leydig cells from intact rats when provided saturating concentrations of pregnenolone *in vitro* (FIGURE 7). This result confirmed that LH withdrawal *in vivo* affected the enzymes of the smooth endoplasmic reticulum that convert pregnenolone to testosterone.[15,27,28]

Protein Synthesis by Percoll-separated Rat Leydig Cells

As shown in FIGURE 8, a number of proteins can be metabolically labeled with [35S]methionine *in vitro* by Percoll-separated rat Leydig cells from normal animals. In preliminary experiments, we have also demonstrated that proteins in Leydig cells isolated from animals after LH withdrawal *in vivo* can be metabolically labeled. Comparative analysis of the two protein profiles indicates quantitative differences in individual polypeptides. At current levels of resolution, we have not been able to detect qualitative differences. Analysis of the effects of LH withdrawal *in vivo* at the molecular level will require the development and application of specific immunological and biochemical (i.e., suicide substrate) probes directed against individual enzymatic or structural proteins of the smooth endoplasmic reticulum. These questions are currently under investigation in our laboratory.

ACKNOWLEDGMENTS

The authors wish to thank Dr. Barry Zirkin for his advice and help with the electron micrographs and their interpretation.

REFERENCES

1. CHRISTENSEN, A. K. & N. R. MASON. 1965. Comparative ability of seminiferous tubules and interstitial tissue of rat testis to synthesize androgens from progesterone-^{14}C in vitro. Endocrinology **76:** 646–656.

2. MENDELSON, C., M. DUFAU & K. J. CATT. 1975. Gonadotropin binding and stimulation of cyclic adenosine 3′:5′ monophosphate and testosterone production in isolated Leydig cells. J. Biol. Chem. **250:** 8818–8823.

3. PODESTA, E. J., M. L. DUFAU & K. J. CATT. 1976. Cyclic adenosine 3′:5′ monophosphate dependent protein kinase of rat Leydig cells: Physical characteristics of two holoenzymes and their subunits. Biochemistry **17:** 1566–1573.

4. COOKE, B. A., M. L. LINDH & F. H. A. JANSZEN. 1976. Correlation of protein kinase activation and testosterone production after stimulation of Leydig cells with luteinizing hormone. Biochem. J. **160:** 439–446.

5. EWING, L. L. & B. BROWN. 1977. Testicular steroidogenesis. In The Testis. A. D. Johnson & W. R. Gomes, Eds. **4:** 239–287. Academic Press. New York.

6. TAMAOKI, B.-I. & M. SHIKITA. 1966. Biosynthesis of steroids in testicular tissue in vitro. In Steroid Dynamics. G. Pincus, T. Nakao & J. F. Tait, Eds.: 493–530. Academic Press. New York.

7. JANSZEN, F. H. A., B. A. COOKE, M. J. A. VAN DRIEL & H. J. VAN DER MOLEN. 1976. LH induction of a specific protein (LH-IP) in rat testis Leydig cells. FEBS Lett. **71:** 269–272.

8. JANSZEN, F. H. A., B. A. COOKE & H. J. VAN DER MOLEN. 1977. Specific protein synthesis in isolated rat testis Leydig cells. Influence of luteinizing hormone and cycloheximide. Biochem. J. **162:** 341–346.

9. NOZU, K., A. DEHEJIA, L. ZAWISTOWICH, K. J. CATT & M. L. DUFAU. 1981. Gonadotropin-induced desensitization of Leydig cells in vivo and in vitro: Estrogen action in the testis. Ann. N. Y. Acad. Sci. **383:** 212–230.

10. NEAVES, W. B. 1973. Changes in testicular Leydig cells and in plasma testosterone levels among seasonally breeding rock hyrax. Biol. Reprod. **8:** 451–466.

11. KNORR, D. W., T. VANHA-PERTTULA & M. B. LIPSETT. 1970. Structure and function of rat testis through pubescence. Endocrinology **86:** 1298–1304.

12. PAHNKE, V. C., F. A. LEIDENBERGER & H. J. KUNZIG. 1975. Correlation between hCG (LH)-binding capacity, Leydig cell number, and secretory activity of rat testis through pubescence. Acta Endocrinol. **79:** 610–618.

13. PIRKE, K. M., H.-J. VOGT & M. GEISS. 1978. In vitro and in vivo studies on Leydig cell function in old rats. Acta Endocrinol. **89:** 393.

14. MERKOW, L., H. F. ACEVEDO, M. SLIFKIN & M. PARDO. 1968. Studies on the interstitial cells of the testis. II. The ultrastructure in the adult guinea pig and the effect of stimulation with human chorionic gonadotropin. Am. J. Pathol. **53:** 989–1007.

15. O'SHAUGHNESSY, P. J. & A. H. PAYNE. 1982. Differential effects of single and repeated administration of gonadotropins on testosterone production and steroidogenic enzymes in Leydig cell populations. J. Biol. Chem. **257:** 11503–11509.

16. EWING, L. L., C. DESJARDINS, D. C. IRBY & B. ROBAIRE. 1977. Synergistic interaction of testosterone and oestradiol inhibits spermatogenesis in rats. Nature **269:** 409–410.

17. EWING, L. L., R. A. GORSKI, R. J. SBORDONE, J. V. TYLER, C. DESJARDINS & B. ROBAIRE. 1979. Testosterone-estradiol filled polydimethylsiloxane implants: Effect on fertility and masculine sexual and aggressive behavior of male rats. Biol. Reprod. **21:** 765–772.

18. ZIRKIN, B. R., D. D. DYKMAN, N. KROMANN, R. C. COCHRAN & L. L. EWING. 1981. Inhibition and recovery of testosterone secretion in rats are tightly coupled to quantitative changes in Leydig cell smooth endoplasmic reticulum. Ann. N.Y. Acad. Sci. **383:** 17–28.

19. EWING, L. L., T.-Y. WING, R. C. COCHRAN, N. KROMANN & B. ZIRKIN. 1983. Effect of luteinizing hormone on Leydig cell structure and testosterone secretion. Endocrinology **112:** 1763–1769.

20. DUFAU, M. L. & K. J. CATT. 1975. Gonadotropic stimulation of interstitial cell functions of the rat testis *in vitro*. Methods Enzymol. **39D:** 252–271.
21. PERTOFT, H., T. C. LAURENT, T. LAAS & L. KAGEDAL. 1978. Density gradients prepared from colloidal silica particles coated by polyvinylpyrrolidone (Percoll). Anal. Biocehm. **88:** 271–282.
22. SCHANBACHER, B. D. & L. L. EWING. 1975. Simultaneous determination of testosterone, 5α-androstan-17β-ol-3-one, 5α-androstan-3α,17β-diol, and 5α-androstan-3β, 17β-diol in plasma of adult male rabbits by radioimmunoassay. Endocrinology **97:** 787–792.
23. PAYNE, A. H., J. R. DOWNING & K. L. WONG. 1980. Luteinizing hormone receptors and testosterone synthesis in two distinct populations of Leydig cells. Endocrinology **106:** 1424–1429.
24. O'FARRELL, P. H. 1975. High resolution two-dimensional electrophoresis of proteins. J. Biol. Chem. **250:** 4007–4021.
25. LAEMMLI, U. K. 1970. Cleavage of structural proteins during the assembly of the head of the bacteriophage. Nature **227:** 680–685.
26. MERRIL, C. R., D. GOLDMAN, S. A. SEDMAN & M. H. EBERT. 1981. Ultrasensitive stain for proteins in polyacrylamide gels shows regional variation in cerebrospinal fluid proteins. Science **211:** 1437–1438.
27. SHIKITA, M. & B.-I. TAMAOKI. 1965. Testosterone formation by subcellular particles of rat testes. Endocrinology **76:** 563–569.
28. PURVIS, J. L., J. A. CANICK, S. A. LATIF, J. H. ROSENBAUM, J. HOLOGGITA & R. H. MENARD. 1973. Lifetime of microsomal cytochrome P-450 and steroidogenic enzymes in rat testis as influenced by human chorionic gonadotropin. Arch. Biochem. Biophys. **159:** 39–46.
29. JANSZEN, F. H. A., B. A. COOKE, M. J. A. VAN DRIEL & H. J. VAN DER MOLEN. 1976. Purification and characterization of Leydig cells from rat testes. J. Endocrinol. **70:** 345–359.
30. VAN BEURDEN, W. M. O., B. ROODNAT, F. H. DE JONG, E. MULDER & H. J. VAN DER MOLEN. 1976. Hormonal regulation of LH stimulation of testosterone production in isolated Leydig cells of immature rats: The effect of hypophysectomy, FSH, and estradiol 17-β. Steroids **28:** 847–866.
31. CONN, P. M., T. TSURUHARA, M. DUFAU & K. J. CATT. 1977. Isolation of highly purified Leydig cells by density gradient centrifugation. Endocrinology **101:** 639–642.
32. DEHEJIA, A., K. NOZU, K. J. CATT & M. L. DUFAU. 1982. Luteinizing hormone receptors and gonadotropic activation of purified rat Leydig cells. J. Biol. Chem. **257:** 13781–13786.
33. BROWNING, J. Y., R. D'AGATA & H. E. GROTJAN, JR. 1981. Isolation of purified rat Leydig cells using continuous Percoll gradients. Endocrinology **109:** 667–669.
34. GALE, J. S., J. STJ. WAKEFIELD & H. C. FORD. 1982. Isolation of rat Leydig cells by density gradient centrifugation. J. Endocrinol. **92:** 293–302.
35. EWING, L. L. & B. ZIRKIN. 1983. Leydig cell structure and steroidogenic function. Rec. Prog. Horm. Res. **39:** 599–635.
36. VAN DER MOLEN, H. J., F. H. DE JONG & F. F. G. ROMMERTS. 1982. Summary of the proceedings of the second European testis workshop. The Netherlands. 11–14 May 1982. Mol. Cell Endocrinol. **28:** 1–11.
37. MORI, R. & A. K. CHRISTENSEN. 1980. Morphometric analysis of Leydig cells in the normal rat testis. J. Cell Biol. **84:** 340–354.

Identification and Possible Function of Pro-opiomelanocortin-derived Peptides in the Testis[a]

C. W. BARDIN, C. SHAHA,[b] J. MATHER, Y. SALOMON,[c]
A. N. MARGIORIS,[d] A. S. LIOTTA,[d]
I. GERENDAI,[e] C.-L. CHEN, and D. T. KRIEGER[d]

The Population Council
New York, New York 10021

[d] *Division of Endocrinology*
Mount Sinai Medical Center
New York, New York 10029

Pro-opiomelanocortin (POMC) is known to serve as a precursor for a variety of peptides including an *N*-terminal fragment, ACTH, the MSHs (α, γ), CLIP (corticotropin-intermediate lobe-like peptide), the lipotropins (β-LPH, γ-LPH), and β-endorphin. β-Endorphin, in turn, contains within it the smaller opioid peptides α- and γ-endorphin and derivatives thereof (FIGURE 1). Although POMC was originally described in the anterior and intermediate lobes of the pituitary, which are still the major source of POMC-derived peptides, it is now clear that this precursor is present and synthesized in a number of nonpituitary tissues. These include the central nervous system,[1-3] placenta,[4-6] and gastrointestinal tract.[7-9] It appears that the processing of the precursor molecule into its component peptides in extrapituitary tissues and in the intermediate lobe differs from that in the anterior pituitary gland. In the anterior pituitary, POMC is processed predominantly to an *N*-terminal fragment, ACTH, and β-LPH. In the intermediate pituitary lobe, ACTH is further processed to α-MSH, [α-N-acetyl ACTH(1–13) NH$_2$] and CLIP, while β-LPH is processed to γ-LPH and β-endorphin (FIGURE 1). In the hypothalamus and in all extrapituitary tissues studied to date, the processing of POMC more closely resembles that in the intermediate lobe.[10,11] In the latter site, however, β-endorphin and α-MSH are present predominantly as α-N-acetylated derivatives, while in the hypothalamus there is little[12,13] or no[14,15] acetylation of these peptides. As will be discussed below, the α-N-acetylation of these peptides may dramatically alter their biological activities.

Following the demonstration of immunoreactive β-endorphin in human semen[16] and rat testicular extracts,[17] our laboratory provided immunologic evidence for the presence of multiple POMC-derived peptides in the male and female

[a] This work was supported by National Institutes of Health Grants NB02893, HD13541, and HD16149 and the Lita Annenberg Hazen Charitable Trust.

[b] The present address of Dr. Shaha is National Institute of Immunology, All India Institute of Medical Sciences, P.O. Box 4922, New Delhi-110029, India.

[c] Dr. Salomon was supported by the Mellon Foundation while a Visiting Scientist on leave from the Department of Hormone Research, Weizmann Institute, Rehovot, Israel.

[e] Dr. Gerendai was supported by the Mellon Foundation while a Visiting Scientist on leave from the 2nd Department of Anatomy, Semmelweis University Medical School, Tulzolto utca 58, 1094 Budapest IX, Hungary.

reproductive tracts.[18,19] The present report summarizes our recent findings in rodent testis. We will review the immunochemical localization of POMC and POMC-derived peptides in Leydig cells, the nature of the immunoreactive POMC-derived peptides in rat testis, the localization of POMC-like mRNA in the testis, the ontogeny of POMC-derived peptides in the testis, factors regulating testicular POMC-derived peptides, possible function of POMC-derived peptides in the testis, and POMC in other steroid-secreting cells.

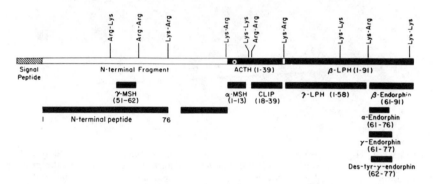

FIGURE 1. Schematic representation of bovine pro-opiomelanocortin (upper horizontal bar). Note that many of the indicated peptide fragments are flanked on both sides by pairs of basic amino acid residues that can potentially be cleaved to yield the component peptides indicated. In the anterior lobe, pro-opiomelanocortin is cleaved to the N-terminal fragment, ACTH, and β-LPH. In the intermediate lobe and brain, ACTH is further processed to α-MSH and CLIP while β-LPH is processed to γ-LPH and β-endorphin. Also indicated are the structures of other opiate peptides contained within the β-endorphin sequence.

THE IMMUNOCYTOCHEMICAL LOCALIZATION OF POMC AND POMC-DERIVED PEPTIDES IN LEYDIG CELLS

Immunoreactive β-endorphin was localized to the Leydig cells of five species including rat, hamster, guinea pig, rabbit, and mouse (FIGURE 2).[18,19] No immunoreactive material was detected in Sertoli, myoid, epithelial, and germ cells in any of these species. In all instances, immunostaining was markedly reduced when the primary antiserum was replaced with absorbed antiserum, preimmune, or hyperimmune sera. When an ACTH antibody (R-1-76) was employed that reacts with determinants within the N- and C-terminal and midportion sequences of synthetic ACTH(1–39), immunoreactive material was seen in Leydig cells but in no other part of the testis. It was of note, however, that no staining was seen with another ACTH antiserum ("West") that cross-reacts predominantly with the midportion determinants of ACTH(1–24). Studies in mouse and hamster testes utilizing an antiserum to γ_3-MSH (a 27 amino acid sequence present in the N-terminal fragment of POMC) revealed staining of Leydig cells.[20] The observation that antisera against peptides derived from the N-terminal, midportion, and C-terminal portions of POMC all demonstrated immunostainable material in Leydig cells raised the question as to whether this precursor and its component peptides were

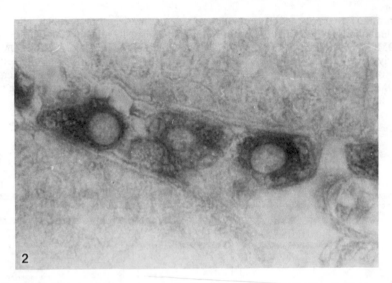

FIGURE 2. High power photomicrograph of mouse Leydig cells showing immunoreactive β-endorphin–like material. The immunostaining was markedly reduced when the primary antiserum was replaced with absorbed antiserum or preimmune serum. A similar staining reaction was also identified with an antibody against $γ_3$-MSH (× 1000).

synthesized in this portion of the testis. We next sought to demonstrate the nature of the immunoreactive material in rat testis using physicochemical characterization.

THE NATURE OF IMMUNOREACTIVE POMC-RELATED PEPTIDES IN RAT TESTIS

Preliminary studies quantified the concentration of immunoreactive POMC-related peptides in acid extracts of rat testis.[19] The tissue was homogenized in acid (0.1 M HCl, 0.1 M HCOOH), centrifuged, and the peptides in the supernatant phase were concentrated on and eluted from SEP-PAK C-18 reverse-phase cartridges. Overall recovery of β-endorphin added to aliquots of testicular tissue was 86%. Immunoreactive peptide concentrations corrected for recovery were: β-endorphin, 0.15 (picomoles g^{-1} wet weight); γ-endorphin, 0.29; N-terminal ACTH, 0.26; and C-terminal ACTH, 0.44. The presence of immunoreactive POMC-derived peptides in testis was in agreement with immunocytochemical findings. Preliminary chromatographic analysis of the immunoreactive β-endorphin-like material indicated that it eluted on gel filtration with a K_{av} similar to authentic β-endorphin(1–31).

A more extensive characterization of POMC-derived peptides was performed on a pool of testes obtained from 75 intact adult male Sprague-Dawley rats.[21] Testes were homogenized as described above and defatted with iso-octane and petroleum ether until lipids were no longer visible at the aqueous–organic phase interface. Supernatants were then extracted with Sep-Pak C-18 reverse-phase cartridges. Recoveries of standard peptides added to representative aliquots of tissue homogenate were: β-endorphin, 90%; α-MSH, 92%; and human β-lipotropin, 55%. The antibodies employed were against: β_c-endorphin; α-N-acetyl β_c-endorphin (which requires the α-acetyl group for recognition), N-terminal ACTH (BF-5a), α-MSH, γ_3-MSH, α-endorphin, and γ-endorphin. A detailed description of these antisera has been presented previously.[21] The concentrations of immunoreactive peptides were determined both in the unfractionated extracts and after gel filtration (Sephadex G-50), reverse-phase high-performance liquid chromatographic (RP-HPLC), and electrophoretic (sodium dodecyl sulfate polyacrylamide gel electrophoresis: SDS-PAGE) fractionation procedures. The mean concentrations of immunoreactive α-endorphin, β-endorphin, and γ-endorphin were 0.07 ± 0.01, 0.18 ± 0.03, and 0.06 ± 0.01 pmol/g (wet wt), respectively. The discrepancies in the concentration of γ-endorphin in this and in the preliminary studies noted above can be explained by the finding that tissue extracts do not produce parallel dilution curves in the γ-endorphin RIA, so that valid quantification could not be performed without prior chromatography. It was shown that the lack of parallelism of the unchromatographed tissue extracts was due to the partial (non-parallel) cross-reactivity of the β-endorphin species present in the extract. Therefore, quantification of immunoreactive γ-endorphin was possible only after RP-HPLC.

On SDS-PAGE, most of the immunoreactive β-endorphin migrated as a single peak, exhibiting the same relative mobility as synthetic β_c-endorphin, which has an identical sequence to rat β-endorphin (FIGURE 3, Left upper). On RP-HPLC (FIGURE 3, Right upper) the major form of immunoreactive β-endorphin detected exhibited the identical retention time as the authentic β-endorphin molecule, with small amounts of later-eluting forms. Only minor amounts of immunoreactive N-acetylated–β-endorphin–like activity were detected. On Sephadex G-50 chromatography (FIGURE 3, lower) of fractions comprising the major β-endorphin–like peaks from RP-HPLC, a single peak of immunoreactive β-endorphin was again found, identical to the K_{av} or authentic β_c-endorphin(1–31). No peptides exhibiting the retention time (t_R) of ACTH(1–39) were detected in the testicular extracts (FIGURE 4). Reverse-phase HPLC analysis (using two different gradient systems exhibiting different selectivities for synthetic POMC-derived peptides) revealed that the majority of the material with N-terminal ACTH immunoreactivity eluted with the same retention time as synthetic des-acetyl α-MSH and that most immunoreactive α- and γ-endorphins displays the retention times of synthetic α-endorphin and des-Tyr^1-γ-endorphin, respectively. No high molecular weight species with the physicochemical properties of POMC was detected. The findings of nearly equimolar concentrations of immunoreactive endorphins [$(\alpha + \beta + \gamma) = 0.31$ pmol/g wet wt] and of immunoreactive N-terminal ACTH activity (i.e., 0.33 ± 0.08 pmol/g wet wt) are consistent with their derivation from a POMC-like molecule.[13]

These studies also indicate that post-translational processing of POMC-like material in rat testes appears to be similar to that in rat pituitary intermediate lobe and hypothalamus, in that peptides similar in size to α-MSH and β-endorphin rather than ACTH(1–39) and β-lipotropin, are major moieties detected in testicular tissue. The present findings differ, however, from those in rat pituitary intermediate lobe in which both α-MSH and β-endorphin are α-N-acetylated and are similar to those in rat brain, where acetylation of these peptides is either substantially reduced[12,13] or absent.[14,15] Therefore, the present findings indicate that the profile of POMC-related peptides in testicular extracts more closely resembles that present in brain rather than in intermediate lobe.

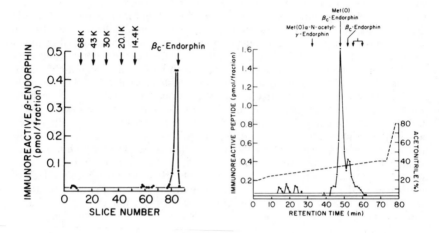

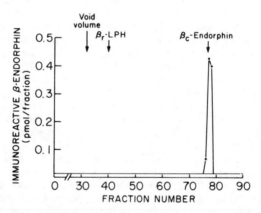

FIGURE 3. (Upper left) Identification of β-endorphin–like material from a testicular extract fractionated on SDS-containing polyacrylamide gels. Migration position of protein molecular weight markers are shown by the arrows. The horizontal line parallel to the abcissa in all figures indicates the sensitivity of the β-endorphin radioimmunoassay. (Upper right) Analysis of testicular immunoreactive β-endorphin by reverse-phase high-pressure liquid chromatography. An aliquot of the testicular extract was oxidized and fractionated on a reverse-phase column. All fractions were assayed in a β-endorphin RIA (●——●) and in an RIA assay that measures only the α-N-acetylated forms of β-endorphin (○——○). (Bottom) Sephadex G-50 superfine chromatography of immunoreactive β-endorphin obtained from the RP-HPLC analysis. All the detectable immunoreactive β-endorphin eluted with the K_{av} of β_c-endorphin is consistent with the results in the upper two panels. (From Magioris *et al.*[21] With permission from *Endocrinology*.).

It should be noted that the concentrations of POMC-related peptides in testes are much lower than those present in pituitary or central nervous system (TABLE 1). It remains to be established whether the low concentrations of these immunoreactive peptides in rat testicular extracts are a true measure of the secretory capacity of this tissue, or whether they reflect a high turnover rate.

THE LOCALIZATION OF POMC-LIKE MRNA IN TESTIS

The studies described above were compatible with POMC synthesis in Leydig cells, but did not exclude the possibility of uptake from blood. It was, therefore, necessary to demonstrate that Leydig cells had the capability of synthesizing this precursor and its derivative peptides. To address this question directly, we sought to demonstrate that Leydig cells contained POMC mRNA. Total RNA was prepared from neurointermediate pituitary, testis, and epididymis of rat, and a mouse Leydig cell line (TM$_3$). RNA was extracted by the urea-lithium chloride procedure[22] and poly A RNA isolated using oligo(dT)cellulose.[23] The RNA was fractionated on denaturing gels and transferred onto nitrocellulose paper. The mRNA was

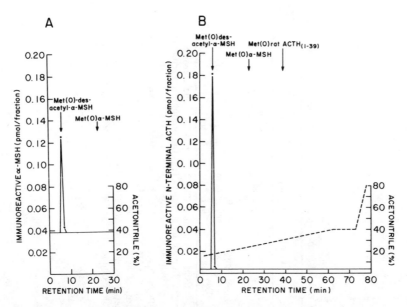

FIGURE 4. Characterization of the α-MSH and the N-terminal ACTH activity in a testicular extract by RP-HPLC. An aliquot of a testicular extract was oxidized and chromatographed. The elution positions of synthetic peptide standards are indicated by the arrows. The horizontal line parallel to the abcissa in each panel indicates the sensitivity of the RIAs. Note there were no immunoreactive peptides with the mobility of ACTH(1–39) or α-MSH. Immunoreactive α-MSH-like material eluted with the same retention time as *des*-acetyl α-MSH. (From Magioris *et al.*[21] With permission from *Endocrinology*.)

TABLE 1. Peptide Content (pmol per organ) and Concentrations (pmol g^{-1} wet weight)

Tissue	Wet Wt.[a]	Immunoreactive β-Endorphin[b]		Immunoreactive ACTH[c]		Immunoreactive α-MSH	
		Content	Conc.	Content	Conc.	Content	Conc.
Hypothalamus	25 mg	3.2 ± 0.6	126 ± 11			3.8 ± 0.3	153 ± 12
Whole Brain	1.5 g	27.0 ± 3.3	18 ± 2.2			21.0 ± 5.1	14 ± 3.4
Pituitary							
Pars distalis	8 mg	204.0 ± 17	25,500 ± 2,175	196 ± 18	24,500 ± 2,250		
Pars intermedia	1 mg	467.0 ± 32	467,000 ± 32,000			398.0 ± 49	398,000 ± 49,000
Testes	2.2 g	0.4 ± 0.3	0.18 ± 0.03			0.72 ± 0.09	0.33 ± 0.08

[a] Average weight, all tissues from male 200–250 g rats (Sprague-Dawley).

[b] Includes β-lipotropin. In pars distalis, β-LPH is the predominant immunoreactive β-Ep-related peptide; in all other tissues listed β-Ep-sized peptides predominate. The antibody employed does not cross-react with α- or γ-endorphin. In all tissues listed, except the testis, α-Ep and γ-Ep-related peptides (α-Ep, γ-Ep, and their des-Tyr^1 derivatives) are present at less than 10% (molar basis) the concentrations of immunoreactive β-Ep, and for the sake of simplicity are not listed. However, in testicular tissue extracts (see text), α-Ep plus γ-Ep-sized peptides are present at about the same molar concentrations as β-Ep.

[c] In all tissues except pars distalis, ACTH(1–39)-sized peptides are minor species and are not cited. In ventral hypothalamus such peptides are present at approximately one fourth the molar concentration of immunoreactive α-MSH.

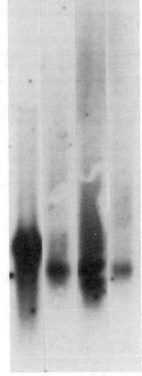

FIGURE 5. Northern blot analysis of polyA mRNA isolated from neurointermediate pituitary (lane 1); the TM$_3$ Leydig cell line (lane 2); testis (lane 3); epididymis (lane 4).

1 2 3 4

then identified using a 550 base-pair rat POMC cDNA probe that had been labeled with ^{32}P.[24] The results of this study demonstrated that POMC-like messenger RNA was present in pituitary, testis, TM$_3$ (Leydig) cells, and epididymis (FIGURE 5) but not in liver (not shown). The size of the POMC-like mRNA is similar in testis, TM$_3$ cells, and epididymis (FIGURE 5) but approximately 150 base pairs shorter than that in pituitary. A similar short POMC-like mRNA has also been demonstrated in portions of the brain other than the hypothalamus, especially the amygdaloid nucleus.[25,26] To determine whether mRNAs from this portion of the brain and testis were of similar size, RNAs from these two organs were compared with those of anterior or neurointermediate pituitary using Northern blot analysis as described above. Testicular POMC-like mRNA was found to be exactly the same size as that found in the amygdaloid nucleus (not shown).

POMC-like mRNA was also localized in rat testes with the technique of *in situ* hybridization.[11] Sections of rat testes were hybridized overnight with [^{3}H]cDNA, coated with emulsion, and exposed for six weeks. After development, silver grains were localized in the cytoplasm of most Leydig cells. There were very few grains over the cells in the seminiferous tubule. These *in situ* studies, as well as those noted above in which Northern blotting was used on poly A RNA from testes and Leydig cell lines, indicate that POMC-like mRNA is present in Leydig cells and suggest that POMC-related peptides may be synthesized in this portion of the testis.

The relative abundance of POMC-like mRNA in the testis and hypothalamus was next compared using dot blot analysis. Total RNA was spotted on nitrocellulose paper and analyzed with the ^{32}P labeled cDNA probe as described above. The results of this study are shown in FIGURE 6. The apparent concentrations of POMC mRNA in hypothalamus and testis were almost identical. Similar results were obtained when this study was repeated using poly A RNA prepared from these two sites (not shown). The finding of comparable amounts of mRNA in testis and in brain was unexpected in view of the fact that the concentration of POMC-derived peptides in the testis is approximately two orders of magnitude less than in whole brain and three orders of magnitude less than in hypothalamus (TABLE 1). The reasons for the apparent discrepancy between the relative amounts of POMC mRNA and peptides in these tissues will require further study.

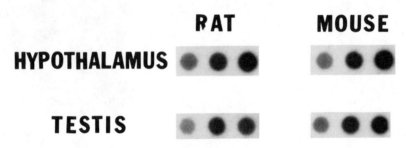

FIGURE 6. Dot-blot analysis of total RNA extracts from rat and mouse hypothalamus and testis. Five, 10, and 20 μg of each RNA preparation were analyzed.

THE ONTOGENY OF POMC-DERIVED PEPTIDES IN LEYDIG CELLS

In view of the immunocytochemical demonstration of multiple POMC antigenic domains in adult Leydig cells, it was of interest to determine whether immunostainable peptides could be demonstrated during fetal and neonatal life when Leydig cell activity is continuously changing.[20] In the fetal mouse, immunoreactive β-endorphin–like material was detected only in a few primitive Leydig cells on day 14 of gestation, the day after testicular differentiation. By day 16, immunostainable material was clearly present in Leydig cells throughout the developing testis (FIGURE 7a). The intensity of staining and the number of staining cells progressively increased throughout fetal life so at the time of birth the immunopositive cells comprised 55% of all interstitial cells (FIGURE 8). This number declined immediately after birth so that staining cells represented only 12% of Leydig cells by 5 days of age. After 10 days of age the number of cells that stained positively with anti–β-endorphin antisera began to increase so that by 40 days of age the number and intensity of staining Leydig cells were comparable to that noted in adult mice (FIGURE 8). Similar findings were observed in studies performed on hamster testis obtained from fetal, neonatal, and pubertal animals.

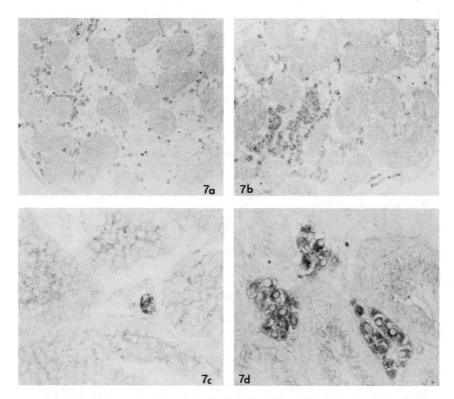

FIGURE 7. Immunoreactive β-endorphin in Leydig cells of mouse testis. (a) Early and (b) late fetal testes (16 and 18 days, respectively); (c) Testis from a 15-day-old mouse that had been treated with saline for 5 days; (d) Testis (comparable to 7c) from a 15-day-old animal that had received hCG for 5 days (× 200).

FIGURE 8. Percentage of interstitial cells that show immunostainable β-endorphin in sections of testis as a function of age and hCG treatment. The dotted line indicates the percentage of immunoreactive cells following 5 days of hCG treatment prior to the age of study. (From Shaha *et al.*[39] With permission from *Endocrinology*.)

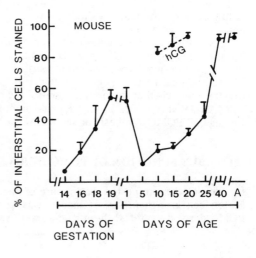

Studies were also performed utilizing an antiserum to γ_3-MSH. With this antiserum similar age-related changes in immunostainable material in Leydig cells was observed as with that against β-endorphin.[20] This is consistent with the post-translational derivation of these peptides from a common precursor. Taken together, these results in mice and hamster suggest that the number and intensity of immunostainable Leydig cells are developmentally regulated, with peaks at birth and after puberty. This time course correlates closely with the acquisition and loss of Leydig cell enzymes required for energy metabolism and steroid synthesis. The amount and intensity of immunoreactive β-endorphin and γ_3-MSH–like material in Leydig cells are also coincident with the morphological differentiation of Leydig cells that is associated with testosterone secretion.

FACTORS REGULATING TESTICULAR POMC-DERIVED PEPTIDES

The fact that immunostainable β-endorphin and other POMC-related peptides in Leydig cells appeared to increase during periods of testosterone synthesis in fetal life and again in puberty suggested that the expression of these peptides might be dependent upon gonadotropin secretion. This possibility was confirmed by the demonstration that there was an increase in the number of cells displaying immunostainable material in neonatal mice following 5 days of hCG treatment.[20] In this experiment hCG treatment was initiated in three groups of mice at 5, 10, and 15 days of age. This treatment resulted in an increase in the percentage of stainable Leydig cells that rose from 20 to 84%, 21 to 87%, and 30 to 93% by 10, 15, or 20 days of age, respectively, (FIGURES 7(c and d) and 8).

Studies were also performed in hypophysectomized rats.[19] Immunostainable β-endorphin and ACTH-like material were still present in Leydig cells 12 days following removal of the pituitary. When acid extracts of testis were prepared from hypophysectomized animals and assayed for POMC-derived peptides, the concentration of such peptides were comparable to those in intact animals. However, the testes of these animals had decreased in size by approximately 50%. As a consequence, the total content of POMC-derived peptides decreased in parallel with testicular weight. Since Leydig cells make up a relatively small portion of the testis and since the dominant loss of weight occurs in the seminiferous tubules following hypophysectomy, this represents a significant decline in Leydig cell immunoreactive material.

Taken together, the studies on the ontogeny of immunostainable POMC-peptides, the response to hCG treatment, and the decline in total immunoassayable peptides following hypophysectomy suggest that the content of Leydig cell POMC and its derivative peptides is under the control of LH. It will be of interest to determine whether factors that control the synthesis and secretion of POMC and its related peptides in anterior and intermediate pituitary lobe also affect Leydig cell POMC synthesis or secretion.

POSSIBLE FUNCTION OF POMC-DERIVED PEPTIDES IN THE TESTIS

In 1980, Mather[27] reported that impure extracts of ACTH increased the rate of Sertoli cell growth *in vitro*. Once it was known that Leydig cells contained POMC-derived peptides, these studies were repeated using synthetic ACTH(1–

24). This peptide also stimulated Sertoli cell growth, eliminating the possibility that trace contaminants in the ACTH of the original study were responsible for the increased cell number.[28] Following these studies, a comprehensive examination of the effect of POMC-derived peptides on primary Sertoli cells and two Sertoli cell lines (TM_4; TRST) was conducted. In a series of experiments, it was shown that ACTH, β-MSH, α-MSH, and *des*-acetyl α-MSH stimulated cyclic-AMP accumulation in Sertoli cells. Representative experiments, shown in TABLE 2, compare the actions of ACTH and β-MSH with those of FSH and isoproterenol on the accumulation of [^{3}H]cAMP in primary Sertoli cells and in two cell lines. The effects of these POMC-derived peptides on Sertoli cell cyclic AMP accumulation were always considerably less than seen with either FSH and isoproterenol (TABLE 2). The action of the peptides, like that of FSH and isoproterenol, was potentiated by forskolin. In the experiment shown in FIGURE 9, forskolin in-

TABLE 2. Stimulation of Adenylate Cyclase by POMC-derived Peptides in Primary Cultures and a Cell Line

Peptide	Concentration	% Conversion	p
Primary Sertoli culture (20 day animals)			
NS control	—	0.07 ± 0.01	—
β-MSH	5.0 μg/ml	0.13 ± 0.01	< 0.025
ACTH(1–24)	0.1 IU/ml	0.08 ± 0.0	> .01
ACTH(1–24)	1.0 IU/ml	0.10 ± 0.01	< .05
ACTH(1–24)	5.0 IU/ml	0.11 ± 0.01	< .025
FSH (NIH S-14)	2.0 μg/ml	0.88 ± 0.1	< .001
TM_4 (clone 1689) cell line			
NS control	—	0.04 ± 0.01	—
ACTH	0.1 IU/ml	0.08 ± 0.01	< .01
Isoproterenol	1.0 μM	2.41 ± 0.29	< .001

Cyclic AMP was determined as amount of [^{3}H]cAMP converted from [^{3}H]adenine. Monolayer cultures were prelabeled with [^{3}H]adenine for 2 hours. Medium was removed and incubation with or without (NS) hormones was carried out for 20 min. The reaction was terminated and [^{3}H]cAMP extracted and purified as previously described.[40] Results are expressed as percentage of cell-associated [^{3}H]adenine converted to [^{3}H]cAMP. Primary Sertoli cultures were prepared from 20-day-old rats and used on day 4 of culture. Values shown are the mean ± SD of triplicate determinations.

creased the apparent potency of ACTH(1–24) for the stimulation of adenylate cyclase in primary Sertoli cell cultures. In this study ACTH was also shown to have a biphasic effect in the presence of forskolin. β-endorphin did not increase Sertoli cell number or stimulate adenylate cyclase activity in any experiment (not shown).

In view of the relatively modest effects of ACTH and the MSHs on Sertoli cells, we thought it pertinent to confirm the biological activity of these peptides on a melanoma cell line (M_2R) that is known to be responsive. It is of note that all four peptides with MSH activity (ACTH, α-MSH, *des*-acetyl α-MSH, and β-MSH) stimulated the melanoma cell line to the same extent at the dose tested (TABLE 3). These observations are of interest and may contrast with the observed effect of α-N-acetylation on the relative biological potency of ACTH(1–13) in stimulating skin darkening activity in frog skin. For example, selective α-N-acetyl-ation of the N-terminal serine residue in ACTH(1–13) increased its melanocyte-stimulating activity three orders of magnitude over that of the unacetylated pep-tide.[29] Although all of the peptides with MSH activity that are present in POMC have some effects on Sertoli cells, their relative biological activities have not been determined. As noted previously, fractionation of adult testes revealed that the unacetylated form of α-MSH (des-acetyl-α-MSH) was the predominant form.[21]

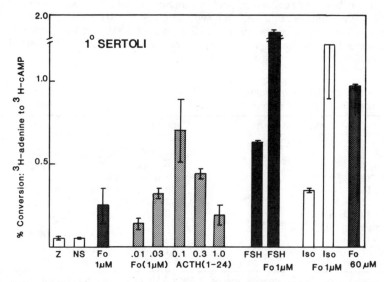

FIGURE 9. Effect of ACTH (U/ml), oFSH (1 μg/ml NIH 5–14), and isoproterenol (1 μM, Iso) with and without forskolin (Fo) on [³H]cyclic AMP formation from [³H]adenine in rat Sertoli cell primary cultures. The effect of suboptimal (1 μM) Fo is to amplify the response to hormones. Z=0 time control; NS=non-stimulated control. Following a 2-hour pre-incu-bation with [³H]adenine (5 μCi/ml), Sertoli cells were washed and further incubated with the various hormones for 20 minutes. Accumulation of [³H]cAMP in the intact cells was mea-sured according to the procedure of Salomon[40] and is expressed as a percent conversion of [³H]adenine into [³H]cAMP.

Since ACTH and the MSHs stimulated Sertoli cells, we wondered whether β-endorphin might be inhibitory in view of the opposing actions of POMC-derived peptides in other tissues (see below). To investigate this possibility we studied the effect of potent opiate antagonists on Sertoli cell function in intact animals at 5 days of age. In these experiments, nalmefene or naloxone[30] were injected intrates-ticularly in neonatal mice that were killed 5 days later (FIGURE 10). Both opiate antagonists increased the compensatory hypertrophy noted following unilateral castration. Treatment with the opiate antagonists was associated with a marked rise in the blood levels of immunoreactive rat androgen binding protein (rABP). At this age, most of the rABP synthesized by the Sertoli cells is secreted into the

TABLE 3. Relative Effectiveness of ACTH, αMSH, and *des*-ac-α-MSH in Stimulating Melanoma Adenyl Cyclase

Peptide	Concentration	[^{32}P]cAMP (pmol/min/mg protein)
Basal	—	143 ± 11
ACTH(1–24)	$1.0 \, \mu M$	500 ± 10
α-MSH	$1.0 \, \mu M$	490 ± 52
des-ac-α-MSH	$1.0 \, \mu M$	527 ± 30

Conversion of [^{32}P]ATP to [^{32}P]cAMP was measured in lysates of the M2R melanoma cell line as previously described.[40] Incubation with peptide was for 10 min. Values shown are the average and range of duplicate determinations.

blood since the blood-testis barrier is not intact.[31] The increase in testicular size and rABP secretion following antagonist administration is consistent with the hypothesis that β-endorphin or other opioids inhibit Sertoli cell growth and secretion during early testicular development and are at this time antagonistic to gonadotropins that stimulate Sertoli cells.[32,33]

Taken together, the results from the *in vitro* and *in vivo* experiments suggest that peptides derived from different portions of POMC may have differential effects on Sertoli cells. ACTH- and MSH-like peptides are stimulatory while β-endorphin is inhibitory. Opposing effects of POMC-derived peptides in other

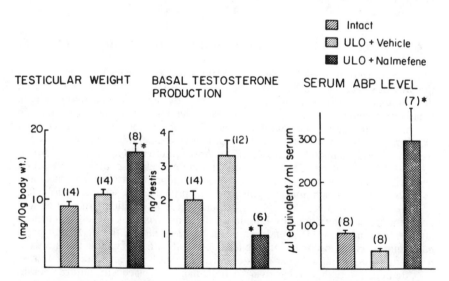

FIGURE 10. Effect of unilateral orchidectomy (ULO) on ABP secretion into blood, testosterone production, and testicular hypertrophy in neonatal animals plus the effect of intratesticular administration of the opiate antagonist, nalmefene, on the remaining testis. Nalmefene increased ABP secretion and compensatory hypertrophy following castration and decreased the basal testosterone secretion from the remaining testes. Animals were operated on and treated at 5 days of age, and killed at 11 days of age.

tissues have previously been reported. For example, ACTH-like peptides and β-endorphin have opposing effects on various types of behavior. This is in keeping with reports that these two types of compounds have opposite effects on the concentration of brain neurotransmitters and cAMP as well as on neuronal firing rates.[34] Furthermore, ACTH and some of its fragments have been reported to bind to opiate receptors,[35] and this peptide is reported to block opiate-induced analgesia in the rat.[36] It has been suggested, however, that such receptors are not specific with regard to opiates as they are naloxone insensitive.[37] Thus, the biological consequences of POMC synthesis in the testis are related not only to the amount of the precursor that is made but which of its component peptides are present in biologically active form.

The effect of opiate antagonist administration on Leydig cell function was also examined in neonatal animals. Results in Figure 10 indicate that nalmefene inhibited basal testosterone secretion from the remaining testes. Naloxone had a similar effect (not shown). In adult animals, in whom compensatory hypertrophy is not seen, intratesticular administration of opiate antagonist had no effect on testicular size and rABP secretion. Intratesticular administration of these agents, however, decreased serum testosterone levels, basal testosterone secretion *in vitro*, and the response of testes to hCG treatment *in vitro*. These effects of opiate antagonists on Leydig cell function were unexpected. They imply that opiates may either directly or indirectly facilitate testosterone secretion. Whether β-endorphin can have an autocrine effect on Leydig cell function or whether it acts by way of a Sertoli cell–produced or myoid cell–produced intermediate remains to be established.

POMC-DERIVED PEPTIDES IN OTHER STEROID SECRETING CELLS

The demonstration of POMC-derived peptides in Leydig cells[18-20] coupled with the previous observation that these agents were also present in placenta[4-6] raised the possibility that they might also be produced by the steroid-secreting cells of the ovary. Previous studies have demonstrated that immunostainable β-endorphin was present in corpora lutea of rat ovaries.[18] This observation was expanded in an experiment in which immunostainable POMC-derived peptides were examined in ovaries of fetal, neonatal, and adult mice. Antisera directed against β-endorphin and γ₃-MSH were used. Unlike the testis, no POMC-related peptides were found in ovaries from embryonic animals. In ovaries from prepubertal animals at 15 and 24 days of age, no staining was observed in primary and secondary follicles; however, weak immunostaining was present in the interstitium. In cycling and pregnant animals the dominant immunoreactive material was present in corpora lutea.[11] Immunoassayable β-endorphin was twice as high in the ovaries of pregnant animals as in those from intact mice consistent with the fact that ovaries from pregnant mice contain a larger mass of corpora lutea.[11] Recent studies of Lim *et al.*[38] demonstrated that ovine ovarian follicular cells placed in culture secrete POMC-derived peptides. The fact that these cells luteinize when placed in culture is consistent with the present observations on intact ovaries.

The fact that immunostainable β-endorphin–like activity in testis increased following hCG administration[20] suggested that a similar situation might exist in ovaries. Administration of hCG to immature animals led to a marked stimulation of immunostainable β-endorphin-like material in the ovarian interstitial area without an increase in follicles. By contrast, PMS administration markedly increased

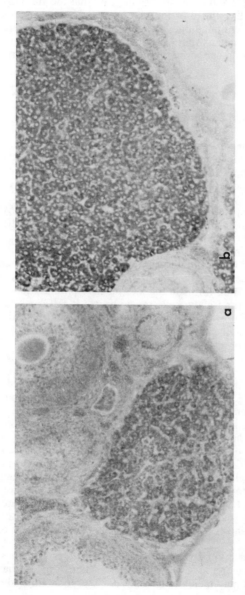

FIGURE 11. Immunoreactive β-endorphin–like material in mouse ovaries showing staining of corpora lutea. (a) Ovary from a normal mouse; (b) ovary from a pregnant mouse (× 100).

immunostainable β-endorphin in both the follicles and interstitium.[31] These findings suggest that the concentration of immunoreactive POMC-derived peptides in
ovary are regulated by gonadotropins.

The results of these and other studies indicate that the steroid-secreting cells
of testis and ovary, like those of the placenta, synthesize and secrete POMC-
derived peptides. Recent immunocytochemical studies of the adrenal cortex indicate that this tissue contains these peptides as well. There observations suggest
that all steroid-secreting endocrine tissues contain this peptide precursor.

SUMMARY AND CONCLUSIONS

(1) Using antibodies against peptides derived from different portions of the POMC
molecule, immunocytochemical evidence suggests that this precursor and/or the
peptides present within it are localized in testicular Leydig cells of at least five
species. There is no evidence for the localization of these peptides or their precursor in any other cell type in this organ.

(2) Examination of testicular extracts by gel filtration, SDS-PAGE, and RP-
HPLC indicate that the testis contains low concentrations of POMC-derived peptides relative to brain. Further analysis indicates that POMC is processed to α-
MSH and β-endorphin similar to its processing in intermediate pituitary lobe and
brain. The relative mobilities of immunoreactive α-MSH and β-endorphin on RP-
HPLC columns indicate that they are in the unacetylated state as in brain and in
contrast to the acetylated forms in the intermediate pituitary lobe.

(3) The potential for Leydig cells to synthesize POMC and its peptides was
suggested by the demonstration of POMC-like mRNA in total testis and Leydig
cell cultures. The size of the POMC-like mRNA is approximately 150 base pairs
shorter than anterior or intermediate pituitary POMC mRNA. POMC-like mRNA
activity has also been localized to Leydig cells in sections of testes using in situ
hybridization.

(4) Immunostainable β-endorphin and other POMC-derived peptides are
present in testicular Leydig cells during fetal life and following puberty at times
when testosterone secretion is maximal.

(5) The accumulation of immunostainable POMC-derived peptides in Leydig
cells is dramatically increased by LH and hCG.

(6) A variety of observations suggests that testicular cells can respond to
POMC-derived peptides. ACTH and the MSHs stimulate growth and cAMP accumulation in Sertoli cells. By contrast, studies using antagonists suggested that β-
endorphin and/or another testicular opioid inhibit Sertoli cell proliferation and
ABP secretion. These observations are consistent with the postulate that different
portions of the POMC molecule may have opposite effects on Sertoli cell function
and suggest a mechanism by which Leydig cells could modulate Sertoli cell activity.

(7) Intratesticular administration of opiate antagonists inhibits testosterone
secretion both in vivo and in vitro. These observations suggest that Leydig cell–
derived β-endorphin may facilitate testosterone secretion either directly or indirectly.

(8) The finding of POMC and its derivative peptides in testis, ovary, adrenal,
and placenta suggests that all steroid hormone–secreting organs in mammals may
utilize this peptidergic system.

REFERENCES

1. KRIEGER, D. T., A. LIOTTA & M. J. BROWNSTEIN. 1977. Proc. Natl. Acad. Sci. USA **74:** 648–652.
2. LIOTTA, A. S., D. GILDERSLEEVE, M. J. BROWNSTEIN & D. T. KRIEGER. 1979. Proc. Natl. Acad. Sci. USA **76:** 1448–1452.
3. LIOTTA, A. S., C. LOUDES, J. F. MCKELVY & D. T. KRIEGER. 1980. Proc. Natl. Acad. Sci. USA **77:** 1880–1884.
4. LIOTTA, A., R. HOUGHTEN & D. T. KRIEGER. 1982. Nature **295:** 593–595.
5. LIOTTA, A. S. & D. T. KRIEGER. 1980. Endocrinology **106:** 1504–1511.
6. LIOTTA, A., R. OSATHANONDH, K. J. RYAN & D. T. KRIEGER. 1977. Endocrinology **101:** 1552–1558.
7. FEURLE, G. E., U. WEBER & V. HELMSTAEDTER. 1980. Biochem. Biophys. Res. Commun. **95:** 1656–1662.
8. LARSSON, L. 1981. Proc. Natl. Acad. Sci. USA **78:** 2990–2994.
9. ORWOLL, E. S. & J. W. KENDALL. 1980. Endocrinology **107:** 438–442.
10. KRIEGER, D. T., A. S. LIOTTA, M. J. BROWNSTEIN & E. A. ZIMMERMAN. 1980. Rec. Prog. Horm. Res. **36:** 272–344.
11. KRIEGER, D. T., A. N. MARGIORIS, A. S. LIOTTA, C. SHAHA, I. GERENDAI, J. PINTAR & C. W. BARDIN. 1984. Proceedings of the First International Meeting of the Italian Society of Endocrinology. Raven Press. New York.
12. O'DONOHUE, T. L., C. G. CHARLTON, M. B. THOA, C. HELKE, T. W. MOODY, A. PERA, A. WILLIAMS, R. L. MILLER & D. M. JACOBOWITZ. 1981. Peptides **2:** 93–100.
13. ZAKARIAN, S. & D. G. SMYTH. 1982. Nature **296:** 250–252.
14. EVANS, C. J., R. LORENZ, E. WEBER & J. D. BARCHAS. 1982. Biochem. Biophys. Res. Commun. **106:** 910–919.
15. WEBER, E., C. J. EVANS & J. D. BARCHAS. 1981. Biochem. Biophys. Res. Commun. **103:** 982–989.
16. SHARP, B. A. & A. E. PEKARY. 1981. J. Clin. Endocrinol. Metab. **52:** 586–588.
17. SHARP, B., A. PEKARY, N. V. MEYER & J. M. HERSHMAN. 1980. Biochem. Biophys. Res. Commun. **95:** 618–623.
18. TSONG, S. D., D. PHILLIPS, N. HALMI, D. T. KRIEGER & C. W. BARDIN. 1982. Biol. Reprod. **27:** 755–764.
19. TSONG, S. D., D. PHILLIPS, N. HALMI, A. S. LIOTTA, A. MARGIORIS, C. W. BARDIN & D. T. KRIEGER. 1982. Endocrinology **110:** 2204–2206.
20. SHAHA, C., A. S. LIOTTA, D. T. KRIEGER & C. W. BARDIN. 1983. Endocrinology. (In press.)
21. MARGIORIS, A. N., A. S. LIOTTA, H. VAUDRY, C. W. BARDIN & D. T. KRIEGER. 1983. Endocrinology **113:** 663–671.
22. AUFFRAY, C. & F. FOUGEON. 1980. Eur. J. Biochem. **107:** 303–314.
23. AVIV, H. & P. LEDER. 1975. Proc. Natl. Acad. Sci. USA **71:** 1408–1412.
24. CHEN, C. L. C., F. T. DIONNE & J. L. ROBERTS. 1982. Proc. Natl. Acad. Sci. USA **80:** 2211–2215.
25. CIVELLI, O., N. BIRNBERG & E. HERBERT. 1982. J. Biol. Chem. **257:** 6783–6787.
26. EVINGER, M. J. Q., J. L. ROBERTS, C. L. C. CHEN & B. S. SCHACHTER. 1983. *In* Gene Expression in Brain. C. Zomzely-Neurath & W. A. Walker, Eds. (In press.)
27. MATHER, J. P. 1980. Biol. Reprod. **23:** 243–252.
28. MATHER, J. P., Y. S. SALOMON, A. S. LIOTTA, A. MARGIORIS, C. W. BARDIN & D. T. KRIEGER. 1982. β-Endorphin and ACTH: Localization of Action in the Testis. European Workshop on the Testis.
29. HOFMANN, K. 1974. The pituitary gland. *In* Endocrinology Section 7, Vol. IV. (part 2) E. Knobil & W. H. Sawyer, Eds.: 29–58. American Physiological Society. Washington, D.C.
30. GERENDAI, I., A. NEMESKERI & V. CSEVRUS. 1983. Andrologia **15:** 398–403.
31. GUNSALUS, G. L., N. A. MUSTO & C. W. BARDIN. 1980. *In* Testicular Development, Structure and Function. A. Steinberger & E. Steinberger, Eds.: 291–297. Raven Press. New York.

32. VOGEL, D., G. L. GUNSALUS, B. B. BERON, N. A. MUSTO & C. W. BARDIN. 1983. Endocrinology **112:** 1115–1121.
33. GUNSALUS, G. L., S. CARREAU, D. L. VOGEL, N. A. MUSTO & C. W. BARDIN. 1984. *In* Sexual Differentiation, Basic and Clinical Aspects. M. Serio, M. Molta, M. Zanisi & L. Martini, Eds.: 53–64. Raven Press. New York.
34. KRIEGER, D. T. 1983. Science **22:** 975–985.
35. TERENIUS, L. 1973. J. Pharm. Pharmacol. **27:** 450–452.
36. SMOCK, T. & H. L. FIELDS. 1981. Brain Res. **212:** 202–206.
37. JACQUET, Y., 1978. *In* Characteristics and Function of Opioids. J. Van Ree & L. Terenius, Eds.:429. Elsevier/North Holland. Amsterdam.
38. LIM, A. T., S. LOOLAIT, J. W. BARLOW, S. O. WAI, I. ZOIS, B. H. TOH & J. W. FUNDER. 1983. Nature **303:** 709–711.
39. SHAHA, C., A. MARGIORIS, A. LIOTTA, D. T. KRIEGER & C. W. BARDIN. 1984. Endocrinology **115:** 378–384.
40. SALOMON, Y. 1979. Adenylate cyclase activity. *In* Advances in Cyclic Nucleotide Research. G. Brooker, P. Greengard & G. A. Robison, Eds.:35–55. Raven Press. New York.

Beta-endorphin, Met-enkephalin, and Calcitonin in Human Semen: Evidence for a Possible Role in Human Sperm Motility

FRANCO FRAIOLI, ANDREA FABBRI, LUCIO GNESSI,
LEOPOLDO SILVESTRONI, COSTANZO MORETTI,
FRANCESCO REDI, and ALDO ISIDORI

V Clinica Medica
Policlinico Umberto I
University of Rome
Rome, Italy

INTRODUCTION

It has recently been demonstrated that a large number of different peptides are present in the testis of several animal species.

In particular, immunoreactive β-endorphin was detected in human semen and rat testicular extracts[1,2] and subsequently localized together with ACTH-like material in the cytoplasm of rat Leydig cells, the epithelia of epididymis, seminal vesicles, and the vas deferens,[3] as well as in the Leydig cells of mouse, hamster, guinea pig, and rabbit.[4]

Moreover high levels of immunoreactive met-enkephalin, leucine enkephalin, β-endorphin, substance P,[5] and calcitonin[6] were found in human spermatozoa and seminal plasma. Immunohistochemical evidence of methionine and leucine enkephalin in nerve fibers related to smooth muscle was also shown for human prostate and seminal vescicles.[7]

These findings suggest that all these peptides may have important regulatory functions in the male reproductive system and the existence of opiate receptors in the mouse vas deferens[8] and calcitonin receptors in rat Leydig cells[9] strengthens this hypothesis. Moreover, the fact that mammalian spermatozoa contain high levels of calmodulin,[10] an intracellular calcium binding protein involved in the mechanisms of sperm motility,[11] coupled with the notion that β-endorphin and calcitonin are potent anticalmodulin drugs,[12–15] indicates a possible action of these substances at sperm level.

In the present study we evaluated the levels of β-endorphin, met-enkephalin, and calcitonin in human semen by radioimmunoassay (RIA), and tested the effects of these peptides on the motility of human spermatozoa.

MATERIALS AND METHODS

Extraction of Peptides from Seminal Fluid

Human semen was obtained by masturbation in eight healthy volunteers, aged between 25 and 35 years, and was processed according to Sharp and Pekary[1] with slight modifications. Briefly, after the semen was combined with an equal volume of 0.5 M acetic acid, boiled for 15 min, and centrifuged at 1,000 rpm for 10 min, the supernatant was separated, adjusted with 1% formic acid, and loaded on octadodecasilyl silica columns (Sep-Pak, Waters Associate, Milford, MA) primed with formic acid, 80% methanol and peptone, and eluted with 5 ml of 90% methanol in formic acid. In a preliminary experiment iodinated β-endorphin, met-enkephalin, and calcitonin, and 5 and 1 ml aliquots of dialysate (free seminal fluid), were loaded on the Sep-Pak cartridges in order to evaluate the respective extraction yields of the three peptides during Sep-Pak extraction.

The methanol eluate was dried under vacuum at 37°C overnight, thereafter the dry residue was reconstituted in distilled water and centrifuged. The clear supernatant was then assayed by RIA.

The overall experimental recovery of ^{125}I-labeled β-endorphin, met-enkephalin, and calcitonin ranged, respectively, from 70–75%, 90–95%, and 65–70%.

RIA for β-Endorphin, Met-Enkephalin, and Calcitonin

The RIA for β-endorphin, met-enkephalin, and calcitonin was carried out using commercial kits supplied, respectively, by the New England Nuclear, Boston, MA, the Immuno Nuclear Co., StillWater, MN, and Byk-Mallinckrodt, Dietzenbach-Steinberg, West Germany.

The antibody for each peptide had 100% cross reactivity with its corresponding antigen peptide and negligible cross-reactivity with other peptides except the antibody for β-endorphin that had 50% cross-reactivity with β-lipotropin.

Intra- and inter-assay coefficient of variation were 7–10% for β-endorphin, 6–8% for met-enkephalin, and 5–9% for calcitonin.

Evaluation of Sperm Motility

Euspermic semen samples were obtained by masturbation following a 4-day period of sexual abstinence. After a standard analysis, the specimen was separated into 0.5 ml aliquots and transferred to plastic sterile tubes. Calcium-free PBS (0.5 ml), 0.03 M, pH 7.6, was carefully layered on the seminal fractions and the preparations were incubated in a vertical position at room temperature for 30–40 min. At the end of incubation time, the buffer phases containing migrated spermatozoa were gently aspirated, pooled, and maintained at room temperature. Aliquots of migrated spermatozoa were thereafter challenged with concentrations ranging from 4×10^{-5} to 4×10^{-10} M of β-endorphin, met-enkephalin, and salmon calcitonin (Bachem) or with buffer alone and subsequently incubated for 5 min prior to measurement of motility. Sperm motility was assessed by a microstrobophotographic method.[16] This type of examination allows the experimenter to record and analyze both the percentage and quality of cell motility. In some experiments naloxone (Sigma), an opiate antagonist, was added to PBS and β-endorphin at the end of the incubation period and sperm motility was assessed after 5 min.

Statistical Analysis

Data were assessed using Student's t-test.

TABLE 1. Immunoreactive β-Endorphin, Met-enkephalin, and Calcitonin Levels in Peripheral Plasma and Seminal Fluid in 8 Normal Subjects (mean ± SE).

	Peripheral Plasma[a]	Seminal Fluid
β-Endorphin (fmol/ml)	2.8 ± 0.4	12.9 ± 1.2[b]
Met-enkephalin (fmol/ml)	41.3 ± 3.8	139.2 ± 8.0[b]
Calcitonin (fmol/ml)	4.5 ± 0.6	14.6 ± 1.0[b]

[a] Blood samples of the subjects were collected and extracted through Sep-Pak cartridges as previously described.[19]
[b] $p < 0.001$.

RESULTS

TABLE 1 shows the levels of immunoreactive β-endorphin, met-enkephalin, and calcitonin present in the seminal fluid of the subjects studied. Detectable amounts of the three peptides were found with levels higher than those found in peripheral plasma (1:3–4.6 ratio).

FIGURE 1 shows the effect of β-endorphin, met-enkephalin, and salmon calcitonin on sperm motility. Met-enkephalin had no effect upon the motility of spermatozoa also at the higher concentration used (4×10^{-5} M) β-endorphin had no effect on motility at concentrations below 10^{-7} M; as the concentration increased

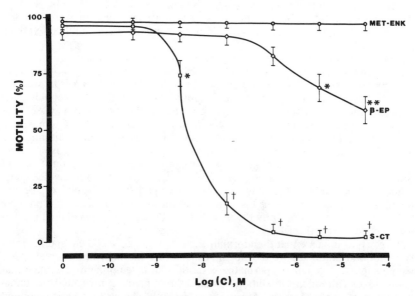

FIGURE 1. Effect of various concentrations of β-endorphin, met-enkephalin, and salmon calcitonin on sperm motility. The cells were incubated with the peptides for 5 min at room temperature prior to measurement of motility. Each point represents the mean ± SE of four determinations, each in triplicate. * = $p < 0.05$; ** = $p < 0.01$; † = $p < 0.001$.

from 4×10^{-7} to 4×10^{-5} M there was a significant rise in the percentage of immotile cells and in cells showing asymmetric beating of the flagella and modification of the waveform. Concentrations of salmon calcitonin ranging from 10^{-9} to 10^{-7} M induced a rapid curling of the sperm tails with complete immobilization of the cells at the latter concentration. Naloxone (10^{-3} M) added to the incubation media did not reverse the inhibition of sperm motility by 4×10^{-6} M β-endorphin (data not shown).

DISCUSSION

Our results, in agreement with other reports,[1,5,6] indicate that human semen contains large amounts of immunoreactive β-endorphin, met-enkephalin, and calcitonin. Furthermore in the present study we show that calcitonin and β-endorphin may act as sperm motility inhibitors.

The seminal levels of β-endorphin, met-enkephalin, and calcitonin were not related to the plasma levels of the substances, suggesting that the male reproductive tract could be an additional source for these peptides. In this line is the observation that in rats hypophysectomy does not induce any change in testicular immunoreactive β-endorphin–sized material,[17] and does not alter the intensity of the immunocytochemical staining localized in the cytoplasm of the Leydig cells.[3]

The finding that rat testis, prostate, and seminal vesicles contain β-endorphin–like material[2,3,5,17] and that human spermatozoa homogenates are particularly rich in β-endorphin immunoreactivity,[5] indicates that these structures are possible production sites of the peptides.

Now, even if in this regard no evidence to date exists for calcitonin, the high blood to seminal fluid ratio observed (1:3.5) kindles the idea that also for this substance a local production in the male reproductive system could be hypothesized.

However, considering the heterogeneity of β-endorphin immunoreactivity in human semen,[1] contrary to rat testicular extracts where the major form of β-endorphin present appears to be β-endorphin (1–31),[17] further work is in progress in our laboratory to separate and better identify β-endorphin, met-enkephalin, and calcitonin immunoreactivity by high pressure liquid chromatography.

What is the physiological meaning for the presence of these peptides in human semen? Paracrine actions on testicular cells can be suggested for calcitonin, as a dose-dependent testosterone production has been demonstrated by isolated rat Leydig cells challenged with salmon calcitonin *in vitro*.[18] In addition it is well established that the vas deferens contains opiate receptors[8] and it has been suggested that opioid peptides may antagonize sympathetic activation of the vas deferens and blood vessels in the penis after an orgasm.[5] Moreover a possible regulation of sperm motility by opioid peptides through a Ca^{2+}-mediated mechanism has been hypothesized.[5]

Our results indicate that β-endorphin and calcitonin act as potent sperm motility inhibitors. Although we did not investigate the mechanism by which these peptides inhibit the human spermatozoa motility, it is tempting to speculate that this involves calmodulin inhibition. Calmodulin is highly represented in human spermatozoa[10] and Tash and Means have recently shown that anticalmodulin drugs are potent sperm motility inhibitors.[11] β-Endorphin has been known to bind specifically to calmodulin[12] and to inhibit the calmodulin activation of phosphodiesterase through a non naloxone-reversible mechanism, while it has been established that met-enkephalin does not interfere with the action of calmodulin.[13] In addition, we previously showed that salmon calcitonin is a very potent antical-modulin peptide with a potency two orders of magnitude higher than β-endorphin (10^{-7} M versus 10^{-5} M maximal inhibition).[15]

Our finding of the failure of met-enkephalin to inhibit sperm motility and of naloxone to reverse the β-endorphin inhibition (data not shown) are consistent with the hypothesis of a calmodulin involvement in the action of this peptide. Interestingly, the ratio of salmon calcitonin versus β-endorphin potencies in inhib-iting sperm motility is similar to the relative potencies of the two compounds in inhibiting the calmodulin-mediated phosphodiesterase activation,[15] also suggest-ing for the former peptide a calmodulin interaction at the sperm level.

In conclusion, high levels of immunoreactive β-endorphin, met-enkephalin, and calcitonin are present in human semen and at least for β-endorphin and calcitonin a possible regulatory role in the motility of human spermatozoa can be suggested.

REFERENCES

1. SHARP, B. A. & A. E. PEKARY. 1981. Endorphin$_{61-91}$ and other β-endorphin-immuno-reactive peptides in human semen J. Clin. Endocrinol. Metab. **52:** 586.
2. SHARP, B., A. PEKARY, N. V. MEYER & J. M. HERSHMAN. 1980. β-Endorphin in male rat reproductive organs. Biochem. Biophys. Res. Commun. **95:** 618.
3. TSONG, S. D., D. PHILLIPS, N. HALMI, A. S. LIOTTA, A. MARGIORIS, C. W. BARDIN & D. T. KRIEGER. 1982. ACTH and β-endorphin-related peptides are present in multi-ple sites in reproductive tract of the male rat. Endocrinology **110:** 2204.
4. TSONG, S. D., D. M. PHILLIPS, N. HALMI, D. T. KRIEGER & C. W. BARDIN. 1982. β-Endorphin is present in male reproductive tract of five species. Biol. Reprod. **27:** 759.
5. RAMA SASTRY, B. V., V. E. JANSON, L. K. OWENS & O. S. TAYEB. 1982. Enkephalin and substance P-like immunoreactivities of mammalian sperm and accessory sex glands. Biochem. Pharmacol. **31:** 3519.
6. ARVER, S., H. E. SJOBERG & E. BUCHT. 1980. Calcitonin, calcium fractions and electrolytes in human semen and breast milk. *In* Calcitonin 1980. A. Pecile, Ed. Suppl. 14, abstract no. 24. University of Milan. Milan.
7. VAALOSTI, A., I. LINNOILA & A. HERRONEN. 1980. Immunohistochemical demonstra-tion of VIP, Met^5- and Leu^5-enkephalin immunoreactive nerve fibers in the human prostate and seminal vesicles. Histochemistry **66:** 89.
8. HUGHES, J., H. W. KOSTERLITZ & F. M. LESLIE. 1975. Effect of morphine on adrener-gic transmission in the mouse vas deferens. Assessment of agonist and antagonist potencies of narcotic analgesics. Br. J. Pharmacol. **53:** 371.
9. CHAUSMER, A. B., M. D. STEVENS & C. SEVERN. 1982. Autoradiographic evidence for a calcitonin receptor on testicular Leydig cells. Science **216:** 735.
10. JONES, H. P., R. W. LENZ, B. A. PALEVITZ & M. J. CORMIER. 1980. Calmodulin localization in mammalian spermatozoa. Proc. Natl. Acad. Sci. USA **77:** 2772.
11. TASH, J. S. & A. R. MEANS. 1982. Regulation of protein phosphorylation and motility of sperm by cyclic adenosine monophosphate and calcium. Biol. Reprod. **26:** 745.
12. MALENCIK, D. A. & S. R. ANDERSON. 1982. Binding of simple peptides, hormones, and neurotransmitters by calmodulin. Biochemistry **21:** 3480.
13. SELLINGER-BARNETTE, M. & B. WEISS. 1982. Interaction of β-endorphin and other opioid peptides with calmodulin. Mol. Pharmacol. **21:** 86.
14. GNESSI, L., A. FABBRI, C. MORETTI, V. BONIFACIO, V. POLITI, G. CAMILLONI, G. DE LUCA, G. DI STAZIO & F. FRAIOLO. 1983. Interaction between calcitonin and calmo-dulin. J. Endocrinol. Invest. **6**(suppl. 1):157.

15. GNESSI, L., G. CAMILLONI, A. FABBRI, V. POLITI, G. DE LUCA, G. DI STAZIO, C. MORETTI & F. FRAIOLI. 1984. In vitro interaction between calcitonin and calmodulin. Biochem. Biophys. Res. Commun. **11:** 648.
16. MAKLER, A. 1978. A new multiple exposure photography method for objective human spermatozoal motility determination. Fertil. Steril. **30:** 192.
17. MARGIORIS, A. N., A. S. LIOTTA, H. VAUDRY, C. W. BARDIN & D. T. KRIEGER. 1983. Characterization of immunoreactive proopiomelanocortin-related peptides in rat testes. Endocrinology **113:** 663.
18. NAKHLA, A. N. & J. P. MATHER. 1983. Calcitonin stimulates cAMP production and alters androgen and estrogen receptor levels in both Leydig and Sertoli cells. Proc. 65th Annual Meeting of the Endocrine Society. San Antonio, June 8–10, abst. No. 106.
19. PANERAI, A. E., A. MARTINI, A. M. DI GIULIO, F. FRAIOLI, C. VEGNI, G. PARDI, A. MARINI & P. MANTEGAZZA. 1983. Plasma β-endorphin, β-lipotropin, and met-enkephalin concentrations during pregnancy in normal and drug addicted women and their newborn. J. Clin. Endocrinol. Metab. **57:** 537.

Studies on the Identification of a LHRH-like Peptide in the Rat Testis

M. P. HEDGER, D. M. ROBERTSON, C. A. BROWNE, and
D. M. DE KRETSER[a]

Departments of Anatomy and Physiology
Monash University
Melbourne, Victoria, Australia

INTRODUCTION

The existence of a LHRH-like peptide in the testis has been adduced in recent years from several lines of evidence. First, the development of agonists of LHRH with increased stability and receptor affinity led to the identification of specific high affinity LHRH receptors on the Leydig cells of the rat testis by several groups of investigators.[1-5] This finding raised the possibility that these receptors exist to detect and thereby modulate direct testicular actions of a LHRH-like peptide.

Secondly, the possibility that a LHRH-like peptide exerted a direct action on the testis was raised by the anti-fertility effects of LHRH agonists on testicular function since they inhibited both spermatogenesis and testosterone production.[6-9] Subsequently, a number of investigators demonstrated inhibitory effects of LHRH agonists on the testis of hypophysectomized rats, thereby confirming that the actions were most likely mediated by the LHRH receptors in the testis.[10,11] Thirdly, the failure of numerous studies to identify significant circulating levels of LHRH in peripheral plasma led to the hypothesis of a testicular source of LHRH. This concept received considerable support from the studies of Sharpe and co-workers,[12] who detected the presence of a LHRH-like material in testicular extracts and interstitial fluid, using a LHRH radioreceptor assay employing rat Leydig cell membranes as a receptor source.[13] Furthermore, they were able to identify the presence of LHRH-like material in media from cultured Sertoli cells using a radioimmunoassay capable of detecting agonist but not native LHRH and suggested that these cells were the source of the material.[14] More recently other groups using different fractionation techniques have provided supportive evidence that a LHRH-like material exists in the testis but it is significant that all used radioimmunoassay procedures to detect the existence of this material.[15,16] The only study that provided evidence for a biologically active LHRH-like peptide was that of Sharpe and colleagues who used an *in vitro* bioassay based on the release of FSH and LH from pituitary halves.[13]

Our interest in this field was derived from our studies that provided evidence that the seminiferous tubules exerted an inhibitory influence on Leydig cell function.[17-20] These results led us to propose that the seminiferous tubules secreted an inhibitor of Leydig cell function, the levels of which were reduced in states of spermatogenic damage, leading to a hypertrophy and hyperresponsiveness of the

---

[a] Address all correspondence to: D. M. de Kretser, Department of Anatomy, Monash University, Clayton, Victoria 3168, Australia.

Leydig cells.[21,22] Sharpe's proposition[12] that a LHRH-like peptide may serve as an intragonadal regulator was therefore of considerable interest since our own data had shown that the function of the Sertoli cell, the purported source of this peptide, was impaired in spermatogenic damage.[17,19] Furthermore, the known effects of LHRH agonists on Leydig cell function were inhibitory and removal of such an inhibitor would be consistent with the hypertrophy seen in our studies. This paper outlines studies aimed at identifying LHRH or LHRH-like materials in the testis. During this work testicular LHRH-peptidase activity was identified, requiring us to modify our purification procedures for the putative LHRH-like substance.

INITIAL STUDIES TO IDENTIFY A TESTICULAR LHRH-LIKE PEPTIDE

In our early studies two methods of detecting LHRH-like activity were used, namely a LHRH radioreceptor assay and a radioimmunoassay utilizing an antiserum (R103) to the LHRH agonist [D-Ser(tBu)^6,desGlyNH$_2^{10}$]LHRH ethylamide (LHRH-A) with nondetectable cross-reactivity to LHRH, kindly provided by Richard Sharpe and Hamish Fraser. Utilizing these methods, LHRH-like activity was detected in testicular cytosols and acetic acid extracts of rat testes (FIGURE 1). Based on these studies it appeared that the rat testis contained 15–50 ng of LHRH-A equivalent activity. When the extract was chromatographed on Sephacryl S-200, the results indicated LHRH-like activity in the molecular weight range of 45,000–50,000, a surprising finding in view of the much lower molecular weight of LHRH (FIGURE 2).

In order to characterize the LHRH-like activity further we utilized an *in vitro* bioassay for LHRH employing pituitary cells in culture as described by Vale and

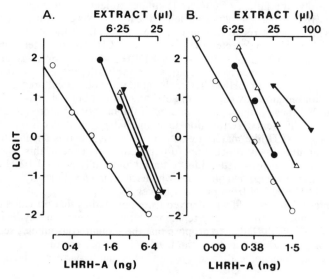

FIGURE 1. Logit-log dose-response curves of LHRH-A standard and testicular acetic acid extracts, as assessed by LHRH-A radioimmunoassay (A) and testicular interstitial cell receptor binding assay (B).

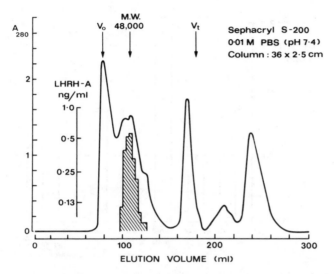

FIGURE 2. Fractionation by gel filtration of apparent LHRH-A immunoactivity in testicular cytosol.

colleagues.[23] Although bioactivity was consistently detected with the LHRH standard in the range of 0.1–35 ng/well, testicular cytosols or acetic acid extracts did not demonstrate bioactivity. In further attempts to delineate the reasons for this inability to demonstrate bioactivity we were able to show that fractions containing the high molecular weight LHRH-like activity, whether from testis cytosols or acetic acid extracts, could antagonize the activity of LHRH (FIGURE 3) and LHRH-A as assessed by *in vitro* bioassay or radioimmunoassay, suggesting the presence of peptidases that degraded LHRH. The presence of peptidase activity was confirmed by the fractionation on HPLC of the iodinated agonist LHRH-A after incubation with testicular cytosol (FIGURE 4).

CHARACTERIZATION OF TESTICULAR LHRH PEPTIDASE

In the majority of these studies LHRH-A was used as the enzyme substrate unless otherwise specified. Peptidase activity was assayed by incubating tissue fractions with LHRH or analogues for 0, 5, 10, and 20 min at 25°C (pH 7.4), conditions under which it had previously been established that degradation was linear in respect to time and tissue-extract concentration. The peptidase activity was stopped by boiling for 5 min prior to the determination of unreacted LHRH or analogue either by bioassay or radioimmunoassay.

Under these conditions, the peptidase activity degraded a number of analogues of LHRH to varying degrees (TABLE 1) but exhibited greatest activity against LHRH. The peptidase activity was inhibited by sulfhydryl-group blocking agents (*N*-ethylmaleimide, *p*-chloromercuriphenyl sulfonic acid, and *p*-chloromercuriphenyl benzoic acid), by the metal-chelating agents 1,10-phenanthroline and EDTA, and by the peptidase inhibitor bacitracin. Additionally a number of inhibitors of trypsin and chymotrypsin failed to inhibit this activity. These findings

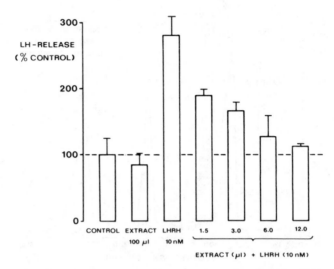

FIGURE 3. Inhibition of LHRH-stimulated LH release from anterior pituitary cells in culture by increasing concentrations of testicular cytosol. Columns and bars are mean ± SD.

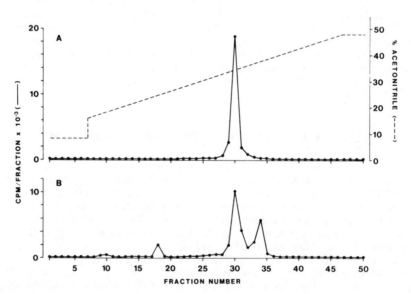

FIGURE 4. Profiles of radioactivity from reverse-phase HPLC of [^{125}I]LHRH-A before and after incubation with testicular cytosol. A: [^{125}I]LHRH-A = 29.4%; B: [^{125}I]LHRH-A incubated with testicular cytosol at 21°C for 2 hr. Note the multiple peaks following incubation with cytosol.

TABLE 1. Specificity of Testicular Peptidase Activity for LHRH and a Range of LHRH Agonists as Measured by *in Vitro* Bioassay (LH Release)[a]

LHRH or Analogue	*In Vitro* Biological Activity[b] (LH release)	Peptidase Activity[c]
[D-Ser(tBu)^6, des-GlyNH$_2^{10}$]LHRH ethylamide	91.9 ± 13.5	0.45 ± 0.17
[D-Leu^6, des-GlyNH$_2^{10}$]LHRH ethylamide	72.8 ± 8.1	0.31 ± 0.15
[D-Ala^6, des-GlyNH$_2^{10}$]LHRH ethylamide	15.5 ± 7.6	0.37 ± 0.15
[D-Lys^6]LHRH	4.6 ± 2.0	0.36 ± 0.14
LHRH	1.0	1.0

[a] Similar results were found for FSH release (data not shown). Initial assay concentration of all analogues was 100 nM.
[b] Mean ± S.E.M. ($N = 4$). Biological activity is expressed relative to LHRH.
[c] Mean ± S.E.M. ($N = 3$). Peptidase activity is expressed relative to LHRH.

indicate that the peptidase activity observed may be due to the presence of one or more proteases in the testicular extract.

Using collagenase-dispersed rat testicular preparations, peptidase activity was predominantly located in the seminiferous tubules (TABLE 2), with essentially undetectable activity in the Leydig cell fraction. However detectable levels of peptidase activity were found in interstitial fluid from the testis collected by the method of Sharpe.[24] It is of interest that the peptidase activity (in pmol/min/g tissue) was predominantly found in the hypothalamus (95.9), testis (seminiferous tubules and interstitial fluid, see TABLE 2), posterior pituitary (167.1), brain (147.9), and liver (411.0) and that the peptidase activity had similar properties to that found in the hypothalamus.[25,26] It has been argued that the hypothalamic peptidases may be biologically important[26,27] and this may also apply within the testis.

The demonstration of peptidase activity in the extracts used to identify the LHRH-like material in the testes raised the question as to whether the entire LHRH radioimmunoassay activity represented an artifact caused by progressive degradation of tracer by increasing quantities of extract. This possibility is of

TABLE 2. Peptidase Activity in Testicular Cytosols, Particulate Fractions, and Interstitial Fluid, Using LHRH-A as Substrate

Tissue	N	Peptidase Activity (pmol/min/mg protein)	(pmol/min/testis)
Cytosols			
Whole testis	11	9.2 ± 0.6[a]	278 ± 33[c]
Seminiferous tubules	10	5.1 ± 0.9[b]	108 ± 16[d]
Interstitial tissue	9	<0.2	<1.1
Particulate fractions			
Whole testis	4	<0.2	<5.1
Seminiferous tubules	4	<0.2	<5.9
Interstitial tissue	3	<1.6	<0.2
Interstitial fluid	3	3.6 ± 0.5	12.5 ± 1.9

Values are mean ± S.E.M. (N = number of preparations).
a vs. b ($p < 0.01$), c vs. d ($p < 0.001$) as assessed by unpaired t-test.

considerable importance since to date attempts to isolate a LHRH-like material have relied almost exclusively on radioimmunoassay data and some studies have identified an LHRH-like material in the same high molecular weight range in which we have shown peptidase activity.[15,16]

FURTHER STUDIES ON THE PURIFICATION OF A TESTICULAR LHRH-LIKE MATERIAL

In view of the presence of peptidase activity in the extracts, attempts were made to neutralize the effect of this activity. Acetic acid extracts, boiled to inactivate peptidase activity, were subsequently found to stimulate both LH and FSH re-

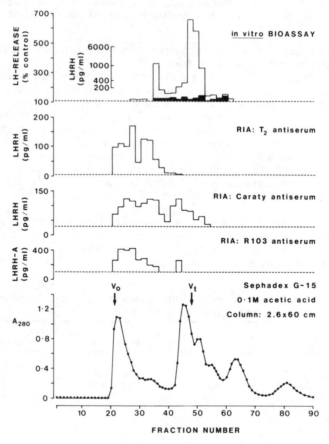

FIGURE 5. Fractionation by gel filtration of LHRH-like activity in testicular acetic acid–boiled extract, as assessed by *in vitro* bioassay, LHRH radioimmunoassays, and LHRH-A radioimmunoassay (open columns) and following extraction of fractions by absorption to ODS-silica as assessed by *in vitro* bioassay (closed columns). (Antiserum T_2: Heber and Odell.[28] Antiserum Caraty: Caraty *et al.*[29] Antiserum R42: Nett *et al.*[30])

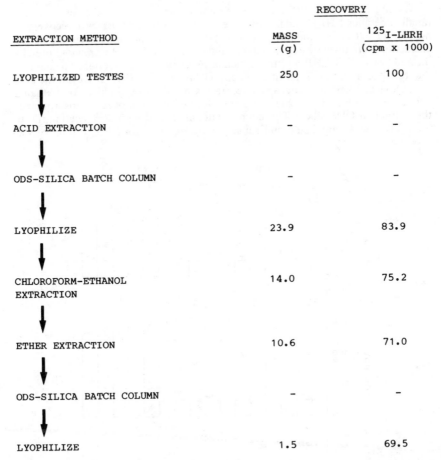

EXTRACTION METHOD	RECOVERY	
	MASS (g)	^{125}I-LHRH (cpm x 1000)
LYOPHILIZED TESTES	250	100
ACID EXTRACTION	-	-
ODS-SILICA BATCH COLUMN	-	-
LYOPHILIZE	23.9	83.9
CHLOROFORM-ETHANOL EXTRACTION	14.0	75.2
ETHER EXTRACTION	10.6	71.0
ODS-SILICA BATCH COLUMN	-	-
LYOPHILIZE	1.5	69.5

FIGURE 6. The LHRH extraction procedure with recovery of mass (g dry wt.) and [^{125}I]LHRH. (Methodology on acid extraction from Bennett *et al.*[31] Methodology on chloroform-ethanol extraction from Bhasin *et al.*[16])

lease *in vitro*. However, absorption of the extract onto octadecylsilyl silica (ODS-silica) cartidges (Sep-Pak, Waters Assoc.), followed by elution with 80% acetonitrile in 0.1% trifluoroacetic acid (TFA), greatly reduced the apparent bioactivity of these extracts (< 20 pg LHRH equivalent/testis). This decrease in activity was attributed to the removal of small molecular weight materials including salts, etc. that interfere in the bioassay. The effect of salts in the sample on the release of FSH and LH was confirmed by chromatography on Sephadex-G-15 (FIGURE 5) whereby the apparent bioactivity was predominantly localized in the salt peak region. The apparent activity in this region could not be absorbed to the ODS-silica, although it had previously been confirmed that native LHRH is retained under these conditions. These extracts also showed a heterogeneous profile of immunoactivity following gel filtration as assessed by various LHRH radioimmunoassays.

Having established the presence of proteolytic activity in the testis, which rapidly degrades LHRH and its analogues leading to possible losses in recovery, a number of extraction methods designed to minimize peptidase activity during extraction were investigated. Recovery and integrity of LHRH were monitored by the addition of [125I]LHRH to the testicular tissue prior to extraction. The method that resulted in optimum purification and yields of [125I]LHRH involved the acid extraction of lyophilized decapsulated testes followed by a chloroform-ethanol extraction step.[16] Salts and highly polar molecules were removed by absorption of the extract to ODS-silica. The bound material, eluted with 80% acetonitrile in 0.1% TFA, was lyophilized and subsequently treated with ether to remove ste-

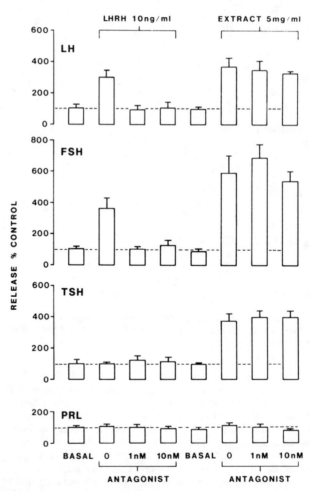

FIGURE 7. Comparison of activity of LHRH and a testicular extract prepared according to FIGURE 6 in the *in vitro* bioassay is shown together with the effect of incubation in the presence of the LHRH antagonist [Ac-Ala¹-pCl-D-Phe²,D-Trp³,⁶]LHRH. TSH: thyroid stimulating hormone: PRL: prolactin. Columns and bars are mean ± SD.

TABLE 3. LHRH Activity of a Partially Purified Testicular Extract, as Assessed by *in Vitro* Bioassay, LHRH Radioimmunoassays, and LHRH-A Radioimmunoassay

	LHRH Activity	
	(pg/mg extract)	(pg/testis)
In vitro bioassay		
LH release	2435[a]	2676
FSH release	1904[a]	2092
Radioimmunoassay		
LHRH antiserum (T_2)	126	138
LHRH antiserum (Caraty)	91[a]	100
LHRH antiserum (R42)	<15	<16
LHRH-A antiserum (R103)[b]	480	520

[a] Preparations give non-parallel dose/response curves when compared with the standard.
[b] Values are pg LHRH-A.

roids. This method resulted in a 100-fold purification of [^{125}I]LHRH with 60–80% recoveries (FIGURE 6).

Using a number of LHRH antisera of different specificities, estimates of the immunoactivity of the partially purified testicular extracts as assessed by RIA varied from <15 to 126 pg LHRH/mg extract (TABLE 3). These results indicate that the levels of LHRH in the testis are very low (approximately 0.1%) when compared with those in the hypothalamus, and there remain a number of substances in the purified extract that are not LHRH, but are immunoreactive in these systems. Furthermore TSH release is also stimulated in the pituitary cell bioassay, although at the same dose level of the extract prolactin release is unaffected (FIGURE 7). In all, these results suggest that the extract is exerting an apparently non-specific effect on the cells, although morphological assessment of the cells in culture did not reveal any obvious signs of toxicity. As a further test of specificity, the ability of an LHRH antagonist ([Ac-Ala^1-pCl-D-Phe^2,D-Trp^{3,6}]LHRH) to inhibit the *in vitro* biological activity of the partially purified testicular extracts to release FSH and LH was evaluated. However, less than 10% of this activity is inhibited by the antagonist of LHRH (FIGURE 7), suggesting that the larger part of the LH and FSH release is caused by mechanisms other than those mediated by the pituitary LHRH receptor.

CONCLUSIONS

It is evident that the isolation and identification of a LHRH-like peptide from testicular tissue is complicated by several problems, one of which is the demonstration of significant LHRH peptidase activity. Unless this peptidase activity is inactivated, the results of radioimmunoassays or radioreceptor assays for the detection of LHRH-like activity must be viewed with caution. Our studies, using modified extraction procedures, indicate that the LHRH-like activity is present in concentrations of less than 15 pg/testis, although LHRH-like proteins with different structures to LHRH may have been excluded by the extraction procedures employed. Our continuing studies suggest that even this level of activity should be viewed cautiously and suggest that further studies in this field should demonstrate that substances claimed to have LHRH-like activity are biologically active and that this activity is abolished by known antagonists of LHRH.

REFERENCES

1. BOURNE, G. A., S. REGIANI, A. H. PAYNE & J. C. MARSHALL. 1980. Testicular GnRH receptors. Characterization and localization on interstitial tissue. J. Clin. Endocrinol. Metab. **51:** 407–409.

2. CLAYTON, R. N., M. KATIKINENI, V. CHAN, M. L. DUFAU & K. J. CATT. 1980. Direct inhibition of testicular function by gonadotropin releasing hormone: mediation by specific gonadotropin releasing hormone receptors in interstitial cells. Proc. Natl. Acad. Sci. USA **77:** 4459–4463.

3. LEFEBVRE, F. A., J. J. REEVES, C. SEGUIN, J. MASSICOTTE & F. LABRIE. 1980. Specific binding of a potent LHRH agonist in rat testis. Mol. Cell Endocrinol. **20:** 127–134.

4. PERRIN, M. H., J. M. VAUGHAN, J. E. RIVIER & W. W. VALE. 1980. High affinity GnRH binding to testicular membrane homogenates. Life Sci. **26:** 2251–2256.

5. SHARPE, R. M. & H. M. FRASER. 1980. Leydig cell receptors for luteinizing hormone releasing hormone and its agonists and their modulation by administration or deprivation of the releasing hormone. Biochem. Biophys. Res. Commun. **95:** 256–262.

6. TCHOLAKIAN, R. K., A. DE LA CRUZ, M. CHOWDHURY, A. STEINBERGER, D. H. COY & A. V. SCHALLY. 1978. Unusual anti-reproductive properties of the analog [D-Leu⁶, des-Gly-NH₂¹⁰]LHRH ethylamide in male rats. Fertil. Steril. **30:** 600–603.

7. PELLETIER, G., L. CUSAN, C. AUCLAIR, P. A. KELLY, L. DESY & F. LABRIE. 1978. Inhibition of spermatogenesis in the rat by treatment with [D-Ala⁶,des-Gly-NH₂¹⁰]LHRH ethylamide. Endocrinology **103:** 641–643.

8. RIVIER, C., J. RIVIER & W. VALE. 1979. Chronic effects of [D-Trp⁶,Pro⁹Net] luteinizing hormone-releasing factor on reproductive processes in the male rat. Endocrinology **105:** 1191–1201.

9. RIVIER, C. & W. VALE. 1979. Hormonal secretion in male rats chronically treated with [D-Trp⁶, Pro⁹Net]-LRF. Life Sci. **25:** 1065–1074.

10. HSUEH, A. J. W. & G. F. ERICKSON. 1979. Extrapituitary inhibition of testicular function by luteinizing hormone releasing hormone. Nature **281:** 66–67.

11. ARIMURA, A., P. SERAFINI, S. TALBOT & A. V. SCHALLY. 1979. Reduction of testicular luteinizing hormone/human chorionic gonadotropin receptors by [D-Trp⁶]-luteinizing hormone releasing hormone in hypophysectomized rats. Biochem. Biophys. Res. Commun. **90:** 687–693.

12. SHARPE, R. M., H. M. FRASER, I. COOPER & F. F. G. ROMMERTS. 1982. The secretion, measurement and function of a testicular LHRH-like factor. Ann. N.Y. Acad. Sci. **383:** 272–292.

13. SHARPE, R. M. & H. M. FRASER. 1980. hCG-stimulation of testicular LHRH-like activity. Nature **287:** 642–643.

14. SHARPE, R. M., H. M. FRASER, I. COOPER & F. F. G. ROMMERTS. 1981. Sertoli-Leydig cell communication via an LHRH-like factor. Nature **290:** 785–787.

15. DUTLOW, C. M. & R. P. MILLAR. 1981. Rat testis immunoreactive LHRH differs structurally from hypothalamic LHRH. Biochem. Biophys. Res. Commun. **101:** 486–494.

16. BHASIN, S., D. HEBER, M. PETERSON & R. S. SWERDLOFF. 1983. Partial isolation and characterization of testicular GnRH-like factors. Endocrinology **112:** 1144–1146.

17. RICH, K. A. & D. M. DE KRETSER. 1977. Effect of differing degrees of destruction of the rat seminiferous epithelium on levels of serum FSH and androgen binding protein. Endocrinology **101:** 959–974.

18. RICH, K. A., J. B. KERR & D. M. DE KRETSER. 1979. Evidence for Leydig cell dysfunction in rats with seminiferous tubule damage. Mol. Cell Endocrinol. **13:** 123–135.

19. KERR, J. B., K. A. RICH & D. M. DE KRETSER. 1979. Alterations of the fine structure and androgen secretion of the interstitial cells in the experimentally cryptorchid rat testis. Biol. Reprod. **20:** 409–422.

20. RISBRIDGER, G. P., J. B. KERR & D. M. DE KRETSER. 1981. Evaluation of Leydig cell function and gonadotrophin binding in unilateral and bilateral cryptorchidism: Evi-

dence for local control of Leydig cell function by the seminiferous tubule. Biol. Reprod. **24:** 534–540.

21. RISBRIDGER, G. P., J. B. KERR, R. A. PEAKE & D. M. DE KRETSER. 1981. An assessment of Leydig cell function after bilateral efferent duct ligation: Further evidence for local control of Leydig cell function. Endocrinology **109:** 1234–1241.

22. DE KRETSER, D. M. 1982. Sertoli cell-Leydig cell interaction in the regulation of testicular function. Int. J. Androl. Suppl. **5:** 11–17.

23. VALE, W., G. GRANT, M. AMOSS, R. BLACKWELL & R. GUILLEMIN. 1972. Culture of enzymatically dispersed anterior pituitary cells: Functional validation of a method. Endocrinology **91:** 562–572.

24. SHARPE, R. M. 1980. Temporal relationship between interstitial fluid accumulation and changes in gonadotropin receptor numbers and steroidogenesis in the rat testis. Biol. Reprod. **22:** 851–857.

25. GRIFFITHS, E. C. & J. A. KELLY. 1979. Mechanisms of inactivation of hypothalamic regulatory hormones. Mol. Cell. Endocrinol. **14:** 3–17.

26. ADVIS, J. P., J. E. KRAUSE & J. F. MCKELVY. 1982. Luteinizing hormone-releasing hormone peptidase activities in discrete hypothalamic regions and anterior pituitary of the rat: Apparent regulation during the prepubertal period and first estrous cycle at puberty. Endocrinology **110:** 1238–1245.

27. ADVIS, J. P., J. E. KRAUSE & J. F. MCKELVY. 1983. Evidence that endopeptidase-catalysed luteinizing hormone releasing hormone cleavage contributes to the regulation of median eminence LHRH levels during positive steroid feedback. Endocrinology **112:** 1147–1149.

28. HEBER, D. & W. D. ODELL. 1978. Development of a GnRH radioimmunoassay utilizing a superactive synthetic GnRH analog: [D-Lys⁶]-GnRH. Proc. Soc. Exp. Biol. Med. **158:** 643–646.

29. CARATY, A., M-M. DE REVIERS, J. PELLETIER & M. P. DUBOIS. 1980. Reassessment of LRF radioimmunoassay in the plasma and hypothalamic extracts of rats and rams. Reprod. Nutr. Develop. **20:** 1489–1501.

30. NETT, T. M., A. M. AKBAR, G. D. NISWENDER, M. T. HEDLUND & W. F. WHITE. 1973. A radioimmunoassay for gonadotropin-releasing hormone (Gn-RH) in serum. J. Clin. Endocrinol. Metab. **36:** 880–885.

31. BENNETT, H. P. J., C. A. BROWNE & S. SOLOMON. 1981. Purification of the two major forms of rat pituitary corticotropin using only reversed-phase liquid chromatography. Biochemistry **20:** 4530–4538.

GnRH-like Factors in the Rat Testis and Human Seminal Plasma[a]

RONALD S. SWERDLOFF, SHALENDER BHASIN, and
REBECCA Z. SOKOL

Department of Medicine
UCLA School of Medicine
Harbor-UCLA Medical Center
Torrance, California 90509

TESTICULAR GnRH-LIKE FACTORS

The search for testicular GnRH-like factors was prompted by observations that GnRH and it agonistic analogs directly inhibit gonadal function in the rat via binding to so-called GnRH receptors on the Leydig cells.[1-3] The presence of these high affinity GnRH receptors on the Leydig cells suggested the possibility that these GnRH-like factor(s) might serve some physiologic function in the normal untreated animal. Since the circulating concentrations of native GnRH are too low to adequately explain these gonadal effects, it was speculated that GnRH-like factors are produced locally in the rat testis. Simultaneous search for these putative factors in several laboratories led to reports that crude testicular extracts displaced $[^{125}I]$GnRH in GnRH radioimmunoassay[4,5] and iodinated GnRH analogs in the GnRH radioreceptor assay.[6-8] GnRH-like substance was demonstrated in the cytoplasm of interstitial cells by immunohistochemical staining.

The term "GnRH-like factor" has been used rather loosely in the literature and this has resulted in considerable confusion. The term has been used to describe factor(s) that interact with certain anti-GnRH sera,[4-6] displace iodinated GnRH analogs in GnRH radioreceptor assays,[6-8] and stimulate LH and FSH in pituitary monolayer cultures.[10] Furthermore, a variety of sources have been used for isolation of these putative factors: these include testicular extracts, seminal plasma, Sertoli cell culture medium, and testicular lymph from several animal species (ovine, bovine, rodent, and human). Depending upon the assay system used and the source of the material, GnRH-like factors have been described with molecular weights varying from 3500 to 100,000. It remains unclear whether these fractions with such diverse molecular weights reflect molecular heterogeneity of a single family of peptides or several unrelated compounds.

Minimal Criteria for the Putative GnRH-like Factor(s) in the Testis

We hypothesized that GnRH and its agonists, because of some structural resemblance, acted as analogs of the endogenous GnRH-like factor and via binding to receptors for this endogenous factor on the Leydig cells, resulted in similar biologic effects. We therefore set up the following criteria for these putative

[a] This work was supported in part by training grant 2 T32 AM07214-06 and National Institutes of Health grants (1 ROI HD17990-01 and 5 ROI HD15132-03).

factors, which we felt were consistent with existing observations relating to direct gonadal effects of GnRH and its agonists. Essential criteria: (1) These factors must bind to GnRH receptors. (2) Their biologic action must resemble the effects of GnRH and its agonist at the gonadal level. (3) Their biologic action must be reversed by an antagonistic analog of GnRH. (4) Synthesis of these factor(s) by the testis should be demonstrable. Non-essential criteria: In addition, these putative factor(s) may interact with certain anti–GnRH antisera, but may or may not have GnRH-like effects at the pituitary level.

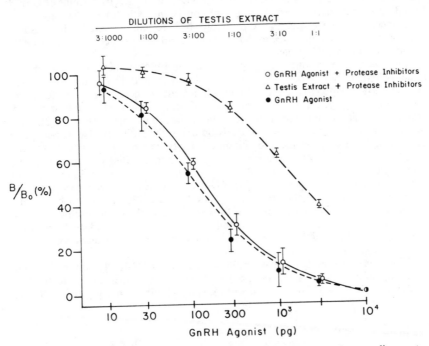

FIGURE 1. Displacement curve of crude ECA extract in pituitary membrane radioreceptor assay in the presence of protease inhibitors and EDTA. Standard curve was established by using serial dilutions of GnRH agonist [D-Leu⁶]des-Gly¹⁰ GnRH EA in the absence (-----) and presence (———) of protease inhibitors and EDTA. (From Bhasin *et al.*[11] With permission from *Endocrinology*.)

Partial Isolation and Biochemical Characterization of GnRH-like Factor(s) from the Rat Testis

Ethanol, chloroform, and acetic acid extracts of rat testes were defatted with ether and treated with charcoal to remove steroids.[11] Defatted and steroid-free extract thus obtained (ECA extract) gave displacement curves that were parallel to that of D-Leu⁶-des-Gly¹⁰ GnRH EA in a GnRH radioreceptor assay (FIGURE 1). The displacement by crude ECA extract was not shifted in the presence of EDTA or protease inhibitors, indicating that the apparent displacement of the iodinated ligand in the radioreceptor assay was not due to divalent cations or cleavage of the ligand by a tissue protease.

In a GnRH radioimmunoassay using an antibody raised against D-Lys[6] GnRH (T$_2$ antibody),[12] serial dilutions of crude ECA extract yielded a displacement curve parallel to that of GnRH, which was not shifted in the presence of 0.1 M EDTA, bacitracin, and soybean trypsin inhibitor. However, no displacement of radiolabeled GnRH by crude ECA extract was seen when antiserum R42 (courtesy of Drs. Nett and Niswender) was used.[13] Antiserum T$_2$ used in these studies recognizes the COOH terminal regions of the native GnRH decapeptide.[12] Antiserum R42, which has been used traditionally to quantify authentic GnRH in biologic specimens, requires both the -NH$_2$, middle, and -COOH termini of GnRH for effective binding.[13] These findings are consistent with those of Dutlow et al. and suggest that these species are probably -NH$_2$ terminally extended forms and may share with the native decapeptide some amino acid sequences in the COOH terminal portion of the molecule.[4]

Immunoaffinity chromatography of the crude ECA extract on cyanogen bromide–activated Sepharose 4B beads covalently bound to T$_2$ antibody raised against D-(lys)[6] GnRH resulted in over a hundredfold increase in specific receptor binding activity. Equivalent amounts of kidney extracts, similarly processed, resulted in insignificant displacement in the radioreceptor assay (FIGURE 2). Acetic acid wash of the Sepharose 4B beads bound to the antibody also displayed no displacement. Thus, the receptor binding activity was relatively tissue specific. Enhancement of receptor binding activity by immunoaffinity chromatography also suggests that at least some of the molecular forms that bind to GnRH receptor are identical to those that interact with GnRH antiserum T$_2$. In separate experiments, coincubation of the tracer [^{125}I]GnRH with material purified by affinity chromatography followed by high performance liquid chromatography of the incubate on reverse-phase ODS column failed to demonstrate peptidase degradation of the tracer indicating that the extract did not have either intrinsic or contaminating proteolytic activity.

High pressure liquid chromatography of the material partially purified by affinity chromatography on a reverse-phase 5 μ ODS column, using an acetonitrile gradient, yielded two discrete peaks of receptor binding activity (FIGURE 3). Gel

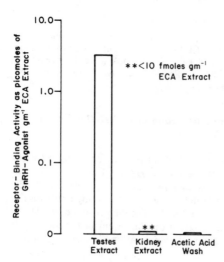

FIGURE 2. Relative amounts of GnRH receptor binding activity in the material purified by immunoaffinity chromatography of 1.0 g of crude ECA extracts of rat testes and rat kidneys. Acetic acid wash of the Sepharose 4B beads covalently linked to the T$_2$ antibody was used as control. The receptor binding activity is described as picomoles of [D-Leu[6]]des-Gly-NH$_2$[10] GnRH EA that displace the same percent of radiolabeled ligand in the radioreceptor assay. (From Bhasin et al.[11] With permission from Endocrinology.)

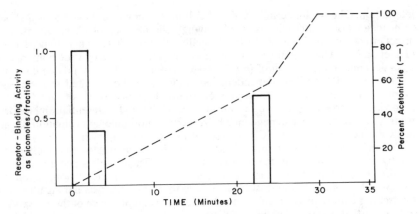

FIGURE 3. Relative amounts of receptor binding activity in various fractions from HPLC of the material partially purified by immunoaffinity chromatography on a reverse-phase 5u ODS column using acetonitrile gradient as shown (From Bhasin *et al.*[11] With permission from *Endocrinology*.)

filtration of the ECA extract on polyacrylamide agarose beads (Ultrogel AcA 202) with linear fractionation range of 1,000–15,000 also resulted in two peaks of receptor binding activity, one in the void volume and the other coeluting with insulin (Ve : Vo is 2.9 : 1).

On SDS polyacrylamide gel electrophoresis in the presence of 10 M urea, a single band was seen with silver stain with an estimated molecular weight of 68,000. The lower molecular weight substance was not detected either because of a very small amount present or because of its failure to interact with silver stain. Thus, the preliminary estimates of molecular weights of these factors are 6,000 and 68,000.

Chromatography on Concanavalin A-Sepharose resulted in retention of a part of the activity on Concanavalin A-Sepharose, which can be eluted with 0.2 M alpha-methylglucopyranoside, suggesting that at least one of the factors may be a glycopeptide.[14] The fraction that was retained on Concanavalin A-Sepharose and then eluted with 0.2 M alpha-methylglucopyranoside was desalted exhaustively and subjected to ion-exchange chromatography on DEAE-Sephacel (Pharmacia). The receptor binding activity was retained on DEAE-Sephacel and eluted with increasing concentrations of NaCl, the peak eluting at 0.2 M NaCl. If further work confirms the glycoprotein nature of this factor, the molecular weight estimates may need to be revised because glycoproteins containing more than 10% carbohydrate behave anomalously during SDS PAGE when compared to standard proteins.[15]

Biologic Effects of the GnRH-like Factors in a Mixed Sertoli–Leydig Cell Culture

Even though GnRH receptors are present only on the Leydig cells, we considered a mixed Leydig-Sertoli cell culture more appropriate bioassay system than an enriched Leydig cell culture because of the possibility that some of the effects of these factors on Leydig cell may require a hitherto undefined Sertoli-Leydig cell interaction. The longer term mixed-cell culture system was chosen over a short term incubation (4 hr) with isolated Leydig cells because of observations that direct effects of GnRH and its agonistic analogs on testis *in vitro* take long periods of incubation. The mixed-cell culture system was validated by demonstrating dose-dependent stimulation of *in vitro* testosterone secretion by graded concentrations of oLH and dose-dependent inhibition of oLH-stimulated testosterone production by graded concentrations of a GnRH agonist D-(Lys)[6] GnRH. The following criteria were devised to ensure specificity and differentiate inhibitory from toxic effects: dose dependence of response, morphologic evaluation of the testicular cells, and use of [51]CR release for assessing cytotoxicity.

In such a bioassay system, serial dilutions of testicular extract partially purified by immunoaffinity chromatography (IC) resulted in dose-dependent inhibition of oLH-stimulated testosterone production over a 48 hr incubation period as shown in FIGURE 4. In contrast, ^{51}Cr release from the cells was not significantly different in culture plates incubated in the absence and presence of the IC extract indicating that apparent inhibition of testosterone production did not represent toxic effects.[16]

In separate experiments simultaneous incubation of IC extract with a GnRH antagonist failed to reverse the inhibitory effects of the IC extract. However, when the cells were preincubated for 24 hr with 10^{-6} M antagonist prior to addi-

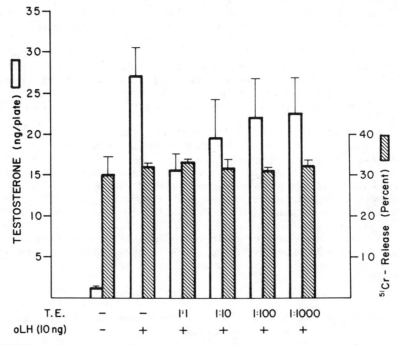

FIGURE 4. Effect of serial dilutions of testicular extract partially purified by immunoaffinity chromatography on oLH-stimulated testosterone secretion in a mixed Sertoli-Leydig cell culture system over a 48 hr incubation period. Data are mean ± 1 S.D. [51]Cr release from the cells was used as a marker of cytotoxicity. (From Bhasin *et al.*[16] With permission from *Biochemical and Biophysical Research Communications.*)

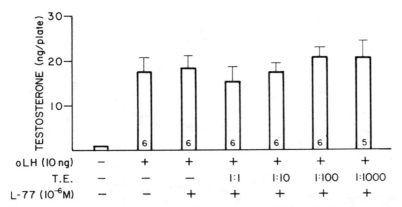

FIGURE 5. Effect of a GnRH antagonist on inhibitory effects of GnRH-like factor(s). The mixed Sertoli-Leydig cell culture plates were preincubated for 24 hr with a potent GnRH antagonist (10^{-6} M) prior to addition of oLH and serial dilutions of testicular extract partially purified by immunoaffinity chromatography. The data are mean ± 1 S.D. The amount of testicular extract added was the same as in previous experiment, shown in FIGURE 4. (From Bhasin *et al.*[16] With permission from *Biochemical and Biophysical Research Communications*.)

tion of serial dilutions of IC extract, no significant inhibition of LH-stimulated testosterone production was seen (FIGURE 5). These observations suggest that GnRH-like factor(s) inhibit LH-stimulated testosterone production via receptor-mediated mechanisms. These factors may thus modulate Leydig cell response to gonadotropins and provide a model for paracrine control of testicular function.

GnRH-LIKE FACTORS IN HUMAN SEMINAL PLASMA

In light of these observations in the rat, we wondered if GnRH-like factors were also present in the human. Because of the difficulties of procuring human testicular tissue, seminal plasma was selected as an alternate source. Two hundred ml of seminal plasma obtained from normal male volunteers was extracted with acetic acid and ethanol and successively filtered through an ultrafiltration system (Amicon) using membranes with exclusion limits of 30,000 and 500 daltons. Aliquots of both lyophilized retentates were assayed for GnRH-like immunoactivity using T_2 antibody raised against D-(lys)[6] GnRH. No displaceable material was found in the retentate containing molecules greater than 30,000 daltons. Serial dilutions of the 30,000-dalton fraction gave displacement curves that were parallel to that of GnRH standard in a GnRH radioimmunoassay. Gel filtration on a molecular sieve (ultrogel AcA 202) identified two peaks with estimated molecular weights of approximately 2600 and 5000.[17]

The immunoaffinity chromatography on Sepharose 4B beads bound to T_2 antibody enhanced the parallel displacement of radiolabeled ligand. Chromatography of extracted seminal plasma on Concanavalin A Sepharose suggested that at least one of the molecular species is a glycoprotein. Preincubation of the seminal plasma with the T_2 antibody decreased the amount of material measured after Concanavalin A chromatography by 300%, indicating neutralization by antibody.

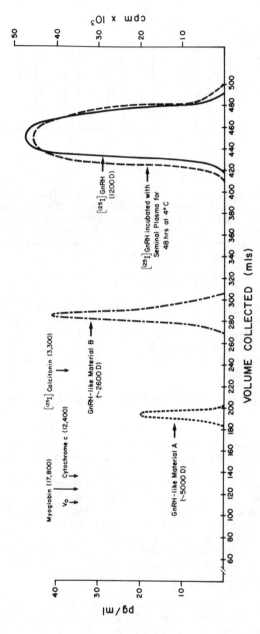

FIGURE 6. Gel filtration of acid-ethanol extract of seminal plasma on a molecular sieve column (ultrogel AcA 202). Eluting buffer was 0.01 M phosphate buffer. Fractions (0.1 ml) were collected and tested in a GnRH radioimmunoassay using T$_2$ antibody. (From Sokol et al.[17])

These data suggest that at least two species of GnRH-like factors are present in human seminal plasma. It remains unclear if these factors are related to those isolated from the rat testis. Since GnRH receptors have not been demonstrated in the human or primate testis, the function and origin of these GnRH-like factors in human seminal plasma remain to be elucidated.

REFERENCES

1. HSUEH, A. J. W. & G. F. ERICKSON. 1979. Extrapituitary inhibition of testicular function by luteinizing hormone-releasing hormone. Nature **281:** 66.
2. CLAYTON, R. N., M. KATIKINENI, V. CHAN, M. DUFAU & K. J. CATT. 1980. Direct inhibition of testicular function by GnRH: Mediation by specific GnRH receptors interstitial cells. Proc. Natl. Acad. Sci. USA **77:** 4459.
3. BOURNE, G. A., S. REGIANI, A. H. PAYNE & J. C. MARSHALL. 1980. Testicular GnRH receptors–characterization and localization on interstitial tissues. J. Clin. Endocrinol. Metab. **51:** 407.
4. DUTLOW, C. M. & R. P. MILLAR. 1981. Rat testis immunoreactive LHRH differs structurally from hypothalamic LH-RH. Biochem. Biophys. Res. Commun. **101:** 486.
5. TURKELSON, C. M., C. R. THOMAS & A. ARIMURA. 1982. Testicular LH-RH like substance. 64th Annual Meeting. The Endocrine Society. Abstract #38.
6. SHARPE, R. M. & H. M. FRASER 1980. hCG Stimulation of testicular LH-RH like activity. Nature **287:** 642.
7. SHARPE, R. M., H. M. FRASER, I. COOPER & F. F. G. ROMMERTS. 1981. Sertoli-Leydig cell communication via an LHRH-factor. Nature **290:** 785.
8. SHARPE, R. M., H. M. FRASER, I. COOPER & F. F. G. ROMMERTS 1982. The secretion, measurement and function of a testicular LH-RH like factor. Ann. N.Y. Acad. Sci. **383:** 272.
9. PAULL, W. K., C. M. TURKELSON, C. R. THOMAS & A. ARIMURA. 1981. Immunohistochemical demonstration of a testicular substance related to luteinizing hormon-releasing hormone. Science **213:** 1263.
10. YING, S. Y., N. LING, P. BOHLEN & R. GUILLEMIN. 1982. Gonadocrinins: Peptides in ovarian follicular fluid stimulating the secretion of pituitary gonadotropins. Endocrinology **108:** 1206.
11. BHASIN, S., D. HEBER, M. PETERSON & R. S. SWERDLOFF. 1983. Partial isolation and characterization of testicular GnRH-like factors. Endocrinology **112:** 1144.
12. HEBER, D. & W. D. ODELL. 1978. Development of a GnRH radioimmunoassay utilizing a superactive synthetic GnRH analog D(lys)⁶ GnRH. Proc. Soc. Exp. Biol. Med. **158:** 643.
13. NETT, T. M., A. M. AKBAR, G. D. NISWENDER, M. T. HEDLUNE & W. F. WHITE. 1973. Radioimmunoassay for GnRH in serum. J. Clin. Endocrinol. Metab. **36:** 880.
14. BHASIN, S., D. HEBER, M. PETERSON & R. S. SWERDLOFF. 1983. Partial isolation and characterization of *in vitro* biosynthesis of GnRH like factors by rat testis. The 65th Annual Meeting. The Endocrine Society. San Antonio, Texas.
15. SEGREST, J. P., R. L. JACKSON, E. P. ANDREWS & V. T. MARCHESI. 1971. Human erythrocyte membrane glycoprotein: A reevaluation of the molecular weight as determined by SDS PAGE. Biochem. Biophys. Res. Commun. **44:** 390.
16. BHASIN, S. & R. S. SWERDLOFF. 1984. Testicular GnRH-like factor(s): Characterization of biologic effects. Biochem. Biophys. Res. Commun. **122:** 1071.
17. SOKOL, R. Z., M. PETERSON & R. S. SWERDLOFF. 1984. GnRH-like factors in human seminal plasma. Science (Submitted for publication.)

LHRH-like Substance in the Rat Testis

AKIRA ARIMURA and CHARLES M. TURKELSON[a]

Laboratories for Molecular Neuroendocrinology and Diabetes
Departments of Medicine and Anatomy
Tulane University Hebert Research Center
Belle Chasse, Louisiana 70037

Although the presence of testicular LHRH-like material, as tested by radiorecep-tor assay or radioimmunoassay (RIA), has been reported by different groups,[1-5] their reports of the chemical characteristics of the LHRH-like materials are vari-ant. Most of those studies suggest that the molecular weight of the testicular LHRH-like substances range from 6,000 to 70,000. In our study,[6] we have demon-strated that the majority of LHRH-like immunoreactivity (LHRH-I) of rat testes extracts elutes immediately after the void volume in gel filtration of Sephadex G-50 column. This apparently large molecular weight LHRH-I is, however, dissoci-ated into a low molecular form by boiling with 8 M guanidine hydrochloride and 5% dithiothreitol, eluting in an area overlapping the salt volume upon gel filtra-tion. Therefore, it is possible that the large molecular weight LHRH-I reported by others is also an aggregated form of small molecular weight LHRH-I material or a small LHRH-I that is bound to a large molecular weight material. In order to provide a clear-cut answer to this problem it is essential to isolate, characterize, and synthesize this material and demonstrate that the synthetic material behaves similarly to that of the natural substance. This report discusses and describes the immunological and biological characteristics of the purified rat testicular LHRH-I, which has been dissociated from the apparently large molecular weight LHRH-I material.

MATERIALS AND METHODS

The acid extracts of rat testes were purified on gel filtration and the fractions were assayed for LHRH by RIA as reported previously.[7] The major peak of LHRH-like immunoreactivity (LHRH-I) was eluted in the area immediately following the void volume. The fractions containing this apparently high molecular weight im-munoreactivity (LHRH-I) were treated with 8 M guanidine hydrochloride and dithiothreitol and rechromatographed on gel filtration.[6] The majority of LHRH-I now eluted in the area overlapping the salt volume, as reported elsewhere.[6]

Dissociated high molecular weight LHRH-I was further purified on reverse-phase high performance liquid chromatography using a Beckman ultrasphere ODS column (0.46 × 25 cm) with acetonitrile by gradients buffered with 40 mM phosphate, pH 2.2. Aliquots of each fraction were evaporated to dryness, recon-stituted in the RIA diluent, and assayed for LHRH by RIA.

LHRH-I was determined by RIA for LHRH using different antisera with defined immunoreactive determinants that are described in RESULTS. Rabbit anti-

[a] Present Address: Harry S. Truman Memorial Veterans Hospital, Research Service (151), 800 Hospital Drive, Columbia, MO 65201.

sera (R422, R743, R744) and ovine antiserum (S772) were used. The extent of immunoreactivity of the extract to each antiserum was expressed so that the mass of LHRH-I observed at logit $B/B_o\% = 50$ with each antiserum expressed as a percentage of the mass for logit $B/B_o = 50$ obtained with R422.

The LH- and FSH-releasing activity of the test materials were determined by an *in vitro* assay using rat pituitary fragments as described elsewhere.[8] The pituitary donors were female adult CD rats (Charles River Breeding Laboratories, Inc.) 12 days post-ovariectomized, estrogen-treated (25 μg estradiol benzoate) and progesterone-treated (25 mg) 48 hours before. LH and FSH were determined by respective RIA using the RIA kits for rat LH and FSH provided by the National Pituitary Agency and NIDDKD. Synthetic LHRH was provided by Peninsula Laboratories (611 Taylorway, Delmont, CA 94002).

RESULTS AND DISCUSSION

HPLC-purified, dissociated LHRH-I was examined for immunoreactivity with different antisera with defined recognition sites. The recognition sites of the antisera are illustrated in FIGURE 1. Antiserum R422 requires the opposing N- and C-terminal of LHRH for full antigen recognition. Antiserum R743 recognizes amino acid positions 3–9, while both R744 and S772 require positions 7–10 amide for recognition. Dilution curves of HPLC-purified and synthetic LHRH were parallel in all RIAs using these four antisera. The relative cross-reactivity of the immunoreactivity in terms of synthetic LHRH, however, was different between these antisera. Assuming the relative immunoreactivity of the HPLC-purified dissociated LHRH-I for R422 is 100%, the cross-reactivity for R743, R744, and S772 were 96%, 57%, and 63%, respectively. Since the material tested was highly purified, the extent of non-specific interference in RIA due to other contaminants may be meager, if at all. Several possible assumptions on the structure of the testicular LHRH-I may be drawn from these results. The C-terminus of the testicular LHRH-I may be Gly-NH$_2$, which is required for recognition by R422, R744, and S772. C-terminal NH$_2$ is essential and required for binding with R744 and S772, and considerably important for R743. The substance must possess pGlu at the N-terminus that R422 requires for binding. The sequence corresponding to C-terminal region, especially from 7 to 10, of LHRH, seems to be particularly more important than the N-terminal region for both antisera R744 and S772. The relatively low cross-reactivity of the testicular LHRH-I with these antisera suggests that the sequence of the corresponding region of this material may differ from that of LHRH. Since the C-terminus Gly-NH$_2$ may be present, the different sequence may be sought in the region between 7 and 9. HPLC revealed that the retention time of testicular LHRH-I was slightly longer than that of LHRH, suggesting that the testicular substance is more lipophilic than hypothalamic LHRH.

The similarity of the testicular LHRH-I with hypothalamic LHRH was also evidenced by the fact that the purified testicular LHRH-I showed a weak LH- and FSH-releasing activity *in vitro*. The addition of 3.2 ng and 0.93 ng of purified testicular LHRH-I (based on RIA quantitation using antiserum R422 and synthetic LHRH as the standard) to the pituitary fragments induced a statistically similar 3- and 2.5-fold increase in LH release, respectively. The addition of 2.1 ng and 0.48 ng synthetic LHRH resulted in statistically similar 8- and 7-fold increase, respectively. Concomitant addition of 2.1 ng synthetic LHRH and 3.2 ng testicular LHRH-I increased LH release by only 2.8-fold, which was not different from

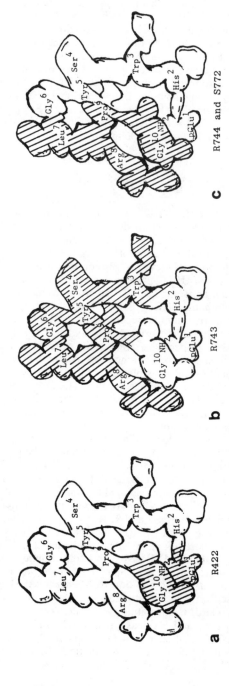

FIGURE 1. Schematic representation of the recognition sites of three rabbit antisera and one sheep antiserum generated against synthetic LHRH, indicated by the shaded areas. (a) R422, (b) R743, and (c) R744, and S772. R422 recognizes the opposing N- and C- terminal of LHRH. R743 recognizes the amino acids sequence from position 3 to 9. R744 and S772 recognizes positions 7 to 10 including C-terminal amide, but the importance of Arg for recognition is unclear.

the LH release stimulated by 3.2 ng testicular LHRH-I, but which was significantly smaller than the LH response to 2.1 ng synthetic LHRH alone. This observation suggests that the testicular LHRH-I is a moderate LHRH agonist and a strong LHRH antagonist. The low agonistic and strong antagonistic actions of this material were also observed for FSH release.

Therefore, the testicular LHRH-I appears to be different from inhibin, which suppresses FSH release without affecting LH release. The chemical structure of inhibin-like material in seminal plasma was recently reported as quite different from hypothalamic LHRH.[9]

Assessment of the actual amount of LHRH-I in the testes by RIA may be difficult, since the estimates may vary considerably with different antisera of different affinity, especially when crude material is assayed. This variation is reduced, however, when LHRH-I is highly purified by HPLC to the extent described before. Since the amino acids corresponding to position 7–9 of LHRH seem to be different from hypothalamic LHRH, an antiserum that does not require this portion for binding, such as R422, may provide a more reasonable estimation of the testicular LHRH-like material. Our estimate of testicular LHRH-I as examined by RIA with antiserum R422 was approximately 7.8 ng per rat testis in terms of synthetic LHRH. This level is similar to the content of LHRH in the hypothalamus and suggests that this substance may be of physiological importance. The presence of LHRH receptors on the Leydig cell, which are similar to those located on the pituitary gonadotroph,[10] and the biological action of the testicular LHRH strongly suggest that the testicular LHRH-I may be the physiological ligand for the testicular LHRH receptor.

REFERENCES

1. SHARPE, R. M. & H. M. FRASER. 1980. hCG stimulation of testicular LHRH-like activity. Nature **287:** 642.
2. DUTLOW, C. M. & R. P. MILLAR. 1981. Rat testis immunoreactive LH-RH differs structurally from hypothalamic LH-RH. Biochem. Biophys. Res. Commun. **101:** 486.
3. SHARPE, R. M., H. M. FRASER, I. COOPER & F. F. G. ROMMERTS. 1981. Sertoli-Leydig cell communication via an LHRH like factor. Nature **290:** 785.
4. SHARPE, R. M., H. M. FRASER, I. COOPER & F. F. G. ROMMERTS. 1982. The secretion, measurement, and function of a testicular LHRH like factor. Ann. N.Y. Acad. Sci. **383:** 272.
5. BHASIN, S., D. HEBER, M. PETERSON & R. SWERDLOFF. 1983. Partial isolation and characterization of testicular GnRH-like factors. Endocrinology **112:** 1144–1146.
6. TURKELSON, C. M., C. R. THOMAS & A. ARIMURA. 1982. Testicular LHRH-like substance. 64th Annual Mtg. The Endocrinology Society Abstract #38.
7. ARIMURA, A., H. SATO, D. H. COY, R. B. WOROBEC, A. V. SCHALLY, C. YANAIHARA & N. SUKURA. 1975. The antigenic determinant of the LH-releasing hormone for three different antiserums. Acta Endocrinol. **78:** 222–231.
8. ARIMURA, A., M. D. CULLER, C. M. TURKELSON, M. G. LUCIANO, C. R. THOMAS, N. OBARA, K. GROOT, J. RIVIER & W. VALE. 1983. In vitro pituitary hormone releasing activity of 40 residue human pancreatic at tumor growth hormone releasing factor. Peptide **4:** 107–110.
9. RAMASHARMA, K., M. R. SAIRAM, N. G. SEIDAH, M. CHRETIEN, P. MANJUNATH, P. W. SAHILLER, D. YAMASHIRO & CHOH HAO LI. 1984. Isolation, structure, and synthesis of a human seminal plasma peptide with inhibin-like activity. Science **223:** 1199–1202.

Tissue Interactions and Prostatic Growth: A New Mouse Model for Prostatic Hyperplasia[a]

LELAND W. K. CHUNG,[b,c] JAMES MATSUURA,[b]
AUDREY K. ROCCO,[b] TIMOTHY C. THOMPSON,[b] GARY J.
MILLER,[c] and MEREDITH N. RUNNER[b]

[b] Department of Pharmacology
School of Pharmacy
University of Colorado
Boulder, Colorado 80309

[c] University of Colorado Health Sciences Center
Denver, Colorado 80262

INTRODUCTION

The pathologic process of human benign prostatic hyperplasia (BPH) has been suggested by McNeal as a reawakening of embryonic growth potential of the adult stroma.[1] The proliferating stromal element in the periurethral region of human prostate can lead to the ingrowth and formation of new epithelial acini and ducts.[2] Experimental support of the reactivation of embryonic growth potential hypothesis was provided by Cunha and his collaborators who showed that embryonic urogenital sinus mesenchyme (equivalent to embryonic prostatic stroma) is a potent inductor for the growth and differentiation of adult bladder epithelia.[3,4] Evidence directly supporting that adult prostatic cells indeed responded to growth induction by fetal urogenital sinus was provided by Chung et al.[5,6] and Rocco et al.[7] They observed extensive overgrowth in chimeric prostates prepared by xenografting fetal urogenital sinus tissues directly into the adult host prostates. These results were confirmed recently by Cunha et al.[8] who demonstrated growth responsiveness of adult mouse dorsolateral prostate to embryonic rat urogenital sinus mesenchyme induction in tissue recombinants.

The purpose of the present study is to document that fetal urogenital sinus tissues have growth-promoting activity both *in situ* and in cultured cells. The respective roles of fetal urogenital sinus mesenchyme (UGM) and its epithelium (UGE) on the overall expression of growth-inductive capability by the intact fetal urogenital sinus (UGS) will be discussed.

The homologous chimeric prostate induced in rodent species (mouse and rat) represents a new model for prostatic hyperplasia.[6] Cellular interactions between fetal and adult prostatic tissues may provide significant insight in elucidating the regulatory mechanisms of adult prostatic growth and differentiation.

[a] This work supported in part by Public Health Service Grant AM-25266 awarded to L.W.K.C.

394

NEW MOUSE MODEL FOR PROSTATIC HYPERPLASIA

FIGURE 1 depicts the typical gross morphology of an adult mouse prostate four weeks following implantation of UGS from three fetal mice (3 × UGS). The wet weight and DNA content of the uninduced prostate ($N=38$, VP_c) increased from 5.8 ± 0.3 mg and 14 ± 0.7 μg to 57.1 ± 9.3 mg and 113.6 ± 18.2 μg ($N = 6$, VP_{UGS}, mean $\pm$ SE), respectively. This accounts for a ten- and eightfold increase over the basal levels of wet weight and DNA content of the adult prostate gland. The size of two other prostate glands with 3 × UGS implants increased to a mean wet weight of 240 mg (mean DNA content was 600 μg) at 25 weeks. This represents an enlargement of the adult prostate gland by 40-fold.

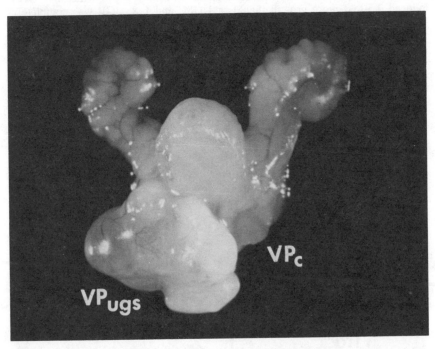

FIGURE 1. Gross morphology of the homologous lobe of chimeric mouse ventral prostate (VP_{UGS}) that was produced by xenografting 3 × UGS from HS mouse fetuses into the VP of an athymic male host (Balb/c-nu). VP_c represents the uninduced lobe of mouse ventral prostate gland.

The fetal UGS-induced adult prostatic hyperplasia can be accounted for by the ability of fetal UGS to induce adult prostatic cells into proliferation. FIGURE 2 shows that the resultant UGS-induced overgrowth of the adult mouse prostate and coagulating gland contains both donor (fetal) and host (adult) glucose phosphate isomerase (GPI) isozymes in about equal proportion. Because GPI isozyme profiles customarily are used to quantify the contribution of donor and host cells in chimeric tissues,[9,10] the equal proportion of GPI isozymes in the resultant UGS-induced overgrowth of the adult prostate indicates that one half of the 113.6 μg

DNA (or 56.8 μg DNA) was derived from the cells of the adult prostate gland proliferating as a result of their interactions with fetal UGS. This amounts to a fourfold increase in DNA content of the host prostate (mean DNA content in adult prostate = 14 μg) after 3 × UGS implantation.

COMPARISON OF THE INDUCTION OF OVERGROWTH OF ADULT PROSTATE GLAND BY FETAL UGS AND FETAL UGM IMPLANTS

The fact that UGS implants induce marked adult prostatic overgrowth prompted an investigation into the role of the individual components of UGS, i.e., UGM and UGE, on growth of the adult prostate gland. FIGURE 3 showed that 1 × UGS induced 2.5-fold more growth than 1 × UGM, and 1 × UGE was completely inactive (top panel). The magnitude of UGS- and UGM-induced prostatic overgrowth was dose-dependent (bottom panel). It is unlikely that differences in efficacy between UGS and UGM may be due to the irreversible loss of growth-inductive substance(s) during tissue isolation, because tissue recombinants consisting of UGM and UGE grew to the same extent as the intact UGS under renal capsules.[11] Alternatively, UGE may modulate the overall expression of the

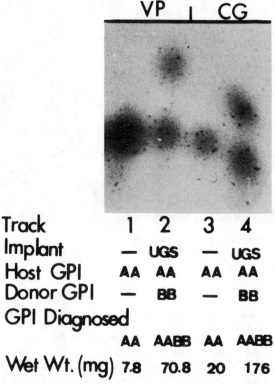

Track	1	2	3	4
Implant	—	UGS	—	UGS
Host GPI	AA	AA	AA	AA
Donor GPI	—	BB	—	BB
GPI Diagnosed	AA	AABB	AA	AABB
Wet Wt. (mg)	7.8	70.8	20	176

FIGURE 2. Glucose phosphate isomerase (GPI) isozyme profiles in the control and UGS-induced growth of adult mouse ventral prostate (VP) and coagulating gland (CG).

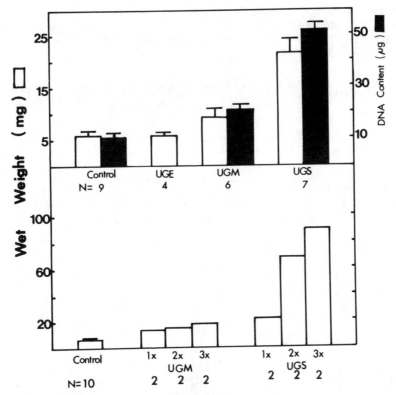

FIGURE 3. Comparison of the growth-promoting effects of intact urogenital sinus (UGS), urogenital sinus mesenchyme (UGM), and urogenital sinus epithelium (UGE). Top panel indicates the net growth (wet weight and DNA content) of the adult mouse VP observed during a four-week growth period following implantation of 1 × UGE, UGM, or UGS (tissues derived from one fetus). Panel B shows a dose-response relationship between the net growth (wet weight) of the adult mouse VP and the dose (1 × to 3 ×) of UGM and UGS during the same growth period. Average or average ± S.E. of 2 to 10 determinations.

inductive capability of UGM, which may determine the ultimate proliferative response of adult prostatic cells. This modulatory role of UGE on the growth-inductive capability of UGM has been demonstrated recently by Rocco *et al.*[7] in tissue recombination experiments. FIGURE 4 shows that rat UGM, when recombined heterospecifically with mouse UGE (Group II), induces two- to fourfold more growth, as measured by total tissue DNA, RNA, and protein content, than when recombined homotypically with rat UGE (Group I). There results suggest that UGM and UGE may exist in a relationship analogous to the paracrine system[12] where UGE modulates the gene expression of its adjacent UGM. We suggest that the greater growth observed in the heterospecific recombinant than that of the homotypic one was due to the regulation to a lesser extent on UGM_{rat} by UGE_{mouse} because of the greatly diminished effectiveness of the negative feedback loop. This may result in overproduction of certain putative mesenchymal growth factor(s) by the heterospecific recombinant that ultimately causes more growth. Preliminary investigation in adult prostatic stroma cells co-cultured with fetal UGS revealed the presence of certain soluble and diffusable fetal UGS-derived growth factor(s).[13] Further characterization of this factor is necessary to validate this suggestion.

REQUIREMENT OF TESTICULAR ANDROGEN FOR BOTH THE INITIATION AND THE MAINTENANCE OF UGS-INDUCED ADULT PROSTATIC OVERGROWTH

To test the androgen dependency of the UGS-induced adult prostatic overgrowth, hosts receiving 3 × UGS either were castrated or treated with estradiol dipropionate (15 μg/mouse every three days) or cyproterone acetate (4 mg/mouse every three days) immediately following 3 × UGS implantation. TABLE 1 shows that the initiation of UGS-induced adult prostatic overgrowth was inhibited as much as 60–70% by these hormonal-depletion regimens. These results suggest that androgenic steroids are required for the initiation of UGS-induced prostatic over-

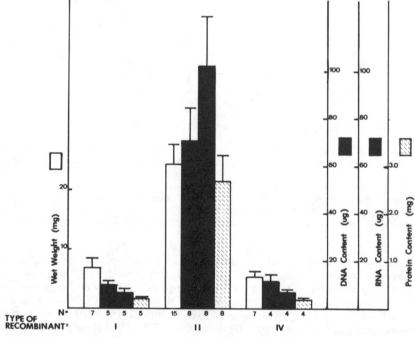

FIGURE 4. Comparison of the net growth (wet weight, DNA, RNA, and protein content) of homotypic (Group I: $UGM_{rat} + UGE_{rat}$) and heterospecific (Group II: $UGM_{rat} + UGE_{mouse}$ and Group IV: $UGM_{mouse} + UGE_{rat}$) tissue recombinants grown under the renal capsules of adult male athymic mice (Balb/c-nu) for an eight-week period. Average ± S.E. of 4 to 15 determinations. Note in the heterospecific recombinants, the growth observed in Group II is greater than that of Group IV. This may be due to the intrinsic difference in the inductive capability between UGM_{rat} and UGM_{mouse}.

TABLE 1. Inhibition of the Initiation of UGS-induced Adult Prostatic Overgrowth by Castration or the Administration of Estrogen or Antiandrogen to Intact Adult Male Hosts.

Condition[a]	N	% Inhibition
Intact control	3	–
Castration	3	70 ± 3.1
Estradiol dipropionate treated	2	61.5
Cyproterone acetate treated	3	59.3 ± 2.4

[a] 3 × UGS (HS mice) were implanted into one lobe of the VP of adult male hosts (Balb/c-nu). The growth of UGS-implanted VP was served as intact controls (0% inhibition). Some hosts were castrated immediately following UGS implantation, and other were treated every three days with either estradiol dipropionate (15 μg) or cyproterone acetate (4 mg) for a period of 10 to 30 days. DNA contents in VP were determined and data were expressed as % inhibition of DNA content ± S.E.

growth. In these experiments, it should be noted, however, that about 30% of the UGS-induced prostatic overgrowth is resistant to inhibition by the hormonal-depletion treatment protocols. These results suggest that UGS implants are capable of inducing androgen-independent prostatic overgrowth in the absence of endogenous testicular androgen.

To determine the requirement of testicular androgen for the maintenance of UGS-induced adult prostatic overgrowth, some male hosts receiving 3 × UGS implants for four weeks were castrated and allowed to grow for two additional weeks. The size of the prostate gland was estimated at the time of castration and was measured at the end of the two-week period. During this period, a 20–30% reduction in the size of the prostate gland was observed. Histological examination revealed typical castration-induced changes, such as atrophic epithelial acini and reduced luminal accumulation of secretory materials as described.[14,15] These results suggest that UGS-induced adult prostatic overgrowth depends upon endogenous testicular androgen for its maintenance.

The suggestion that UGS-induced prostatic overgrowth is androgen-dependent is further supported by the assessment of cytosolic androgen receptors in the UGS-induced adult mouse prostate. Scatchard analysis of cytosolic androgen receptors in the UGS-induced overgrowth of adult mouse prostate gland showed the presence of high affinity (K_d=0.73 nM) and low capacity (B_{max}=4.7 fmole/mg) androgen binding (R1881 binding) resembling that detected in the host prostate glands.[16] These results again are consistent with the suggestion that an androgen-dependent chimeric prostate was induced by fetal UGS implants.

SPECIFICITY OF UGS-INDUCED OVERGROWTH OF ADULT MOUSE PROSTATE

Donor Tissue Specificity

TABLE 2 shows that the implantation of live fetal bladder, fetal skin, fetal salivary gland, or adult prostate gland, of comparable size with 3 × UGS, results

TABLE 2. Donor Tissue Specificity for the Induction of Adult Mouse Prostatic Overgrowth

Donor Tissue[a]	N	Wet Weight (mg)	DNA Content (μg)
None (sham-operated)	6	5.7 ± 0.4	11.1 ± 0.3
3 × UGS	6	40.4 ± 5.3	80.0 ± 5.5
Adult ventral prostate	3	5.2 ± 0.6	15.0 ± 1.1
Fetal urinary bladder	3	4.5 ± 0.4	11.0 ± 1.4
Fetal skin	3	5.4 ± 1.1	13.4 ± 2.3
Fetal salivary gland	3	4.9 ± 1.0	13.2 ± 3.1

[a]Donor tissues were obtained from HS mice. Adult male hosts (Balb/c-nu) were implanted with either adult (50–90 day) or fetal tissues (16-day) and were allowed to grow for four weeks. Wet weight and DNA content in the control (sham-operated) and implanted lobe of mouse VP were determined.

in no overgrowth of the adult host prostate gland. Induction of adult prostatic overgrowths depends upon the implantation of live urogenital sinus tissues. Fetal UGS subjected to either heat (100°C for 5 min), freeze (−20°C) and thaw (room temperature), or radiation (5,000 rad for 4.1 min) was completely inactive (TABLE 3).

Implantation Site Specificity

Implanting fetal UGS into all of the mouse male accessory sex organs, such as the prostate, coagulating gland, and seminal vesicles,[5] induces the overgrowth of adult male accessory sex organs. Implantation of fetal UGS or tissue recombinants composed of UGM and UGE under the renal capsules, however, does not induce the overgrowth of the mouse kidneys.[11] These results suggest that the fetal UGS-induced overgrowth of adult organs is implantation-site specific.

Strain and Species Specificity

TABLE 4 shows that the phenomenon of UGS-induced adult prostatic overgrowth is not limited to Balb/c-nu mice. UGS isolate from C3H or Babl/c mice was

TABLE 3. Effects of Heat, Freeze and Thaw, and Radiation on the Growth-inductive Capability of Fetal UGS on Adult Mouse Ventral Prostate Gland

Donor Tissue[a]	N	Wet Weight (mg)	DNA Content (μg)
None (sham-operated)	6	5.7 ± 0.4	11.1 ± 0.3
3 × UGS (untreated)	6	40.4 ± 5.3	80.0 ± 5.5
3 × UGS (heat-treated)	4	7.5 ± 0.5	—
3 × UGS (freeze and thaw–treated)	2	3.8	—
3 × UGS (radiation-treated)	2	3.8	10.1

[a]Total growth period for the chimeric prostate (UGS implants isolated from HS mice into the adult prostate of Balb/c-nu mice) was four weeks (see TABLE 1).

found to induce adult prostatic overgrowth in their respective inbred strains of mice. In addition, fetal UGS isolated from Nb rats also was found to be capable of inducing adult prostatic overgrowths in both adult male syngeneic (Nb) and nude (Hooded-nu) rats.

PROGRESSION OF UGS-INDUCED ADULT PROSTATIC HYPERPLASIA

Adult mouse ventral prostate glands after UGS induction were isolated at three different intervals (15, 30, and 180 days) and were analyzed by histological methods. At 15 days following the implantation of 3 × UGS, the UGS implants ap-

TABLE 4. Strain and Species Specificity for UGS-induced Overgrowth of the Adult Prostate Gland

Donor[a]	Host	N	Ventral Prostatic Wet Weight (mg)	Ventral Prostatic DNA Content (μg)
Mouse				
None	C3H	4	12.6 ± 2.4	19.7 ± 2.5
C3H	C3H	4	24.9 ± 2.7	45.7 ± 1.9
None	Balb/c-nu	2	5.4	—
C3H	Balb/c-nu	2	72.4	—
None	Balb/c	2	3.5	3.2
Balb/c	Balb/c	2	49.5	79.8
None	Balb/c-nu	2	7.8	11.9
Balb/c	Balb/c-nu	2	51.0	80.3
Rat				
None	Nb	4	157.8 ± 21.2	—
Nb	Nb	4	439.7 ± 45	—
None	Hooded-nu	1	70	—
Nb	Hooded-nu	1	350	—

[a]Donor UGS isolated from 16- or 18-day-old embryos of mice and rats, respectively, were used in these studies. One lobe of the ventral prostate of the adult male host was implanted with 3 × UGS and the other lobe was sham-operated. Ventral prostates were harvested from the hosts at the end of the 30-day period. Wet weight and DNA content were expressed as average or average ± S.E. of 1 to 4 determinations.

peared to be markedly swollen and can be clearly identified. Thirty days after the initiation of the growth period, areas containing mixed adult and fetal cell populations were identified. Abundant new prostatic acini were found in many of the enlarged glands. Nests of cell aggregates that have the appearance of immatured prostate glands and/or urethral glands were observed. However, when the UGS-induced growth was allowed to proceed for 180 days, there are three distinct morphologies that can be identified in the histological specimens: (1) the pre-existing adult prostate gland, (2) the hyperplastic adult prostate gland with area of nodular hyperplasia resembling that observed in human and atrophic cystic acini filled with secretory products, and (3) the persistence and proliferation of small nests of cell aggregates that resemble the immatured prostate glands and/or the prostatic urethral glands. Total areas occupied by the pre-existing glands, the hyperplastic/cystic acini, and the immatured prostate glands and/or the prostatic urethral glands in the largest cross-sectional area of the specimen were approximately 25, 50, and 25%, respectively. As described earlier, typical castration-induced histological changes were apparent in UGS-induced prostatic growth following castration.[15]

TISSUE INTERACTIONS AND THE DEVELOPMENT OF PROSTATIC HYPERPLASIA IN RODENT

The present study has established the importance of tissue interactions, the inter-actions between fetal and adult prostatic cells, in the development of prostatic hyperplasia in the rodent species. We have developed a new mouse model for prostatic hyperplasia. This model was developed on the basis that fetal and adult prostatic cells interact, which resulted in the induction of adult prostatic cells into

TABLE 5. Comparison Between Dog and Mouse BPH as Potential Models for Screening Anti-BPH Compounds

	Dog Prostatic Hyperplasia[a]	Mouse Prostatic Hyperplasia[b]
Induction period	Long (3–6 mo)	Short (1 mo)
Fold of induced growth	2–4 fold	20–60 fold[15]
Factors regulating the magnitude of prostatic overgrowth	Genetic (?)	Number of UGS or UGM implanted
Requirement of exogenous hormones	Yes	No
Potential interference of anti-BPH compounds in bioassay	Yes	No
Ease of handling	More difficult	Less difficult
Expense of maintenance	More expensive	Less expensive

[a] Dog model of prostatic hyperplasia was established by Walsh and Wilson.[17]
[b] Mouse model of prostatic hyperplasia was developed by Chung et al.[15]

proliferation. A 10- to 20-fold overgrowth of the adult mouse prostate gland can be induced in one month by implantation of fetal UGS directly into the adult prostate gland. Both components of UGS, the fetal UGM and the fetal UGE, may be involved in the regulation of adult prostatic overgrowth. The androgen dependency and the specificity (donor tissue, site of implantation, and strain and species) of UGS-induced adult prostatic overgrowth have also been established.

The question remains whether the prostatic hyperplasia seen in this mouse model may be representative of human BPH. At present it is not possible to answer this question. However, it has been known for decades in developmental biology that tissue interactions occurred between species. Using fetal UGM_{mouse} as an inductor, Cunha et al.,[8] have presented evidence to show that prostatic morphogenesis occurred in fetal human bladder epithelium (as that of the mouse bladder epithelium) upon cellular interactions with fetal UGM_{mouse}. These results supported the relevance of mouse prostatic hyperplasia for future exploration of the disease processes in human BPH.

The observation that fetal UGS implants induce adult prostatic overgrowth in the complete absence of exogenous sex steroids supports the hypothesis of McNeal that human BPH may develop as a result of the reactivation of fetal growth potential in the periurethral area of the adult prostate gland.[1] The present mouse model offers several advantages, such as the predictably greater induction that occurs in a shorter period, the non-interference with the testing of anti-BPH drugs, and the ease of animal handling, over the canine prostatic hyperplasia model (Walsh and Wilson[17] and TABLE 5). This mouse model of prostatic hyperplasia may be used as a new test system for the future development of anti-BPH drugs.

REFERENCES

1. MCNEAL, J. E. 1978. Origin and evolution of benign prostatic enlargement. Invest Urol. **15**: 340–345.
2. WILSON, J. D. 1980. The pathogenesis of benign prostatic hyperplasia. Am. J. Med. **68**: 745–756.
3. CUNHA, G. R. & B. LUNG. 1978. The possible influence of temporal factors in androgenic responsiveness of urogenital tissue recombinants from wild-type and androgen-insensitive (Tfm) mice. J. Exp. Zool. **205**: 181–194.
4. CUNHA, G. R. & L. W. K. CHUNG. 1981. Stromal-epithelial interactions. I. Induction of prostatic phenotype in urothelium of testicular feminized (Tfm/y) mice. J. Steroid Biochem. **14**: 1317–1321.
5. CHUNG, L. W. K., J. MATSUURA, T. C. THOMPSON & R. C. F. Y. CHAO. 1982. A new approach to regulation of prostatic growth: Interactions between embryonic urogenital sinuses and adult prostate in situ. Proc. West Pharmacol. Soc. **25**: 141–145.
6. CHUNG, L. W. K., J. MATSUURA, A. K. ROCCO, T. C. THOMPSON, G. J. MILLER & M. N. RUNNER. 1984. A new mouse model for prostatic hyperplasia: induction of adult prostatic overgrowth by fetal urogenital sinus implants. *In* New Approaches to the Study of Human Benign Prostatic Hyperplasia. Buhl, Carter & Kimball, Eds.: 291–306. Alan R. Liss, Inc. New York.
7. ROCCO, A., J. MATUSUURA, M. RUNNER & L. W. K. CHUNG. 1983. Biochemical characterization of growth induction by fetal urogenital sinus: A new mouse model for studying prostatic hyperplasia. Fed. Proc. **42**: 1768 (Abstract).
8. CUNHA, G. R., L. W. K. CHUNG, J. M. SHANNON, O. TAGUCHI & H. FUJII. 1983. Hormone-induced morphogenesis and growth: role of mesenchymal-epithelial interactions. Rec. Prog. Horm. Res. **39**: 559–598.
9. ILLMENSEE, K. & B. MINTZ. 1976. Totipotency and normal differentiation of single terato-carcinoma cells cloned by injection into blastocysts. Proc. Natl. Acad. Sci. USA **73**: 549–553.
10. GOOTWINE, E., C. G. WEBB & L. SACHS. 1982. Participation of myeloid leukemic cells injected into embryos in haematopoietic differentiation in adult mice. Nature **299**: 63–65.
11. CHUNG, L. W. K. & G. R. CUNHA. 1983. Stromal-epithelial interactions. II. Regulation of prostatic growth by embryonic urogenital sinus mesenchyme. The Prostate **4**: 503–511.
12. HAKANSON, R. & F. SUNDLER. 1983. The design of the neuroendocrine system: A unifying concept and its consequence. Trends Pharmacol. Sci. **4**: 41–43.
13. THOMPSON, T. C. & L. W. K. CHUNG. 1984. Evidence for the fetal urogenital sinus-derived growth factor(s). Ann. N.Y. Acad. Sci. This volume.
14. CHUNG, L. W. K. & D. K. MCFADDEN. 1980. Sex steroids imprinting and prostatic growth. Invest. Urol. **17**: 337–342.
15. CHUNG, L. W. K., J MATSUURA & M. N. RUNNER. 1984. Tissue interactions and prostatic growth. I. Adult prostatic overgrowth induced by fetal urogenital sinus implants. Biol. Reprod. **31**: 155–163.

16. THOMPSON, T. C., L. W. K. CHUNG, G. R. CUNHA, B. L. NEUBAUER & J .M. SHANNON. 1983. Biochemical characterization of tissue recombinants composed of wild-type fetal urogenital sinus mesenchyme (UGM) and Tfm/y adult bladder epithelium (ABLE). Fed. Proc. **42**: 1769 (Abstract).
17. WALSH, P. C. & J. D. WILSON. 1976. The induction of prostatic hypertrophy in the dog with androstanediol. J. Clin. Invest. **57**: 1093–1097.

Extracellular Matrix in Testicular Differentiation[a]

LAURI J. PELLINIEMI,[b,c] JORMA PARANKO,[d]

SILVIA K. GRUND,[e]

KIM FRÖJDMAN,[c] JEAN-MICHEL FOIDART,[f]

and TAINA LAKKALA-PARANKO[d]

[c]Laboratory of Electron Microscopy
[d]Department of Anatomy
University of Turku
SF-20520 Turku 52, Finland

[e]Institut für Humangenetik und Anthropologie
Albert-Ludwigs-Universität
D-7800 Freiburg, Federal Republic of Germany

[f]Clinique Gynécologique et Obstétricale
Université de Liège
B-4020 Liège, Belgium

INTRODUCTION

The crucial and definitive event in the formation of a testis from a sexually indifferent gonad is the organization of epithelial testicular cords.[1] The indifferent gonad consists of histologically unorganized gonadal blastema in the medulla and a cortex of stratified surface epithelium, which at places is continuous with the medullary blastema.[1,2] The earliest signs of the initiation of epithelial cord formation are the attachment of adjacent cells by plasma membrane apposition and the appearance of basement membrane–like material along the future basal surface of the cord.[2,3] Ever since the introduction of the H-Y theory about the mechanisms of the testis cord formation by Wachtel et al.[4] the cell surface events have received the most attention among the interested investigators.[1,5] However, an epithelium is not only defined by close mutual adherence of particular cells but rather by production of a basement membrane as a physicochemical barrier against the surrounding tissue. Any regulatory factor involved in the epithelial organization must therefore account for one or both of these events. The temporal

[a] Financial support received from Sigrid Jusélius Foundation, the Academy of Finland, and Turku University Foundation. S. K. G. was a recipient of a European Molecular Biology Organization short-term fellowship.
[b] Editorial correspondence to: Dr. Lauri J. Pelliniemi, Laboratory of Electron Microscopy, University of Turku, Kiinamyllynkatu 10, SF-20520 Turku 52, Finland.

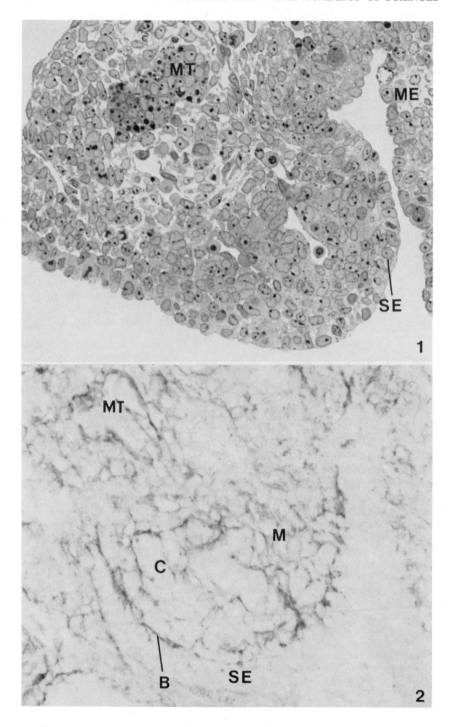

relationship of the cell attachment and the onset of basement membrane production is not known. A cell surface–associated glycoprotein, fibronectin has been found to play a role in cell-cell adhesion as well as cell–basement membrane relations.[6] Based on these considerations, we have analyzed basement membrane components and fibronectin, both related to the formation of the testicular cords in differentiating rat embryos, by light and electron microscopy and by immunocytochemical methods.[2]

EXTRACELLULAR MATRIX IN EMBRYONIC DIFFERENTIATION

Fibronectin is a dimer of two 220 kilodalton glycoprotein chains connected with disulfide bridges, and it has binding sites for cell surface, collagen, fibrin, heparin, and hyaluronic acid.[6] This adhesive molecule is present in extracellular matrix, basement membranes, and cell surface. Biological activities include cell-cell aggregation, reversion of transformed phenotype, increased cell motility, and specific binding to macromolecules of the extracellular matrix and the cell surface.[21] Fibronectin appears first in late blastocyst inner cell mass, and later on in endoderm and mesoderm, but not in the ectoderm.[7] Characteristically, fibronectin disappears from differentiating mesenchymal cells in many organs.[6] The basement membranes consist of a net-like matrix of type IV collagen associated with laminin, heparan sulfate proteoglycan, entactin, type V collagen, and fibronectin.[8] Analysis of these components has become an important method in studies of epithelial differentiation and morphogenetic tissue interactions in several tissues such as the salivary gland[9] and kidney.[10] During the growth of salivary epithelium into the mesenchyme the basement membrane is selectively degraded and remodeled.[11] In this regard the behavior of normal embryonic epithelium resembles that of malignant invasive tissue.

Extracellular matrix components are linked to intracellular structural and contractile filaments and in this way they form an interacting functional unit.[12] The importance of the extracellular matrix in developing embryonic organ systems has been well documented in several animal species.[12]

FIGURE 1. Indifferent male gonad of rat fetus (age 13.5 days). Light micrograph of a cross section from the gonadal ridge. Gonadal cords can not yet be observed. The specimen was fixed in glutaraldehyde and osmium, and embedded in epon.[2] SE, surface epithelium; MT, mesonephric tubule; ME, mesentery. Scale 360:1.

FIGURE 2. Developing male gonad of rat fetus (age 13.5 days). Fibronectin is localized as a black meshwork in the mesenchyme of gonadal ridge (M) and along the basement membrane (B) of the surface epithelium (SE). Small cords (C) of fibronectin-negative cells are already present and delineated with fibronectin. The specimen was fixed with periodate-lysine-paraformaldehyde and peroxidase-antiperoxidase was used for the immunocytochemical reaction.[2] MT, mesonephric tubule. Scale 330:1.

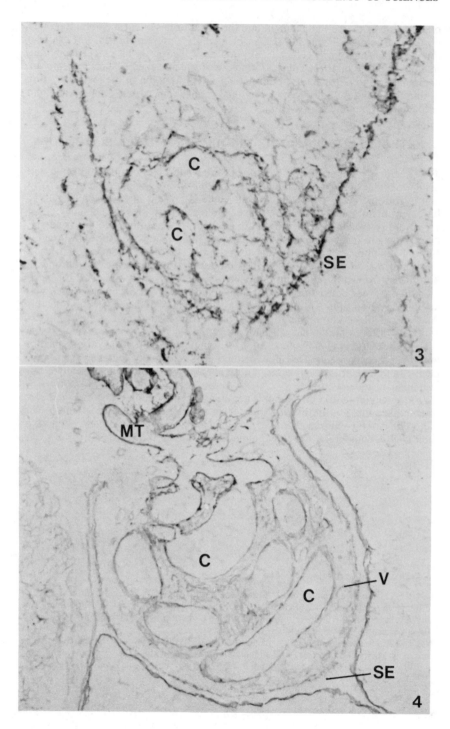

DIFFERENTIATION *IN VIVO*

The morphological basis of gonadal differentiation has been well documented in several species at light and electron microscope level as summarized in our previous publication.[2] Extracellular matrix is intimately involved in the organization of the testicular cords. The basement membrane under the surface epithelium of the early undifferentiated gonad (FIGURE 1) becomes discontinuous and epithelial cell cords appear connecting the medulla and the surface epithelium. Simultaneously, new cords appear in the medulla. In our own analysis of rat embryos, disappearance of fibronectin from the presumptive testicular cord cells at the age of 13.5 days (FIGURE 2) is the first sign of gonadal differentiation. The fibronectin-negative cord cell groups become at the same time surrounded by a thin layer of basement membrane components: laminin (FIGURE 3), collagen type IV and V, and heparan sulfate proteoglycan. Fibronectin is also present along the developing basement membrane (FIGURE 2).

The regulatory factors responsible for the disappearance of fibronectin from the extracellular space inside the cords are not known. Fibronectin is depleted from the surface of cells undergoing mitosis or malignant transformation.[21] The possible mechanisms are decrease in synthesis and secretion, proteolytic degradation, or both. The regulatory linkages of the fibronectin gene[22] with general and sex-specific genes guiding testicular differentiation are tempting challenges for future research.

The formation of the basement membrane around the new testicular cords as an initially interrupted layer of its components is in agreement with observations in other organ systems.[23] The appearance of different antigenically active components of the basement membrane before a continuous lamina is seen at the ultrastructural level suggests that the final membrane is assembled in the extracellular space from complete component molecules.

Subsequent events in the developing rat testis are completion of the basement membrane around the cords at the age of 14 to 15 days (FIGURES 4–6), growth of the cords in thickness and length, and disconnection of the continuity with the surface epithelium. The latter event is specific for the male sex and apparently involves selective proteolysis of basement membrane adjacent to the surface epithelium.

In view of the H-Y theory of testicular differentiation and the accumulated information obtained by different serological methods,[5] there is a lack of direct evidence from the actual histological formation of the testicular cords. After the basic analysis of the extracellular matrix and the differentiating testicular cords, we wanted to establish a simplified *in vitro* model for testicular differentiation in a chemically defined environment.

FIGURE 3. Developing testis of rat fetus (age 13.5 days). Laminin is localized as black deposits in the basement membrane of the surface epithelium (SE) and around irregular cell cords (C) inside the gonadal ridge. The method was the same as in FIGURE 2. Scale 380:1.
FIGURE 4. Developing testis of rat fetus (age 15.5 days). Laminin is localized as black deposits in the basement membranes of the testicular cords (C), the surface epithelium (SE), and the vascular wall (V). The method was the same as in FIGURE 2. MT, mesonephric tubule. Scale 140:1.

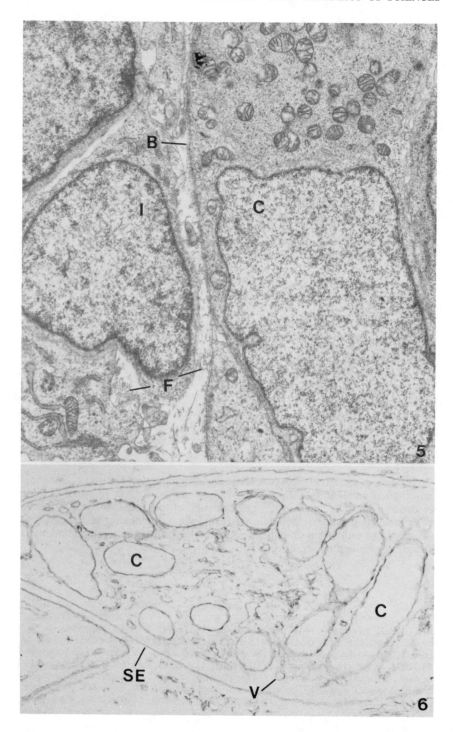

DIFFERENTIATION *IN VITRO*

Organ culture experiments aiming at the sexual differentiation of the male gonad have produced important, but sometimes controversial information about the process in different species. In the rat, serum has been shown to inhibit testicular cord formation in culture, whereas in a serum-free medium the cords developed like those *in vivo*.[13,14] In the mouse, mesonephric tissue inhibited testicular differentiation *in vitro* in one experiment[16] but failed to do so in another similar system.[15]

We set out to test whether the gonadal explants differentiated in a defined medium without serum would be suitable models for testicular differentiation. Our results confirmed the reported inhibition of cords by serum,[14] and in a serum-free medium the cords organized like those *in vivo* (FIGURE 7). Light and electron microscopic analysis revealed that the cultured cords consisted of fetal Sertoli cells and were surrounded by a basal lamina and some peritubular cells (FIGURE 8). Morphologically the cords in culture were similar to those developed *in vivo*.[2]

A new dimension to the culture system was opened when dissociated immature rat testis cells were found to form tubular aggregates when plated in high density.[17] Separated 20-day-old rat Sertoli and myoid cells cultured together also formed nodules resembling seminiferous tubules.[18] Reaggregation experiments of testicular cells in rotation culture have given promising results when analyzed in paraffin sections with a light microscope.[19,20]

The enzymes used to dissociate the cells degrade the extracellular matrix and apparently modify the cell surface components. This treatment brings the cells down to a very primitive stage and during the subsequent culture period they have to reconstitute both their matrices and the surface molecules before they are able to reorganize histotypic structures. These properties make dissociation-reaggregation experiments very useful for differentiation experiments because the different stages of reorganization can be monitored by morphological and immunocytochemical methods without disturbing the tissue organization.

For our purposes as described before we dissociated newborn rat testes and cultured the total suspension in a serum-free medium for four days (FIGURE 9). The formed reaggregates were found to contain several cords that were histologically similar to those in the original newborn testis (FIGURE 9). Electron microscopic analysis revealed typical Sertoli cells inside the cords, a basal lamina, and flattened myoid-like cells around the cord (FIGURE 10). Even at the ultrastructural level the cords in the reaggregates were similar to those in the intact neonatal testis and in the cultured explants. There results indicate that dispersed newborn testis cells separated from their extracellular matrix are able to maintain their positional information and reconstitute the proper extracellular matrix as well as cellular relations. The reaggregation of newborn testis in culture resembles closely the differentiation of the embryonic testis *in vivo*.[2]

FIGURE 5. Developing testis of rat fetus (age 16.5 days). Electron micrograph of testicular cord (C) and interstitium (I) interface. The basal lamina (B) of the cord is continuous and collagen fibers (F) have appeared in the extracellular space. Method was the same as in FIGURE 1. Scale 9,000:1.

FIGURE 6. Developing testis of rat fetus (age 17.5 days). Type IV collagen was localized in the basement membrane of the surface epithelium (SE), the testicular cords (C), and vascular wall (V). The method was the same as in FIGURE 2. Scale 130:1.

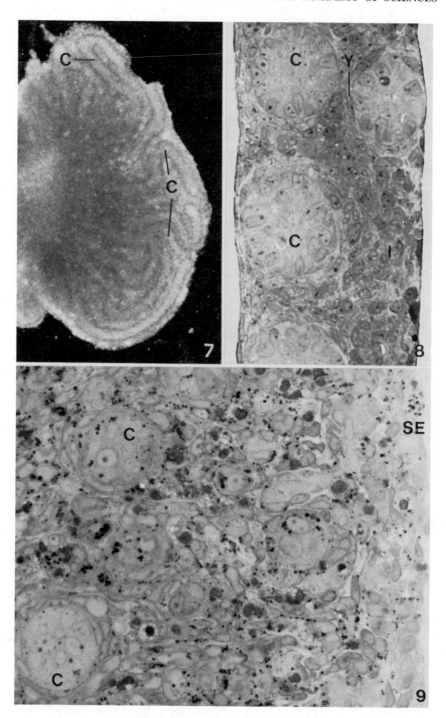

CONCLUDING REMARKS

The present experiments have shown that the analysis of developing gonads at three different levels of initial organization: the normal gonad *in vivo*, gonadal explants, and dissociated gonadal cells *in vitro* provides a useful model of testicular differentiation. The effects of different regulatory factors on matrix synthesis and organization can be tested at various defined stages of testicular differentiation and this should bring us one step closer to the final understanding of the regulatory mechanisms involved.

ACKNOWLEDGMENTS

The skillful contributions of Mrs. Raija Andersen, Mrs. Sirpa From, Mrs. Marja Huhtinen, Mr. Mauno Lehtimäki, and Mr. Urpo Reunanen in laboratory and secretarial work are gratefully acknowledged. The authors thank Dr. Jennie P. Mather for practical advice and many helpful discussions about the culture techniques.

FIGURE 7. Developing male gonad of rat fetus (age 13.5 days, compare FIGURES 1–3) cultured for 5 days. A survey dark-field light micrograph of the gonad after culture shows the loop-like testicular cords (C). The gonadal ridge with mesonephros was cultured on agar-coated metal grid in a petri dish with medium 199 + glutamine (100 mg/l). Scale 70:1.

FIGURE 8. Developing male gonad of rat fetus (age 13.5 days) cultured for 5 days. Same specimen as in FIGURE 7. Light micrograph of an epon section after testicular differentiation for 5 days in culture. The cylindrical testicular cords (C) are clearly delineated from the interstitium (I) and surrounded by some developing myoid cells (Y). The specimen was prepared as in FIGURE 1. Scale 430:1.

FIGURE 9. Newborn rat testis reaggregate after culture of separated single cells for 4 days. The surface epithelium (SE) is flat and testicular cords (C) have reorganized. The testis was dissociated into single cells with collagenase-dispase and filtered through a tissue sieve (pore-size 10 μm). Cells were cultured on a grid in a petri dish with minimum essential medium (Eagle) with Earle's salts and L-glutamine. Scale 510:1.

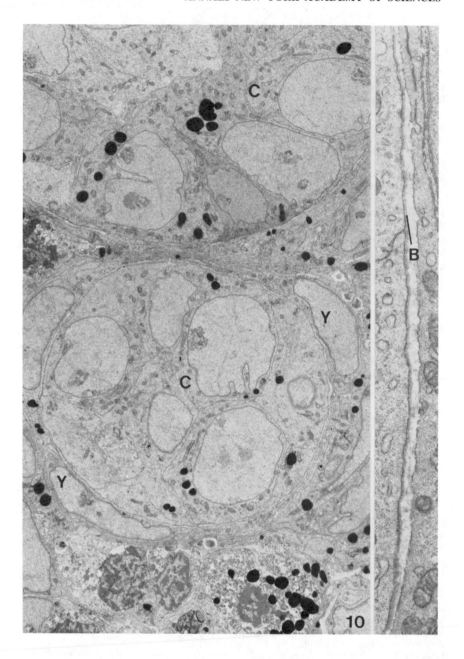

REFERENCES

1. PELLINIEMI, L. J. & L. LAUTEALA. 1981. Development of sexual dimorphism in the embryonic gonad. Hum. Genet. **58:** 64–67.
2. PARANKO, J., L. J. PELLINIEMI, A. VAHERI, J-M. FOIDART & T. LAKKALA-PARANKO. 1983. Morphogenesis and fibronectin in sexual differentiation of rat embryonic gonads. Differentiation **23** (Suppl.): S72–S81.
3. PELLINIEMI, L. J. 1976. Ultrastructure of the indifferent gonad in male and female pig embryos. Tissue Cell **8:** 163–174.
4. WACHTEL, S. S., S. OHNO, G. C. KOO & E. A. BOYSE. 1975. Possible role for H-Y antigen in the primary determination of sex. Nature **257:** 235–236.
5. WACHTEL, S. S. 1983. H-Y antigen and the biology of sex determination. Grune & Stratton, Inc. New York
6. RUOSLAHTI, E., E. ENGVALL & E. G. HAYMAN. 1981. Fibronectin: current concepts of its structure and functions. Collagen Res. **1:** 95–128.
7. WARTIOVAARA, J., I. LEIVO & A. VAHERI. 1979. Expression of the cell surface-associated glycoprotein, fibronectin, in the early mouse embryo. Dev. Biol. **69:** 247–257.
8. RISTELI, L. & J. RISTELI. 1981. Basement membrane research. Med. Biol. **59:** 185–189.
9. BANERJEE, S. D., R. H. COHN & M. R. BERNFIELD. 1977. Basal lamina of embryonic salivary epithelia. Production by the epithelium and role in maintaining lobular morphology. J. Cell Biol. **73:** 445–463.
10. EKBLOM, P. 1981. Deterination and differentiation of the nephron. Med. Biol. **59:** 139–160.
11. SMITH, R. L. & M. BERNFIELD. 1982. Mesenchyme cells degrade epithelial basal lamina glycosaminoglycan. Dev. Biol. **94:** 378–390.
12. HAY, E. D. 1981. Extracellular matrix. J. Cell Biol. **91:** 205–223.
13. MAGRE, S. & A. JOST. 1980. The initial phases of testicular organogenesis in the rat. An electron microscopy study. Arch. d'Anat. Microsc. **69:** 297–318.
14. JOST, A., S. MAGRE & R. AGELOPOULOU. 1981. Early stages of testicular differentiation in the rat. Hum. Genet. **58:** 59–63.
15. TAKETO, T. & S. S. KOIDE. 1981. In vitro development of testis and ovary from indifferent fetal mouse gonads. Dev. Biol. **84:** 61–66.
16. BYSKOV, A. G. & J. GRINSTED. 1981. Feminizing effect of mesonephros on cultured differentiating mouse gonads and ducts. Science **212:** 817–818.
17. ERICKSON, L. A., J. C. DAVIS, P. R. BURTON & J. SNYDER. 1980. Correlative light and electron microscopy of dissociated immature rat testicular cells undergoing morphogenesis in vitro. J. Embryol. Exp. Morph. **60:** 283–293.
18. TUNG, P. S. & I. B. FRITZ. 1980. Interactions of Sertoli cells with myoid cells in vitro. Biol. Reprod. **23:** 207–217.
19. ZENZES, M. T. & W. ENGEL. 1981. The capacity of testicular cells of the postnatal rat to reorganize into histotypic structures. Differentiation **20:** 157–161.
20. MÜLLER, U. & E. URBAN. 1981. Reaggregation of rat gonadal cells in vitro: experiments on the function of H-Y antigen. Cytogenet. Cell Genet. **31:** 104–107.
21. YAMADA, K. M. & K. OLDEN. 1978. Fibronectins—adhesive glycoproteins of cell surface and blood. Nature **275:** 179–184.

FIGURE 10. Newborn rat testis reaggregate after culture of separated cells for 4 days. Electron micrograph of reorganized testicular cords (C) and developing myoid cells (Y) around the cords. The inset shows the cord-interstitial interface with a basal lamina (B) and flocculent extracellular material. The culture was performed as in FIGURE 9 and the specimen was prepared as in FIGURE 1. Scale 3300:1, inset 11,000:1.

22. ZARDI, L., M. CIANFRIGLIA, E. BALZA, B. CARNEMOLLA, A. SIRI & C. M. CROCE. 1982. Species-specific monoclonal antibodies in the assignment of the gene for human fibronectin to chromosome 2. EMBO (European Molecular Biology Organization) J. **1:** 929–933.
23. EKBLOM, P., K. ALITALO, A. VAHERI, R. TIMPL & L. SAXEN. 1980. Induction of a basement membrane glycoprotein in embryonic kidney: possible role of laminin in morphogenesis. Proc. Natl. Acad. Sci. USA **77:** 485–489.

Effect of Substrate on the Shape of Sertoli Cells *in Vitro*[a]

CARLOS A. SUÁREZ-QUIAN,[b] MARK A. HADLEY, and
MARTIN DYM

Georgetown University
School of Medicine-School of Dentistry
Washington, D.C. 20007

INTRODUCTION

The importance of the extracellular matrix (ECM) as an essential component of normal cellular function has been recognized only recently. ECM is composed of three basic classes of compounds: collagen molecules; other glycoproteins, including fibronectin and laminin; and glycosaminoglycans.[1,2] At present, five genetically distinct types of collagen molecules have been characterized based on their biochemical and antigenic properties. Labeled I to V, each collagen type is generally associated with certain classes of tissue.[1,2] For example, type I collagen is a component of skin, bone, tendon, and cornea, whereas type IV collagen comprises the lamina densa of typical endothelial and epithelial basal laminae. In all likelihood, the diversity of collagen molecules and their segregation into different microenvironments suggest a specialization in collagen molecules to facilitate their interaction with diverse cell types. In turn, this interaction may regulate cellular activity.

The metabolic activity of cultured cells varies with cell shape. In fact, it has been proposed that normal *in vitro* cell growth requires a delicate balance between cell-cell contact and between cells and substrate.[3] The effect of a collagen substrate in influencing the biochemical activity and shape of cells *in vitro* is amply documented. Liver parenchyma cells cultured on collagen-coated plates or floating collagen membranes, mimicked morphological and metabolic features of *in vivo* cells.[4] In response to lactogenic hormones, mammary epithelial cells plated

[a] This research was supported by National Institutes of Health supported by Grant #HD16260 and by a Mellon Foundation grant. This work was submitted in partial fulfillment for the Ph.D. degree at Harvard University by CASQ.

[b] Present Address: National Institute of Child Health, Cell Biology, and Metabolism Branch, Bldg. 10, Room 9N-204, Bethesda, MD.

417

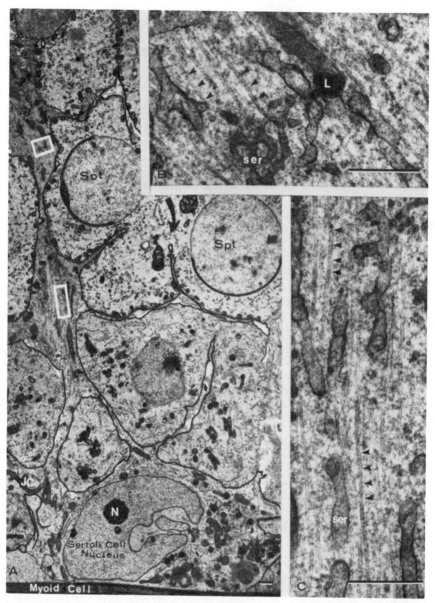

FIGURE 1. (A) Profile of a Sertoli cell sectioned along its longitudinal axis. The plasma membrane has been artificially darkened to demarcate its boundary. Note lateral processes embracing round spermatids (Spt). Cytoplasmic bridges between spermatids resulting from incomplete cytokinesis are indicated by curved arrows. A junctional complex (JC) between adjacent Sertoli cells is labeled. Bar = 1.0 μm. (B and C) Enlarged views of the two rectangles contained in the Sertoli "trunk" portion of (A). Both images have been mounted

onto floating collagen membranes acquire ultrastructural and biochemical characteristics reminiscent of cells *in vivo*.[5] Cultures of human epidermal keratinocytes on collagen-coated plastic surfaces or on a collagen gel, reassemble into a stratified epithelium.[6] Moreover, avian corneal fibroblasts and flattened gerbil fibroma fibroblasts generate a typical bipolar morphology when grown in hydrated collagen gels.[7]

In the case of epithelial cells, laminin and collagen are capable of influencing adhesion and cell shape.[1,8-10] Laminin is secreted only by epithelial cells and does not exhibit any affinity for fibroblasts.[2,8] In the presence of laminin, epithelial cells *in vitro* express a certain polarity with respect to their basal and apical surfaces comparable to the polarity exhibited by *in vivo* cells.[11]

The cytoskeleton of epithelial cells appears disorganized when cells are dissociated from their basal lamina.[9] Addition of soluble ECM components reorganizes the cytoplasmic fibers of epithelial cells. Similar results have been obtained in primary cultures of hepatocytes plated onto collagen gels.[12] These results may explain the enhanced biochemical activity of cells grown on collagen, since the cytoskeleton has been implicated in protein synthesis.[13,14]

Sertoli cells have been successfully cultured for some time on plastic or type I collagen, but their morphology does not closely resemble the *in vivo* cell. Various attempts to improve the morphology and secretion of biological markers have involved altering the composition of nutrients in the culture medium. In particular, Sertoli cells have been successfully cultured in serum-free media.[15] Recent attempts have included co-culture of Sertoli cells with peritubular myoid cells from testes. In this case, the Sertoli cells display a less flattened morphology and an enhanced rate and duration of androgen-binding protein (ABP) secretion.[16] A similar study confirmed the stimulatory effects of the myoid cells on ABP secretion, but showed that conditioned media from monocultures of these same myoid cells did not contain this stimulatory effect.[17] Moreover, in parabiotic cultures, where myoid and Sertoli do not come in contact with each other, ABP secretion was not enhanced.[18] Careful inspection of electron micrographs published by Tung and Fritz[16] revealed a well-developed ECM. Consequently, the effects of native components of Sertoli cell basal lamina, type IV collagen, and laminin, were assessed as to their effect on the morphology of *in vitro* cells.

MATERIALS AND METHODS

Culture of Sertoli cells and preparation for electron microscopy was carried out as described previously[19] but with the following modifications: (1) collagen type I, rat tail collagen (Collaborative Research, Inc., Waltham, MA), was dissolved in 0.1 M acetic acid, applied (10 $\mu g/cm^2$) to plastic coverslips, and sterilized overnight under UV light; (2) collagen type IV and laminin, previously character-

---

such that they remain in register with the base of the Sertoli cell in (A). Smooth endoplasmic reticulum (ser) and lipochrome granules (L) are labeled. Microtubules are indicated by arrowheads. Note that the microtubules are aligned perpendicularly to the base of the seminiferous tubule. (B and C) Bar = 0.5 μm.

ized,[20] were gifts of Dr. Hynda Kleinman (NIH; Dental Inst.–LDBA; Bethesda, MD 20205): (3) type IV collagen (10 μg/cm^2) was applied to coverslips and laminin (100 μg/ml) was added to the settled collagen on the coverslips. Tannic acid fixative for cytoskeleton was as follows: 2 mM MgSO$_4$, 50 mM MgCl, 0.01% saponin, 0.1% tannic acid, 3.0% glutaraldehyde in 0.1 M sodium phosphate, pH 7.0.

RESULTS

In vivo the Sertoli cell has been described as an irregularly columnar cell that extends from the base of the seminiferous tubule to the tubule lumen (FIGURE 1). The base of the Sertoli cell rests on a typical basement membrane and the basal cytoplasm, adjacent to the plasma membrane, contains numerous cytoskeletal elements, including microtubules, intermediate filaments, and a cortical mat of f-actin. Generally, the Sertoli cell nuclei adopt one of two configurations: tall and slender (or almost pyramidal) with the base resting on the lamina propria or flattened against the basement membrane. Thus the polarity of the longitudinal axis of the nucleus compared to its parallel axis length varies from cell to cell. The supranuclear cytoplasm, considered the "trunk" of the Sertoli cell, sends out lateral processes that engulf developing germ cells. Within the supranuclear cytoplasm numerous microtubules are generally found that are oriented perpendicularly to the base of the seminiferous tubule. In fact, based on its morphology, the Sertoli cell "trunk" portion has been likened to a neuronal axon and may serve both a support and transport function.[21]

Profiles of Sertoli cells *in vitro* plated onto plastic or collagen type I substrates, cultured from 16-day-old rat pups, are shown in FIGURE 2. The morphology of *in vitro* Sertoli cells may be discerned following sectioning of cells either perpendicularly or horizontally to the plane of the substrate. Characteristic Sertoli cell features are noted in both: nuclear infoldings are clearly visible, the nuclear density is that exhibited by euchromatin in plastic 1 μm sections, and favorable profiles display only one nucleolus within each nuclei. In sections cut parallel to the substrate, large numbers of cells are illustrated and show that only one cell type is present. Myoid cells and fibroblasts were found infrequently in such sections. The typical morphology of Sertoli cells *in vivo*, however, is not maintained in the cultured state. *In vivo*, the Sertoli cell supranuclear cytoplasm extends 80 μm or more towards the seminiferous tubule lumen. In Sertoli cells *in vitro* plated onto collagen type I, on the other hand, the supranuclear region is almost totally absent. Further, *in vitro* Sertoli cells sectioned perpendicularly to the substrate fail to display any polarity with respect to the nuclei.

Low power electron micrographs of cultured Sertoli cells, cut perpendicularly or horizontally to the plane of growth are shown in FIGURE 3. Typical Sertoli cell characteristics exhibited by cultured cells include the following: nuclei contain mainly euchromatin, only one nucleolus is present, and inter-Sertoli junctional complexes are revealed. Mitochondria are similar in configuration and matrix density to those of *in vivo* Sertoli cells. In addition, germ cells remain attached to the Sertoli cell; apparently, lateral processes, presumed to grasp germ cells during their differentiation *in situ*, are sometimes maintained by Sertoli cells *in vitro*. Additional Sertoli cell properties illustrated by cells *in vitro* include a dispersed Golgi, various organelles exhibiting differential densities, assumed to be lysoso-

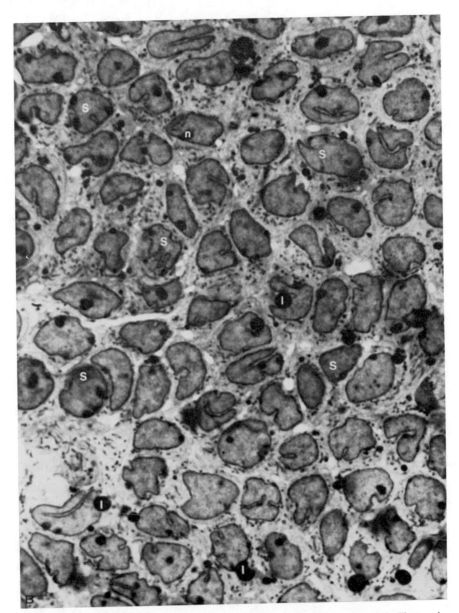

FIGURE 2. (A) Sertoli cells sectioned perpendicularly to their plane of growth. Flattened, Sertoli cell nuclei (S) and a large lipid granule (l) are labeled. Arrow points to processes extending from the apical surface of Sertoli cells. A germ cell (G) is shown. Asterisk indicates empty space occupied by media bathing the cells. Magnification = 1,100×. (B) Sertoli cells sectioned parallel to their plane of growth. Irregularly shaped nuclei (S), nucleoli (n), and lipid granules (l) are indicated. Magnification = 1,100×.

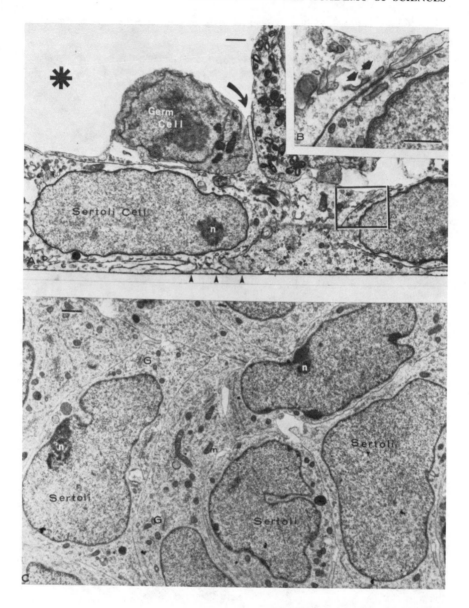

mal in character, and rough and smooth endoplasmic reticulum. Also, the reticular network of the singular nucleolus and few peripheral clumps of heterochromatin in the nuclei is maintained (FIGURE 3).

Although cells *in vitro* may be identified as Sertoli cells, it is readily apparent that little if any polarity of cytoplasmic organelles remains. The inter-Sertoli junction, for example, is situated in the apical cytoplasm, not the basal portion. Presumed lateral processes, recognized to intertwine between germ cells, extend apically. In short, it appears as though the Sertoli cells fell onto their lateral borders during the *in vitro* studies.

Tannic acid fixation was used to enhance the visualization of cytoplasmic filaments in cultured Sertoli cells. Cortical bundles of filaments close to the plasma membrane, however, are not common features of Sertoli cells *in vitro* plated onto collagen type I. Furthermore, unlike Sertoli cells *in vivo,* juxtanuclear microtubules of Sertoli cells *in vitro* do not appear perpendicular to the plane of growth (FIGURE 4). In sections of *in vitro* Sertoli cells cut perpendicular to the substrate, microtubules are aligned parallel to the substrate (FIGURE 4, A–C). In sections cut parallel to the plane of the substrate, microtubules are seen randomly aligned within the plane of section (FIGURE 4, D and E). Further, examination of the supranuclear cytoplasm of *in vitro* Sertoli cells failed to reveal the presence of microtubules to the extent that they appear in Sertoli cells *in vivo.*

The height of *in vitro* Sertoli cells varies depending on the type of substrate used to plate the cells. A comparison between *in vitro* Sertoli cells grown on different collagen substrates as discerned at the resolution provided by the light microscope is shown in FIGURE 5. Two features are immediately obvious: the height of Sertoli cells is greater when plated onto type IV collagen and laminin and nuclei appear oriented with their longer axis perpendicular to the plane of growth. In addition, germ cells appear to remain more viable in primary cultures of Sertoli cells plated onto collagen type IV and laminin (data not shown).

Not all Sertoli cells, however, form a monolayer when plated onto components of their natural substrate. Often, Sertoli cell aggregates form that resemble a cryptorchid testes (FIGURE 5). Within the clump, Sertoli cells retain their characteristic morphology, but their *in vivo* orientation no longer exists.

Ultrastructural studies of Sertoli cells plated onto collagen type IV plus laminin are presented in FIGURES 6–9. In all instances, Sertoli cells were sectioned perpendicularly to their plane of growth, thin sections were transferred to Formvar-coated slotted grids and examined with the electron microscope.

FIGURE 3. (A) Sertoli cells sectioned perpendicularly to their plane of growth. Asterisk indicates empty space occupied by media bathing the cells. Arrowheads point to collagen type I substrate. Nucleolus (n), contained within flattened Sertoli cell nucleus, is labeled. Curved arrow points to a presumed lateral process. Bar = 1.0 μm. (B) Enlarged view of rectangle in (A). Thick arrows point to an inter-Sertoli junctional complex located near apical surface. Bar = 0.5 μm. (C) Sertoli cells sectioned parallel to their plane of growth. Irregularly shaped nuclei, nucleolus (n), Golgi (G), and mitochondria (M) are labeled. Bar = 1.0 μm.

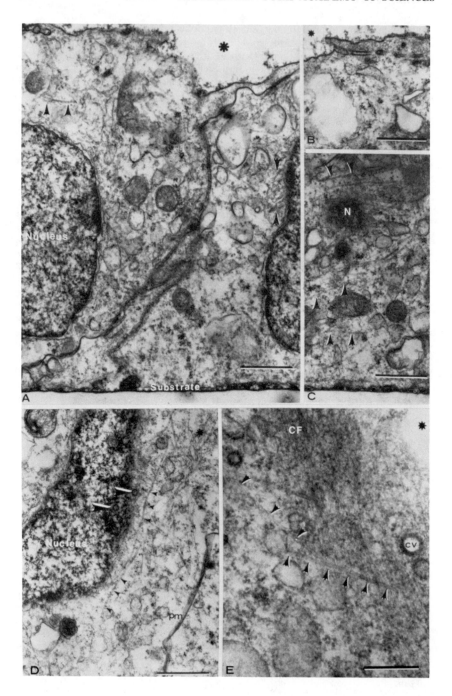

Sertoli cells plated onto collagen type IV plus laminin resemble more closely their *in vivo* counterparts. For example, the supranuclear cytoplasm extends apically and is greater in length than in Sertoli cells plated onto collagen type I or plastic (compare FIGURE 7 with FIGURE 3). Further, Sertoli cells resting on the collagen type IV plus laminin substrate often maintain a perpendicularly oriented nucleus, even if the supranuclear cytoplasm resides within a cell aggregate and is not exposed to the media (FIGURES 7 and 9).

Cytoplasmic organelles of cultured Sertoli cells plated onto collagen type IV plus laminin display a certain polarity reminiscent of *in vivo* Sertoli cells. The supranuclear cytoplasm, for example, contains areas rich in Golgi and smooth endoplasmic reticulum. Also, mitochondria appear more elongated and oriented in groups in the supranuclear cytoplasm (FIGURE 7, A).

Ultrastructural studies of Sertoli cell cytoskeleton plated onto collagen type IV plus laminin revealed that microtubules within the supranuclear cytoplasm appeared aligned close to the longitudinal axis of the cell (FIGURES 7–9). Often, several microtubules were noted coursing perpendicularly to the plane of growth. This microtubule orientation is similar to the orientation displayed by microtubules of Sertoli cells *in vivo*. Further, a cortical mat of filaments, subjacent to the plasma membrane, was discerned in the basal cytoplasm.

DISCUSSION

These results clearly illustrate that the substrates used to culture Sertoli cells affect their shape. Sertoli cells grew well on either rat tail collagen or collagen type IV plus laminin. However, Sertoli cells *in vitro* resembled the morphology of their *in vivo* counterparts most closely when plated onto type IV collagen plus laminin (constituents of native basal laminae). Sertoli cells were much taller, the nuclei displayed a polarity (horizontal versus perpendicular), and the microtubules inhabited the supranuclear cytoplasm in a fashion akin to the *in vivo* situation. Although the data are not shown, laminin plus collagen type I had the same effect on Sertoli cell shape as collagen type I alone. These results concur with previous investigations that suggest the organization of the cytoskeleton of epithelial cells is dependent on laminin and collagen.[9,10] And, in particular, laminin interaction with basal lamina requires the presence of type IV collagen, not type I.[1]

FIGURE 4. The cytoskeleton of Sertoli cells as maintained with tannic acid fixation (see MATERIALS AND METHODS for further details) is shown in (A–E). (A–C) Sertoli cells sectioned perpendicularly to plane of growth. Collagen type I substrate is labeled. Asterisk indicates empty space occupied by media bathing cells. Black-on-white arrowheads point to microtubules lying parallel to the plane of the substrate. (D and E) Cells sectioned parallel to their plane of growth. (D) Shows a tangentially sectioned nucleus. Black-on-white arrowheads point to nuclear pores cut in cross section. Small arrowheads point to microtubules and asterisk shows area of intermediate filaments. Plasma membrane (pm) is labeled. (C) shows cortical cytoplasm of a Sertoli cell. Cortical filaments (CF) and coated vesicle (CV) are illustrated. Microtubules are indicated by black-on-white arrowheads. Asterisk marks empty space occupied by media. (A–E) Bar = 0.5 μm.

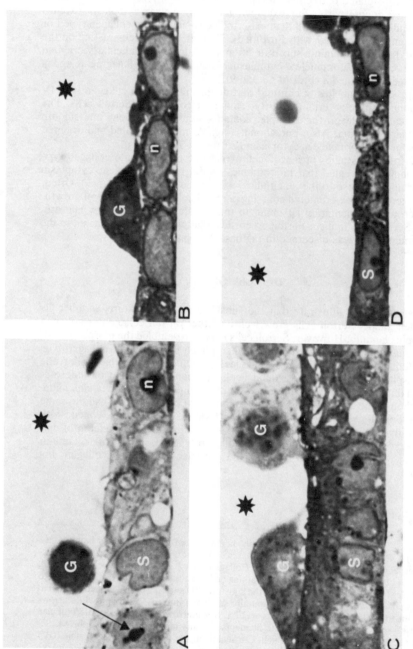

FIGURE 5. (A–D) Profiles of cultured Sertoli cells sectioned perpendicularly to their plane of growth. (A and C) Sertoli cells plated onto collagen type IV plus laminin and cultured for either three or five days, respectively. (B and D) Sertoli cells plated onto collagen type I. Note that Sertoli cell nuclei (S), containing a single nucleolus (n), remain oriented perpendicularly to the substrate in (A) and (C), but have become flattened in (B) and (D). Germ cells (G) are generally more numerous in Sertoli cell primary cultures plated onto type IV collagen and laminin. Asterisks mark empty space occupied by media. Arrow in (A) points to a class tripartite nucleolus. (A–D) Magnification = 1,100×.

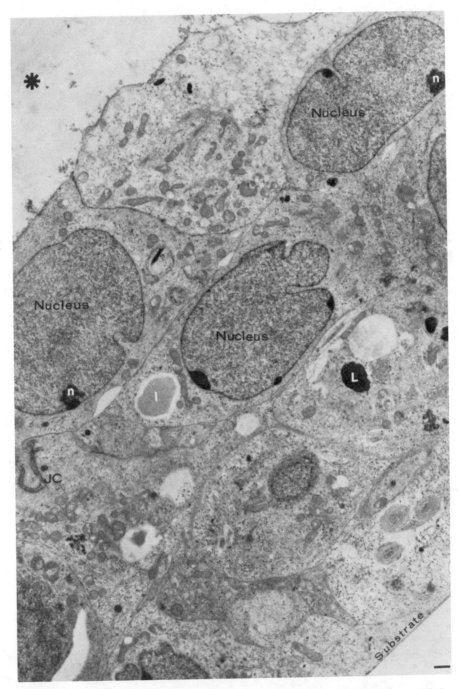

FIGURE 6. An aggregate of Sertoli cells after five days in culture, resembling the stratified epithelium morphology of a cryptorchid testes, is shown. Note, however, that peripheral heterochromatin clumps are scarce. The amorphous collagen type IV plus laminin substrate is illustrated. Lipochrome bodies (L), lipid granules (l), and junctional complexes are labeled. Asterisk marks empty space occupied by media. Bar = 1.0 μm.

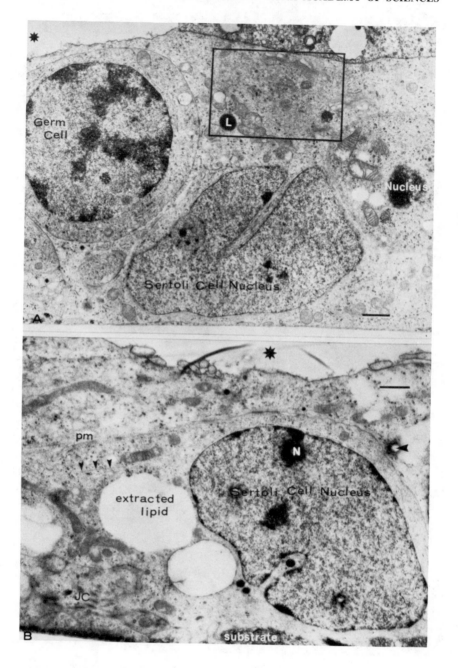

Sertoli cells *in vitro* plated onto type IV collagen plus laminin orient their cytoplasmic organelles into a more polarized state. *In vivo,* the orientation of Sertoli cell nuclei varies during different stages of the cycle of the seminiferous epithelium: approximately 50% of nuclei throughout the cycle will exhibit a perpendicular orientation.[22] Sertoli cells grown *in vitro* and plated onto type I collagen, however, rarely exhibit a nuclear orientation perpendicular to the substrate. Sertoli cells plated onto collagen type IV plus laminin, on the other hand, often revealed nuclei oriented perpendicularly to the substrate.

The presence of a cortical mat of filaments subjacent to the plasma membrane was also noted when Sertoli cells were plated onto collagen type IV plus laminin. Further, the supranuclear cytoplasm of Sertoli cells plated onto collagen type IV plus laminin was generally filled with Golgi, microtubules, and various membrane-bound vesicles. In particular, the microtubules contained in the Sertoli cell "trunk" resemble the *in vivo* situation.

Epithelial cells *in vivo* rest on a basal lamina composed of collagen type IV, glycoproteins, and glycosaminoglycans.[1,2] The basal lamina provides the means by which *in vivo* epithelial cells anchor to a substrate.[10] Part of the anchorage is presumably mediated via a high molecular weight glycoprotein, laminin, that acts as a link between the collagen molecules and the basal plasma membrane.[1,8] Furthermore, a carpet of cortical filaments is found in the basal cytoplasm of epithelial cells subjacent to the plasma membrane. Although the mechanism of interaction between the cortical filaments and the basal cytoplasm is still uncertain, one can speculate that the appearance of a basal cortical bundle of filaments in association with a basal lamina is a prerequisite to normal cell function.

Sertoli cells *in vivo* are not unlike other epithelial cells in that they rest on a typical basal lamina and exhibit a cortical mat of filaments subjacent to the basal plasma membrane.[21,23] Further, the supranuclear cytoplasm contains numerous microtubules aligned perpendicularly to the lamina propria of the seminiferous tubules.[24] From the supranuclear cytoplasm (the "trunk" portion of the Sertoli cell), lateral processes of cytoplasm project outwards to engulf germ cells. Undoubtedly, the shape of the Sertoli cell *in vivo,* and consequently its height, are mediated by the cytoskeleton, including the supranuclear microtubules. However, it seems likely that the germ cells, embedded within the "trunk" region and

FIGURE 7. (A) Sertoli cell, plated onto collagen type IV plus laminin, sectioned perpendicularly to its plane of growth and having its apical surface exposed to the media (asterisk) is shown. Note that the nucleus is not flattened and that the cell contains a cytoplasmic "trunk" portion with projecting lateral processes engulfing a germ cell. A tangentially sectioned Sertoli cell nucleus is also shown. An enlarged view of the enclosed rectangle is shown in FIGURE 8 (A). Bar = 1.0 μm. (B) An image of a Sertoli cell nucleus maintaining a perpendicular polarity with the substrate. Cell has been sectioned perpendicularly to its plane of growth. The plasma membrane (pm) does not appear to reach the apical surface exposed to the media (asterisk). Internalized junctional complexes and extracted lipid are labeled. Small arrowheads point to microtubules coursing along the longitudinal axis of the Sertoli cell cytoplasmic "trunk" portion. Large arrowhead indicates hole in Formvar plastic used to prepare cells for electron microscopy examination. Bar = 1.0 μm.

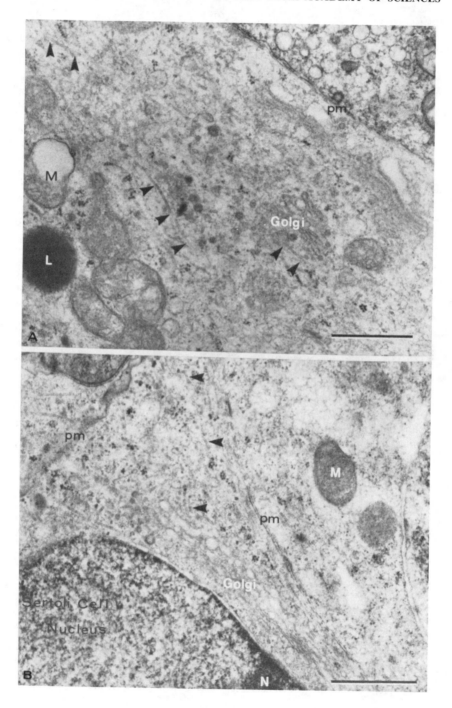

the lateral processes of the Sertoli cells, generate a reciprocal action on the sustentacular cells, providing an additional support on the lateral borders. This latter point may explain why Sertoli cells *in vitro,* even if plated onto type IV collagen plus laminin, do not obtain the optimum height of Sertoli cells *in vivo.*

Together, however, the supranuclear cytoskeleton and the reciprocal support provided by germ cells do not appear sufficient to maintain the normal morphological appearance of the Sertoli cells *in vivo.* For example, a thickening of the basal lamina is a common feature in damaged testes. In these instances, ultrastructural studies have revealed that the Sertoli cell cytoskeleton is modified considerably.[25,26] In particular, the cortical bundle of filaments in the basal cytoplasm disappears. In turn, the morphology of Sertoli cells is dramatically altered. Based on the results presented in this investigation, it is suggested that modification of basal lamina constituents by disease, in particular the interaction of laminin with collagen type IV, will affect Sertoli cell function severely. Further, it is shown for the first time that the substrate used to prepare primary cultures is a prerequisite in the normal expression of Sertoli cell structure and that the structure may be maintained by microtubules.

The results presented in this study are intriguing and may belie previous biochemical studies obtained from Sertoli cells plated onto plastic substrates. In this regard it becomes important to note that ABP secretion by Sertoli cells *in vitro* is enhanced when Sertoli cells are plated onto myoid cells.[16] In this case, the morphology of *in vitro* cells resembles more closely the appearance of Sertoli cells *in vivo.* Presumably, this enhanced resemblance is mediated by the cytoskeleton. Similar results in other cell types have suggested that protein synthesis appears to require a normal cytoskeleton.[13,14] Therefore, biochemical data generated by Sertoli cells plated onto artificial substrates should be re-examined.

FIGURE 8. (A) Enlarged view of rectangle in FIGURE 7 (A). The plasma membrane (pm), mitochondria (m), lipid granule (L), and Golgi are labeled. Arrowheads point to microtubules. Note that the polarity of the microtubules runs along the longitudinal plane of the Sertoli cell cytoplasmic "trunk" portion (compare with FIGURE 7 A). Bar = 1.0 μm. (B) Image of a Sertoli cell supranuclear cytoplasm and the beginning of the "trunk" portion. The limiting plasma membrane (pm) is labeled. Note the abundance of Golgi profiles. Arrowheads point to microtubules oriented along the longitudinal axis of the Sertoli cell. Bar = 1.0 μm.

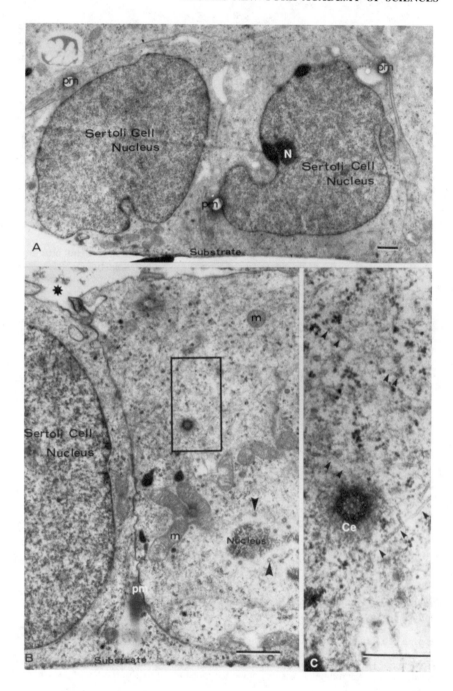

REFERENCES

1. KLEINMAN, H. K., R. J. KLEBE & G. R. MARTIN. 1981. Role of collagenous matrices in the adhesion and growth of cells. J. Cell Biol. **88:** 473–485.
2. HAY, E. D. 1982. Interaction of embryonic cell surface and cytoskeleton with extracellular matrix. Am. J. Anat. **165:** 1–12.
3. FOLKMAN, J. & A. MOSCONA. 1978. Role of cell shape in growth control. Nature **273:** 345–349.
4. MICHALOPOULOS, G. & H. C. PITOT. 1975. Primary culture of parenchymal liver cells on collagen membranes. Exp. Cell Res. **94:** 70–78.
5. EMERMAN, J. T., J. ENAMI, D. R. PITELKA & S. NANDI. 1977. Hormonal effects on intracellular and secreted casein in cultures of mouse mammary epithelial cells on floating collagen membranes. Proc. Natl. Acad. Sci. USA **74:** 4466–4470.
6. LIU, S.-C. & M. KARASEK. 1978. Isolation and growth of adult human epidermal keratinocytes in cell culture. J. Invest. Dermatol. **71:** 157–162.
7. TOMASEK, J. J., E. D. HAY & K. FUJIWARA. 1982. Collagen modulates cell shape and cytoskeleton of embryonic corneal and fibroma fibroblast distribution of actin, actinin, and myosin. Dev. Biol. **92:** 107–122.
8. TERRANOVA, V. P., D. H. ROHRBACH & G. R. MARTIN. 1980. Role of laminin in the attachment of PAM 212 (Epithelial) cells to basement membrane. Cell **22:** 719–726.
9. SUGRUE, S. P. & E. D. HAY. 1981. Response of basal epithelial cell surface and cytoskeleton to solubilized extracellular matrix molecules. J. Cell Biol. **91:** 45–54.
10. SUGRUE, S. P. & E. D. HAY. 1982. Interaction of embryonic corneal epithelium with exogenous collagen, laminin, and fibronectin. Role of endogenous protein synthesis. Dev. Biol. **92:** 97–106.
11. HAY, E. D. 1982. Collagen and embryonic development. *In* Cell Biology of Extracellular Matrix. E. D. Hay, Ed.: 379–409. Plenum Press. New York.
12. SATTLER, C. A., G. MICHALOPOULOS, G. L. SATTLER & H. C. PITOT. 1978. Ultrastructure of adult rat hepatocytes cultured on floating collagen membranes. Cancer Res. **38:** 1539–1549.
13. LENK, R., L. RANSON, Y. KAUFMAN & S. PENMAN. 1977. A cytoskeletal structure with associated polyribosomes obtained from HeLa cells. Cell **10:** 67–78.
14. FULTON, A. B., K. M. WAN & S. PENMAN. 1980. The spatial distribution of polyribosome in 3T3 cells and the associated assembly of proteins into the skeletal framework. Cell **20:** 849–857.
15. MATHER, J. P. & G. H. SATO. 1979. The growth of mouse melanoma cells in hormone supplemented serum-free medium. Exp. Cell Res. **120:** 191–200.
16. TUNG, P. S. & I. B. FRITZ. 1980. Interaction of Sertoli cells with myoid cells *in vitro*. Biol. Reprod. **23:** 207–217.
17. HUTSON, J. C. & D. STOCCO. 1981. Peritubular cell influence on the efficiency of androgen-binding protein secretion by Sertoli cells in culture. Endocrinology **108:** 1362–1368.

FIGURE 9. (A) Image of two adjoining Sertoli cells in an aggregate, sectioned perpendicularly to the plane of growth, whose nuclei are oriented perpendicularly to the substrate. The plasma membrane (pm) delineates the boundary of the two cells. Bar = 1.0 μm. (B) Image of two adjoining Sertoli cells sectioned perpendicularly to the plane of growth. The amorphous substrate is labeled and the asterisk marks the apical free surface of the cells. The intervening plasma membrane (pm) and typical mitochondria (m) are illustrated. Arrowheads point to cross sections of nuclear pores from a tangentially sectioned nucleus. Enlarged view of rectangle is shown in (C). Bar = 1.0 μm. (C) Profile of a centriole (Ce) cut in cross section. Microtubules closely aligned perpendicularly to the plane of growth are marked by small arrowheads. Bar = 0.5 μm.

18. HUTSON, J. C. 1983. Metabolic cooperation between Sertoli cells and peritubular cells in culture. Endocrinology **112:** 1375–1381.

19. SUÁREZ-QUIAN, C. A., M. DYM, A. MAKRIS, J. BRUMBAUGH, K. J. RYAN & J. A. CANICK. 1983. Estrogen synthesis by immature rat Sertoli cells *in vitro*. J. Androl. **4:** 203–209.

20. KLEINMAN, H. K., M. L. MCGARVEY, L. A. LIOTTA, P. G. ROBEY, K. TRYGGVASON & G. R. MARTIN. 1982. Isolation and characterization of type IV procollagen, laminin, and heparan sulfate proteoglycans from EHS sarcoma. Biochemistry **21:** 6188–6193.

21. FAWCETT, D W. 1975. Ultrastructure and function of the Sertoli cell. *In* Handb. Physiol. **5:** 21–55.

22. LEBLOND, C. P. & Y. CLERMONT. 1952. Definition of the stages of the cycle of the seminiferous epithelium in the rat. Ann. N.Y. Acad. Sci. **55:** 548–572.

23. DYM, M. & J. C. CAVICCHIA. 1978. Functional morphology of the testis. Biol. Reprod. **18:** 1–15.

24. CHRISTENSEN, A. K. 1965. Microtubules in Sertoli cells of guinea pig testis. Anat. Rec. **151:** 335.

25. CHEMES, H. E., M. DYM, D. W. FAWCETT, N. JAVADPOUR & R. J. SHERINS. 1977. Pathophysiological observations of Sertoli cells in patients with germinal aplasia or severe germ cell depletion. Ultrastructural findings and hormone levels. Biol. Reprod. **17:** 108–123.

26. KERR, J. B., K. A. RICH & D. M. DE KRETSER. 1979. Effects of experimental cryptorchidism on the ultrastructure and function of the Sertoli cell and peritubular tissue of the rat testis. Biol. Reprod. **21:** 823–838.

Cooperativity between Sertoli Cells and Peritubular Myoid Cells in the Formation of the Basal Lamina in the Seminiferous Tubule

PIERRE S. TUNG, MICHAEL K. SKINNER, and
IRVING B. FRITZ

Banting and Best Department of Medical Science
University of Toronto
Toronto M5G 1L4, Canada

INTRODUCTION

When Sertoli cell–enriched aggregates are plated on top of a layer of peritubular myoid cells, the properties of each of the two cell types are very different from those observed in cells in monoculture. In the co-cultured system, both cell populations survive for months in a serum-free medium. In contrast, peritubular myoid cells in monoculture detach from the plate within days when they are plated in the absence of serum, and primary cultures of Sertoli cells do not remain functional beyond three weeks. In the co-cultured system, Sertoli cells and peritubular cells interact, undergoing a morphological rearrangement to form a structure resembling the seminiferous tubule, and a basement membrane is laid down between the two cell types.[1] In addition, the production of androgen binding protein (ABP) by Sertoli cells is enhanced in the presence of peritubular cells, and ABP formation is maintained for longer periods in the co-cultured system.[1,2]

It appeared possible that separate extracellular matrix (ECM) components synthesized by Sertoli cells and peritubular myoid cells in co-culture may interact to permit the formation of a basement membrane that cannot be elaborated by either cell type alone. We offer the speculation that cooperativity between Sertoli and peritubular cells may be required for the synthesis of all ECM components needed for basal lamina organization and formation. In initial attempts to examine these possibilities, we have investigated the synthesis of specific ECM components by each cell type. In addition, we have explored the effects of various ECM components on the histotype of Sertoli cells and peritubular cells maintained in monoculture. Results to be presented demonstrate that the two cell types secrete different ECM components, and that the nature of the substratum upon which the cells are cultured greatly influences the histotype expressed.

MATERIALS AND METHODS

Procedures for the preparation and culture of conventional rat Sertoli cell–enriched aggregates,[3,4] of hyaluronidase-treated purified Sertoli cell–enriched aggregates,[5] and of primary and secondary cultures of peritubular cells[1,4] were the same as those previously described. All cells were maintained and cultured in Eagle's modified essential minimal medium (MEM), containing either no serum or 10% calf serum, (GIBCO, Grand Island, NY) as specified in the legends to figures. All cells were prepared from testes of 20-day-old Wistar rats unless specified otherwise.

We employed fluorescent microscopic procedures for the localization of laminin or fibronectin by indirect immunofluorescent techniques, using the same procedures as those described elsewhere.[5,6] Antisera employed included rabbit antiserum against laminin, kindly provided by Drs. George Martin and Hynda Kleinman (National Institutes of Health, Bethesda, MD); goat antiserum directed against human or rat fibronectin, purchased from Calbiochem (La Jolla, CA); and a mouse monoclonal IgG directed against porcine fibronectin, kindly provided by Dr. J. Aubin (University of Toronto, Toronto, Canada). Bulk adsorption techniques with lyophilized laminin and fibronectin were performed as described elsewhere,[5] and morphological techniques were the same as those previously employed.[5,7,8]

Techniques for the culture of cells on various substrata, including seminiferous tubule biomatrix (ST-matrix), were the same as those recently described.[9]

RESULTS

Detection of Fibronectin and Laminin in Peritubular Boundary Tissue

We employed indirect immunofluorescent microscopy to localize fibronectin and laminin in cryostat sections of testes from 20-day-old rats. Experiments with antisera to these glycoproteins revealed that fibronectin and laminin were each distributed primarily in or along the basal lamina of the seminiferous tubule boundary tissue (FIGURE 1). Neither of these ECM components was detectable within the luminal compartment. Antibodies against fibronectin and laminin preadsorbed with fibronectin or laminin, respectively, did not react. In contrast, fibronectin antibody preadsorbed with laminin, or laminin antibody preadsorbed with fibronectin, retained full activity (data not shown).

Fibronectin is Detectable in Cultures of Peritubular Cells but not in Cultures of Sertoli Cells

Peritubular myoid cells in culture for 24 hr or longer have a positive reaction to fibronectin antibodies, whereas purified populations of Sertoli cells do not.[5] The nature of the fibronectin localization depends upon the culture conditions, with a fibrillar-like extracellular arrangement in preparations cultured in the presence of serum, and predominantly a perinuclear distribution in peritubular cells cultured in serum-free medium for four days (see FIGURES 2 and 3 of Tung *et al.*[5]). Primary cultures of peritubular cells show occasional areas free of fibronectin antibody-reactive material (FIGURE 2 A,B), associated with the inclusion of a few Sertoli cell aggregates in the preparation. In contrast, almost all peritubular cells in secondary cultures are positive for fibronectin (FIGURE 2 C and D).

To extend these observations obtained with indirect immunofluorescent microscopy, we have investigated the synthesis of fibronectin by cells cultured in medium containing [^{35}S]methionine. Proteins immunoprecipitated with fibronec-

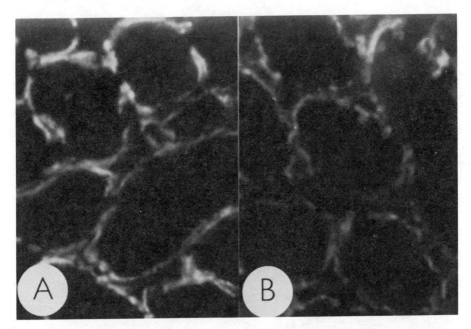

FIGURE 1. Immunofluorescent micrographs of cryostat sections of testis from a 20-day-old rat. (A) A section initially reacted with goat antiserum against human fibronectin (1 : 20), and then with FITC-conjugated rabbit anti-goat IgG (1 : 30 with PBS). (B) A section initially reacted with rabbit antiserum against laminin (1 : 10), followed by incubation with FITC-conjugated goat-anti-rabbit IgG (1 : 30). Immunofluorescence was not detected with antisera previously adsorbed with fibronectin or laminin, respectively (data not shown). (300 ×).

tin antibodies were subjected to slab gel electrophoresis. The gels were then fluorographed or they were stained with Coomassie blue. Peritubular cells secreted a labeled protein, immunoprecipitated with a fibronectin antibody, that had a molecular mass (220,000) indistinguishable from that of authentic fibronectin (FIGURE 3). In contrast, a protein having these characteristics was not detectable in secretions from Sertoli cell–enriched aggregates that had been treated with hyaluronidase (FIGURE 3).

Conventional Sertoli cell–enriched aggregates not treated with hyaluronidase during the isolation procedure are contaminated by peritubular cells (7.6 ± 0.9%). These cells readily proliferate when cultured in the presence of 10% calf serum unless an inhibitor of DNA synthesis is added.[10] After four days in medium containing serum but no inhibitor, the percentage of peritubular cells in conventional Sertoli cell–enriched aggregates increases to 23 ± 1.7%.[5] This is correlated with the presence of fibronectin in conventional Sertoli cell preparations, which are cultured in medium containing 10% calf serum (FIGURE 4 A and C). We have used the detectability of fibronectin as a criterion for improving procedures for isolating Sertoli cell–enriched aggregates free of containing peritubular cells, and have observed that treatment with hyaluronidase diminishes the number of peritubular cells in the preparation. Such purified Sertoli cell preparations have no

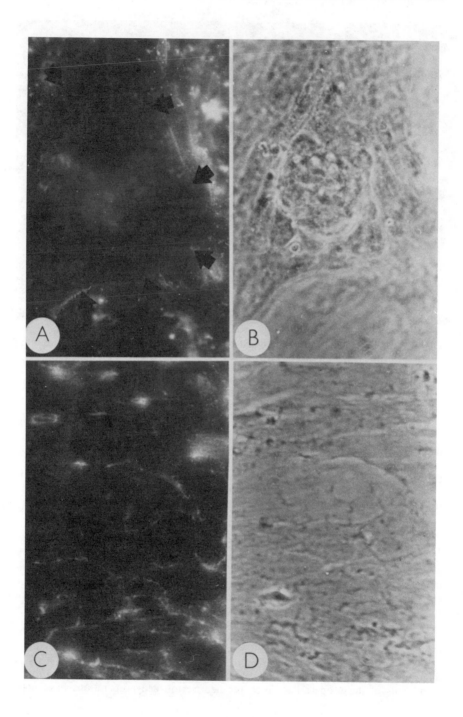

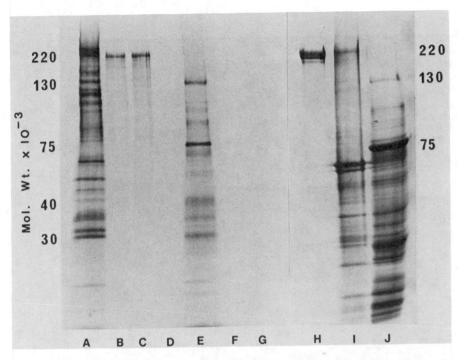

FIGURE 3. Electrophoretic analysis of radiolabeled proteins synthesized by cultures of Sertoli or peritubular cells, and immunoprecipitation by fibronectin antibody. An SDS 5 to 15% polyacrylamide gradient slab gel was either stained with Coomassie blue (lanes H to J), or radiolabeled proteins were fluorographed (lanes A through G). The fluorograph lanes are (A) peritubular cell–secreted radiolabeled proteins, (B) goat anti-rat fibronectin immunoprecipitate of peritubular cell–secreted proteins; (C) mouse anti-pig fibronectin immunoprecipitate; (D) control non-immune serum immunoprecipitates of peritubular cell–secreted proteins; (E) Sertoli cell–secreted proteins; (F) goat anti-rat fibronectin immunoprecipitate of Sertoli cell–secreted proteins; and (G) control non-immune immunoprecipitate of Sertoli cell–secreted proteins. (From Tung *et al.*[5] With protein lanes are: (H) rat fibronectin, (I) peritubular cell–secreted proteins; and (J) Sertoli cell–secreted proteins. (From Tung *et al.*[5] With permission from *Biology of Reproduction*.)

FIGURE 2. Immunofluorescent micrographs (A and C) and phase-contrast micrographs (B and D) of representative fields of primary peritubular cell cultures (A and B) and secondary cultures (C and D). The primary culture (A,B) had been maintained on glass coverslips in modified MEM containing 10% calf serum for 6 days. Cells were then fixed (3% paraformaldehyde in Ca^{2+}- and Mg^{2+}-free Hanks' buffer for 20 min at room temperature, followed by immersion in acetone at $-10°C$ for 7 min) and reacted with goat antiserum against fibronectin (1 : 25). Arrows in (A) point to a fibronectin-negative area associated with unidentified cell contaminants, possibly Sertoli cells. The secondary culture (C,D) had been prepared by plating trypsinized primary cultures of peritubular cells onto glass coverslips, and then treating these cells (after maintenance for 6 days in culture) in a manner identical to that described above for cells in primary culture. (750 ×).

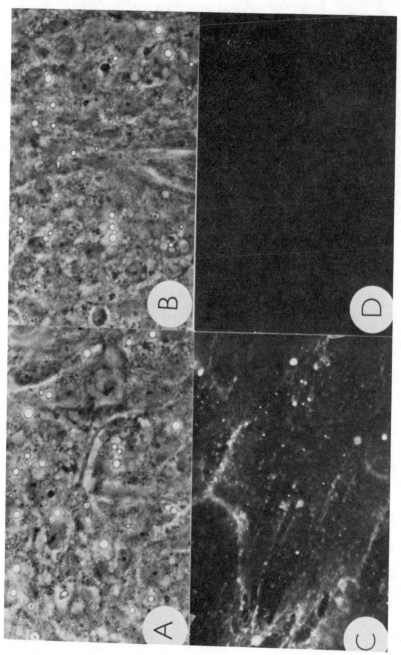

FIGURE 4. Phase-contrast micrographs (A,B) and immunofluorescent micrographs (C,D) of confluent cultures of Sertoli cells. (A) and (C) show a representative field of a dense culture (1,500 aggregates/100 mm²) from a conventional Sertoli cell–enriched preparation not subjected to hyaluronidase treatment. (B) and (D) show a representative field of a comparably dense culture from a purified Sertoli cell–enriched preparation that had previously been digested with hyaluronidase, as described in METHODS. All cells had been cultured for 6 days in modified MEM containing 10% calf serum, fixed, and reacted with fibronectin antiserum as described in the legends to FIGURES 1 and 2. Similar observations have been made in cells plated at lower density (200 aggregates/100 mm²). (750 ×). (From Tung *et al.*[5] With permission from *Biology of Reproduction*.)

detectable fibronectin, even when cultured for four days in medium containing 10% calf serum (FIGURE 4 B and D), and the number of microscopically recognizable peritubular cells is less than 1%.[5]

These data demonstrate that fibronectin is a suitable marker for the presence of peritubular cells in testicular cell cultures. Determination of rates of fibronectin synthesis may be expected to provide a more quantitative measure of the degree of contamination of Sertoli cell–enriched preparations by peritubular cells.

Laminin is Detectable in Cultures of Sertoli Cells but not in Cultures of Peritubular Cells

Newly isolated aggregates of conventional or purified Sertoli cell–enriched preparations did not initially react with laminin antiserum (data not shown). Shortly after conventional Sertoli cell–enriched aggregates attached to the polystyrene surface (3 to 4 hr after plating), cells within the aggregate began to migrate, frequently assuming a fibroblast-like appearance as they spread beyond the initial aggregates. These rapidly migrating cells failed to show any reaction to laminin antibodies. In contrast, cells within the aggregate reacted positively with laminin antibodies. The strongest reactions appeared in cells around the periphery of the aggregates (FIGURE 5 A and C). The location of fluorescence in the indirect immunofluorescent microscopic assay for laminin precisely followed the shape of the colonies of aggregated Sertoli cells, and this remained evident in purified Sertoli cell–enriched preparations maintained in culture for periods up to 14 days (data not shown). Peritubular cell preparations in culture did not react with laminin antibodies (FIGURE B and D). Laminin was undetectable in peritubular or interstitial cells maintained in culture for periods up to 10 days.

Seminiferous Tubule Biomatrix Promotes Rat Sertoli Cell Histotypic Expression in Vitro

We have investigated the possible effects of altering the substratum upon which Sertoli cell–enriched preparations are plated on the properties of these cells in culture. Various substrata examined included uncoated polystyrene, polystyrene coated with seminiferous tubule biomatrix (ST-biomatrix), and polystyrene coated with Type I collagen or polylysine. Sertoli cells maintained their normal *in vivo* histotype best when cultured on the ST-biomatrix (FIGURES 6 and 7). The most striking differences consisted of the taller columnar-shaped appearance of Sertoli cells maintained on ST-biomatrix. These cells had an average height of 8.7 μM, whereas Sertoli cells cultured on uncoated plastic for 6 days under otherwise comparable conditions had an average thickness of only 2 μm (FIGURE 6). In addition, basolateral tight junctions were maintained in cells in culture on the ST-biomatrix but not on the other substrata employed (FIGURES 6 and 7). The percentage of cells surviving at 21 days after plating was increased from about 25% of cells plated on polylysine-coated polystyrene to 80% of cells plated on ST-biomatrix.[9]

Peritubular cells cultured on each of these substrata in MEM containing 10% calf serum readily spread to form monolayers. We are currently investigating the differences in morphology of peritubular cells maintained on ST-biomatrix, Type I collagen, or uncoated plastic (Tung and Fritz[9] and unpublished observations).

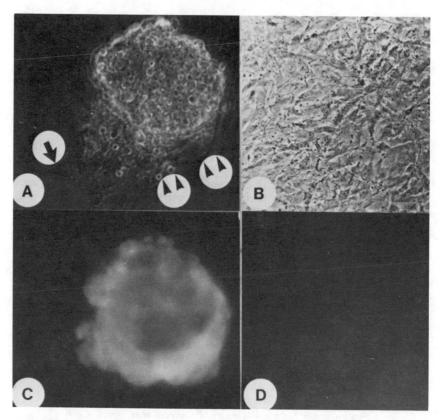

FIGURE 5. Phase-contrast micrographs (A,B) and immunofluorescent micrographs (C,D) of Sertoli cell–enriched preparations (A,C) and peritubular cells (B,D) reacted with rabbit antiserum against laminin (1 : 15). (A) and (C) show a representative aggregate of a conventional Sertoli cell–enriched preparation maintained for 6 hr in modified MEM containing 10% calf serum. The preparation was fixed 6 hr after plating and incubated with laminin antiserum. Note that only the fibroblast-like cells in (A) (arrows) that have migrated away from the Sertoli cell aggregate are negative for laminin-dependent immunofluorescence (C). (B) and (D) show a representative portion of a primary culture of peritubular cells maintained for 6 days in modified MEM containing 10% calf serum, and demonstrate the absence of laminin-dependent immunofluorescence in peritubular cells (D). Sertoli cells at the periphery of the aggregate (C) have strongest reactions with laminin antibody. (350 × figure reduction, 70%).

DISCUSSION

Data presented indicate that fibronectin and laminin are distributed primarily in or along the basal lamina of the seminiferous tubule (FIGURE 1), and that these ECM components are most probably derived from different cell types. Sertoli cells in culture synthesize laminin but not fibronectin, while peritubular cells in culture produce fibronectin but not laminin (FIGURES 2–5). In experiments in progress, we have observed other differences between the two cell types with respect to the

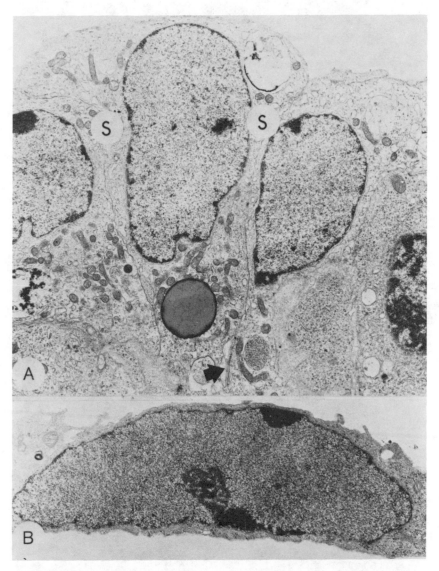

FIGURE 6. Transmission electron micrographs of vertical sections of Sertoli cells prepared from testes of 20-day-old rats, and maintained for 6 days in serum-free MEM. In (A), the substratum for the cells was ST-biomatrix, and in (B) the substratum was uncoated polystyrene. Note taller cell shape of cells cultured on ST-biomatrix (average thickness of 8.7 μm) than of cells cultured on plastic (average thickness of 2.0 μm) S represents adjacent Sertoli cells, and the arrow indicates junctional complex in basolateral region ($\times$ 18,400, figure reduction, 95%). (From Tung & Fritz.[9] With permission from *Biology of Reproduction*.)

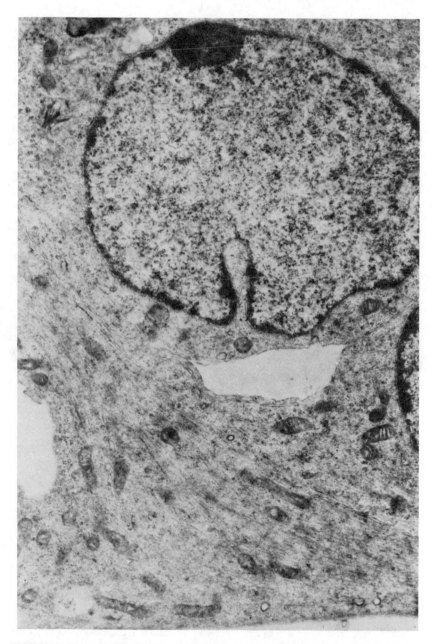

FIGURE 7. Transmission electron micrograph of a vertical section of Sertoli cells prepared from testes of 20-day-old rats, and maintained for 6 days in serum-free MEM. Note presence of abundant microtubules and microfibrils, oriented vertically ($\times$ 19,600, figure reduction, 95%).

nature of ECM components synthesized. For example, each of the two cell types synthesize proteoglycans, but the nature of the proteoglycans is different (Skinner and Fritz, in preparation). The proteoglycans formed by Sertoli cells in culture are of different molecular mass than those synthesized by peritubular cells. We think it highly probable that the formation of the basement membrane that takes place in co-cultures of Sertoli cells and peritubular cells[1] is dependent upon contributions of different ECM components by each cell type. The physiological significance of these interactions in basal lamina formation and maintenance *in vivo* remains to be determined. The data, however, are consonant with the speculation that the basal lamina of the seminiferous tubule boundary tissue is deposited as a consequence of cooperativity between Sertoli cells and peritubular cells.

Hyaluronidase treatment of Sertoli cell–enriched aggregates greatly diminishes the number of contaminating peritubular cells in the preparation. Addition of this step to the isolation procedure permits the culture of purified populations of Sertoli cell aggregates in medium containing 10% calf serum without the overgrowth of peritubular cells that otherwise would occur.[5,9] Some of the proteins reported to be synthesized by conventional preparations of Sertoli cell–enriched preparations cultured in the presence of serum could have been produced by peritubular cells. The synthesis of fibronectin provides a suitable marker to evaluate this possibility.

The functions of the basal lamina in the seminiferous tubule are not established. It provides a structural support that separates the basal surfaces of Sertoli cells from adjacent peritubular cells, but it may also have other functions. The normal *in vivo* histotype of Sertoli cells is remarkably well maintained in cells plated on seminiferous tubule biomatrix as substratum. Sertoli cell aggregates plated on this substratum retain a cuboidal to columnar shape, with numerous and complex surface projections. They manifest a normal polarity as indicated by the presence of tight junctional complexes in the basolateral regions; and they have an abundance of microtubules and microfibrils in vertical bundles perpendicular to the basal surface of the columnar cells (Tung and Fritz,[9] and FIGURES 6 and 7). The ST-biomatrix was observed to be superior to other substrata examined (uncoated polystyrene or polystyrene coated with Type I collagen or polylysine) in maintaining the unique histotypic features of Sertoli cells.[9] These data suggest that the seminiferous tubule basal lamina may play an important role in orienting the structure of Sertoli cells, and thereby indirectly influencing the architecture of the seminiferous tubule. Further studies are in progress to determine factors that modulate the synthesis of specific ECM components by each cell type and to evaluate the control of the deposition of ECM components during the *in vitro* formation of the basal lamina–like structure. We are evaluating the hypothesis that Sertoli cells and peritubular cells act synergistically to generate the basal lamina of the seminiferous tubule.

REFERENCES

1. TUNG, P. S. & I. B. FRITZ. 1980. Biol Reprod. **23:** 207–217.
2. HUTSON, J. C. & C. M. STOCCO. 1981. Endocrinology **108:** 1362–1368.
3. DORRINGTON, J. H., N. F. ROLLER & I. B. FRITZ. 1975. Molec. Cell Endocrinol. **3:** 57–70.
4. TUNG, P. S. & I. B. FRITZ. 1977. Isolation and culture of testicular cells. A morphological characterization. *In* Techniques of Human Andrology. E. S. E. Hafez, Ed.: 125–146. Elsevier/North Holland Biochem. Amsterdam.

5. TUNG, P. S., M. K. SKINNER & I. B. FRITZ. 1984. Biol. Reprod. **30:** 199–211.
6. TUNG, P. S. & I. B. FRITZ. 1978. Dev. Biol. **64:** 297–315.
7. TUNG, P. S., J. H. DORRINGTON & I. B. FRITZ. 1975. Proc. Natl. Acad. Sci. USA **72:** 1838–1842.
8. TUNG, P. S., E. Y. C. LIN & I. B. FRITZ. 1976. A scanning electron microscopic study of cultured cells prepared from rat seminiferous tubules. *In* Scanning Electron Microscopy, Part VI. Proceedings of the Workshop on SEM in Reproductive Biology IIT Res. Inst. pp. 417–424.
9. TUNG, P. S. & I. B. FRITZ. 1984. Biol. Reprod. **30:** 213–229.
10. TUNG, P. S., M. LACROIX & I. B. FRITZ. 1980. Biol. Reprod. **22:** 1255–1261.

Therapeutic Considerations and Results of Gonadotropin Treatment in Male Hypogonadotropic Hypogonadism

HENRY G. BURGER and H. W. G. BAKER

Medical Research Centre
Department of Endocrinology
Prince Henry's Hospital, Melbourne
Howard Florey Institute of Experimental
Physiology and Medicine
University of Melbourne
Victoria, Australia

INTRODUCTION

Patients with hypogonadotropic hypogonadism (HH) may be classified into several etiological groups, as shown in TABLE 1, the major distinction being made by whether the deficiency had its onset before or after puberty. The miscellaneous group includes patients with apparently partial gonadotropin deficiency. Prepubertal gonadotropin deficiency is termed Kallmann's syndrome if clinical evidence of a disordered sense of smell is present, and is termed idiopathic in the absence of such evidence and of any other causes. Gonadotropin deficiency may be of varying degrees of severity, although absolute measurement of the degree has proved difficult, due in part to the relatively poor discrimination of gonadotropin assays at the lower end of the normal male ranges. The deficiency may involve FSH and/or LH, and may result from a primary disorder of the gonadotroph or from a deficiency of gonadotropin-releasing hormone (GnRH). We have observed a high frequency of patients of Mediterranean origin (11 of 17) among those with idiopathic HH (TABLE 2).

HORMONAL MANAGEMENT OF DEFICIENT VIRILIZATION

The choice of therapy to induce and/or maintain virilization and normal sexual functioning lies between gonadotropin and androgen.

Human chorionic gonadotropin (hCG) is now recognized to have a relatively prolonged effect on plasma testosterone and can often be given conveniently in a once-weekly dosage schedule. We have evidence[1,2] that, in normal men, 3,000 IU by intramuscular injection gives a maximal testosterone response, seen at 72–96 hours, and sustained for 6–7 days. A similar response has been reported in HH.[2] However, occasional patients require a twice-weekly regimen in order to maintain normal testosterone levels. There is no consensus as to the indications to use hCG in prepubertal HH. However, because the injection can be given in a mixture with growth hormone, it is the treatment of choice in inducing puberty in patients with combined growth hormone and gonadotropin deficiency. Our current practice is to commence hCG in low dosage (500 IU weekly) at age 12–13 years in such patients, in order to maximize synergism between growth hormone and androgen.

447

TABLE 1. Etiologic Classification of Hypogonadotropic Hypogonadism

I.	Pre-pubertal gonadotropin deficiency
	Idiopathic
	Isolated
	With other deficiencies
	Associated with anosmia or hyposmia
	Organic, e.g. post-trauma, craniopharyngioma,
	chromophobe adenoma, granuloma etc.
II.	Post-pubertal gonadotropin deficiency
	Idiopathic
	Organic
III.	Miscellaneous varieties difficult to classify

Testosterone may be given orally, by intramuscular injection of long-lasting esters, or by implant. Until recently, oral testosterone, in the form of 17-alkylated derivatives, was not favored because of lack of efficacy and concern about cholestatic jaundice. Recently, a lipophilic ester, testosterone undecanoate, has become available for oral use, and does not carry risks to hepatic function as it is not 17-alkylated. We have found it to provide satisfactory virilization in a group of 21 hypogonadal men, 5 of whom had HH. In a daily dose of 160 mg, mean plasma testosterone levels in the latter were increased from 3.0 to 6.9 nmol/l ($p < 0.05$), while dihydrotestosterone rose from 0.54 to 1.82 nmol/l ($p < 0.01$).

Long-acting testosterone esters have been widely and successfully used to induce virilization. However, the injections are sometimes painful and beard growth is often less than what is desired by the patient. Testosterone implants have been used relatively infrequently.

Our previous data[3] suggest that induction of puberty with exogenous testosterone does not impair subsequent stimulation of spermatogenesis.

HORMONAL TREATMENT OF INFERTILITY

Any consideration of the hormonal management of HH must take account of the uncertainty that surrounds the precise roles of FSH, LH, and testosterone in the

TABLE 2. Ethnic Characteristics of Hypogonadotropic Hypogonadism[a]

Classification	Number	Mediterranean[b]	Anglo-Saxon
Prepubertal deficiency			
Idiopathic			
Isolated	6	6	0
Multiple	2	1	1
Kallmann's	7	3	4
Organic	—	—	—
Post-pubertal deficiency (idiopathic)	1	1	0
Miscellaneous	1	0	1
Total	17	11	6

[a] Only patients seen by the Melbourne group.

[b] This group represented approximately 6.8% of the population of Victoria in the 1981 census. (Birthplace: Italy 2.9%, Greece 1.8%, Yugoslavia 1.5%, Lebanon 0.4%, Turkey 0.2%).

initiation and maintenance of spermatogenesis. Data have been presented suggesting that spermatogenesis, suppressed by testosterone administration to normal men, can be qualitatively restored with hCG,[4] whilst FSH also produces this effect.[5] Furthermore, Marshall et al.[6] have shown that in stalk-sectioned rhesus monkeys, testosterone was capable of restimulating spermatogenesis. It could be expected that results of therapy in men with HH could therefore be conflicting with regard to the effects of FSH, LH, and testosterone.

GONADOTROPINS

Although HH is one of the few specifically treatable forms of male infertility, results of therapy fall well short of the ideal. TABLES 3 and 4 summarize data

TABLE 3. Results of Therapy for Infertility: Hypogonadotropic Hypogonadism[a]

Classification	Number	Number with at Least One Pregnancy	Sperm Production— No Pregnancy	Failure to Induce Sperm Production	Incomplete Data
I. Prepubertal deficiency					
Idiopathic					
Isolated	23	10	2	5	6
With other deficiencies	2	1	0	0	1
Kallmann's	11	1	1	4	5
Organic	1	0	0	1	0
Subtotal	37	12 (32%)	3	10	12
II. Post-pubertal deficiency					
Idiopathic	6	4	1	0	1
Organic	11	5	3	0	3
Subtotal	17	9 (53%)	4	0	4
III. Miscellaneous	8	6	1	0	1
Total	62	27 (44%)	8	10	17

[a] Data by courtesy of the Human Pituitary Advisory Committee, Australian Commonwealth Department of Health, Canberra. Analyzed September, 1983.

obtained by courtesy of the Human Pituitary Advisory Committee, Australian Commonwealth Department of Health, to which applications are made for the use of hCG and/or human pituitary gonadotropin (hPG, a clinical grade mixture of FSH and LH, ampuled in fractions of a pituitary gland equivalent, and ranging in potency from 130 to 300 IU FSH and 100 to 500 IU LH per pituitary). Local practice has been to give hCG, in doses of 1,500–3,000 IU once to twice weekly for an initial four- to six-month period. Failure to observe sperm in the ejaculate or severe oligospermia (< 1 million sperm/ml) persisting despite more prolonged hCG has been the indication to add hPG. The variety of dosage schedules used over the past 15 years renders conclusions about the required dose of FSH difficult, but the majority of patients successfully treated have required the equivalent of one to two pituitaries three times per week, giving a total dose of 400 to 1,800

IU FSH, 300 to 3,000 IU LH, plus 3,000 to 9,000 IU hCG per week. Some post-pubertal HH patients have responded to 0.5 pituitaries three times per week (200–400 IU FSH per week). Adequacy of dosage has been monitored by regular testosterone measurements, measurements of testicular volume with an orchido-meter, and semen analyses at one to two month intervals. Changes in dosage have usually been performed at three to six month intervals.

For patients with prepubertal HH, 12 of 25 for whom data are complete, have impregnated their wives, whilst 10 others failed to produce sperm, and three produced no pregnancy, although sperm appeared in the ejaculate. This indicates only an approximately 50% successful treatment rate. All these patients in whom treatment has been completed required both hCG and hPG, although one patient achieved low sperm numbers on hCG alone.

The ten subjects treated with hCG and hPG for 6–28 (mean 13.5) months who failed to produce sperm in their ejaculate had diagnoses as follows: Kallmann's syndrome (4), idiopathic HH (5), and prepubertal hypopituitarism from chromophobe adenoma (1). Other features in this group that may have been adverse were previous bilateral undescended testes and varicocele, unilateral ectopic testis, and varicocele and past unilateral acute epididymitis in three of the patients with Kallmann's syndrome. The fourth was aged 40 and at the start of treatment had

TABLE 4. Results of Therapy: Completed Courses of Gonadotropins

Classification	Number	Number Successfully Treated	Failed Therapy[a]
Prepubertal HH	25	12	13
Post-pubertal HH	13	9	4
Miscellaneous	7	6	1
Total	45	27	18

[a] No sperm output or no pregnancy.

tiny testes (0.5 and 1 ml). Poor testosterone responses (maximal serum concentrations 7.3 and 10.9 nmol/l) were seen in two subjects, but the others had normal adult male testosterone levels and clinical virilization. The most notable feature of this group was the small increase in testicular volume during treatment in most subjects. Eight patients with pretreatment mean testicular volumes between 1 and 5 ml had maximal testicular volumes between 3 and 10 ml (mean 6 ml), whereas our 6 successfully treated patients had mean maximum testicular volumes between 10 and 21 ml (mean 15 ml). The patient with the chromophobe adenoma had an increase in testicular volume during 9 months of treatment from 5 to 20 ml. There was no record of testicular volume for the tenth patient. Testicular biopsies were performed during treatment in five patients and showed hypospermatogenesis in three, mixed germ cell aplasia and arrest at primary spermatocyte stage in one, and germ cell arrest at the secondary spermatocyte stage in another. Three of these men had pretreatment testicular biopsies showing immature testis. The patient with the chromophobe adenoma had been treated previously with hCG and menopausal gonadotropins and sperm appeared in his ejaculate in low numbers (less than 2 million/ml); a biopsy performed some time after this treatment showed some development up to the primary spermatocyte stage.

Thirteen patients completed treatment for post-pubertal HH. Six had developed isolated gonadotropin deficiency for no obvious reasons. Three responded to hCG alone and one required both hCG and hPG to achieve pregnancy. Of the remaining two, one was treated with hCG for only three months and the other had near-normal semen quality on hCG/hPG, but no pregnancy occurred. Six men had hypopituitarism after surgery for pituitary tumors or trauma, three responded to hCG alone, one required both hCG and hPG, and two produced no pregnancies despite achieving normal sperm outputs with hCG/hPG. One man had hemochormatosis and produced a pregnancy after treatment with hCG/hPG. In summary, nine of the 13 patients with post-pubertal HH were treated successfully (70%) and six of these required only hCG. Of the four failures, three had good sperm production but no pregnancy resulted.

There was a miscellaneous group of eight patients, seven of whom have completed treatment. Four had histories of delayed puberty treated with hCG and testosterone before presenting for induction of spermatogenesis. Testosterone replacement was stopped and sperm appeared during treatment with hCG alone. Semen quality persisted, and in some cases improved, and pregnancies occurred after cessation of all treatment. Three men maintained normal androgen production, but one man had low serum testosterone levels (5 nmol/l) when not receiving hCG, but at a time when his semen analyses were normal. Some of these subjects may have had an extreme form of constitutional delayed puberty complicated by gonadotropin suppression from administered androgens. Alternatively, they may have low gonadotropin secretion insufficient to initiate spermatogenesis and Leydig cell maturation, but sufficient to maintain these after initiation by exogenous hormones.

In the other three patients, the relevance of gonadotropin deficiency to their infertility was doubtful. One presented with delayed puberty, hyposmia, and low androgen and gonadotropin levels. After several years treatment with hCG or androgens, his testes were 12 ml in volume, there were a few sperm in the ejaculate, and a testicular biopsy showed germ cell arrest. Treatment with hCG and hPG for one year did not increase sperm output. The second man had a prolactinoma and oligospermia. Treatment with hCG/hPG produced little improvement in semen quality whereas addition of bromocriptine resulted in a dramatic improvement and a pregnancy followed. The last man had hemosiderosis from multiple blood transfusions for thalassemia major, oligospermia, and low testosterone and gonadotropin levels. Treatment with hCG reduced the sperm concentration further, but despite this his wife conceived.

Factors that appeared to affect prognosis for successful therapy included absence of other testicular pathology, particularly past undescended testes, a rapid increase in testicular volume to above 10 ml, appearance of sperm in the ejaculate within nine months, and a stable marriage. It is our impression that response to treatment is quicker in subsequent courses of therapy for prepubertal HH patients and that post-pubertal HH patients are also more responsive. Some patients have maintained sperm production on hCG alone after initiation with hCG and hPG and occasionally a second pregnancy has been achieved. However, there were also several failures of hCG to maintain sperm production after initiation with hPG.

It is noteworthy that 11 conceptions occurred in the wives of six of our patients treated with hCG and hPG at sperm concentrations ranging from less than 1 million to 21 million/ml (TABLE 5). These results were for either a single semen analysis performed in the same month as, or the mean of two analyses within two months before and after conception. In our experience, few men achieve "normal" semen quality and attempts to store semen frozen for later artificial insemination are usually unsuccessful.

GONADOTROPIN RELEASING HORMONE

GnRH has been used successfully in the induction and maintenance of spermatogenesis in HH,[7,8] but we have not used this form of therapy to date. Such treatment requires pumps programmed to administer the peptide in a pulsatile manner. Optimal regimens have yet to be defined; dosage has varied from 25 ng/kg/2 hours (approximately 20 μg per day)[7] to 90–160 μg/day, given hourly.[8] Data so far obtained suggest that the likelihood of stimulating spermatogenesis may be similar to that achieved with gonadotropins.

TABLE 5. Semen Quality at Time of Conception[a]

Sperm Concentration ($\times 10^6$/ml)	Number	Sperm Motility (%)	Number
<1	1	<50	6
1.1–5	2	>50	5
5.1–10	4		
		Normal Morphology (%)	Number
10.1–20	3	<50	6
>20	1	>50	4
		Mean	Range
Sperm Concentration ($\times 10^6$/ml)		8.7	<1–21
Sperm Motility (%)		49	<10–72
Normal Morphology (%)		50	17–74

[a] Eleven courses of hCG/hPG in six men.

CONSIDERATIONS FOR THE FUTURE

Issues that require further investigation and resolution in the management of HH include: (1) choice of an appropriate regimen for achievement and maintenance of virilization, (2) choice of an appropriate regimen of gonadotropin replacement to induce fertility, (3) definition of the relative roles of gonadotropin and GnRH in induction of fertility, and (4) more precise definition of the types of HH.

REFERENCES

1. PADRON, R. S., J. WISCHUSEN, B. BURGER & D. M. DE KRETSER. 1980. Prolonged biphasic response of plasma testosterone to single intramuscular injections of human chorionic gonadotropin. J. Clin. Endocrinol. Metab. **50:** 1100.
2. BURGER, H. G., W. J. BREMNER, D. M. DE KRETSER, D. L. HEALY, B. HUDSON, G. T. KOVACS, R. PADRON & J. D. WILSON. 1981. Hypogonadotrophic hypogonadism in male and female. *In* Endocrinology of Human Infertility—New Aspects. P. G. Crosignani & B. L. Ruben, Eds.: 185. Academic Press. London.
3. BURGER, H. G., D. M. DE KRETSER, B. HUDSON & J. D. WILSON. 1981. Effects of preceding androgen therapy on testicular response to human pituitary gonadotrophin (HPG) in hypogonadotrophic hypogonadism (HH): A study of three patients. Fertil. Steril. **34:** 341.

4. BREMNER, W. J., A. M. MATSUMOTO, A. M. SUSSMAN & C. A. PAULSEN. 1981. Follicle-stimulating hormone and human spermatogenesis. J. Clin. Invest. **68:** 1044.
5. MATSUMOTO, A. M., A. E. KARPAS, C. A. PAULSEN & W. J. BREMNER. 1983. Reinitiation of sperm production in gonadotropin suppressed normal men by administration of FSH. J. Clin. Invest. **72:** 1005.
6. MARSHALL, G. R., E. J. WICKINGS, D. K. LUDECKE & E. NIESCHLAG. 1983. Stimulation of spermatogenesis in stalk-sectioned rhesus monkeys by testosterone alone. J Clin. Endocrinol. Metab. **57:** 152.
7. HOFFMAN, A. R. & W. F. CROWLEY. 1982. Induction of puberty in men by long-term pulsatile administration of low-dose gonadotropin-releasing hormone. N. Eng. J. Med. **307:** 1237.
8. KEOGH, E. J., A. DUNN, S. MALLAL, C. SOMERVILLE, S. McCOLM, T. MARSHALL, J. ATTIKIOUZEL, R. HAGUE & N. BATESON. 1982. Induction of spermatogenesis by pulsatile administration of GnRH. Proc. 25th Annual Meeting. The Endocrine Society of Australia. Sydney, August, 1982. (Abstract No. 37).

Gonadotropin Replacement Therapy in Patients with Hypogonadotropic Hypogonadism[a]

E. VICARI, A. MONGIOI', and R. D'AGATA

Endocrine Unit
Institute of Internal Medicine
University of Catania
Catania, Italy

Patients with the syndrome of idiopathic hypogonadotropic hypogonadism (HH) are clinically characterized by the absence of sexual development, inability to achieve adult testicular size, and more or less severe impairment of germinal cell maturation in the testis. Lack of androgen secretion, secondary to impairment of gonadotropin release, accounts for the symptoms found. Deficiency of FSH and LH secretion in these patients is commonly due to the selective absence of hypothalamic GnRH release.[1]

Gonadotropin therapy has been found to achieve virilization and induction of spermatogenesis. The ultimate HH choice of treatment, of course, depends on many factors of which the patient's goal and wishes are foremost.

TREATMENT WITH hCG: DOSE AND INTERVALS OF ADMINISTRATION

The Leydig cells of HH respond to long-course hCG administration with a prompt and sustained release of testosterone. These adult levels can be maintained even after long-term drug administration.[2] In five patients with selective HH, aged 18 to 31 years, in chronic treatment with hCG (1,500 U hCG, three times a week), the kinetics of steroid responsiveness was evaluated after a bolus of 2,000 U hCG given during month 23 of therapy. Serum testosterone concentrations remained in plateau for at least 72 hr after the hCG bolus, then started falling below the pre-administered levels (FIGURE 1).

We concluded, thus, that a dose of 2,000 U hCG is sufficient to maintain stimulated levels of testosterone in physiological range for at least three days. So it appears that this dose should be given at intervals of two to three days to obtain maximal testosterone stimulation, to keep testosterone levels at steady levels, during the long-term HH therapy with hCG required to achieve spermatogenesis, and to obtain full virilization as well.

Higher doses of hCG may not be necessary since some of these patients seem to be maximally stimulated by this regimen of hCG. In two patients, aged 19 to 21 years, for instance, in chronic treatment with hCG (16–36 months), 5,000 and 10,000 U hCG given as bolus 48 hr after the daily injection of 1,500 U did not further stimulate testosterone release (FIGURE 2). This suggests that the Leydig

[a] Supported by grants from CNR (820215104) and the Ministero P.I. (20120104.26).

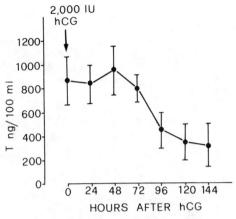

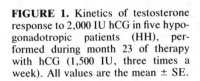

FIGURE 1. Kinetics of testosterone response to 2,000 IU hCG in five hypogonadotropic patients (HH), performed during month 23 of therapy with hCG (1,500 IU, three times a week). All values are the mean ± SE.

cells in these patients were already maximally stimulated with 2,000 U hCG and would not release more testosterone in response to higher hCG doses. It is well documented that hCG, besides stimulating testosterone release, induces augmented serum concentrations of 17β-estradiol (E_2) in normal men,[3,4] and estrogens seem to exert a negative effect on the germinal epithelium.[5,6] The use of chronic

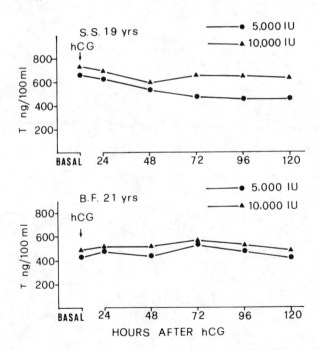

FIGURE 2. Testosterone responsivenesses to 5,000 and 10,000 IU hCG in two patients with HH during long-term treatment with hCG (16–36 months).

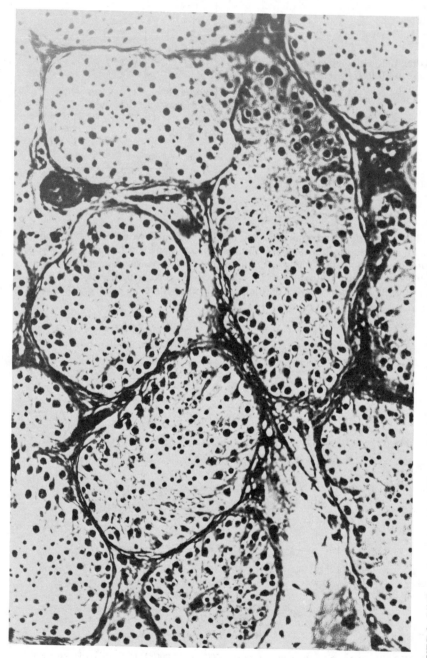

FIGURE 3. Microscopic appearance of biopsy of right testis in a HH subject after he has been treated for as long as 18 months with hCG alone. Note the almost total absence of elongated spermatids. H.E. × 400.

high-dose hCG may, therefore, through a stimulation of E_2 levels, have a negative effect on the maturation of the germinal epithelium.

The concentration of serum testosterone and its relationship with the appearance and maintenance of sperm output in the semen of these patients have yet to be defined.

One has to assume that physiological concentrations of testosterone must be achieved during chronic hCG administration in HH in order to assure the elevated intratesticular testosterone concentrations needed for induction and maintenance of germinal maturation.

ROLE OF hCG IN INDUCTION OF GERMINAL MATURATION IN HYPOGONADOTROPIC HYPOGONADISM

The hypogonadotropic syndrome represents a large spectrum of disorders ranging from complete to partial gonadotropin insufficiency. Consequently, HH patients can present any of the intermediate stages of tubular maturation, from the least developed, with total absence of germinal cells, to the opposite extreme, characterized by the presence of spermatid stage in the seminiferous tubules.

Therapy with hCG alone, therefore, might suffice to trigger full spermatogenesis and adequate sperm output in some patients with adequate tubular maturation, which would reflect the presence of either a partial gonadotropin deficiency or a sufficient endogenous production of FSH.

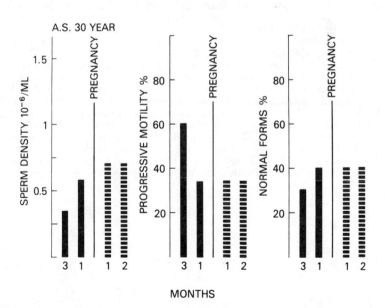

FIGURE 4. Semen characteristics of a HH patient who fathered a child after treatment with hCG + hMG regimen. Several semen analyses have been carried out in this patient at various intervals around the time of conception.

In two HH subjects, treatment with hCG alone brought about full germinal maturation and induced appearance of spermatozoa with ejaculate after 12–24 months of therapy.[7] Testicular biopsies evaluated before hCG regimen showed in one of the two subjects the presence of primary spermatocytes in some tubules, which indicates a partial germinal maturation of the tubular epithelium. However, germinal maturation in HH does not usually progress beyond the spermatid stage with hCG treatment alone (FIGURE 3). In this patient, a supplemented dose of FSH was necessary to complete spermatogenesis and obtain adequate sperm output.

Use of hCG + hMG in HH induced sperm output adequate to achieve pregnancy, although HH patients usually exhibit only 2 to 5 million sperm per ejaculate. One HH patient of ours impregnated his spouse with a sperm density of only 0.5 million (FIGURE 4).

This indicates that our concept of the minimum adequate sperm output required for impregnation should be revised. Sperm function might not correlate with sperm number and percentage motility.

REFERENCES

1. SHERINS, R. 1982. Hypogonadotropic hypogonadism. *In* Current Therapy of Infertility 1982–1983. C. R. Garcia, L. Mastroianni, R. D. Amelar & L. Rubin, Eds.: 10–14 B.C. Decker Inc. Trenton, N.J.
2. D'AGATA, R., E. VICARI, A. ALIFFI, G. MAUGERI, A. MONGIOI' & S. GULIZIA. 1982. Testicular responsiveness to chronic human chorionic gonadotropin administration in hypogonadotropic hypogonadism. J. Clin. Endocrinol. Metab. **55:** 76–80.
3. FOREST, M., A. LECOCQ & J. M. SAEZ. 1979. Kinetics of human chorionic gonadotropin-induced steroidogenic response of the human testis. II. Plasma 17-hydroxyprogesterone, Δ^4-androstenedione, estrone and 17β-estradiol: evidence for the action of human chorionic gonadotropin on intermediate enzymes implicated in steroid biosynthesis. J. Clin. Endocrinol. Metab. **49:** 284–291.
4. WANG, C., R. W. REBAR, B. R. HOPPER & S. S. C. YEN. 1980. Functional studies of the luteinizing hormone-Leydig cell-androgen axis: exaggerated response in C-18 and C-21 testicular steroid to various modes of luteinizing hormone stimulation. J. Clin. Endocrinol. Metab. **51:** 201–208.
5. KALLA, N. R., B. C. NISULA, R. MENARD & D. L. LORIAUX. 1980. The effect of estradiol on testicular testosterone biosynthesis. Endocrinology **106:** 35–39.
6. VIGERSKY, R. A. & A. R. GLASS. 1981. Effects of Δ^1-testolactone on the pituitary-testicular axis in oligospermic men. J. Clin. Endocrinol. Metab. **52:** 897–902.
7. D'AGATA, R., J. J. HEINDEL, E. VICARI, S. GULIZIA & P. POLOSA. 1983. hCG-induced maturation of the seminiferous epithelium in hypogonadotropic men. Horm. Res. **17:**

Relevance of Sperm Maturity Detection in Gonadotropin Treatment

GAETANO FRAJESE[a]

Reproductive Medicine Section
Clinica Medica V
University of Rome
Rome, Italy

While sperm structural maturity is not synonymous with fertilizing ability, the two are closely linked inasmuch as in order for a sperm to fertilize it must be structurally mature. The most up-to-date sperm maturity evaluation methods are: sperm DNA determination, sperm nuclear protein (SNP) analysis, and sperm arginine content evaluation. The normal values of such indexes of sperm maturity are DNA: approximately 1.4 pg/spermatozoon (indole microchemical technique);[1] SNP: an almost exclusive presence of protamines (polyacrylamide gel electrophoresis technique);[2] and high arginine content (histochemical technique).[3]

Gonadotropin therapy is well suited for hypogonadotropic hypogonadism and is most effective in inducing or restoring spermatogenesis. Yet, it is commonly observed that, even with a good sperm output induced by gonadotropin treatment, very seldom is the previously azoospermic patient able to fertilize.

The fertilizing capacity of a man is assessable only when he is married or, in any case, has a partner whom he may and wants to fertilize. However, clinically proven hypogonadotropic patients with a partner are not easily found. In the last eight years we have come across only three married, clinically evident hypogonadotropic patients. Gonadotropin therapy successfully induced sperm output up to an average of 32×10^6 sperm/ml in these patients. Nonetheless, no pregnancies were achieved.

On the other hand, the same treatment improved sperm output and pregnancies were achieved in seven previously oligozoospermic patients affected with partial hypogonadotropism.

In an attempt to verify differences in the quality of sperm in these two groups of positive responders to gonadotropin treatment, one of previously azoospermic patients and the other of previously oligozoospermic patients, we carried out DNA determination on the sperm of both groups. The determination of DNA content of spermatozoa was made using the following method: the number of spermatozoa in 1.0 ml of seminal fluid was determined with a Thomas-Zeiss hemocytometer. To spermatozoa isolated by centrifugation (four times at 1,500 rpm) from 1.0 ml of seminal fluid, 0.5 ml of 0.6 M KOH was added to obtain a cell lysate that was incubated with 0.35 ml of 1.2 M perchloric acid in an ice bath for 30 minutes to precipitate nucleoproteins.

Subsequently, 3.0 ml of 2.0 M perchloric acid were added and, after centrifugation at 4000 rpm for 30 minutes, the supernatant containing the acid-soluble fractions extracted from the spermatozoa was discarded. To the pellet were added 1.0 ml of 0.3 M KOH, 0.5 ml of 12 M HCl, and 0.5 ml of 0.06% indole solution in water. This preparation was incubated in a screw-cap tube at 100° C for 15 min-

[a] Address correspondence to: Via di Porta Pinciana, 34, 00187 Roma (Italy).

utes in order to obtain complexes between the indole and the polysaccharide fractions. After cooling under running tap water, 2.0 ml of amylacetate were added to the sample, which was then thoroughly mixed and centrifuged at 5000 rpm for 5 minutes. Thus, an aqueous phase containing the stable indole-deoxyribose complexes, the amylacetate with the lipidic fractions, and an interface gel containing the proteins was obtained. The aqueous phase was extracted again with 2.0 ml of amylacetate and the resulting aqueous phase was read at 480 to 490 nm in a Unicam SP800 spectrophotometer with 0.5-cm quartz cuvettes. The results were expressed as micrograms of DNA per milliliter. Blanks consisted of 1.0 ml of 0.3 M KOH, 0.5 ml of 12 M HCl, and 0.5 ml of 0.06% aqueous indole solution. They were processed like the samples, taking as time zero the addition of indole. The standard curve was prepared with aqueous solutions of calf thymus DNA (Merck).

The results of this study are: (1) sperm DNA determination in the three cases of hypogonadotropic hypogonadism, positive responders to gonadotropin treatment, revealed a mean value of 2.78 ± 0.52 pg/cell (FIGURE 1). (2) The same determination made on the sperm of seven previously oligozoospermic patients after gonadotropin treatment showed a mean value of 1.42 ± 0.18 pg/cell (FIGURE 2), that is a value that almost matches that found in the sperm before the beginning of treatment (1.41 ± 0.23)—values that fall, in any case, within the area of DNA sperm distribution considered physiological.

These observations suggest that in complete hypogonadotropic hypogonadism the spermatogenesis induced by gonadotropin treatment presents a tendency towards a maturational defect at the meiotic level resulting in a failure of reduction of DNA content. As a consequence, the "spermatozoa" found in these patients were such only morphologically, while nuclear maturation was typical of that of primary spermatocytes. This observation could be sustained by the frequent pres-

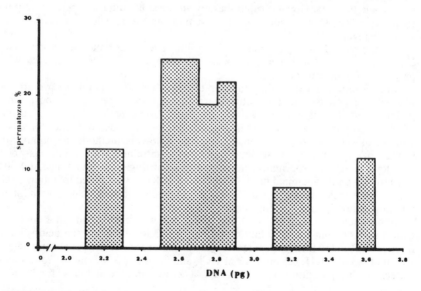

FIGURE 1. Distribution of DNA in sperm population obtained in three infertile, previously azoospermic hypogonadotropic patients after gonadotropin treatment.

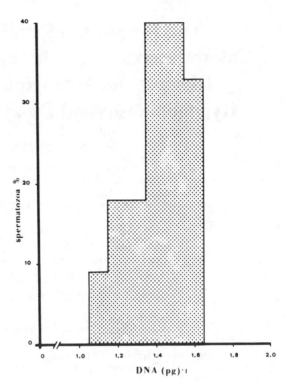

FIGURE 2. Distribution of DNA in sperm population obtained in seven fathers previously oligozoospermic subclinical hypogonadotropic patients after gonadotropin treatment.

ence of numerous atypical forms and the abnormal motility often found in such peculiar germ cells. This maturational defect does not seem to occur during gonadotropin treatment–induced spermatogenesis in partial hypogonadotropism. In conclusion, it would appear that the infertility of the previously azoospermic hypogonadotropic hypogonadal patients, in spite of a good sperm output induced by gonadotropin treatment, might be explained by a greatly reduced fertilizing capacity of the sperm themselves. Evidence of abnormal nuclear structure of these sperm upholds such a hypothesis.

Following this line of reasoning, we might also hypothesize that in hypogonadotropic hypogonadism not only is there a deficiency in gonadotropins, but also in other factors involved in sperm maturation. The detection of some structural sperm indexes could be used by the clinician not only as a diagnostic tool, but also as a means of verifying the effectiveness of the therapy.

REFERENCES

1. FRAJESE, G., L. SILVESTRONI, F. MALANDRINO & A. ISIDORI. 1976. High deoxyribonucleic acid content of spermatozoa from infertile, oligospermic human males. Fertility Sterility **1:** 14–19.
2. SILVESTRONI, L., G. FRAJESE & F. MALANDRINO. 1976. Histones instead of protamines in terminal germ cells of infertile, oligospermic men. Fertility Sterility **27:** 1428–1437.
3. SILVESTRONI, L., G. FRAJESE & C. CONTI. 1978. Arginine evaluation to verify sperm maturation in man. Arch. Andrology **1:** 363–365.

The Response of Prolactin to Chlorpromazine: Use in the Differential Diagnosis of Hypogonadotropic Hypogonadism and Delayed Puberty

STEPHEN J. WINTERS

Department of Medicine
Montefiore Hospital
University of Pittsburgh School of Medicine
Pittsburgh, Pennsylvania 15213

RICHARD J. SHERINS

Developmental Endocrinology Branch
National Institute of Child Health and Human Development
Bethesda, Maryland 20205

ROGER E. JOHNSONBAUGH

Department of Pediatric Endocrinology
Department of Pediatrics
National Naval Center and
Uniformed Services University of the Health Sciences
Bethesda, Maryland 20814

The distinction between patients with delayed puberty and those with idiopathic hypogonadotropic hypogonadism (IHH) remains difficult. The presence of midline defects, such as anosmia, and a positive family history are helpful, but these findings are limited to approximately 50% of cases of IHH. In both disorders serum gonadotropin and testosterone levels are low and neither group responds to clomiphene with an increase in gonadotropin secretion. Presence of sleep-associated increases in LH and testosterone levels and a maturing response of LH to luteinizing hormone–releasing hormone are sometimes, but not consistently useful in this differential diagnosis.[1]

Previous investigators found that the release of prolactin (PRL) following stimulation with chlorpromazine was diminished in untreated patients with IHH.[2-4] In contrast, we observed that PRL responded normally to chlorpromazine stimulation in men with IHH who were receiving treatment with testosterone or human chorionic gonadotropin.[5] Together, these findings suggested that a lack of steroid exposure, rather than a specific hypothalamic abnormality, was responsible for the failure of chlorpromazine to increase PRL levels in untreated subjects. A normal PRL response to chlorpromazine persists for several months following cessation of testosterone therapy, indicating that the steroid requirement for sustaining this response is small. In light of recent observations that reveal that the prepubertal testis produces testosterone,[6] it was attractive to postulate that boys with delayed puberty would respond to chlorpromazine whereas patients with IHH do not.

Six boys, aged 10½ to 14⁸/₁₂ years, sought medical attention for evaluation of gonadal function; none had received prior treatment. Five of these boys had Stage 1 pubic hair development and one boy was Stage 2. The testis size was 2–6 ml. Morning serum testosterone levels were less than 40 ng/dl. These boys proved to be normal when clinical and hormonal evidence for spontaneous pubertal progression became evident on reexamination during the next 6–24 months. Seven previously untreated subjects with complete IHH, age 17–24, were also studied. Anosmia was present in three. Serum testosterone levels were less than 30 ng/dl.

FIGURE 1 demonstrates the increase in serum PRL levels following the intramuscular administration of chlorpromazine (0.33 mg/kg). The increment in prolactin ranged from 15 to 52 ng/ml in the early pubertal boys, but was less than 5 ng/ml in each untreated subject with complete IHH. This figure also includes data from ten men with treated hypogonadotropism, whose PRL responses were similar to those of normal men.[5]

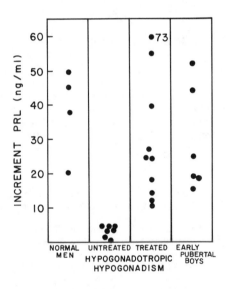

FIGURE 1. Increment in serum PRL concentration after chlorpromazine administration (0.33 mg/kg i.m.) to normal men, previously untreated patients with complete idiopathic hypogonadotropic hypogonadism, and a comparable group receiving therapy with hCG or testosterone, and early pubertal boys who ultimately proved to be normal. (From Winters *et al.*[9] With permission from *Clinical Endocrinology*.)

Although the precise mechanism to explain the difference in response to chlorpromazine is unknown, it is clearly related to sex steroids. Data *in vitro* and *in vivo* indicate that estrogens influence the mammotrophs to produce PRL.[7,8] As such, the estradiol derived by peripheral or central nervous system aromatization of administered or testicular testosterone could play a role in modulating these responses. However, current radioimmunoassay methods are insufficiently sensitive to differentiate between the low levels of testosterone and estradiol in peripheral blood among these subjects.

Our observations are preliminary but, may be of clinical importance, as they suggest that study of PRL response to chlorpromazine could be used to differentiate simple delayed puberty from IHH. A representative case study is shown in FIGURE 2. This 10½ year old obese white male was referred for evaluation of a microphallus. His testes were each 2 ml, measured with a calibrated orchidometer; his phallus was 4.5 cm in length. Blood samples drawn every 2 hr for 24 hr

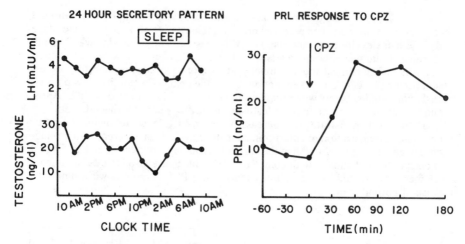

FIGURE 2. Serum LH and testosterone levels determined every 2 hr for 24 hr and the PRL response to chlorpromazine in a 10½ year old boy.

revealed that serum testosterone levels were consistently less than 30 ng/dl and that there was no sleep-associated increase in LH and testosterone secretion. Following chlorpromazine administration serum PRL levels increased by 19 ng/ml. Based upon the normal PRL study we predicted that normal sexual development would occur, a prediction that proved to be correct.

REFERENCES

1. KULIN, H. E. & R. J. SANTEN. 1982. Normal and aberrant pubertal development in man. *In* Clinical Reproductive Neuroendocrinology. J. L. Vaitukaitis, Ed.: 19–68. Elsevier Biomedical. New York.
2. ANTAKI, A., M. SOMMA, H. WYMAN & J. VAN CAMPENHOUT. 1974. Hypothalamic-pituitary function in the olfacto-genital syndrome. J. Clin. Endocrinol. Metab. **38:** 1083–1089.
3. SPITZ, I. M., V. ALMALIACH, E. ROSEN, W. POLISHUK & D. RABINOWITZ. 1977. Dissociation of prolactin responsiveness to TRH and chlorpromazine in women with isolated gonadotropin deficiency. J. Clin. Endocrinol. Metab. 45: 1173–1178.
4. TURKSOY, R. N. 1979. Dissociation of prolactin responsiveness to thyrotropin-releasing hormone and chlorpromazine in a female with Kallmann's syndrome. Fertil. Steril. **32:** 228–229.
5. WINTERS, S. J., R. S. MECKLENBURG & R. J. SHERINS. 1978. Hypothalamic function in men with hypogonadotrophic hypoganadism. Clin. Endocrinol. **8:** 417–426.
6. FORTI, G., S. SANTORO, G. A. GRISOLIA, F. BASSI, R. BONINSEGNI, G. FIORELLI & M. SERIO. 1981. Spermatic and peripheral plasma concentrations of testosterone and androstenedione in prepubertal boys. J. Clin. Endocrinol. Metab. **53:** 883–886.
7. BUCKMAN, M. T. & G. T. PEAKE. 1973. Estrogen potentiation of phenothiazine-induced prolactin secretion in man. J. Clin. Endocrinol. Metab. **37:** 977–980.
8. GUDELSKY, G. A., O. D. NANSEL, J. REYMOND & J. C. PORTER. 1981. Role of estrogen in the dopaminergic control of prolactin secretion. Endocrinology **108:** 440–444.
9. WINTERS, S. J., R. E. JOHNSONBAUGH & R. J. SHERINS. 1982. The response of prolactin to chlorpromazine stimulation in men with hypogonadotropic hypogonadism and early pubertal boys: relationship to sex steroid exposure. Clin. Endocrinol. **16:** 321–330.

Gonadotropin Control of Spermatogenesis in Man: Studies of Gonadotropin Administration in Spontaneous and Experimentally Induced Hypogonadotropic States[a]

WILLIAM J. BREMNER,[b] A. M. MATSUMOTO,[b] and
C. A. PAULSEN[c]

Endocrinology Section
[b] VA Medical Center
[c] Pacific Medical Center
[b,c] Population Center for Research in Reproduction
[b,c] Department of Medicine
University of Washington School of Medicine
Seattle, Washington 98108

It is clearly established in man, as in other mammalian species, that normal spermatogenesis requires the stimulatory actions of pituitary gonadotropins.[1] Both luteinizing hormone (LH) and follicle-stimulating hormone (FSH) exert effects on testicular function, but the specific role played by each in controlling spermatogenesis is unclear.

We have performed a series of studies both in spontaneously occurring hypogonadotropic eunuchoidism and in normal men made hypogonadotropic by the administration of exogenous testosterone. We have used these two types of hypogonadotropic men to assess the effects of administering purified preparations of gonadotropins to help understand the normal physiology of the control of human spermatogenesis.

METHODS

Study 1

This study was designed to determine whether normal blood levels of FSH are necessary for human spermatogenesis. Five normal men were studied.

The first three months of the study constituted a control period during which observations and measurements (*see below*) were performed in each subject, but no hormones were administered. After the control period, testosterone enanthate (T) (Delatestryl, E. R. Squibb and Sons, Princeton, NJ) administration was begun (200 mg i.m. weekly). The injections of T alone were continued until three successive seminal fluid analyses (obtained every 2 wk) revealed sperm counts <5 million/ml. At this point, while the injections of T were continued, administration

[a] Supported by National Institutes of Health grants P-50-HD 12629 and P-32-AM 07247 and by the Veterans Administration.

of hCG (Profasi, Serono Laboratories, Inc., Braintree, MA), 5000 IU i.m. three times weekly, was added. The combination of hCG and T injections was continued in all five men until three successive sperm counts were within the individual's control range or a minimum of 17 wk.

At this time, to demonstrate that the increases in sperm counts found were due to hCG and not to a decline in the suppressive effect of testosterone, hCG injections were stopped in two subjects and T alone was continued until sperm counts were again suppressed to very low levels. Then T was discontinued and the two subjects entered a post-treatment control period lasting until three successive sperm counts were within the subject's control range.

During each month of the study, each subject submitted two seminal fluid specimens obtained by masturbation after two days of abstention from ejaculation. In addition, monthly venous blood samples were obtained for measurement of LH, FSH, and testosterone levels.

Study 2

This study was designed to determine whether normal blood levels of FSH are sufficient to stimulate human spermatogenesis.

Four normal men underwent a three-month period of control observation during which no hormones were administered. During this time, clinical observations, hormonal measurements, and seminal fluid analyses were performed at regular intervals as described below.

After the control period, each subject began receiving 200 mg i.m. of testosterone enanthate (Delatestryl, E. R. Squibb and Sons, Princeton, NJ) weekly. T alone was administered until three successive sperm counts (performed twice monthly) became <5 million/cm^3.

After this initial T-alone period, while continuing T at the same dosage, the men simultaneously received 100 IU FSH s.c. daily for a period of 13 to 15 weeks to replace FSH activity. The FSH preparation used in these selective replacement studies (LER 1577, Lot No. 4) was kindly provided by the National Pituitary Agency, Baltimore, MD. This preparation contained <1% LH activity in the ovarian ascorbic acid depletion and ventral prostate weight bioassays, reported by the National Pituitary Agency, as well as in the *in vitro* mouse Leydig cell bioassay performed in our laboratory. However, this FSH preparation contained significant amounts (17%) of immunoreactive, nonbioactive LH-like material. As a result, monitoring of LH activity during the study required the measurement of LH bioactivity using the *in vitro* mouse Leydig cell bioassay (*described below*) instead of LH by radioimmunoassay (RIA). On the other hand, close correspondence of FSH measured by RIA and bioassay permitted the use of RIA to monitor FSH activity during the study.

After the FSH-plus-T period, FSH injections were stopped in all four subjects and T alone was continued until three successive sperm counts were again suppressed to <5 million/cm^3. The resuppression of sperm counts with continued administration of T alone after discontinuation of FSH was used to demonstrate that any rise in sperm counts observed during the FSH-plus-T period was due to FSH administration and not to a decline in the suppressive effect of exogenous T with time.

During each month of the study, each subject submitted two seminal fluid specimens obtained by masturbation after two days of abstention from ejaculation. In addition, monthly venous blood samples were obtained for measurement of LH by bioassay and FSH and T by radioimmunoassay.

Study 3

In this study, 13 men with hypogonadotropic eunuchoidism were treated with hCG, 2,000–5,000 three times weekly. We assessed the effect on sperm production of the hCG administration alone, without the addition of FSH.

Measurement Techniques

LH, FSH, and T were measured by previously described radioimmunoassays.[2,3] LH was measured in some samples by the *in vitro* Leydig cell bioassay.[2] Seminal fluid analysis was performed as described previously.[2]

RESULTS

Study 1

Following the three-month control period, administration of testosterone led to severe inhibition of sperm production (FIGURE 1). Three subjects became azoospermic, whereas two consistently exhibited sperm counts of <3 million/ml. While the testosterone injections were continued, hCG was added (5,000 IU i.m., three times weekly). Sperm counts (FIGURE 1) increased markedly during hCG administration ($p < 0.001$ compared with testosterone injections alone). In two subjects, sperm counts during hCG plus T injections returned into the normal control range for each man. In the other three men, although sperm counts increased markedly on hCG plus T, reaching mean levels of 12, 13, and 94 million/ml, they did not consistently reach the men's control ranges. Medication records revealed that the two men with the lowest counts did not receive all their scheduled hCG injections. Serum FSH values (FIGURE 1) were normal (111 ± 10 ng/ml) in the control period and were suppressed to undetectable levels (<25 ng/ml) in the T alone and in the hCG-plus-T phases of the study.

Following the hCG-plus-T phase of the study, in which all men participated, two men received only T injections for 2.5 and 4.0 months. Sperm counts during the T injections alone returned to azoospermic or severely oligospermic levels.

Study 2

After the three-month control period, exogenous T administration (200 mg i.m. weekly) resulted in marked suppression of sperm production (FIGURE 2). Sperm counts after two months of initial T administration alone were reduced to 0.3 ± 0.2 million/ml (mean ± SEM) compared with 94 ± 12 million/ml during the control period. Two subjects had sperm counts consistently suppressed to <2 million/ml.

While T injections were continued, all subjects received FSH (100 IU s.c. daily) simultaneously with T. Sperm counts (FIGURE 2) increased significantly

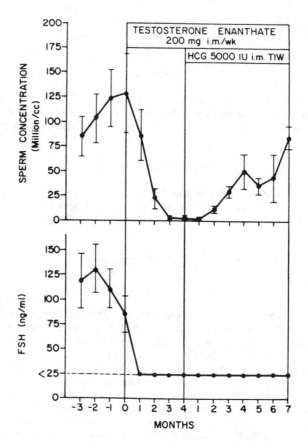

FIGURE 1. Monthly sperm concentrations and serum FSH data in five normal men during the control, testosterone administration alone, and hCG-plus-testosterone phases of the study (mean ± SE). Note the increase in sperm concentration induced by hCG in spite of very low serum levels of FSH. (From Bremner *et al.*[2] By permission of Rockefeller University Press.)

with the addition of FSH to T, reaching a mean of 33 ± 7 million/ml after two months of FSH-plus-T ($p < 0.02$ compared with T alone). Although sperm concentrations increased markedly on FSH-plus-T, they did not consistently reach the individuals' control ranges. The mean sperm concentrations achieved after three months of FSH-plus-T treatment were 34, 43, 29, and 9 million/ml. The maximum sperm concentrations achieved on FSH-plus-T were 88, 51, 35, and 13 million/ml.

After the FSH-plus-T period, all four men continued to receive T alone after FSH injections were stopped. Sperm counts were again severely suppressed in all subjects, reaching a mean of 0.2 ± 0.1 million/ml after two months of T treatment alone (FIGURE 2). Two subjects became azoospermic, whereas two subjects had sperm counts suppressed to <0.7 million/ml after two months of T alone.

Serum FSH levels (FIGURE 2), normal during the control period (98 ± 21 ng/ml), were suppressed to undetectable levels (<25 ng/ml) during the initial T-alone period. With the addition of FSH to T, serum FSH levels increased to a mean of 273 ± 44 ng/ml, just above the upper limits of the normal range for FSH levels (30–230 ng/ml). After discontinuation of FSH injections, continued T injections alone again suppressed FSH levels to <25 ng/ml, the limit of detectability of FSH in our assay.

Serum LH bioactivity was markedly suppressed during initial T administration alone (140 ± 7 ng/ml) compared with the control period (373 ± 65 ng/ml, $p <$ 0.03). With the addition of FSH injections to T administration, serum LH bioactivity was not significantly changed compared with the initial T-alone period (147

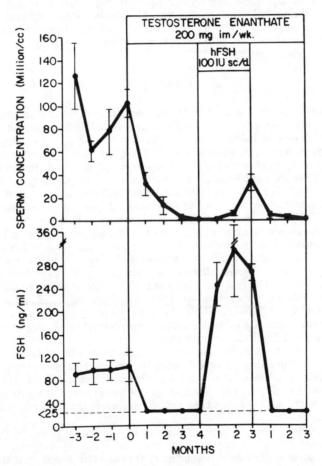

FIGURE 2. Mean monthly sperm concentrations (million per cubic centimeter) and serum FSH levels (in nanograms per milliliter) in four normal men during the control, initial T-alone, FSH-plus-T, and second T-alone periods of the study (mean ± SE). Exogenous T administration markedly suppresses sperm concentrations to severely oligospermic levels and serum FSH to undetectable levels. Note FSH replacement at a slightly supraphysiological dosage increases sperm concentration. (From Matsumoto *et al.*[3] By permission of Rockefeller University Press.)

± 9 ng/ml). LH bioactivity remained unchanged after FSH injections were stopped during the second T-alone period (153 ± 5 ng/ml).

Serum T levels increased from 6.5 ± 0.4 ng/ml during the the control period to 13.7 ± 1.9 ng/ml during the initial T alone period. T levels during the FSH-plus-T period (13.1 ± 3.1 ng/ml) and the second T-alone period (11.0 ± 2.2 ng/ml) were not significantly differently from the initial T-alone period.

Study 3

All hypogonadotropic men receiving hCG demonstrated increases of serum T levels into the normal range. Four of the 13 hypogonadotropic men receiving hCG alone began to produce sperm in their ejaculates. The highest sperm counts attained by these men were 0.1, 1.1, 6.1, and 42 million/ml.

DISCUSSION

Our results in Study 1 demonstrate that spermatogenesis as assessed by sperm counts may be reinitiated and maintained at normal levels in men with undetectable FSH levels in blood. Similarly, the results of Study 3 demonstrate that spermatogenesis may be stimulated by hCG alone in some patients with congenital hypogonadotropic eunuchoidism. These results demonstrate that normal blood levels of FSH are not absolutely necessary for human spermatogenesis.

Two of our five subjects in Study 1 demonstrated sperm counts that were indistinguishable from their own control values during the period that they were receiving hCG-plus-T and had undetectable serum FSH levels. The other three subjects reinitiated spermatogenesis in spite of undetectable serum FSH levels and demonstrated mean sperm counts within the normal adult male range. However, they did not achieve mean counts within their own control range during the time of hCG-plus-T administration in this study. In two of these subjects, irregular administration of hCG may have been important in their failure to achieve complete normalization of sperm counts. The limited duration of hCG-plus-T phase of this study may also have contributed to the failure to achieve full normalization of sperm counts. Alternatively, this incomplete spermatogenic response could be due to the low FSH levels in these men.

In two men, stopping the administration of hCG after the hCG-plus-T phase of the study and continuing only the T injections led to suppression of sperm production equally as complete as when T was first administered alone. These results demonstrated clearly that the reinitiation and maintenance of sperm production were due to the hCG injections and not to a decline in the suppressive effect of T with time.

Our results in Study 2 demonstrate that in a setting of markedly suppressed gonadotropin levels induced by T, exogenous FSH administration alone can reinitiate sperm production in normal men. These results demonstrate that FSH is sufficient to stimulate human spermatogenesis in the setting of very low LH levels. Exogenous T administration in our subjects resulted in a severe reduction in LH and FSH levels. In this setting of T-induced endogenous hypogonadotropism, our subjects received highly purified hFSH to replace FSH alone, leaving LH levels suppressed. All four men demonstrated significant stimulation of sperm production on FSH plus T. Three of the four subjects attained mean sperm counts within the normal adult male range and achieved at least one sperm count in their control range. The remaining subject, who was azoospermic during the initial T alone period, demonstrated a definite rise in sperm counts with the addition of FSH to T. However, his mean sperm concentration remained in the oligospermic range. None of the subjects achieved sperm counts consistently within his own control range.

In none of our studies has selective FSH or hCG replacement returned sperm production fully to normal levels in all men studied. We feel that although it is possible to demonstrate a stimulatory role for either FSH or hCG alone on human spermatogenesis, neither gonadotropin may be sufficient by itself to induce quantitatively normal sperm production in all men. It is likely that normal levels of both LH and FSH are necessary to maintain quantitatively normal spermatogenesis. Since each gonadotropin, in the near absence of the other, is capable of at least a partial stimulatory effect on sperm production, it seems very unlikely that selective suppression of either gonadotropin alone would be an effective method of suppressing sperm production to the extent necessary to cause infertility. Therefore, our results do not lend support to the concept that selective gonadotropin suppression might be an effective technique for male contraceptive development.

ACKNOWLEDGMENTS

We are grateful for the assistance of Patricia Payne, Judy Tsoi, Vasumathi Sundarraj, Patricia Gosciewski, Florida Flor, Lorraine Shen, Elaine Rost, Connie Pete, Marian Ursic, Louise Parry, Anne Bartlett, Patricia Jenkins, and Maxine Cormier. We appreciate the gifts of assay reagents and clinical grade FSH from the National Pituitary Agency and of assay reagents from the World Health Organization.

REFERENCES

1. diZEREGA, G. S. & R. J. SHERINS. 1980. Endocrine control of adult testicular function. *In* The Testis. H. Burger & D. DeKretser, Eds.: 127–140. Raven Press. New York.
2. BREMNER, W. J., A. M. MATSUMOTO, A. M. SUSSMAN & C. A. PAULSEN. 1981. Follicle-stimulating hormone and human spermatogenesis. J. Clin. Invest. **68:** 1044–1052.
3. MATSUMOTO, A. M., A. E. KARPAS, C. A. PAULSEN & W. J. BREMNER. 1983. Reinitiation of sperm production in gonadotropin-suppressed normal men by administration of follicle-stimulating hormone. J. Clin. Invest. **72:** 1005–1015.

An Ultrastructural Study of the Cytoplasmic Bridges between Germ Cells of the Canine Testis

CAROLYN J. CONNELL

Department of Anatomy
Colorado State University
Fort Collins, Colorado 80523

The regulation of mitotic and meiotic divisions in germ cell lines remains one of biology's unsolved problems. In their 1955 paper, Burgos and Fawcett[1] described pairs of differentiating spermatids connected by a narrow protoplasmic bridge. The bridge itself was marked by a ring of granular, osmiophilic material in the cytoplasm adjacent to the plasma membrane. They noted that organelles seem to span the bridge between germ cells, indicating that there was a continuity of cytoplasm. The work of McGregor[2] in 1899 was cited by the authors. In this work McGregor had noted in Amphiuma that "spindle remnants" persisted as delicate bridges between daughter cells in spermatogenesis, and that these structures persisted between spermatogonia, primary, and secondary spermatocytes, and connected spermatids until late in development. Dym and Fawcett[3] extended the information on the intercellular bridges and noted that the bridges are retained throughout spermatogenesis and at spermiation these bridges are retained in the residual cytoplasm. These intercellular or cytoplasmic bridges are ubiquitous in insects, birds, and mammals and exist in both male and female gonads.[4] Fawcett suggested that these bridges could function to maintain synchrony of germ cell clones during development and maturation. Other possible roles that have been put forth are nutrition, restriction of motility, genetic regulation in maintaining gametic neutrality, and finally the possibility that cytoplasmic bridges may prevent unlimited divisions of germ cells and the formation of neoplasms.[4]

The tissues and the method of preparation of the tissues have been described previously[5] for canine testicular tissue.

In the canine tests the intercellular bridges largely resemble those described by Dym and Fawcett.[3] However, there appear to be some unique characteristics of the bridge in this species. In transmission electron micrographs, the bridges are characterized by punctate accumulations of electron-dense material. In glancing sections the electron-dense material is seen in parallel rows extending from germ cell to germ cell forming a rib-like cage for the narrow bridge cytoplasm. In cross-section the electron-dense material has a punctate appearance (FIGURE 1). In freeze-fracture replicas, raised ridges of membrane extend from germ cell to mid region of the bridge. These ridges from each cell may be separated by a band of unsculptured membrane or the ridges may interdigitate. These ridges run in the same direction as the electron-dense material just below the inner plasma membrane (FIGURE 2). The number of intramembranous particles may be similar on the joined cells or quite different. A variable condition is the presence of parallel cisternae connecting the "sides" of the bridge arranged perpendicular to the rows of electron-dense material and the intramembranous ridges (FIGURES 3 and 4). These cisternae are continuous with the endoplasmic reticulum system of the cell.

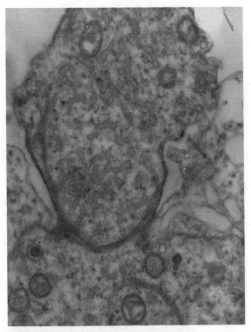

FIGURE 1. In this oblique section through a cytoplasmic bridge between two germ cells, the punctate arrangement of the "rods" of electron-dense material in the cytoplasm beneath the plasma membrane are seen. The smooth endoplasmic membranes are closely applied to the electron-dense material. 15,600 ×.

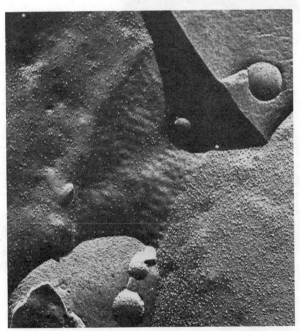

FIGURE 2. In this image of a freeze-fracture replica the intramembrane structure of the cytoplasmic bridge is revealed as ridges and furrows. Intramembranous particles are associated with the exposed P-face membrane. The number of particles on the P face of the germ cell to the left is similar to the number of particles present on the bridge. However, the P face of the germ cell on the right has many more intramembranous particles. 47,635 ×.

473

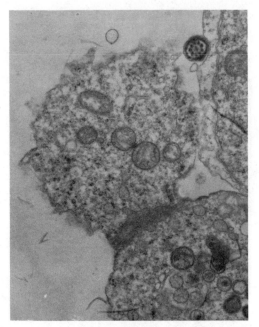

FIGURE 3. Components of the smooth membrane system of the germ cells joined by this bridge traverse the long axis of this bridge. Note the punctate appearance of the electron-dense material of the bridge component adjacent to the plasma membrane, 15,350 ×.

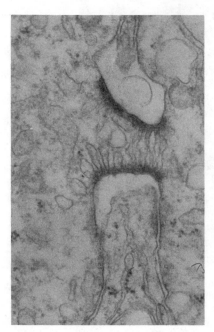

FIGURE 4. The electron-dense material of the inner plasma membrane region of the bridge appears to be continuous with the lumen of the cisternae of the smooth membranes in this view of the cytoplasmic bridge. 14,000 ×.

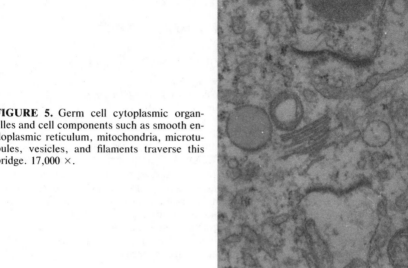

FIGURE 5. Germ cell cytoplasmic organelles and cell components such as smooth endoplasmic reticulum, mitochondria, microtubules, vesicles, and filaments traverse this bridge. 17,000 ×.

The electron-dense material of the bridge sometimes extends into the lumen of the smooth endoplasmic reticulum. Microtubules span across the bridge and other images show microtubules passing from one cell to the other parallel to the bridge. This arrangement resembles a spindle body. Interspersed between the microtubules are ribosomes and smooth endoplasmic reticulum (FIGURE 5).

A highly sculptured structure surrounds the cytoplasm that bridges between germ cells. This framework has both a cytoplasmic and an intramembranous component. The role that this structure plays in maintaining the necessary environment for the orderly development of the germ cells is largely inferential. However, it is possible to envisage the germ cell clone rigidly maintained in a precise relationship by these girdles of structural material. The experimental testing of this role awaits the development of new probes.

REFERENCES

1. BURGOS, M. H. & D. W. FAWCETT. 1955. J. Biophys. Biochem. Cytol. **1:** 287–315.
2. McGREGOR, J. G. 1899. J. Morph. **15:** suppl., 57.
3. DYM, M. & D. W. FAWCETT. 1971. Biol. Reprod. **4:** 195–215.
4. GONDOS, B. Ultrastructure of Reproduction and Early Development. J. Van Blerkon & P. M. Motta, Eds. Martinus Nijhoff. The Hague.
5. CONNELL, C. J. 1978. J. Cell Biol. **76:** 57–75.

Further Observations on the Microfilament Bundles of Sertoli Cell Junctional Complexes[a]

CARLOS A. SUÁREZ-QUIAN[b] and MARTIN DYM

Department of Anatomy
Georgetown Medical School-School of Dentistry
Washington, D.C. 20007

Part of the morphological basis of the blood-testis barrier, which subdivides the seminiferous epithelium into basal and adluminal compartments, is the inter-Sertoli junction.[1] These junctional complexes consist of apposing plasma membranes between adjoining Sertoli cells, a subjacent layer of microfilament bundles, and cisterns of endoplasmic reticulum. Compartmentalization of the seminiferous epithelium presupposes opening and closing of the barrier to permit entry of spermatocytes into the adluminal compartment. Using heavy meromyosin, it was shown that the microfilament bundles contain f-actin, suggesting that they may be contractile, and thus provide the motive force necessary to open and close the barrier.[2]

This report re-examines the composition of microfilaments contained within inter-Sertoli junctional complexes but suggests an alternative function as to their role. The ultrastructural characterization of microfilaments was carried out on Sertoli cells *in vivo* and their identity revealed as actin on Sertoli cells *in vitro* using the S1 fragment of skeletal muscle myosin. Changes in the microfilament bundles at different stages of the seminiferous cycle were observed using NBD-phallicidin, a fluorescent probe that binds specifically to f-actin.[3]

MATERIALS AND METHODS

Tissue was prepared for electron microscopy as described previously.[1] Sertoli cells were cultured using previously published methods.[4] Decoration of f-actin with S1 was done as described elsewhere.[5] Staining of filaments with NBD-phallicidin (Molecular Probes; Junction City, OR) was carried out in 6 μm frozen sections of testes fixed in 3.7% formalin in PBS. Images were obtained using epifluorescence.

RESULTS AND DISCUSSION

Ultrastructurally, junctional complexes cut in cross section reveal the typical punctate pattern of microfilaments (FIGURE 1, A), whereas profiles of longitudi-

[a] This work was funded by National Institute of Health grant #HD16260 and by a Mellon Foundation Grant. This work was submitted to Harvard University as partial fulfillment for the Ph.D. degree by C. A. S.-Q.
[b] Present Address: National Institute of Health, NICHD; Bldg. 10, Rm. 9N 204; Bethesda, MD.

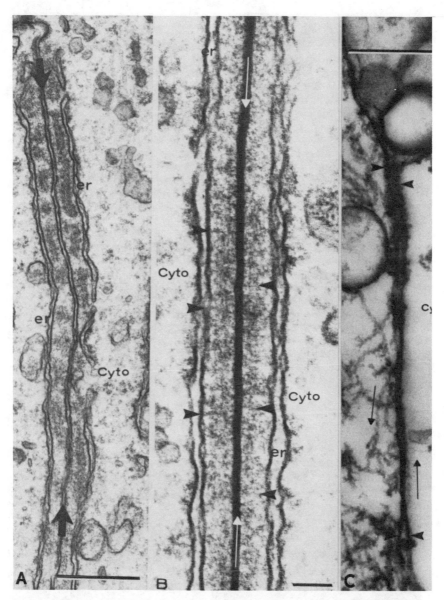

FIGURE 1. Tissue illustrated in A and B was post-fixed in OsO_4-potassium ferrocyanide. Image in B is from a thin section cut at a purple to dark gold interference color. A, shows microfilaments cut in cross section in the cytoplasm between the plasma membrane and the cistern of endoplasmic reticulum (er) of a junctional complex. The apposing plasma membranes of the two Sertoli cells are marked by thick arrows. B is the same as A except the microfilaments were sectioned in longitudinal fashion. Apposing plasma membranes are indicated by white arrows. Arrowheads point to cross-bridges. C, a presumed junctional complex is illustrated. Arrowheads point to the two apposing plasma membranes giving rise to the junctional complex. The polarity of the decorated microfilaments, sectioned longitudinally, on either side of the junction, is marked by the direction of the arrows. Magnification: A, bar = 0.5 μm; B, bar = 0.1 μm; C, bar = 0.5 μm.

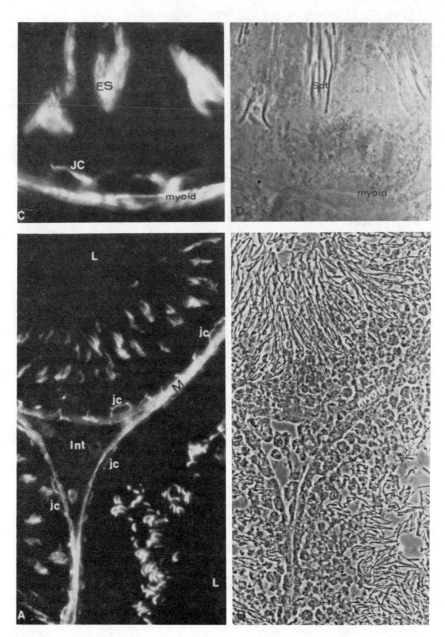

FIGURE 2. NBD-phallicidin staining of 6 μm frozen sections of testes is shown in A and C, and the corresponding phase images are shown in B and D, respectively. A survey light micrograph, A, illustrates that fluorescent staining is limited to Sertoli cell junctional complexes (jc), ectoplasmic specializations (ES), and myoid cells (M). The lumen (L) of the seminiferous tubules and interstitial tissue are labeled for reference. Magnification, A and B = 200×. C illustrates a higher magnification view of a similar area as shown in A. Note that the junctional complex (jc) is only one cell layer away from the myoid cell. D is the corresponding phase image. Note that the elongated spermatids (Spt) in D correspond to the fluorescent staining on the ectoplasmic specializations (ES) in C. Magnification: C and D = 504×.

nally sectioned junctional complexes exhibit microfilaments aligned parallel to the plasma membrane (FIGURE 1, B). In these latter images, cross-bridges between microfilaments, between microfilaments and plasma membranes, and between microfilaments and endoplasmic reticulum were noted. The identity of junctional complex microfilaments as actin was ascertained in cultured Sertoli cells using S1. The polarity of microfilaments on either side of the junctional complex was random, but all microfilaments within the same bundle were oriented in the same direction (FIGURE 1, C). NBD-phallicidin permitted visualization of junctional complex microfilaments in Sertoli cells *in situ* (FIGURE 2). In frozen sections of testes, fluorescent staining was distinctly localized in myoid cells, at ectoplasmic specializations and at junctional complexes. Staining characteristics of junctional complexes varied during the different stages of the seminiferous cycle. A clear "intermediate compartment" was readily delineated by the NBD-phallicidin staining of microfilaments at stage IX of the cycle, during which time spermatocytes enter the adluminal compartment. Further, although myosin could be detected immunocytochemically in myoid cells, it was not found in junctional complexes (data not shown).

The sliding-filament theory of sarcomere motility in skeletal muscle has often prejudiced investigators into thinking that the presence of f-actin is always associated with some sort of action. In the case of junctional complex microfilaments, however, no evidence of myosin has been obtained. Further, the presence of cross-bridges bundling the microfilaments probably provides a steric hindrance to contraction.

At present, evidence has been obtained that correlates the conspicuous presence of microfilament bundles in sessile cells *in situ* subjected to turgor pressure. These include epithelial cells of fish scales, vascular endothelial cells, and in the microvilli of cells lining the gut epithelia.[6-8] Presumably, the microfilaments provide support rather than force in these instances. Experimental evidence also suggests that the junctional specializations surrounding the acrosomal region of elongated spermatids (not unlike half of an inter-Sertoli junction in appearance) provide support to the plasma membrane.[9] Similarly, we propose that microfilaments of junctional complexes act to stabilize the plasma membrane of these regions and thereby enhance the integrity of the blood-testis barrier.

REFERENCES

1. DYM, M. & D. FAWCETT. 1970. The blood-testis barrier in rat and the physiological compartmentation of the seminiferous epithelium. Biol. Reprod. **3:** 308–326.
2. TOYAMA, Y. 1976. Actin-like filaments in the Sertoli cell junctional specializations in the swine and mouse testis. Anat. Rec. **186:** 477–492.
3. ESTES, J. D., L. A. SELDEN & L. C. GERHSAN. 1981. Mechanism of action of phalloidin on the polymerization of muscle actin. Biochemistry **20:** 708–712.
4. SUÁREZ-QUIAN, C. A., M. DYM, A. MAKRIS, J. BRUMBAUGH, K. J. RYAN & J. A. CANICK. 1983. Estrogen synthesis by immature rat Sertoli cells *in vitro.* J. Androl. **4:** 203–209.
5. BEGG, D. A., R. RODEWALD & L. I. REBHUN. 1978. Visualization of actin filament polarity in thin-section. J. Cell Biol. **79:** 846–852.
6. BYERS, H. R. & K. FUJIWARA. 1982. Stress fibers in cells *in situ:* immunofluorescence visualization with antiactin, antimyosin, and anti-alpha actinin. J. Cell Biol. **93:** 804–811.
7. WONG, A. J., T. D. POLLARD & I. M. HERMAN. 1983. Actin filament stress fibers in vascular endothelial cells *in vivo.* Science **219:** 867–869.

8. MOOSEKER, M. S., E. M. BONDER, B. G. GRIMWADE, C. L. HOWE, T. C. S. KELLER
    III, R. J. WASSERMAN & K. A. WHARTON. 1982. Regulation of contractility, cytoske-
    letal structure, and filament assembly in the brush border of intestinal epithelial cells.
    Cold Spring Harbor Symp. Quant. Biol. **46:** 855–870.
9. ROMRELL, L. J. & M. H. ROSS. 1979. Characterization of Sertoli-germ cell junctional
    specializations in dissociated testicular cells. Anat. Rec. **193:** 23–42.

A Simple Method for Quantitative Analysis of Human Testicular Biopsies from Epon Sections[a]

J. CHAKRABORTY, A. P. SINHA-HIKIM, and
J. JHUNJHUNWALA[b]

Department of Physiology
[b] Department of Surgery (Urology)
Medical College of Ohio
Toledo, Ohio 43699

INTRODUCTION

The apparent disorderly arrangement of human germ cell populations during the spermatogenic cycle poses great difficulty for the accurate estimation of various cell types at their particular stages of differentiation.[1-3] Moreover, an accurate identification and estimation of these cell types at a particular stage of their cellular association are both time consuming and confusing. Therefore, although the usefulness of quantitative analysis of human testicular biopsy materials has been emphasized by several investigators for better understanding of the pathology of human testis, it is almost impossible to adopt this technique using paraffin-embedded blocks for routine pathological evaluation. We proposed a simplified approach to overcome these difficulties: quantitative analyses of three major groups of germ cells from small biopsy samples embedded in epon.

MATERIALS AND METHODS

Bilateral testicular biopsies from three healthy, young kidney donors were fixed in 2.5% glutaraldehyde, post-fixed in 1% OsO_4, dehydrated, and embedded in epon, following the usual procedure. Semithin sections (1 μm) were cut from five blocks of each biopsy specimen and stained with 1% toluidine blue. A Nikon Optiphot light microscope was used for routine examination and for quantitative analytical purposes. Cross sections and oblique sections of seminiferous tubules with full view of the lumen, were chosen at random for cell counting. Numbers of spermatogonia (sum of dark-type A, pale-type A, and B spermatogonia), spermatocytes (sum of preleptotene, leptotene, zygotene, and pachytene stages), and spermatids (sum of early and late), relative to the number of Sertoli cells nuclei were counted. Total number of germ cells, for at least 500 Sertoli cells, were counted from each biopsy specimen. Ratios of germ cells to Sertoli cell were finally calculated and presented in the tabular form (TABLE 1)

[a] Supported by National Institutes of Health grant #14774.

481

TABLE 1. Differential Cell Counts of the Germinal Epithelium Expressed per Sertoli Cell

Biopsy Number	Side	Cell Type		
		Spermatogonia	Spermatocytes	Spermatids
137	Lt	1.07	1.95	2.45
	Rt	0.99	2.20	3.03
231	Lt	1.32	1.85	2.68
	Rt	1.23	1.96	2.49
243	Lt	1.05	2.10	2.35
	Rt	1.04	2.08	2.44
Mean ± SE		1.11 ± 0.05	2.02 ± 0.05	2.57 ± 0.10
Range		(0.99–1.32)	(1.85–2.20)	(2.35–3.03)

RESULTS AND DISCUSSIONS

Paraffin-embedded tissue sections had variable degree of shrinkage, artifactual damage, and loss of compactness, causing difficulty in identification and accurate estimation of various cell types. These problems were easily avoided in the epon-embedded tissue sections (FIGURE 1 A and B). The major concern regarding the epon-embedded tissue sections was whether such small pieces of tissues would provide reliable quantitative estimation of differentiating germ cells. Data obtained from our investigation on germ cell–Sertoli cell ratios, based on epon sections from six biopsy specimens, revealed an intriguing similarity with the data obtained by the previous investigators (TABLE 2) from paraffin sections. Moreover, our preliminary data on cell counts from large paraffin versus epon sections yielded a similar range of spermatogonia, spermatocytes, and spermatids counts (1.35, 2.09, and 2.3 in epon sections in comparison to 1.18, 1.88, and 2.42 in paraffin sections). The deviations in counts between the two preparations were not significant.

The present method is relatively simple and does not require the complicated identification of "staging" during spermatogenesis. Finally, based on our present data, as well as our work on an animal model,[4] it can be safely concluded that

TABLE 2. Quantitative Analysis of the Human Seminiferous Epithelium[a]

Authors	Number of Biopsies	Cell Types		
		Spermatogonia	Spermatocytes	Spermatids
Present study (epon section)	6	1.11(0.99–1.32)	2.02(1.85–2.20)	2.57(2.35–3.03)
Rowley and Heller[5] [c]	100	1.47	2.43	4.66
Skakkebaek and Heller[6] [c]	39	1.77(1.05–2.83)	2.43(1.17–3.68)	5.19(3.03–8.50)
Zukerman et al.[7c]	12[b]	1.14(0.6–2.20)	2.16(1.20–3.50)	3.59(1.2–7.8)

[a] Cell counts are expressed as number/Sertoli cell. Values are given as mean (range).
[b] From subjects with sperm count ranges from 16.0 to 89.0 × 10[6]/ml.
[c] Paraffin sections.

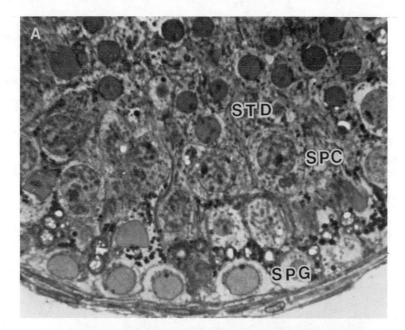

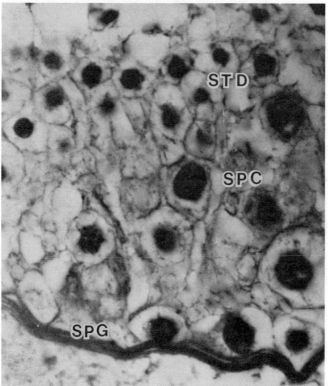

FIGURE 1. (A) Semithin section (1 μm) of a portion of human seminiferous tubule, embedded in epon, showing the compactness and better preservation of the tissue. Spermatogonia (SPG), spermatocytes (SPC), and spermatids (STD) can be easily identified in epon sections. ×960. (B)Paraffin section of the same biopsy specimen, showing poor preservation of the tissue. Although spermatogonia (SPG), spermatocytes (SPC), and spermatids (STD) can be identified, the damage in cellular morphology is evident. ×1,200.

epon-embedded small biopsy materials of human tissues may be effectively used for quantitative analysis of germ cell populations for better understanding of the testicular pathology.

REFERENCES

1. ROOSEN-RUNGE, E. C. & F. D. BARLOW. 1953. Am. J. Anat. **93:** 143–169.
2. HELLER, C. G. & Y. CLERMONT. 1964. Rec. Prog. Horm. Res. **20:** 545–575.
3. CHOWDHURY, A. K. 1971. Anat. Rec. **169:** 296 (abstr).
4. SINHA-HIKIM, A. P. & J. CHAKRABORTY. 1984. Arch Androl. (In press.)
5. ROWLEY, M. J. & C. G. HELLER. 1971. Z. Zellforsch. **115:** 461–472.
6. SKAKKEBAEK, N. E. & C. G. HELLER. 1973. J. Reprod. Fert. **32:** 379–389.
7. ZUKERMAN, Z., L. J. RODRIGUEZ-RIGAU, D. B. WEISS, A. K. CHOWDHURY, K. D. SMITH & E. STEINBERGER. 1978. Fertil. Steril. **30:** (4) 448–455.

Modulation of the Pulsatile Release of Biologically Active Luteinizing Hormone by Endogenous Opiates[a]

JOHANNES D. VELDHUIS,[b,c] ALAN D. ROGOL,[d]
MICHAEL L. JOHNSON,[e] and MARIA L. DUFAU[f]

[d,e]Department of Pharmacology
Division of Endocrinology and Metabolism
[b]Departments of Internal Medicine and
Obstetrics and Gynecology
[e]Biomathematics Core Laboratory
Diabetes Research and Training Center
The University of Virginia Medical Center
Charlottesville, Virginia 22908

[f]Section on Molecular Endocrinology
Endocrinology and Reproduction Research Branch
National Institute of Child Health and Human Development
National Institutes of Health
Bethesda, Maryland 20205

INTRODUCTION

The preferential release of pools of luteinizing hormone (LH) enriched in biologically activity has been difficult to demonstrate in humans when single bolus or continuous low dose infusions of exogenous GnRH have been used.[1,2] As an alternative experimental approach to characterize physiological release of immunoactive and bioactive LH in humans, we chose to enhance endogenous GnRH pulses by administering an opiate-receptor antagonist (Naltrexone, Endo Labs, Inc.)

MATERIALS AND METHODS

Blood was drawn at 20-minute intervals for eight hours in eight healthy men, after oral ingestion of placebo or Naltrexone (1 mg/kg). The samples were assayed for testosterone and immunoactive LH by RIA[1,2] and for bioactive LH using the rat interstitial cell testosterone assay (RICT).[1,2] Pulsatile LH secretion profiles were analyzed as described earlier.[3] A chi-square table was constructed to analyze the

[a] This work was supported in part by a Research Career Development Award AM 00153 (ADR), by National Institutes of Health Biomedical Research Support Award 5S07RR05431, a University of Virginia Computer Services Grant, and National Institute of Alcohol & Drug Abuse grant #1R03DA03315-01 (JDV), by US Public Health Service General Clinical Research Grant RR-847, and by the Diabetes Research and Training Center Grant 5 P60 AM 22125-05.
[c] Address all requests for reprints to: Dr. Johannes Veldhuis, Box 202, Department of Internal Medicine, University of Virginia Medical School, Charlottesville, Virginia.

TABLE 1. Pulsatile Secretion of Bioactive Luteinizing Hormone in Humans

Subject	Treatment	Mean LH[a]	Area[b]	Pulses/8 hours	Incremental[c]	Peak[d]	Fractional (%)[e]	Mean Periodicity[f]
A	Placebo	13.71 ± 4.96	6623	2	14.0	25.9	80	220
	Naltrexone	14.16 ± 3.07	6850	5	7.3	18.9	65	100
B	Placebo	24.86 ± 7.02	11992	3	12.1	30.3	87	180
	Naltrexone	29.21 ± 7.59	14101	4	24.2	42.2	72	125
C	Placebo	10.50 ± 3.43	5032	2.5	9.8	17.2	149	200
	Naltrexone	19.64 ± 7.08	9644	6	13.4	27.4	92	63
D	Placebo	38.77 ± 6.27	18682	3	15.0	43.8	55	180
	Naltrexone	47.38 ± 7.84	22968	4.5	17.2	57.2	65	115
E	Placebo	33.90 ± 6.57	17041	2	19.6	46.3	39	220
	Naltrexone	46.64 ± 11.86	22588	4	16.9	59.8	69	125
F	Placebo	30.86 ± 3.47	14820	1	5.9	39.6	38	–
	Naltrexone	36.40 ± 7.41	17564	3	23.6	47.0	63	180
G	Placebo	40.62 ± 17.4	19657	3	28.2	60.1	79	180
	Naltrexone	42.92 ± 15.6	20479	5.5	29.3	61.4	110	100
H	Placebo	16.21 ± 5.43	7877	2	12.1	29.3	57	220
	Naltrexone	28.23 ± 8.06	13550	3	24.	41.4	70	180
Means ± SD	Placebo	26.18 ± 10.90	12175 ± 5327	2.31 ± 0.66	14.6 ± 6.34	38.6 ± 13.2	73 ± 34	200 ± 19
	Naltrexone[g]	33.07 ± 11.5	15954 ± 5583	4.375 ± 1.02	19.5 ± 6.64	44.4 ± 14.4	76 ± 16	124 ± 37
p value (Placebo vs Naltrexone)		<0.001	<0.002	<0.001	NS	<0.01	NS	<0.002

[a] mIU/ml, mean ± SD (N = 25 samples).
[b] Area in mIU/ml × min (over eight hours of sampling).
[c] mIU/ml increment from nadir to peak.
[d] Maximal absolute LH value achieved in the pulse (mIU/ml).
[e] Percent increase above nadir.
[f] Minutes.
[g] Naltrexone 50 μg/l was devoid of effect in the RICT bioassay in vitro.

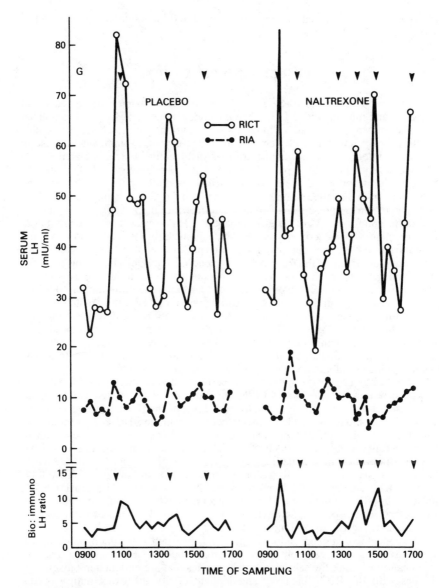

FIGURE 1. Pulsatile secretion of bioactive and immunoactive LH in one normal man following the administration of placebo or Naltrexone (1 mg/kg) at 0800. As shown on the horizontal axis, blood samples were drawn at 20-minute intervals beginning at 0900. Blood was assayed for immunoactive (RIA) and bioactive (RICT) LH, from which the corresponding profiles of LH release were constructed and the associated bioactive and immunoactive LH ratios (bio : immuno) computed. Significant bioactive LH pulses are designated by the arrows (three pulses after placebo and four pulses after Naltrexone). Note the tendency of increased bio : immuno LH ratios (lowermost curve) to accompany LH pulses after either placebo or Naltrexone ingestion.

expected versus observed distribution of increased bioactive and immunoactive LH ratios within LH pulses.[3]

RESULTS AND DISCUSSION

We have been able to characterize for the first time changes in the release of bioactive and immunoactive LH, when the endogenous GnRH signal is amplified by opiate-receptor blockade. Under these conditions, in which no discernible opiate agonist action can be demonstrated, there was a significant increase in mean and integrated serum concentrations of bioactive LH, associated with a striking accentuation in the pulsatile pattern of LH release ($p<0.01$) (TABLE 1). Since the pituitary gland is devoid of intrinsic periodicity for LH release, the enhancement in bioactive LH pulse frequency must reflect an amplification of the endogenous GnRH pulse signal. In association with this presumptive augmentation of the endogenous GnRH signal, bioactive LH pulses demonstrated preferential enrichment in bioactivity, reflected by significantly increased bioactive and immunoactive LH ratios compared with interpulse baseline ratios ($p<0.001$). We infer that modulation of the frequency of the endogenous GnRH stimulus provides one hypothalamic mechanism by which to control net pituitary release of LH molecules that retain high biological activity. This inference was supported by our demonstration of acutely increased mean or integrated serum testosterone concentrations in these men after Naltrexone administration (mean testosterone levels rose from 570 ± 151 to 645 ± 120 ng/dl, $p<0.05$). Thus, the apparent increase in bioactive LH quantitated by the RICT assay *in vitro* correctly reflects an increase in circulating concentrations of biologically effective LH with consequent significant effects upon target cells in the gonad *in vivo*.

Our studies do not permit us to ascertain whether increased testosterone secretion represents a response to the increase in LH pulse frequency, the increase in LH pulse amplitude, or both. However, further investigations using the *in vitro* RICT bioassay to quantitate effective circulating LH concentrations in subjects in whom the frequency and amplitude of LH pulses can be experimentally controlled will be able to clarify which attributes of the pulsatile LH signal are most important in stimulating Leydig cell steroidogenesis. Use of the RICT bioassay of LH (rather than RIA alone) provides an important investigative tool, because RIA estimates of LH pulses were 29% discordant with bioactive LH pulses, while 17% of bioactive LH pulses occurred without significant immunoactive pulses. Thus, some bioactive LH pulses could not be detected from analysis of immunoactive LH data alone.

We conclude that neuroendocrine mechanisms, such as the endogenous opiate system studied here, can control the pulsatile mode of LH release and thereby significantly regulate the secretion of LH species that are enriched in bioactivity. Studies with the RICT bioassay should help clarify the exact nature of the pulsatile bioactive LH signal that is most effective in enhancing trophic and steroidogenic functions of the gonad in health and disease.

ACKNOWLEDGMENTS

We are grateful for the expert technical support of Mercedes A. Serabian and our nurses in the Clinical Research Center of the University of Virginia. We thank

Doctor Richard Santen and Doctor Robert A. Steiner for provision of the computer programs. Reagents for the LH assay were donated by the National Institute of Arthritis, Metabolic, & Digestive Diseases, National Institutes of Health, Bethesda MD.

REFERENCES

1. DUFAU, M. L., I. Z. BEITINS, J. W. MCARTHUR & K. J. CATT. 1976. Effects of luteinizing hormone releasing hormone (LHRH) upon bioactive and immunoreactive serum LH levels in normal subjects. J. Clin. Endocrinol. Metab. **43:** 658–665.
2. BEITINS, I. Z., M. L. DUFAU, K. O'LOUGHLIN, K. J. CATT & J. W. MCARTHUR. 1977. Analysis of biological and immunological activities in the two pools of LH released during constant infusion of luteinizing hormone-releasing hormone (LHRH) in men. J. Clin. Endocrinol. Metab. **45:** 605–611.
3. DUFAU, M. L., J. D. VELDHUIS, F. FRAIOLI, M. L. JOHNSON & I. Z. BEITINS. 1983. Mode of bioactive luteinizing hormone secretion in man. J. Clin. Endocrinol. Metab. **57:** 993–1000.

Leydig Cell Cytoplasmic Mass, Daily Sperm Production, and Serum Gonadotropin Levels in Aging Men[a]

WILLIAM B. NEAVES,[b] LARRY JOHNSON, JOHN C. PORTER, C. RICHARD PARKER, JR., AND CHARLES S. PETTY

Departments of Cell Biology,
Obstetrics and Gynecology, and Pathology
The University of Texas Health Science
Center at Dallas
Dallas, Texas 75235

Our study defined Leydig cell mass and sperm production rates in testes of aging men while examining relevant hormone levels in the serum. Our previous work[1] showed that Leydig cell mass diminished with increasing age but did not address the impact of this loss on androgen status, as reflected in circulating levels of testosterone. Nor did that work examine circulating levels of gonadotropin for insight into extratesticular factors associated with aging. The present study was designed to address these points while yielding new evidence on the spermatogenic function of aging human testes.

We studied 17 men between 20 and 50 years of age (33 ± 2 yr, mean and S.E.) and 16 men between 51 and 85 years of age (60 ± 3 yr). Testes and blood samples were obtained at autopsy in less than 15 hours after sudden, unattended death. Leydig cell cytoplasmic mass was determined by quantitative histometric estimation of the proportion of glutaraldehyde-perfused, decapsulated testicular parenchyma (weighed to the nearest 0.01 g) occupied by Leydig cell cytoplasm in both testes of each subject. Daily sperm production was determined by phase-contrast cytometry of round spermatids in homogenates of both fixed testes from each individual. LH and FSH in serum of blood from the heart or large veins of the subjects were quantified by radioimmunoassay, and the values were unrelated to postmortem time (rho $= +0.06$, $p > 0.7$ and $+0.05$, $p > 0.8$ for LH and FSH, respectively).

Total Leydig cell cytoplasmic mass was 63% greater in the younger men (1.74 ± 0.14 g versus 1.07 ± 0.10 g, $p < 0.005$) than in the older men and showed a significant negative correlation with increasing age in all 33 men (rho $= -0.60$, $p < 0.001$). The mean LH level in the older men was more than twice that in the younger men (135 ± 20 ng/ml versus 55 ± 18 ng/ml, p < 0.01), and serum LH was positively correlated with increasing age (rho $= +0.47$, $p < 0.01$). Total daily sperm production in the older men was less than half that in the younger men ($130 \pm 18 \times 10^6$ versus $274 \pm 27 \times 10^6$, $p < 0.001$) and was negatively correlated with

[a] Supported by National Institutes of Health grant AG 02260.

[b] Address correspondence to: Dr. W. B. Neaves, Department of Cell Biology, The University of Texas Health Science Center at Dallas, 5323 Harry Hines Blvd., Dallas, Texas 75235.

increasing age (rho = -0.72, $p < 0.001$). The mean FSH level in the older men was more than twice that in the younger men (209 ± 56 ng/ml versus 85 ± 18 ng/ml, $p < 0.001$), and serum FSH was positively correlated with increasing age (rho = $+0.57$, $p < 0.001$). Neither prolactin nor testosterone levels were significantly different in the two age groups. The highest FSH levels (914 and 652 ng/ml) were observed in two men who were 72 and 73 years old and who had the lowest daily sperm production recorded in the study (25×10^6 and 41×10^6, respectively). Hence, it appears that the decline in Leydig cell cytoplasmic mass and in daily sperm production in aging men is accompanied by increasing blood levels of LH and FSH.

This work confirms the age-related decline in Leydig cell cytoplasm described in an earlier study of similar subjects.[1] It also shows that aging is associated with elevated levels of serum LH and with undiminished levels of serum testosterone. Hence, the loss of substantial Leydig cell mass in older men does not necessarily result in reduced levels of testosterone in the circulation.

This study also shows that daily sperm production declines in aging men and that the decline is accompanied by marked elevation of serum FSH. Extremely high levels of serum FSH in men with the lowest daily sperm production indicate a sensitivity of the pituitary to a primary testicular defect in spermatogenesis.

REFERENCE

1. KALER, L. W. & W. B. NEAVES. 1978. Attrition of the human Leydig cell population with advancing age. Anat. Rec. **192:** 513–518.

Effect of Age and Illness on LH Bio/Immuno Ratio[a]

B. WARNER,[b] M. DUFAU,[c] and R. J. SANTEN[d]

[b]Department of Medicine
Wright State University School of Medicine
Dayton, Ohio 45428

[c]Section on Molecular Endocrinology
Endocrinology and Reproduction Research Branch
National Institute of Child Health and Human Development
National Institutes of Health,
Bethesda, Maryland 20205

[d]Department of Medicine
Division of Endocrinology
The Milton S. Hershey Medical Center
The Pennsylvania State University
Hershey, Pennsylvania 17033

INTRODUCTION

Decreased testicular function occurs as a concomitant of aging in men and is accentuated by the presence of systemic illness.[1] Previous studies identified an intrinsic Leydig cell defect as reflected by high LH/testosterone ratios and impaired hCG responsiveness in older men.[1,2] No quantitative impairment of gonadotropin secretion, apparent upon study of integrated LH levels, pulse amplitude, or frequency, and LHRH responsiveness has been consistently identified.[2] This study questioned whether a qualitative change in LH secretion, as reflected by altered bio/immuno LH ratios, might occur during aging and be accentuated by systemic illness.

MATERIALS AND METHODS

Eighty-seven men were included in the study: 18 non-castrate prostate cancer patients older than 40 years old; 23 men more than 40 years old and free of systemic illness (i.e., general medical clinical patients without acute illness, medical school faculty volunteers, and hospitalized patients without systemic illness); 27 men more than 40 years old but with systemic illness (including hospitalized patients actively being treated for both acute and chronic problems other than prostate cancer) and 18 young well volunteers who were less than 40 years of age. Specific methodologies for the rat interstitial cell testosterone (RICT) assay (i.e., bioassayable LH) and LH and testosterone radioimmunoassays have been previously published.[3,4] Unpaired two-tailed t tests with unequal variances as well as linear regression analyses were performed.

[a] Supported in part by Grant No. RU1 CA35816 to R. J. S. from the National Cancer Institute.

RESULTS

LH by RIA increased as a function of age ($r = 0.39$, $p < .001$) and testosterone fell ($r = -.34$, $p < .001$) as expected. The surprising finding, however, was the lack of an increase in biologically active LH with aging. Men younger than 40 years old (pre-40) had LH levels of 37 ± 3.3 mIU/ml ($N = 18$) whereas those older than 40 (post-40) had concentrations of 35 ± 5.8 mIU/ml ($N = 69$) (FIGURE 1). The rise in LH by RIA with no change by RICT resulted in a marked drop in the

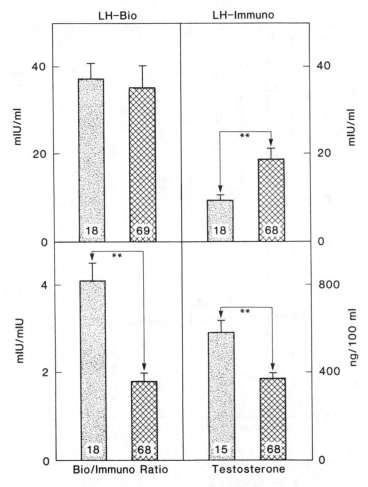

FIGURE 1. Mean ($\pm$ SEM) levels of serum LH by bioassay (LH-Bio) and radioimmunoassay (LH-Immuno), mean ratios of bioassayable to radioimmunoassayable LH (Bio/Immuno Ratio), and mean testosterone concentrations. The bars with random dots indicate normal men less than 40 years old and the double cross-hatched bars indicate the group of men over 40 who are both sick or well. The number within the bar designates the number of men whose data were available for analysis. *$p < .05$, **$p < .01$, ***$p < .001$.

bio/immuno LH ratio with aging ($r = -.53$, $p < .001$). Expressed as group means, a significantly lower ratio was observed in the post-40 group (1.79 ± 0.15) than in the men pre-40 (4.10 ± 0.34, $p < .01$). This change in bio/immuno ratio strongly suggested that a qualitative change in the circulating form of LH occurs with aging. To dissect out the effects of aging from those of illness, subsets of well

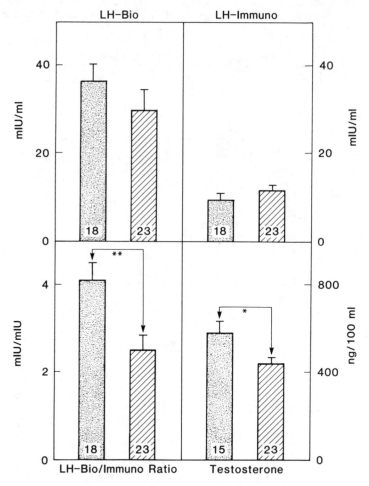

FIGURE 2. Similar to FIGURE 1 but the single hatched bars indicate the subset of 23 men over 40 who were well.

and sick men were analyzed. Both increasing age and systemic illness independently lower bio/immuno LH ratios. For example, well men over 40 had lower bio/immuno LH ratios (2.50 ± 0.32, $N = 23$) than well men less than 40 (4.10 ± 0.34, $p < .01$, $N = 18$) (FIGURE 2). The regression analysis also revealed a significant linear decline in bio/immuno LH ratio with age ($r = -.47$, $p < .01$). Sick men over 40 had lower ratios (1.44 ± 0.14, N = 45) than their well counterparts who were also over 40 years of age (2.50 ± 0.32, p < .01). The lowered bio/ immuno ratios predominantly reflected significant rises in immunologically measured LH with variable changes in biological active LH. For example, the subgroup of intact men with prostatic carcinoma (N = 18), average age 67, exhibited an increase in bioactive LH (74 ± 17 mIU/ml) whereas the intact, sick men without prostatic cancer (N = 27), average age 56, had levels of LH by bioassay of only 11.7 ± 1.1 mIU/ml. Despite the variable levels of bioactive LH, the bio/ immuno ratio in both groups was significantly lower than those observed in normal, young subjects (prostate cancer intact, 2.02 ± 0.27; intact sick men, 1.05 ± 0.08; normal young subjects, 3.95 ± 0.97).

DISCUSSION

From these data, we conclude that in addition to the Leydig cell dysfunction that occurs with aging, a qualitative abnormality of LH secretion is present. This contention is supported by direct studies in the rat[5] that demonstrated that a higher molecular weight, more sialylated form of LH is secreted by aged as opposed to young rats. Both pituitary and circulating plasma LH in the old animals studied appeared in earlier fractions eluted from gel filtration columns in young rats and this difference disappeared after neuraminidase treatment. In addition, Winters et al.[2] found a slower apparent rate of decline of LH after LHRH-induced peaks in elderly men, a finding consistent with a qualitative change in LH (as well as with other possibilities).

Based upon these studies, we suggest that regulation of the qualitative type of the LH molecule secreted could provide an additional level of control of the reproductive system in men. Qualitative changes in LH have now been demonstrated during the fall of LH during infancy and the rise during puberty, during LH pulse peaks as opposed to interpulse intervals, and during the process of aging and with systemic illness.[6-8]

REFERENCES

1. BREMNER, W. J., M. V. VITIELLO & P. N. PRINZ. Loss of circadian rhythmicity in blood testosterone levels with aging in normal men. J. Clin. Endocrinol. Metab. 56: 1278–1281.
2. WINTERS, S. J. & P. TROEN. 1982. Episodic luteinizing hormone secretion and the response of LH and follicle-stimulating hormone to LH-releasing hormone in aged men: Evidence for coexistent primary testicular insufficiency and an impairment in gonadotropin secretion. J. Clin. Endocrinol. Metab. 55: 560–565.
3. DUFAU, M., I. BEITINS, J. McARTHUR & K. CATT. 1977. Bioassay of serum LH concentrations in normal and LHRH-stimulated human subjects. In The Testis in Normal and Infertile Men. P. Troen & H. Nankin, Eds.: 309–325. Raven Press. New York.
4. DUFAU, M. L., R. POCK, A. NEUBAUER & K. J. CATT. 1976. In vitro bioassay of LH in human serum: the interstitial cell testosterone (RICT) assay. J. Clin. Endocrinol. Metab. 42: 958–968.
5. CONN, P. M., R. COOPER, C. McNAMARA, D. C. ROGERS & L. SHOENHARDT. 1980. Qualitative change in gonadotropin during normal aging in the male rat. Endocrinology 106: 1549–1553.

6. TORRESANI, T., E. SCHUSTER & R. ILLIG. 1983. Bioactivity of plasma luteinizing hormone in infants and young children. Acta Endocrinol. **103:** 326–330.
7. REITER, E. O., I. Z. BEITINS, T. OSTREA & J. P. GUTAI. 1982. Bioassayable luteinizing hormone during childhood and adolescence and in patients with delayed pubertal development. J. Clin. Endocrinol. Metab. **54:** 155–161.
8. DUFAU, M. L., J. D. VELDHUIS, F. FRAIOLI, M. L. JOHNSON & I. Z. BEITINS. 1983. Mode of secretion of bioactive luteinizing hormone in man. J. Clin. Endocrinol. Metab. **57:** 993–1000.

Idiopathic Post-pubertal LH Deficiency

GLENN R. CUNNINGHAM

Departments of Medicine and Cell Biology
Baylor College of Medicine
Veterans Administration Medical Center
Houston, Texas 77211

INTRODUCTION

Post-pubertal deficiency of LH in the absence of a pituitary, parasellar, or hypothalamic tumor, hyperprolactinemia, or trauma is said to be rare. During the past two years, we have evaluated four men with complaints of sexual dysfunction who were found to be androgen deficient and to have unexplained deficiency of LH.

PATIENT POPULATION AND RESULTS

Historical and physical findings are indicated in TABLE 1. None of the men were diabetic and screening chemistries revealed normal renal and liver function. Serum iron was not elevated. Each man had normal thyroid tests and basal prolactin levels (<10 ng/ml). Patient 4 had an 8 A.M. cortisol level of 7.4 μg/dl, but it rose to 30 μg/dl following insulin-induced hypoglycemia. Patient 2 had a basal cortisol value of 14 μg/dl. Although his serum glucose fell from 78 to 44 mg/dl following the administration of insulin, there was no GH or cortisol response. Serum prolactin and TSH increased normally after the administration of TRH.

Evaluation of the hypothalamic-pituitary-testicular axis is shown in TABLE 2. Basal serum values were determined using pooled aliquots from three specimens obtained at 15-minute intervals. Basal LH levels were inappropriately low for the reduced levels of testosterone, indicating hypothalamic or pituitary disease. None of the men had normal testosterone values after taking clomiphene citrate; however, patients 1 and 3 had some response. The discrepancies in gonadotropin and testosterone responses for patient 4 are unexplained. Patient 2 had no rise in LH or FSH following LHRH treatment.

None of the men had radiographic evidence of a pituitary, parasellar, or hypothalamic tumor. Each man underwent computerized tomography (CT) with axial and direct coronal views of the sella turcica and the parasellar and hypothalamic areas. A partially empty sella of normal size was observed in patient 1. The multiple endocrine deficiencies of patient 2 resulted in extensive radiological studies. A CT scan using 3-mm cuts indicated that the sella was normal, and no suprasellar lesion was noted when metrizamide was used to outline the parasellar structures. Polytomography of the sella demonstrated calcification of the carotid siphon, but cerebral angiography indicated no aneurysm or displacement of the vascular structures.

Each of these men has experienced dramatic subjective resolution of the presenting complaints during treatment with testosterone cypionate (200 mg i.m. every two or three weeks) and no new symptoms have evolved. The duration of treatment ranged from 3 to 22 months.

TABLE 1. Clinical Data

Patient	Age	Presenting Symptoms	Married (yrs)	Children (ages)	Medicines	Testis Size (cm)	Signs of Androgen Deficiency	Other Medical Problems
1	29	No ejaculate ×5 yr Intercourse 1×/wk	3 Divorced 4 mo.	Wife had tubal ligation	None	L–4.6×2.0 R–4.6×2.2	Hair–light Prostate–0	
2	60	Impotent <10 yr	40	39 37 27	Ascriptin Sulandec	L–4.5×2.1 R–4.4×2.0	Hair–light ♀ escutcheon Face–fine wrinkles Prostate–1+	Rheumatoid Arthritis Antithyroglobulin Antibody titer (+) 1:5120
3	46	↓Libido × 1 yr Intercourse 1×/mo	22	19 16	Nicotinic acid	L–4.7×2.3 R–4.6×2.6	Hair–Nl Prostate–2+	Hypertriglyceridemia
4	55	↓Libido × 1.5 yr Intercourse 1×/mo	30	29 27 22	Ventolin Chlortrimeton	L–5.5×3.0 R–4.6×3.0	Hair–Nl Prostate–2+	Obesity (+47%) Asthma CA Parotid–(12 yr post-op, post-radiation)
Normal						>4.0×>2.0	Prostate–2+	

TABLE 2. Evaluation of the Hypothalamic-pituitary-testicular Axis

Patient	Testosterone (ng/dl)		LH (ng/ml)[b]		FSH (ng/ml)[b]		LH (ng/ml)	
	Basal	Clomiphene[a]	Basal	Clomiphene[a]	Basal	Clomiphene[a]	Basal	Peak[c]
1	60	100	<16	<16	<31	<31		
2	65		<16		<31		<16	<16
3	152	309	<16	18.0	76.4	110.9		
4	319	263	<16	37.0	<77	116.0	<16	74
Normal	350–1000		<16–70		<31–260		<16–70	

[a] Clomiphene citrate 50 mg p.o. bid × 7 days.
[b] Standard LER-907.
[c] LHRH 100 μg given as an i.v. bolus.

DISCUSSION

The four men presented in this report developed symptoms and signs of androgen deficiency many years after normal sexual maturity was achieved. All four have gonadotropin deficiency in the absence of hyperprolactinemia. Patient 2 also has loss of GH and ACTH reserve. The pathogenesis of the LH deficiency in these men is unresolved since the usual etiologies of acquired LH deficiency have been excluded. Patient 2 has rheumatoid arthritis and a significant titer of anti-thyro-globulin antibodies. Thus, autoimmune hypophysitis is a consideration. Patient 4 is 47% overweight. This could result in a low total testosterone value and a low normal free testosterone, but it should not cause an abnormal response to clomiphene citrate. His pituitary may have been exposed to some radiation when the parotid bed was previously irradiated for treatment of a parotid tumor. This would appear to be an unlikely cause of isolated gonadotropin deficiency. Thus, we have no explanation for the LH deficiency in patients 1 and 3, and can only speculate on the etiology in patients 2 and 4. Detection of four patients with idiopathic post-pubertal LH deficiency by a single physician over a two-year interval suggests that this condition may not be so rare.

Circulating Immune Complexes and Antisperm Antibodies in Vasectomized and Vasovasostomized Rhesus Macaques[a]

NANCY J. ALEXANDER,[b,d] THOMAS B. CLARKSON,[c] and
DAVID L. FULGHAM[b]

[b]Reproductive Biology and Behavior
Oregon Regional Primate Research Center
Beaverton, Oregon 97006

[c]Department of Comparative Medicine
Bowman Gray School of Medicine
Wake Forest University
Winston-Salem, North Carolina 27103

Sperm contain many antigens that can elicit autoantibody production. After a vasectomy, spermatozoa are confined to the epididymis and vas deferens, where they degenerate and release antigens that enter the circulation directly or are phagocytosed by macrophages. A humoral immune response is initiated and circulating antibodies to sperm develop in both men and animals.

We measured the levels of circulating antibodies to spermatozoa in 51 vasectomized rhesus monkeys (*Macaca mulatta*), some of whom had been vasectomized for as long as 14 years, and compared these values to data on control monkeys. Antibodies to sperm, measured by immobilization[1] and sperm agglutination,[2] developed in 43% of the vasectomized monkeys but in none of the controls (FIGURE 1). We gave 15 monkeys vasectomy reversals six months after their initial operation. One year later, 53% (8/15) remained positive for circulating antibodies to sperm.

Spermatozoa produced after a vasectomy are a constant source of antigen that results in antibody production. The presence of antigen and persistent antibody may result in immune-complex disease. We have postulated that the increase in atherosclerosis found in vasectomized monkeys is due to injury of the arterial wall by immune-complex deposition.[3,4] To test this hypothesis, we evaluated the levels of circulating immune complexes in the same 51 vasectomized monkeys. We measured the circulating immune complexes either by a *Staphylococcus aureus* binding assay[5] or a Clq solid-phase assay.[6] Circulating immune complexes were present in 57% of the vasectomized monkeys but in only 15% of the control group ($p < 0.005$ by χ^2) (FIGURE 1). There was no association between the presence of antibodies and circulating immune complexes. Before reversal, circulating immune complexes were present in 10 of the 15 monkeys; 6 had antibodies. One year

[a] The work described in this article, Publication No. 1336 of the Oregon Regional Primate Research Center, was supported by National Institute of Child Health and Human Development contract N01-HD-8-2827 and National Institutes of Health grant RR-00163.

[d] Address correspondence to: Nancy J. Alexander, Ph.D. Oregon Regional Primate Research Center, 505 N.W. 185th Avenue, Beaverton, OR 97006.

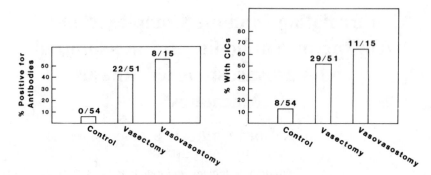

FIGURE 1. Percentages of control, vasectomized, and vasovasostomized rhesus macaques with antisperm antibodies (left). On the right, the percentages of monkeys with circulating immune complexes (CIC) are compared. The fraction above each bar is the number positive/ the number tested.

TABLE 1. Relationship of the Presence or Absence of Antisperm Antibody and Circulating Immune Complexes to the Extent of Atherosclerosis

Monkey Number	Time Post Vasectomy (years)	Antisperm Antibodies	Circulating Immune Complexes	Extensive Abdominal Aorta Atherosclerosis
1062	14	−	+	+
1065	14	−	+	+
1067	14	−	+	+
3148	10	−	−	+
3152	10	−	−	+
3157	10	−	−	+
3150	10	+	−	−
3151	10	+	−	−
5316	9	+	+	−
5532	9	+	+	−
7938	4	+	+	−
7939	4	−	+	+
7940	4	+	+	−
7946	4	+	+	−
7948	4	+	+	−
7138	3	+	+	−
Controls				
1207		−	−	−
1636		−	−	−
1658		−	−	−
5020		−	−	−
5530		−	−	−
5531		−	−	−
7158		−	−	−

after the vasovasostomy, 11 of 15 had circulating immune complexes. There was no correlation between the presence of antibodies and the presence of circulating immune complexes.

We compared the extent of the atherosclerotic lesions in control and vasectomized monkeys. Plaques in the control animals occupied an average of 4.5% of the intimal surface, whereas those in the long-term–vasectomy group had a mean intimal surface involvement of 34.6% ($p < 0.001$).[4] We sought to determine if there was any relationship between the extent of abdominal atherosclerosis in the vasectomized monkeys and the presence of antisperm antibodies or circulating immune complexes. There was more extensive atherosclerosis in animals whose vasectomies had been performed years earlier (TABLE 1). Extensive atherosclerosis seemed to develop more often in monkeys lacking antisperm antibodies than in monkeys with antisperm antibodies. Furthermore, there was no correlation between the presence or absence of circulating immune complexes measured at the time of necropsy and the presence of atherosclerosis; the reason may be the fact that all immune complexes do not damage the endothelium. Complexes of a certain size may be particularly detrimental. Other unknown factors may also play an important role in plaque formation.

Vasectomy reversal did not cause a reduction in the percentage of monkeys with circulating immune complexes. It is not clear whether this is because certain histopathologic phenomena, once initiated, are continued, or because vasectomy reversal does not eliminate sperm leakage. We do know that in a study on vasectomized cynomolgus macaques castration resulted in a rapid diminution of circulating immune complexes and, at a later date, a loss of antisperm antibody activity (data not presented).

In summary, vasectomy in rhesus monkeys results in an immune response to sperm antigen, i.e., in the development of circulating immune complexes and antisperm antibodies that persist after vasectomy reversal. There is no one-to-one association between circulating immune complexes and the severity of abdominal atherosclerosis. In some cases, the presence of antisperm antibodies seems to protect against the development of atherosclerosis.

REFERENCES

1. ISOJIMA, S., T. S. LI & Y. ASHITAKA. 1968. Immunologic analysis of sperm-immobilizing factor found in sera of women with unexplained sterility. Am. J. Obstet. Gynecol. **101:** 677–683.
2. KIBRICK, S., D. L. BELDING & B. MERRILL. 1952. Methods for the detection of antibodies against mammalian spermatozoa. II. A gelatin agglutination test. Fertil. Steril. **3:** 430–438.
3. ALEXANDER, N. J. & T. B. CLARKSON. 1978. Vasectomy increases the severity of diet-induced atherosclerosis in *Macaca fascicularis*. Science **201:** 538–541.
4. CLARKSON, T. B. & N. J. ALEXANDER. 1980. Long-term vasectomy: Effects on the occurrence and extent of atherosclerosis in rhesus monkeys. J. Clin. Invest. **65:** 15–25.
5. BARKAS, T. 1981. A simple, rapid and sensitive assay for immune complexes using a *Staphylococcus aureus* immunoadsorbent. J. Clin. Lab. Immunol. **5:** 59–65.
6. HUNT, J. S., M. P. KENNEDY, K. E. BARBER, & A. R. McGIVEN. 1980. A microplate adaptation of the solid-phase Clq immune complex assay. J. Immunol. Methods **33:** 267–275.

Detection of Spontaneously Occurring Sperm-directed Antibodies in Infertile Couples by Immunobead Binding and Enzyme-linked Immunosorbent Assay

RICHARD BRONSON, GEORGE COOPER, and
DAVID ROSENFELD

Department of Obstetrics and Gynecology
North Shore University Hospital
Long Island, New York

STEVEN S. WITKIN

Department of Obstetrics and Gynecology
New York Hospital
Cornell University Medical College
New York, New York 10021

Those early events leading to fertilization (capacitation, the acrosome reaction, and gamete membrane fusion) are associated with alterations in the sperm cell surface. It has been our premise that antibodies directed against antigens of the sperm surface would have the potential to impair fertilization.[1] As sera of fertile men and women also possess naturally occurring antibodies directed against internal components of spermatozoa,[3] tests utilized to detect the presence of antisperm antibodies must distinguish between these two groups. Immunobead binding utilizes the interaction of test serum with living, motile sperm[3] and an antibody detector (Immunobeads, Bio-Rad), in contrast to most enzyme-linked immunosorbent assays (ELISA), where spermatozoa or sperm extracts are fixed by different methods to microtiter wells. Our concern was that denaturation and loss of surface antigens might occur during fixation, and in addition, breakdown of the sperm plasma membrane might lead to exposure of intracellular antigens that would be expected to play no role in reproduction.

Five sera were initially studied that possessed antisperm antibodies of known immunoglobulin classes directed against different regions of the sperm surfaces, as detected by immunobead binding. These results were compared with those obtained by an enzyme-linked immunosorbent assay that utilized (1) live motile sperm glutaraldehyde-fixed to wells following their interaction with antibodies in test serum; (2) fresh sperm pre-fixed by glutaraldehyde to wells followed by reaction with serum; (3) fresh sperm air-dried to wells subsequently reacted with test serum; or (4) frozen spermatozoa. Alkaline phosphatase–conjugated Ig class–specific swine antiglobulins were used as second antibodies. The patterns of immunoglobulin classes of sperm-reactive antibodies detected were comparable only when live sperm were incubated in test serum prior to their fixation. Certain antibody classes were missing and new antibody classes detected in each of the three other categories (TABLE 1).

In a larger group of sera tested, utilizing live sperm for ELISA, 78% of the sera were judged positive for sperm-reactive antibodies by both methods, while for

TABLE 1. Comparison of Antisperm Antibodies Detected by Immunobead Binding Versus ELISA

Patient Sera	Immunobead Binding			Sera Reacted First With Live Motile Sperm Then Glutaraldehyde Fixed to Wells			Sera Reacted With Fresh Sperm Glutaraldehyde Fixed to Wells			Sera Reacted With Fresh Sperm Air Dried to Wells			Sera Reacted With Frozen Sperm Glutaraldehyde Fixed to Wells		
	IgG	A	M	IgG	A	M	IgG	A	M	IgG	A	M	IgG	A	M
R	+	+	−	+	+	−	+	−	+	+	+	+	+	+	+
M	+	+	+	+	+	+	+	−	+	+	+	−	+	−	+
Rm	+	+	−	+	+	−	+	−	−	+	+	−	−	−	−
E	+	+	−	+	+	−	+	−	+	−	+	−	−	−	−
B	+	+	−	+	+	−	+	+	+	+	+	−	+	−	+

The patterns of immunoglobulin classes of sperm-reactive antibodies detected were comparable only when live sperm were incubated in test serum prior to fixation. Certain antibody classes were missing and new antibody classes detected in each of the other three test categories, indicating that fixation of spermatozoa had altered their antigenicity.

fixed sperm, the assays were in agreement only 47% of the time. When the assays disagreed, serum was often judged to be negative for sperm-reactive antibodies by ELISA but positive by immunobead binding, occurring in 18% and 38% of sera when live or fixed sperm were used, respectively. When live spermatozoa were used, 83% of the IgG classes detected by immunobead binding were also detected by ELISA. Seventy percent of the IgAs were also detected. However, only 36% of IgMs were detected by ELISA when compared with immunobead binding. The dropout rate was even higher when fixed sperm were used in the enzyme-linked immunosorbent assay. Only 13% of IgGs, 44% of IgAs, and 36% of IgMs were detected (TABLE 2).

TABLE 2. Comparison of Antisperm Antibodies Detected in 45 Sera by Immunobead Binding Versus ELISA

Ig Classes Detected by Immunobeads in Positive Sera	Ig Classes Detected by ELISA (Live Sperm)							
	G	A	M	G M	A M	A G	G A M	Negative
G	1	1						
A		1						
M			1		1			3
AM		1			1	1		2
AG	2		1			4	1	1
GM	2						1	
GAM	1			1		4	1	2

Summary Immunoglobulin Classes Detected	Immunobead Binding	ELISA
G	23	19 (83%)
M	22	8 (36%)
A	25	17 (70%)

Comparison is made of the Ig classes detected by both techniques. When live sperm were used, 83% of the IgG classes detected by immunobead binding were also detected by ELISA. Seventy percent of the IgAs were also detected. However, only 36% of IgMs were detected by ELISA when compared with immunobead binding.

The dropout rate was even higher when fixed sperm were used in the enzyme-linked immunosorbent assay. Only 13% of IgGs, 44% of IgAs, and 36% of IgMs were detected.

These results lend credence to our concern that use of non-living or fixed spermatozoa exhibit altered antigenicity, leading to an inability to detect large classes of antibodies.

Sources of error that might account for the disagreement between assays include (1) varying incubation time of test serum and target sperm during passive antibody transfer; (2) varying sensitivity and specificity of detector antiglobulins; (3) the amount of reaction product produced in the enzyme-linked immunosorbent assay would be expected to vary with the extent of binding to the sperm surface of the enzyme-linked second antibody. ELISA may then be insensitive to the presence of those antibodies directed against limited specific regions of the sperm surface, such as the tail end-piece. (4) Expression of antigens on the sperm surfaces may vary between individuals, an important consideration in tests utilizing spermatozoa from unselected donors, as would be the case both in ELISA and radiolabeled antiglobulin assays.

In summary, these results emphasize the importance of using living spermatozoa in the detection of sperm-reactive antibodies. They indicate that antigens may be altered or lost during fixation processes leading to false negative or positive results. Defined populations of motile sperm, preferably from the husband of the involved infertile couple, should be utilized for testing if clinical judgement is to be made concerning the relevance of such antibodies to altered reproduction.

REFERENCES

1. BRONSON, R. A., G. COOPER & D. ROSENFELD. 1983. Complement-mediated effects of sperm head-directed human antibodies on the ability of human sperm to penetrate zona-free hamster eggs. Fertil. Steril. **40:** 91–95.
2. TUNG, K., W. D. COOK, JR., T. A. MCCARTY & P. ROBITAILLE. 1976. Human sperm antigens and antisperm antibodies. II. Age-related incidence of antisperm antibodies. Clin. Exp. Immunol. **25:** 73.
3. WITKIN, S. S. & A. M. BONGIOVANNI. Enzyme-linked immunosorbent assay for antibodies to spermatozoa. WHO Workshop on Antibodies to Reproductive Tract Antigens. (Tokushima, August 13–15, 1983.)

Characterization of Human Sperm Antigens Using Monoclonal Antibodies[a]

MARK D. HIRSCHEL, MOHAMED A. ISAHAKIA, and
NANCY J. ALEXANDER[b]

Reproductive Biology and Behavior
Oregon Regional Primate Research Center
Beaverton, Oregon 97006

Department of Anatomy
Oregon Health Sciences University
Portland, Oregon 97201

Investigators have attempted to identify the intrinsic or sperm-coating antigens that elicit an iso- or autoantibody response. Despite their efforts, difficulties in using sera from infertile men and women have prevented a solution. In our study, we sought to develop monoclonal antibodies that agglutinated or immobilized sperm in a manner similar to that of serum from patients believed to be immunologically infertile. Using these monoclonal antibodies, we have identified and partially characterized sperm surface antigens that generate a response resembling the iso- or autoimmune response.

METHODS

Monoclonal antibodies to human sperm were produced by fusion of NS-1 myeloma cells to spleen cells of BALB/c mice[1] (immunized with washed ejaculated sperm). We screened the initial clones in an enzyme-linked immunosorption assay (ELISA) involving whole sperm and Triton X-100 or lithium 3,5-diiodosalicylate sperm membrane extracts.[2] We subsequently screened the recloned lines with ELISA, indirect immunofluorescence,[3] and Western blot techniques;[4] these involved seminal plasma from vasectomized men, sperm, and extracts of peripheral blood lymphocyte membranes. The immunoglobulin classes of the monoclonals were determined by immunodiffusion in agar.[5] Human sperm were used in the agglutination[6] and immobilization tests.[7] The zona-free hamster egg sperm penetration assay (SPA) was performed as described by Rogers *et al.*[8] We incubated capacitated sperm with antibody for 30 min at 37°C prior to combining them with the oocytes.

[a] The work described in the article, Publication No. 1337 of the Oregon Regional Primate Research Center, was supported by National Institutes of Health grants HD-14572 and RR-00163, U.S. Public Health Service training grant 2-T32 HD-07133, and the World Health Organization (WHO-HRP).

[b] Address correspondence to: Nancy J. Alexander, Ph.D., Oregon Regional Primate Research Center, 505 N.W. 185th Avenue, Beaverton, OR 97006.

TABLE 1. Characteristics of Monoclonal Antibodies to Human Sperm

Monoclonal Antibody	Immunoglobulin Class	Immunofluorescence Pattern	Sperm Agglutinating Activity	Sperm Immobilizing Activity[c]	SPA[a] (ova penetrated)
MA 3	IgG	Acrosomal	H-H	+	5% (2/39)
MA 4	IgG	Midpiece	—	—	ND[b]
MA 5	IgM	Equatorial	—	+	89% (30/34)
MA 8	IgG	Acrosomal	—	+	ND
MA 11	IgG	Acrosomal	H-H	—	ND
MA 12	IgG	Neck	—	—	0% (0/34)
MA 13	IgM	Acrosomal	—	+	ND
MA 18	IgG	Acrosomal	H-H	—	ND
MAH 24	IgG	Tail	ND	ND	0% (0/33)

[a] Zona-free hamster egg sperm penetration assay.
[b] ND = not determined.
[c] MA 3, MA 5, MA 8, and MA 13 immobilize live sperm in the presence of guinea pig complement.

RESULTS AND DISCUSSION

Of 24 hybridoma cell lines quantitatively assessed for antibody binding, nine were defined as sperm specific. Antigenic sperm specificity was based on a lack of cross-reactivity with seminal plasma from vasectomized men and with the lymphocyte membrane extract.

Characteristics of these sperm-specific antibodies are summarized in TABLE 1. Seven were IgG and two were IgM. Indirect immunofluorescence showed that each antibody was localized on the sperm surface. The predominant fluorescence pattern was acrosomal (diffuse and speckled, similar to that observed by Tung[3]); however, some lines reacted with the sperm midpiece, equatorial region, and tail. Six of these antibodies were positive in one or both of the tests used for sperm immobilization or agglutination. Monoclonals MA 3, 11, and 18 caused sperm to agglutinate head to head; MA 3, MA 5, MA 8, and MA 13 immobilized live sperm in the presence of guinea pig complement. Three of four monoclonals tested in the SPA blocked sperm penetration (MA 3, MA 12, and MAH 24). This finding suggests that the respective antigens are directly involved in processes essential to normal fertilization.

Sodium dodecyl sulfate–polyacrylamide gel electrophoresis and Western blotting were used to determine the molecular weights of antigens recognized by corresponding monoclonal antibodies. Antibodies MA 3, MA 4, MA 5, MA 8, MA 11, and MA 18 recognized single antigens with molecular weights of 240 K, 30 K, 71 K, 115 K, 34 K, and 53 K, respectively. Antibodies MA 12 and MA 13 recognized antigenic determinants present on multiple bands less than 21 K and 40 K, respectively. Monoclonal antibody MAH 24 gave a negative result in this procedure. MA 3, MA 11, and MA 18 recognized three different acrosomal antigens involved in head-to-head agglutination of live sperm. Poulsen and Hjort[9] used sera from infertile patients, known to contain sperm-agglutinating and -immobilizing autoantibodies, to identify two 77 K molecular weight and one 40 K molecular weight iso- or autoantigenic polypeptides. They reported that additional sera with equally strong antibody activities did not implicate similar antigens. On the basis of these findings and our monoclonal results, we think several sperm-specific antigens are involved in agglutination.

One sperm-specific monoclonal antibody, MA 4, was bound to the midpiece of dog, rabbit, rat, and mouse sperm. Indirect immunofluorescence involving mouse testis revealed this antigen on spermatids, an indication that it may appear during spermatogenesis. Furthermore, this cross-reactivity suggests that similar antigenic determinants have been conserved through evolution on sperm of several mammalian species.

In summary, monoclonal antibodies directed against human sperm can be used to evaluate and partially characterize the specific antigens involved in sperm agglutination or immobilization. Additionally, these reagents are valuable probes for the investigation of sperm function.

REFERENCES

1. FAZEKAS DE ST. GROTH, S. & D. SCHEIDEGGER. 1980. Production of monoclonal antibodies: Strategy and tactics. J. Immunol. Methods 35: 1–21.
2. ALEXANDER, N. J. & D. BEARWOOD. 1984 An immunosorption assay for antibodies to spermatozoa: Comparison with agglutination and immobilization tests. Fertil. Steril. 41: 270–276.

3. TUNG, K. S. K. 1975. Human sperm antigens and antisperm antibodies. I. Studies on vasectomy patients. Clin. Exp. Immunol. **20:** 93–104.

4. TOWBIN, H., T. STAEHELIN & J. GORDON. 1979. Electrophoretic transfer of proteins from polyacrylamide gels to nitrocellulose sheets: Procedure and some applications. Proc. Natl. Acad. Sci. USA **76:** 4350–4354.

5. OUCHTERLONY, O. 1958. Diffusion-in-gel methods for immunological analysis. Prog. Allergy **5:** 1–78.

6. KIBRICK, S., D. L. BELDING & B. MERRILL. 1952. Methods for the detection of antibodies against mammalian spermatozoa. II. A gelatin agglutination test. Fertil. Steril. **3:** 430–438.

7. ISOJIMA, S., T. S. LI & Y. ASHITAKA. 1968. Immunologic analysis of sperm-immobilizing factor found in sera of women with unexplained sterility. Am. J. Obstet. Gynecol. **101:** 677–683.

8. ROGERS, B. J., H. VAN CAMPEN, M. UENO, H. LAMBERT, R. BRONSON & R. HALE. 1979. Analysis of human spermatozoal fertilizing ability using zona-free ova. Fertil. Steril. **32:** 664–670.

9. POULSEN, F. & T. HJORT. 1981. Identification of auto-antigens of the human sperm membrane. J. Clin. Lab. Immunol. **6:** 69–74.

Evaluation of Serum Antisperm Antibodies in Infertile Patients by Means of an Enzyme-linked Immunoabsorption Assay[a]

NANCY J. ALEXANDER[b] and DANA BEARWOOD

Reproductive Biology and Behavior
Oregon Regional Primate Research Center
Beaverton, Oregon 97006

Currently used tests for evaluating immunologic infertility generally rely on fresh motile sperm. Some, i.e., the sperm agglutination test (SAT)[1] and the mixed antiglobulin reaction,[2] are qualitative. Recently, the assessment of antisperm antibody titers by means of radioimmunoassays and enzyme-linked immunosorption assays (ELISA) has been reported.[3,4] These assays have been an important step in the development of a test for antisperm antibodies, but the need for fresh sperm specimens, specimen-to-specimen variability, and a changing background value, which makes it difficult to determine the baseline over which levels are clinically significant, remain problems. We report the use of a sperm membrane preparation to evaluate patients and a comparison to assays involving whole sperm. For a more complete description see Alexander and Bearwood.[5]

We used 50-ml aliquots of thawed sperm ejaculates that had been thrice-washed in 0.01 M phosphate-buffered saline (PBS). The 2 ml of packed, washed sperm were resuspended in 5 ml of 0.3 M lithium 3,5-diiodosalicylate (LIS) (Eastman Kodak, Rochester, NY) in tris(hydroxymethyl)aminomethane (Tris) buffer (pH 7.4), left at room temperature for 30 min, and then centrifuged at $15,000 \times g$ and 4°C for 30 min. The supernatant was saved. The pellet was resuspended in Tris buffer, and centrifugation was repeated. The pooled supernatants were dialyzed against several changes of Tris buffer and stored at $-20°C$. Proteins were determined with the Lowry method, and the soluble extracts were diluted to a concentration of 15 $\mu g/ml$ in carbonate buffer (pH 9.6). The diluted extract was added to each well of microtiter plates, and the trays were stored at $-4°C$. The wells were washed twice in Tween buffer (0.05% Tween 20 [Sigma Chemical Company, St. Louis, MO] in PBS). The wells were filled with a 1% wt/vol solution of polyvinyl alcohol (Sigma Chemical Company, St, Louis, MO) in Tween buffer. After 30 min, the wells were washed twice in the same buffer. The serum samples, diluted 1:20 in 4% polyethylene glycol 6000 in Tween buffer, were added to wells in triplicate, incubated at 37°C, and then washed three times in Tween buffer. The β-D-galactosidase–protein A conjugate (Zymed Laboratories, Inc., Burlingame, CA) was diluted 1:500 in Tween buffer, and 150 μl were added to

---

[a] The work described in this article, Publication No. 1335 of the Oregon Regional Primate Research Center, was supported by Syva Company and National Institutes of Health grant RR-00163.

[b] Address correspondence to: Nancy J. Alexander, Ph.D., Oregon Regional Primate Research Center, 505 N.W. 185th Avenue, Beaverton, OR 97006.

each well. After 60 min, the wells were washed five times in PBS, and then p-nitrophenyl-β-D-galactopyranoside in buffer was added to each well and the contents were incubated. Optical densities were determined.

The data on 159 serum samples from infertile patients already demonstrated to have antibodies by the sperm immobilization test (SIT) or SAT were compared to those on 18 controls (FIGURE 1). TABLE 1 summarizes a study on 186 patients, only 7 of whom were incorrectly categorized on the basis of ELISA results. The predictive value was 96%. The association between the ELISA and currently accepted tests was $p < 0.0001$.

When replicate measurements of a single serum sample were made, the coefficient of variation was less than 7%.

Serum samples from a group of infertile couples revealed that antibody values determined by the ELISA are similar for both males and females. The antigen preparation therefore seems effective for antibody screening in both male and female partners.

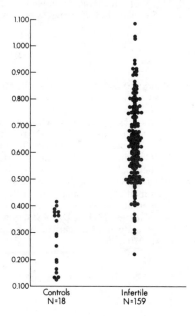

FIGURE 1. Scattergram of lithium 3,5-diiodosalicylate enzyme-linked immunosorption assay results on serum samples from infertility patients (with antibodies to sperm; determinations based on current methods) and a group of controls. All samples were run with the same lot of conjugate. The ordinate represents the optical density (opt dens) at 405 nm after incubation at 37°C for 2 hours. (From Alexander & Bearwood.[5] With permission from *Fertility and Sterility*.)

The results do not give a one-to-one correspondence with SAT or SIT results, but there is an excellent correlation between samples positive by the SAT and those positive by the ELISA ($p < 0.001$) and likewise those positive by the SIT and those positive by the ELISA ($p < 0.001$).

The sperm membrane ELISA has many advantages. It obviates the need for fresh semen and prevents a factor from any one ejaculate from being a major influence. It requires less expensive equipment and no radioactivity is involved. It can be performed as a qualitative test through naked-eye checking of samples against a color chart, or as a quantitative test through measurement of absorption units. We think the use of a sperm membrane extract fixed to the wells eliminates many problems associated with previous antisperm antibody tests, and results in values that correlate well with currently accepted SAT and SIT results.

TABLE 1. Correlation of Sperm Agglutination and Sperm Immobilization Tests with the Enzyme-linked Immunosorption Assay[a]

Category	Negative ELISA Results		Positive ELISA Results	
	Number of Persons	% of Total Population	Number of Persons	% of Total Population
SAT and SIT both negative	30	16.1	3	1.6
SAT or SIT positive	7	3.7	54	29.0
SAT and SIT both positive	4	2.2	88	47.3

[a] Total number of samples = 186. Chi square = 111.80365 with 3 degrees of freedom, $p \leq 0.0001$. Kendall's correlation coefficient, SAT and SIT, = 0.3895; ELISA and SAT = 0.2580; ELISA and SIT = 0.3214. Abbreviations: SAT, sperm agglutination test, positive ≥ 20; SIT, sperm immobilization value ≥ 2.0; ELISA, enzyme-linked immunosorption assay with 3,5-diiodosalicylate antigen.

REFERENCES

1. KIBRICK, S., D. L. BELDING & B. MERRILL. 1952. Methods for the detection of antibodies against mammalian spermatozoa. II. A gelatin agglutination test. Fertil. Steril. **3:** 430–438.
2. STEDRONSKA, J. & W. F. HENDRY. 1983. The value of the mixed antiglobulin reaction (MAR test) as an addition to routine seminal analysis in the evaluation of the subfertile couple. Am. J. Reprod. Immunol. **3:** 89–91.
3. BROWNLEE, K. A. 1953. The analysis of variance. *In* Industrial Experimentation. P. 51. Chemical Publishing Company, Inc. New York.
4. WITKIN, S. S. 1983. Enzyme-linked immunosorbent assay (ELISA) for detection of antibodies to spermatozoa. *In* Research in Reproduction. R. G. Edwards, Ed.: 1–2. International Planned Parenthood Federation. London, England.
5. ALEXANDER, N. J. & D. BEARWOOD. 1984. An immunosorption assay for antibodies to spermatozoa: Comparison with agglutination and immobilization tests. Fertil. Steril. **41:** 270–276.

Rat Spermatogenesis *in Vitro* Traced by Live Cell Squashes and Monoclonal Antibodies

JORMA TOPPARI,[a] WILLIAM R. A. BROWN,[b] and
MARTTI PARVINEN[a]

[a]*Institute of Biomedicine*
Department of Anatomy
University of Turku
SF-20520 Turku 52, Finland

[b]*MRC Reproductive Biology Unit*
Centre for Reproductive Biology
Edinburgh EH 3 9 EW, United Kingdom

The only method for follow-up of spermatogenesis *in vitro* has been the labeling of the preleptotene spermatocytes with [³H]thymidine and tracing their differentiation by autoradiography. These cells reach late pachytene in organ culture, but meiotic divisions or spermatid differentiation have never been observed in mammals.[1] We have used a new approach based on the fact that spermatogenesis in the seminiferous tubule proceeds in a wave-like fashion. Defined segments of the rat seminiferous tubules with accurately known cellular composition can be isolated for culture from any stage of the epithelial cycle by transillumination combined with phase-contrast microscopy. With this approach, it was first observed that late pachytene and diakinetic primary spermatocytes are able to differentiate up to step 5 of spermiogenesis in chemically defined conditions *in vitro*.[2] This study has now been continued in order to clarify how some critical stages of spermatogenesis proceed *in vitro*. In addition to morphological criteria, monoclonal antibodies against acrosomal glycoproteins have been used as markers for certain steps of differentiation.

Segments of the rat seminiferous tubules (2 mm) from desired stages of epithelial cycle were isolated using transillumination-assisted microdissection and placed in culture. Adjacent segments were squashed for accurate staging by phase-contrast microscopy and then frozen in liquid nitrogen. The coverslips were removed and the cells were fixed in acetone for immunoperoxidase staining. Tubular segments were incubated in 96-well tissue culture plates in 200 μl of M-199 supplemented with 1-glutamine (2 mM) and antibiotics (penicillin 100 IU/ml and streptomycin 50 μg/ml) at 32°C in a water-saturated atmosphere of 5% CO_2 and 95% air. After the culture each segment was cut into two parts, one of which was squashed and the other fixed for light or electron microscopy. The squash preparations were examined by phase-contrast microscope and immunoperoxidase stained with monoclonal antibodies CRB 8, CRB 11, CRB 13, or CRB 14, which were raised in a ten-week-old female (Balb/c $\times$ DBA/2)F_1 mouse against lentil lectin binding glycoproteins purified from rat epididymal spermatozoa.[3] The expression of antibodies was revealed by immunoperoxidase staining of precisely staged squash preparations from all stages of the epithelial cycle. The expression is as follows: CRB 8, zygotene (stage XIII) through late pachytene (stage XII)

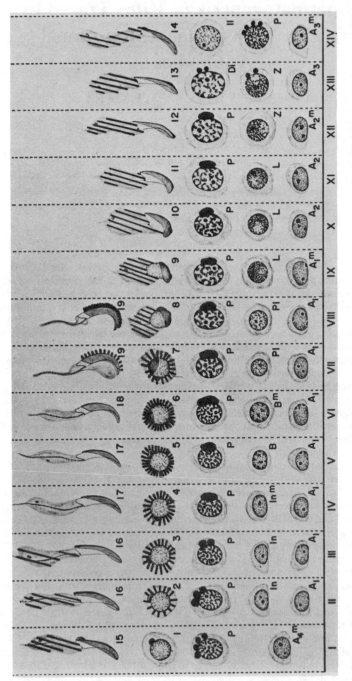

FIGURE 1. Schematic drawing of the expression of the acrosomal antigen detected by monoclonal antibody CRB 8 superimposed on a map of rat spermatogenesis. CRB 8 is a marker for zygotene primary spermatocytes (stage XIII) and steps 2 and late 19 (stages VII_c–VIII) spermatids. (From Dym & Clermont.[4] With permission from the *American Journal of Anatomy*.)

primary spermatocytes and steps 2–16 and late step 19 (stages VII$_c$–VIII) spermatids (FIGURE 1); CRB 11, steps 3–16 and late step 19 (stage VIII) spermatids; CRB 13, steps 8–19 spermatids; and CRB 14, steps 3–19 spermatids.

The differentiation of leptotene primary spermatocytes to zygotene was traced by CRB 8. The cultures were started from stages IX–XI, and continued for two days. After the culture, the chromosomes showed rotational movement typical

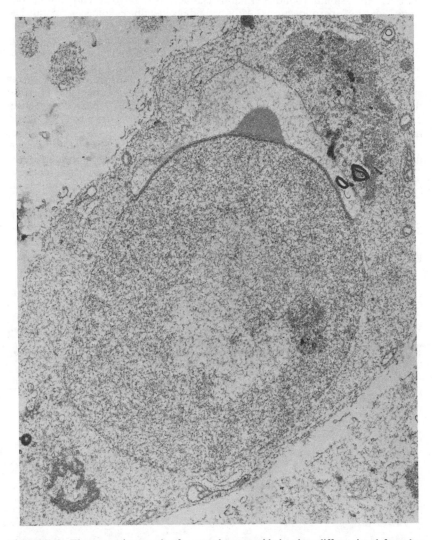

FIGURE 2. Electron micrograph of a round spermatid that has differentiated from late pachytene primary spermatocyte (stage XII) during eight days *in vitro* in chemically defined medium without added hormones or growth factors. The acrosomic system is typical for step 6 of spermiogenesis. Magnification 12,000×.

for zygotene, but not found in leptotene. In the cytoplasm of these cells, faint CRB 8–positive granules had appeared as signs of differentiation to zygotene.

The progression of early spermiogenesis was traced by monoclonal antibodies CRB 8, CRB 11, and CRB 14. Cultures were started from stages XII–XIII of the cycle, carefully controlling the absence of the round spermatids in the preparations at the onset of the culture by phase-contrast microscopy of live cell squashes from adjacent following segments. After seven days in culture, all three antigens showed expression in round spermatids characteristic for differentiation beyond steps 2 and 3 of spermiogenesis. After eight days in culture, some spermatids had acrosomic systems typical for step 6 of spermiogenesis (FIGURE 2).

The elongation of the spermatids was studied by starting the cultures from stages VII$_{a-b}$ of the cycle. After four days in culture, no nuclear elongation was observed, and only occasionally the expression of CRB 13 was detected.

The maturation of step 18 spermatids was studied by starting the cultures from stage VI of the cycle and tracing the differentiation by CRB 8 and CRB 11. After three days in culture, the expression of both antigens had appeared typical for differentiation to late step 19 of spermiogenesis. Spermiation was, however, never observed *in vitro*.

These observations suggest that spermatogenic cells that show morphological differentiation *in vitro* are able to express at least some of their specific antigens. This is particularly valuable, since in several important steps of spermatogenesis morphology of the cells does not change enough to allow precise identification.

REFERENCES

1. STEINBERGER, A. & E. STEINBERGER. 1970. In vitro growth and development of mammalian testes. *In* The Testis. A. D. Johnson, W. R. Gomes & N. L. Vandemark, Eds. **2:** 363–391. Academic Press. New York.
2. PARAVINEN, M., W. W. WRIGHT, D. M. PHILLIPS, J. M. MATHER, N. A. MUSTO & C. W. BARDIN. 1983. Spermatogenesis in vitro: completion of meiosis and early spermiogenesis. Endocrinology **112:** 1150–1152.
3. BROWN, W. R. A. & M. NIEMI. 1984. Acrosomal antigens are markers of spermatogenic differentiation in the rat. (Submitted for publication.)
4. DYM, M. & Y. CLERMONT. 1970. Role of spermatogonia in the repair of the seminiferous epithelium following X-irradiation of the rat testis. Am. J. Anat. **128:** 265–282.

Genetic Control of Steroidogenesis and Spermatogenesis in Inbred Mice[a]

CURTIS CHUBB and CATHERINE NOLAN

Department of Cell Biology
The University of Texas Health Science Center at Dallas
Dallas, Texas 75235

Genetically defined mice bearing a single gene mutation provide an experimental tool for deciphering the genetic control of testicular function. In the current studies, we investigated the reproductive effects of atrichosis (*at*), a recessive gene mutation that induces male sterility.[1] The specific effects of the mutation on spermatogenesis and testicular steroidogenesis were defined by comparisons of inbred mice that were genetically identical except at the *at* gene locus.

MATERIALS AND METHODS

Inbred male mice (F33) were purchased from the Jackson Laboratory, Bar Harbor, ME. The mice were siblings and were either mutants homozygous for the *at* gene mutation (*at/at*) or normal controls (?/+). Sibling mice were housed together and supplied with feed and water *ad libitum*. The animal room was maintained at $23 \pm 2°C$ with 14 hr light/24 hr.

Mice (9–14 weeks old) were sacrificed by cervical dislocation, selected organs weighed, and the testes trimmed of adnexa. Intact testes were either perfused *in vitro*[2] or perfusion-fixed with 2% glutaraldehyde in 0.1 M cacodylate buffer and embedded in methacrylate.[3] Randomly selected sections of testes were stained with toluidine blue.

In vitro perfused testes were utilized to assess the steroidogenic potential of mutant and control testes. The secretion profile of nine steroids was quantitatively assessed with a capillary gas chromatographic method.[4]

Spermatogenesis was evaluated by morphometric analyses of methacrylate-embedded testes. The nuclear volume fractions of Leydig cells and germ cells were determined by a point-counting method.[5] A total of 20,000 points was evaluated at $1,000\times$ magnification for each of four testes.

Significant differences were determined by Student's *t* test for unpaired samples.

RESULTS AND DISCUSSION

The atrichosis gene mutation induces sterility in male mice by depopulating the seminiferous epithelium of spermatogonia via an unknown mechanism.[1] The

[a] Supported in part by US Public Health Service Grant HD15594 from the National Institute of Child Health and Human Development.

present study confirmed the complete absence of spermatogonia in mutant mouse testes (FIGURE 1). However, the diminutive testes of atrichosis mutant mice contained abundant Sertoli and Leydig cells (FIGURE 1). Handel and Eppig[6] have previously reported that Sertoli cells of *at/at* mice differentiate normally.

The steroidogenic potential of testes was assessed by *in vivo* and *in vitro* parameters. Seminal vesicle weights of mutant and control mice were not significantly different ($p > 0.5$) (FIGURE 1). This result suggests that hypothalami were secreting LH and that Leydig cells of mutant mice were metabolically active *in vivo*. Although the morphometric studies (FIGURE 1) suggested a decrease in the relative mass of Leydig cell nuclei in mutant mice, microscopic analyses revealed a hypertrophied Leydig cell cytoplasm filled with lipid droplets. These observations support the hypothesis[7] that the degeneration of germinal epithelium stimulates Leydig cell activity. Steroid secretion rates of testes perfused *in vitro* demonstrated that mutant and control testes were comparable in their steroidogenic potential and their response to LH stimulation (FIGURE 2). Significantly, mutant and control testes secreted similar amounts of steroids although mutant testes weigh only 13% of control testes.

We conclude that the genetic controls of testicular steroidogenesis and spermatogenesis are separate. In the present case, the atrichosis gene mutation ex-

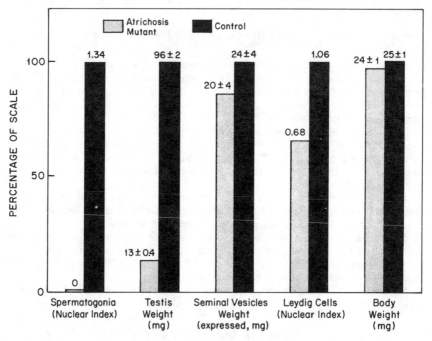

FIGURE 1. Measurements of selected reproductive parameters of atrichosis mutant mice (*at/at*) and their normal siblings (?/+). The results are expressed as a percentage of scale with the control measurements equal to 100% of scale. Nuclear indices of spermatozoa and Leydig cells were determined morphometrically according to the following formula: (volume fraction × testicular weight) · 100. The nuclear index is an estimate of the relative mass of each component. The values above the bars represent the mean ± SEM. [N = 16–22 (testis), 10–14 (seminal vesicles), 9–12 (body)].

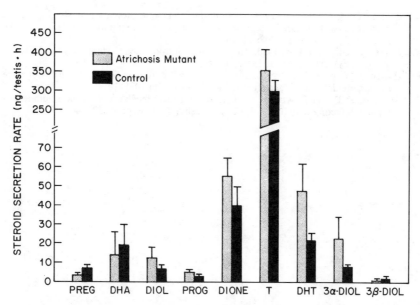

FIGURE 2. Steroids secreted by LH-stimulated testes of atrichosis mutant (*at/at*) and control (?/+) mice. The testes were perfused *in vitro* for 4 hr. DHT secretion exhibited the only significant difference ($p < 0.05$). The abbreviations and trivial names for the measured steroids are: PREG (pregnenolone), DHA (dehydroepiandrosterone), DIOL (androstene-diol), PROG (progesterone), DIONE (androstenedione), T (testosterone), DHT (dihydrotes-tosterone), 3α-DIOL (3α-androstanediol), and 3β-DIOL (3β-androstanediol). Each value represents the mean ± SEM. ($N = 4$–6).

erted a specific effect on spermatogenesis since the Leydig cells secreted normal levels of steroids in the complete absence of spermatogenesis. The results support the atrichosis mutant mouse as a genetically defined animal model of male infertility characterized by the Sertoli cell–only syndrome.

ACKNOWLEDGMENTS

Luteinizing hormone, NIAMMD-oLH-24, was provided by the National Pituitary Agency, National Institute of Arthritis, Metabolism, and Digestive Diseases, National Institutes of Health, Bethesda, MD.

REFERENCES

1. HUMMEL, K. P. 1966. Mouse News Lett. **34:** 31.
2. CHUBB, C. & C. DESJARDINS. 1983. In vitro perfusion of isolated mouse testes: a model system for investigating testicular steroidogenesis. Comp. Biochem. Physiol. **74A:** 231–237.
3. RUDDELL, C. L. 1967. Embedding media for 1–2 micron sectioning. 2. Hydroxyethyl methacrylate combined with 2-butoxyethanol. Stain Technol. **42:** 253–255.

4. CHUBB, C. & C. NOLAN. 1984. Quantitative metabolic profiling of testicular steroid secretions with bonded-phase capillary gas chromatography: validation of the method. J. Chromatogr. **308:** 11–18.
5. ELIAS, H. & D. M. HYDE. 1980. An elementary introduction to stereology (quantitative microscopy). Am. J. Anat. **159:** 411–445.
6. HANDEL, M. A. & J. J. EPPIG. 1979. Sertoli cell differentiation in the testes of mice genetically deficient in germ cells. Biol. Reprod. **20:** 1031–1038.
7. AOKI, A. & D. W. FAWCETT. 1978. Is there a local feedback from the seminiferous tubules affecting activity of the Leydig cells? Biol. Reprod. **19:** 144–158.

The Expression of Haploid-specific Genes Including an α Tubulin During Spermatogenesis in the Mouse[a]

ROBERT J. DISTEL, KENNETH C. KLEENE, and
NORMAN B. HECHT

Department of Biology
Tufts University
Medford, Massachusetts 02155

At least 10% of the proteins synthesized during spermiogenesis in the mouse are not synthesized in meiotic testicular cells or Sertoli cells.[1,2] To determine whether some of these temporal differences in protein synthesis can be attributed to haploid gene expression, we have isolated cDNA clones for several haploid-specific genes including an α tubulin and a group of translationally regulated proteins.

Using a rat brain cDNA plasmid (pILαT1) that contains both the coding and 3' untranslated regions from α tubulin, we have screened a mouse testis cDNA library and isolated a testis α tubulin cDNA (pRDαTT1). Since pRDαTT1 does not hybridize to the 3' untranslated region of pILαT1, but does hybridize to other regions of the rat α tubulin gene, we conclude it encodes a different α tubulin gene than that recognized by the brain probe. Subcloning a 360 base pair fragment from the 3' end of pRDαTT1 yields a plasmid (pRDαTT.3) that has no homology to the rat α tubulin clone, pILαT1. The remainder of pRDαTT1 was renamed pRDαTT.7. Following digestion of mouse sperm DNA with a restriction enzyme such as PstI, both pRDαTT.7 and pRDαTT.3 hybridize to many DNA fragments indicating homology to multiple mouse α tubulin genes (FIGURE 1). Similar results were obtained following digestion of genomic DNA with other enzymes such as Bam H1 and Ava 1. In addition, pRDαTT.3 hybridized to several fragments of mouse genomic DNA not detected by pRDαTT.7 or pILαT1 suggesting this clone recognizes one or more "unique" mouse α tubulin genes (note DNA fragments of 4.0, 1.8, and 1.3 kb in FIGURE 1c).

To discover the tissues and cell types that express RNA(s) homologous to pRDαTT.3, RNA blot hybridizations were performed (FIGURE 2). pRDαTT.3 hybridized to two transcripts of 2100 and 1550 bases in total of poly(A)$^+$RNA from mouse testis but no homologous transcripts could be detected in poly(A)$^+$ RNA from brain or total RNA from kidney, spleen, ovary, and liver. Hybridization of poly(A)$^+$ testis RNA with pRDαTT.7 or pILαT1 revealed an additional homologous RNA sequence of 1650 bases while two sequences of 2200 and 1750 bases were found in poly(A)$^+$ brain RNA. The 1,650 base transcript was found in both meiotic and post-meiotic cells. The haploid round spermatids and elongating spermatids but not the meiotic pachytene spermatocytes contained both the 2100 and 1550 base transcripts. These results indicate that novel α tubulin RNA transcripts are expressed in haploid testicular cells, a time during spermatogenesis when "unique" tubulins may be required in the formation of the manchette or flagellar

[a] Supported by National Institutes of Health Grant GM 29224.

axoneme. The absence of transcripts homologous to pRDαTT.3 in mouse brain suggests that the haploid testicular α tubulin(s) and the brain α tubulin(s) are transcripts from different genes. Evidence from two-dimensional gel electrophoresis of the radiolabeled polypeptides found in pachytene spermatocytes, round spermatids, and elongating spermatids supports the contention that multiple isoforms of α and β tubulin exist and that a new isoform of α tubulin (and perhaps β tubulin) is synthesized in post-meiotic cells.[3]

Several additional cDNA clones specifying poly(A)[+] mRNA whose abundance increases at least tenfold in post-meiotic cells have been isolated.[4] Two, pIC3-2 and pAH11, hybridize to mRNAs of about 580 and 900 bases, respectively. For each, the intensity of hybridization was at least tenfold greater with RNA from round and elongating spermatids than with RNA from pachytene spermatocytes. Hybridization to cytoplasmic poly(A)[+] RNA from the testes of 16-day-old mice (a developmental stage before haploid cells have differentiated) or total cytoplasmic RNA from Sertoli cells, brain, or liver failed to detect these RNA sequences. Although the mRNA encoded by pIC3-2 is present at high and constant levels throughout spermiogenesis, the expression of the encoded protein, protamine, has been demonstrated to be regulated translationally during the haploid phase of spermatogenesis.[4-6] Studies of the distribution of the protamine mRNA in polysomal and non-polysomal fractions of round spermatids and elongating spermatids demonstrated that protamine mRNA first accumulates as an untranslated ribonucleoprotein in round spermatids and is initially translated in elongating spermatids. Coincident with its translation, the 3′ poly(A) tail is shortened markedly. Although we do not know yet the protein encoded by pAH-11, these results demonstrate the existence of additional poly(A)[+] mRNAs that are absent during meiosis, present in high abundance in post-meiotic cells, and translationally regulated during spermiogenesis. The existence of haploid-specific

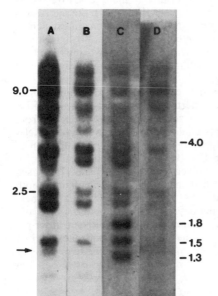

FIGURE 1. Hybridization of Pst I-digested mouse sperm DNA with tubulin cDNA clones. Mouse sperm DNA was isolated from epididymal sperm and digested with Pst I. Ten micrograms of DNA were loaded in each lane and electrophoresed in a 1% agarose gel. DNA was transferred to nitrocellulose filters, hybridized in 0.4 M sodium phosphate buffer (pH 7.0) 2× Denhardt's solution and 100 μg/ml salmon sperm DNA at 65°C, for 16 hours and washed in several changes of 0.4 M phosphate buffer, 1% SDS at 65°C, followed by a one-hour wash in 0.04 M phosphate buffer, 1% SDS at 65°C. Each lane was hybridized to a different ^{32}P-labeled α tubulin probe: (A) pI-LαT1, (B) pRDαTT.7, (C) pRDαTT.3, and (D) 195 bp of the 3′ end of pILαT1 derived by digestion with Mbo II (pILαT111).

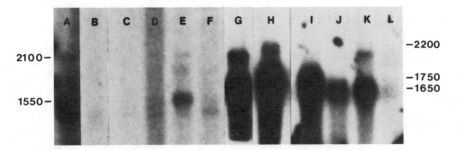

2100—

1550—

—2200

—1750
—1650

FIGURE 2. Estimate of the size of α tubulin mRNA recognized by mouse testicular and rat brain cDNA probes. Six micrograms of RNA from each tissue or cell type were denatured with glyoxal, electrophoresed in a 1.5% agarose gel, and transferred to nitrocellulose. Filters were hybridized to pRDαTT.3 as described in Figure 1, washed by the Thomas method, and rehybridized to pILα1. The sources of RNA were: (A) total testis poly(A)$^+$, (B) brain poly(A)$^+$, (C) 16-day-old prepuberal testis, (D) pachytene spermatocyte, (E) round spermatid, and (F) elongating spermatid. Lanes A–F were hybridized to pRDαTT.3, lanes G–L were rehybridized to pILαT1.

genes for protamine and α tubulin presents compelling evidence for the haploid genome to play an essential role in post-meiotic gamete differentiation.

REFERENCES

1. STERN, L., B. GOLD & N. B. HECHT. 1983. Gene expression during mammalian spermatogenesis. I: Evidence for stage-specific synthesis of polypeptides "in vivo." Biol. Reprod. **28:** 483–496.
2. GOLD, B., L. STERN & N. B. HECHT. 1983. Gene expression during mammalian spermatogenesis II: Evidence for stage-specific differences in mRNA populations. J. Exp. Zool. **225:** 123–134.
3. HECHT, N. B., K. C. KLEENE, R. J. DISTEL & L. M. SILVER. 1984. The differential expression of the actins and tubulins during spermatogenesis in the mouse. Exp. Cell Res. **153:** 275–280.
4. KLEENE, K. C., R. J. DISTEL & N. B. HECHT. 1983. cDNA clones encoding poly (A)$^+$ RNAs which first appear at detectable levels in haploid phases of spermatogenesis in the mouse. Dev. Biol. **98:** 455–464.
5. KLEENE, K. C., R. J. DISTEL & N. B. HECHT. 1984. Translational regulation and coordinate deadenylation of a haploid mRNA during spermiogenesis in the mouse. Dev. Biol. **105:** 71–79.
6. KLEENE, K. C., R. J. DISTEL & N. B. HECHT. 1985. The nucleotide sequence of a cDNA clone encoding mouse protamine I. Biochemistry. (In press.)

Sequential Analysis of the Epididymal Sperm Maturation Process in the Boar

J. L. DACHEUX,[a] M. PAQUIGNON [b] and M. LANNEAU

Institut National de Recherche Agronomique
Physiologie de la Reproduction
37380 Nouzilly, France

[a]*Centre National de la Recherche Scientifique*
Faculté des Sciences
37000 Tours, France

[b]*Institut Technique du Porc*
149 rue de Bercy
75595 Paris Cedex 12, France

Sperm maturation in the epididymis is the result of many morphological and metabolic changes.[1,2] However, no relation has been shown between such changes and the acquisition of motility and fertilizing ability by the gamete. Here we report a study in the boar in which we analyzed the transformations occurring in the spermatozoa and their corresponding epididymal fluids in order to obtain a topographic localization in the epididymis of these different phenomena.

Sexually mature boars (Large White) were used throughout the studies. Spermatozoa and fluid were collected from the testis and the 10 regions (R1 to R10) of the epididymis as previously described[3] by cannulation[4] and microperfusion.[5] In the fluid (rete testis or epididymal) obtained after several centrifugations, protein composition was analyzed by SDS-PAGE. In spermatozoa, migration of cytoplasmic droplets, number of immunoglobulin receptors,[6] percentage motile, head-to-head agglutination, heterologous sperm binding to zona-free hamster eggs,[3] and sperm cell surface were examined.

IN SPERM

The migration of the cytoplasmic droplets begins in R2 and is maximum in R4 (post part of the caput). The percentage of agglutination after incubation in Krebs Ringer Bicarbonate (KRB) is maximum in R5 (corpus). The greatest number of sperm with immunoglobulin receptors is seen in R4 and R10 (caput and post part of cauda). The capacity of sperm to bind zona-free hamster egg appeared in R4–R5 and is maximum in R7. The percentage of motile sperm (after 10 min incubation at 37°C in KRB estimated by laser doppler velocimetry) increased in R3–R4 and is maximum in R7.

SPERM SURFACE MEMBRANE

Spermatozoa were radioiodinated (^{125}I) in the presence of chloroglycoluril incubated in KRB.[7] The labeled proteins (FIGURE 1) were fractionated on an 8–16%

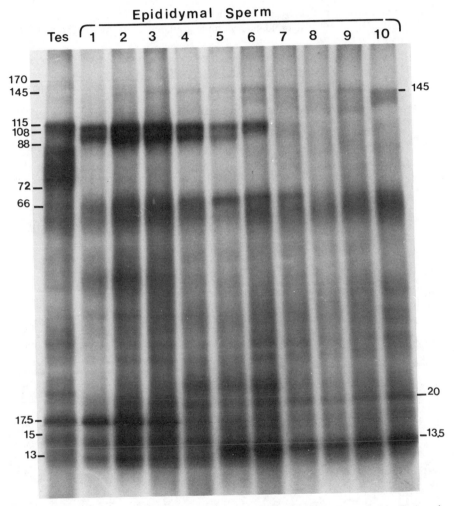

FIGURE 1. Electrophoretic analysis of ^{125}I-labeled components of testicular (Tes) and epididymal spermatozoa from 10 regions.

sigmoïdal acrylamide gradient. Major surface components of testicular spermatozoa (115–108, 88–72, and 17.5 Kd) disappear successively in the epididymis: region 1 = 88–72 Kd components, region 4–5 = 17.5 Kd components, and region 6 = 108–115 Kd components. New proteins are labeled on the epididymal sperm surface membrane: region 3 = 145 Kd components, region 5–6 = 66 Kd (transient), and region 5 = 13.5 Kd.

EPIDIDYMAL FLUID

Protein composition of rete testis fluid (RTF) and epididymal fluid was analyzed on SDS-PAGE (8–16%) sigmoïdal acrylamide gradients (FIGURE 2). The majority

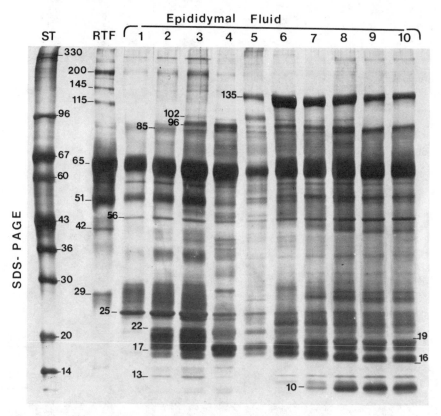

FIGURE 2. Staining pattern of fractionated fluid proteins from RTF and 10 regions (1 to 10) of the epididymis (st: standard for molecular weight calibration).

of the proteins from the RTF disappears successively in the epididymis: in R1, 125, 51, 42, and 29 Kd components and in R4–R5, the 200 Kd protein. New components are seen in epididymal fluid: region R1, 25 Kd protein or subunit; R1–R2, 22–17 Kd, which disappears in R4–R5; R5, 135 Kd; and region R6–R7, 19–16 Kd.

This analysis clearly shows the localization and the succession of the studied parameters. In epididymal regions R3 and R4, all the parameters used to estimate the maturation process in these studies begin to change; this region seems to play an important role.

However, the evolution of the sperm cell surface membrane shows very rapid transformations as soon as the cell enters the epididymis. Such striking changes are also seen between protein composition of fluid from the rete testis and the first part of epididymis.

These results show that the surface-labeled pattern of the spermatozoa cannot be exclusively related to the major exogenous epididymal proteins surrounding the cell. Such results have also been obtained in the ram.[8]

The importance of these successive transformations either on the sperm or in the epididymal fluid on maturation remains unknown.

REFERENCES

1. DACHEUX, J. L. & M. PAQUIGNON. 1980. Relation between the fertilizing ability, motility and metabolism of epididymal spermatozoa. Reprod. Nutr. Develop. **20:** 1085–1099.
2. ORGEBIN-CRIST, M. C. & M. T. HOCHEREAU-DE REVIERS. 1980. Sperm formation and maturation role of testicular and epididymal somatic cells. 9th Int. Cong. Artificial Insemination (Madrid), pp. 59–82.
3. DACHEUX J. L., M. PAQUIGNON & Y. COMBARNOUS. 1983. Head-to-head agglutination of ram and boar epididymal spermatozoa and evidence for an epididymal antagglutin. J. Reprod. Fert. **67:** 181–189.
4. DACHEUX J. L., T. O'SHEA & M. PAQUIGNON. 1979. Effects of osmolality bicarbonate and buffer on the metabolism and motility of testicular, epididymal and ejaculated spermatozoa of boars. J. Reprod. Fert. **55:** 287–296.
5. DACHEUX, J. L. 1980. An *in vitro* luminal perfusion technique to study epididymal secretion. IRCS. Med. Sci. **8:** 137.
6. SUAREZ, S. S., B. T. HINTON & G. OLIPHANT. 1981. Binding of a marker for immunoglobulins to the surface of rabbit testicular, epididymal and ejaculated spermatozoa. Biol. Reprod. **25:** 1091–1097.
7. VOGLMAYR, J. K., G. FAIRBANKS, M. A. JACKOWITZ & J. R. COLELLA. 1980. Posttesticular developmental changes in the ram cell surface and their relationship to luminal proteins of the reproductive tract. Biol. Reprod. **22:** 655–667.
8. VOGLMAYR, J. K. & J. L. DACHEUX. 1983. Surface change sequence in ram spermatozoa during epididymal transit. Biol. Reprod. **28** (Suppl. 1): 136 (Abstr.).

Rat and Bull Sperm Immobilization in the Caudal Epididymis: A Comparison of Mechanisms

MARION C. USSELMAN,[a] DANIEL W. CARR, and
TED S. ACOTT

Department of Biophysics
The Johns Hopkins University
Baltimore, Maryland 21218

Departments of Ophthalmology and Biochemistry
School of Medicine
Oregon Health Sciences University
Portland, Oregon 97201

One of the primary functions of the mammalian caudal epididymis is to maintain sperm viability prior to ejaculation. As part of this storage process, sperm of many species are completely immobilized in the caudal epididymis and do not initiate motility until they are ejaculated or diluted into isotonic buffers. Mechanisms proposed in the literature for maintaining this quiescence include low oxygen tension in the epididymis,[1] low concentrations of calcium[2] or sodium[3] in cauda epididymal (CE) fluid, mechanical inhibition caused by sperm-sperm contact,[4] inhibition by an ion or small molecule in CE fluid (e.g., carnitine[5] or potassium[6]), and the presence of a sperm-immobilizing protein in the CE fluid.[7] We have independently investigated the mechanisms of sperm immobilization in rat (Usselman) and bull (Carr and Acott) and here compare the two.

The sperm from both rat and bull are quiescent when highly diluted with oxygenated, neat CE fluid: rat sperm are completely immotile whereas bull sperm exhibit a slight quivering motion. This implies that neither sperm-sperm contact nor oxygen deprivation is responsible for sperm quiescence in these species. Sperm from both species become vigorously motile when diluted into isotonic buffers, including solutions that provide only osmotic support (e.g., sucrose in distilled water). CE sperm, therefore, do not require any added activators to initiate motility, and instead are immobilized by inhibitors in the CE fluid. The inhibitor in rat CE fluid is not sperm specific, since rat CE fluid suppresses the motility of the bacteria *E. coli*. In contrast, bull CE fluid has little effect on *E. coli* motility. The initiation of sperm motility is completely reversible since motile sperm from both bull and rat become immotile again when resuspended in neat CE fluid.

The motility inhibiting factor in rat CE fluid can be purified by centrifuging diluted CE fluid for one hour at 80,000 g. The sedimented pellet contains primarily "immobilin," a highly viscoelastic mucus glycoprotein (FIGURE 1). Immobilin completely immobilizes sperm by increasing the viscoelastic drag of the CE fluid to a level comparable to glycerol and 1,000 times the drag of water.[8] Enzymatic

---

[a] Current address: Marion C. Usselman, Laboratory of Human Reproduction and Reproductive Biology, Harvard Medical School, 45 Shattuck St., Boston, MA 02115.

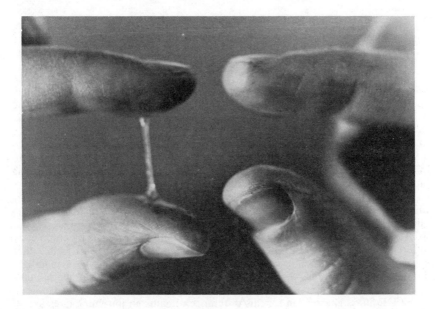

FIGURE 1. The viscoelasticity of rat CE fluid (left fingers) and 5% bovine serum albumin (right fingers).

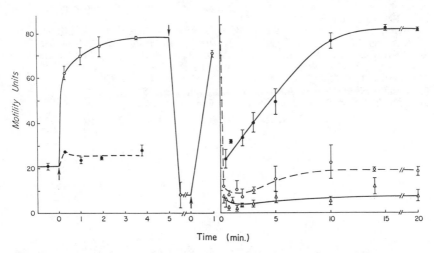

FIGURE 2. Time courses for bull sperm motility changes in bull CE fluid in response to changes in pH and dilution. The motility of CE sperm diluted with CE fluid (left panel) after addition (first arrow) of NaOH (open circles) or NaCl (closed circles). HCl was added at the second arrow and NaOH at the third arrow. CE sperm were diluted (right panel) into CE fluid (triangles) or buffer (closed circles). Motile sperm were resuspended in CE fluid (open circles).

digestion, sonication, or slight dilution of CE fluid decreases the drag of the fluid, and concurrently allows for the initiation of motility. Rat sperm are therefore immobilized in the caudal epididymis mechanically and not by a specific biochemical inhibitor.

Bull sperm are not mechanically immobilized in the epididymis, since the viscoelasticity of bull CE fluid is near that of water, not glycerol. Instead, bull sperm quiescence is maintained by a pH-dependent factor in the CE fluid.[9] The pH of neat bull CE fluid is 5.86 ± 0.1 ($N = 110$). Increasing the pH of bull CE fluid to 7.6 without significant dilution reversibly eliminates the immobilizing capability of the fluid (FIGURE 2). In contrast, reducing the pH of assay buffers from 7.6 to 5.5 has only minimal effect on sperm motility. However, buffers containing 10 mM lactate (or other permeant weak acids) mimic CE fluid by reversibly inhibiting bull sperm motility at pH 5.5 but not at pH 7.6. Glycerylphosphorylcholine, carnitine, and impermeant weak acids have no effect of sperm motility at either pH. This suggests that there is a factor in bull CE fluid that maintains sperm quiescence by decreasing the intracellular pH.

Although rat and bull sperm are immobilized in the epididymis by completely different mechanisms, both mechanisms can immobilize the sperm from either species. Bull sperm are quiescent in rat immobilin, and although rat sperm initiate motility in bull CE fluid, their motility is greatly suppressed within five minutes after dilution. In contrast to rat and bull, rabbit sperm are vigorously motile in rabbit CE fluid. The reason for this difference remains an intriguing question.

REFERENCES

1. REDENZ, E. 1924. Arch. F. Mikrosk. Anat. U. Ent. Mech. **103:** 593.
2. MORTON, B., J. HARRIGAN-LUM, L. ALBAGLI & T. JOOSS. 1974. Biochem. Biophys. Res. Commun. **56:** 373.
3. WONG, P. Y. D., W. M. LEE & A. Y. F. TSANG. 1981. Exp. Cell. Res. **131:** 97.
4. CASCIERI, M., R. P. AMANN & R. H. HAMMERSTEDT. 1976. J. Biol. Chem. **251:** 787.
5. HINTON, B. T., R. W. WHITE & B. P. SETCHELL. 1980. J. Reprod. Fertil. **58:** 395.
6. WONG, P. Y. D. & W. M. LEE. 1983. Biol. Reprod. **28:** 206.
7. TURNER, T. T. & R. D. GILES. 1982. Am. J. Physiol. **242:** R199.
8. USSELMAN, M. C. & R. A. CONE. 1983. Biol. Reprod. **29:** 1241.
9. ACOTT, T. S. & D. W. CARR. 1984. Biol. Reprod. **30:** 926.

Localization of a Sperm Surface Molecule in the Epididymis[a]

CHARLES H. MULLER[b][c] and E. M. EDDY[c][d]

Population Center for Research in Reproduction
[b] *Department of Obstetrics and Gynecology*
[c] *Department of Biological Structure*
University of Washington
Seattle, Washington 98195

The mechanisms involved in the maturation of spermatozoa in the epididymis are numerous, but one likely process is the synthesis and secretion of sperm-binding molecules by the epididymal epithelium. Evidence for this process in the rat and mouse has been obtained by immunohistochemical techniques employing antisera[1-4] or a monoclonal antibody.[5] These antibodies recognize determinants distributed over the sperm surface or restricted to the tail. In contrast, we have produced a mouse anti-mouse sperm monoclonal antibody that binds to a determinant restricted to the sperm surface overlying the acrosome.[6,7] This determinant-bearing molecule, sperm maturation antigen #6 (SMA 6), appears on sperm during maturation in the epididymis, is androgen dependent, and changes in distribution on the sperm head during capacitation. SMA 6 overlies the acrosome of mouse and rat epididymal sperm, but is not present on testicular cells or human, rabbit, or guinea pig sperm. On the sperm surface and in sperm extracts, SMA 6 has the extraction and partitioning characteristics of a ganglioside.

Two approaches were used to test the hypothesis that SMA 6 is of epididymal origin. First, immunohistochemistry using an indirect avidin-biotin-peroxidase procedure was employed. Epididymides from control and experimentally manipulated mice were processed for either frozen sectioning with or without prior fixation, or the paraffin method after fixation in one of seven fixatives. Best results were obtained with unfixed, frozen tissue, and 0.1% glutaraldehyde-fixed, paraffin-embedded tissue. Anti-SMA 6 bound only to sites in the apical cytoplasm (resembling Golgi apparatus) of the distal caput to proximal corpus epididymidis. Other areas of the epididymis were negative. More reaction product was present in sections from intact or ductuli efferentes-ligated mice than in those from mice castrated for four days.

Second, an enzyme immunoassay was used to detect the molecule in tissue homogenates. Caput, corpus, and cauda epididymides were isolated from control and experimental mice and homogenized in 50 mM Tris (pH 7.4 at 4°C) containing 0.5% NP-40 and 0.2 mM PMSF. Protein concentration in the $11,500 \times g$ supernatant was determined by a modified micro Bradford method. Dilutions of supernatant were placed into wells of polystyrene enzyme immunoassay plates

[a] Supported by U.S. Public Health Service Grant HD-14054 to E.M.E. and grants HD-16211 and HD-12629 to C.H.M.

[b] Send correspondence to: Charles H. Muller, Obstetrics and Gynecology, RH20, University of Washington, Seattle, WA 98195.

[d] Present address: Laboratory of Reproductive and Developmental Toxicology, National Institute of Environmental Health Sciences, NIH, Research Triangle Park, NC 27709.

and incubated overnight. After blocking with phosphate-buffered saline–gelatin, dilutions of anti-SMA 6 were added, followed by peroxidase-conjugated rabbit anti-mouse IgM as second antibody and o-phenylenediamine as substrate. Absorbance at 492 nm was recorded. Dilutions of either homogenate or primary antibody yielded linear decreases in absorbance; maximal binding occurred at 1 μg homogenate protein/well. Homogenates of caput epididymidis contained the most immunoreactivity, about 40 times more SMA 6 than corpus; no SMA 6 was detected in cauda epididymidis. Ligation of the ductuli efferentes resulted in a less than twofold decrease in SMA 6, while castration for four days abolished SMA 6 reactivity in the caput and corpus.

These results show that a determinant shared by the maturing spermatozoon and a discrete portion of the epididymal epithelium is recognized by monoclonal antibody anti-SMA 6. In either location, the presence of SMA 6 is dependent on circulating androgens; ductuli efferentes ligation has little effect compared with castration. A significant portion of SMA 6 reactivity in epididymal homogenates can be ascribed to epithelium and luminal contents since spermatozoa were absent from the caput and proximal corpus four days after ductuli efferentes ligation.

Spermatozoa first express SMA 6 in the caput (12% of sperm are positive) and corpus epididymidis (42%). Thus, it is tempting to speculate that SMA 6 is synthesized by the androgen-stimulated epididymal epithelium, secreted into the lumen (perhaps with a carrier protein), and bound to or inserted into the maturing sperm membrane. Studies of the synthesis and biochemical properties of SMA 6 will help clarify the role of this molecule in sperm maturation and the events leading to fertilization.

REFERENCES

1. LEA, O. A., P. PETRUSZ & F. S. FRENCH. 1978. Purification and localization of Acidic Epididymal Glycoprotein (AEG): A sperm coating protein secreted by the rat epididymis. Int. J. Androl. (Suppl. 2): 592–607.
2. FAYE, J. C., L. DUGUET, M. MAZZUCA & F. BAYARD. 1980. Purification, radioimmunoassay, and immunohistochemical localization of a glycoprotein produced by the rat epididymis. Biol. Reprod. 23: 423–432.
3. KOHANE, A. C., M. S. CAMEO, L. PIÑEIRO, J. C. GARBERI & J. A. BLAQUIER. 1980. Distribution and site of production of specific proteins in the rat epididymis. Biol. Reprod. 23: 181–187.
4. KIERSZENBAUM, A. L., O. A. LEA, P. PETRUSZ, F. S. FRENCH & L. L. TRES. 1981. Isolation, culture, and immunocytochemical characterization of epididymal epithelial cells from pubertal and adult rats. Proc. Natl. Acad. Sci. USA 78: 1675–1679.
5. VERNON, R. B., C. H. MULLER, J. C. HERR, F. A. FEUCHTER & E. M. EDDY. 1982. Epididymal secretion of a mouse sperm surface component recognized by a monoclonal antibody. Biol. Reprod. 26: 523–535.
6. MULLER, C. H. & E. M. EDDY. 1983. Androgens regulate the appearance of sperm surface molecules recognized by monoclonal antibodies. Endocrinology 112 (Suppl.): 249.
7. MULLER, C. H. & E. M. EDDY. 1983. Androgen-dependence and properties of a mouse sperm surface component defined by a monoclonal antibody. Biol. Reprod. 28 (Suppl. 1): 135.

Evidence for a Protease Involvement in Sperm Motility[a]

CLAUDE GAGNON,[b] EVE DE LAMIRANDE, and
MARTHE BELLES-ISLES

Unité de Biorégulation cellulaire et moléculaire
Centre hospitalier de l'Université Laval
Sainte-Foy, Québec, Canada G1V 4G2

Département de Pharmacologie
Faculté de Médecine, Université Laval
Québec, Canada G1K 7P4

Demembranated reactivated sperm models from primitive organisms have been extensively used in the past to study the energetics and mechanics of sperm motility.[1-3] While studying a similar model system, but with mammalian spermatozoa, we observed that two protease inhibitors, aprotinin and leupeptin, prevented the motility of demembranated spermatozoa incubated with Mg·ATP (TABLE 1). Aprotinin not only blocked the reinitiation of movement but also the motility of reactivated spermatozoa. On a molar basis, aprotinin was 400-fold more potent than leupeptin. Other protease inhibitors, such as phenylmethlysulfonyl fluoride (PMSF), α-1-antitrypsin, pepstatin, and antithrombin III, had no or only marginal effects on motility. On the other hand, soybean trypsin inhibitor (STI) increased sevenfold the length of reactivation, probably by interacting with a protease hydrolyzing essential axonemal components.[4] Thus the effects of aprotinin on sperm motility were rather specific.

Since the inhibitory effects of aprotinin on sperm motility were reversed by Mg·ATP,[5] we investigated the effect of aprotinin on the force-generating dynein ATPase. For this purpose, bull sperm dynein was extracted by low ionic strength and the 19S particle was isolated on sucrose density gradient. This particle had two peptides with molecular weight above 400,000, characteristic of dynein ATPase. Aprotinin, even at a concentration 60-fold higher than that needed to inhibit sperm motility, had only a marginal effect on dynein ATPase activity.

The possibility that aprotinin affects sperm motility by acting on a specific protease was investigated. Various serine protease substrates were tested on the motility of demembranated reactivated rabbit spermatozoa. Substrates with arginine ester bonds, such as benzoyl-phe-val-arg-*p*-nitroanilide and carbobenzoxy-val-gly-arg-*p*-nitroanilide, inhibited motility while others, such as *N*-benzoyl-tyr-*p*-nitroanilide, had no effect on motility (TABLE 2). Moreover, when benzoyl-phe-val-arg-*p*-nitroanilide and carbobenzoxy-val-gly-arg-*p*-nitroanilide were hydrolyzed by trypsin prior to their addition to motile spermatozoa, both substances lost their inhibitory effects on motility. Similar results were obtained with rat and bull spermatozoa.

[a] Supported by the Medical Research Council of Canada and The Population Council (New York).

[b] Address correspondence to: Dr. Claude Gagnon, Urology Research Laboratory, Royal Victoria Hospital, 687 Pine Avenue West, H6, Montréal, Québec H3A 1A1, Canada.

TABLE 1. Effects of Protease Inhibitors on Motility of Demembranated Reactivated Rabbit Spermatozoa

Protease Inhibitors[a]	Reactivation Duration (min)[b]
Control medium	5.8 ± 0.4
STI (100 μg/ml)	41.7 ± 1.6
PMSF (40 μg/ml)	5.0 ± 0.8
Antithrombin III (100 μg/ml)	3.9 ± 0.6
α-1-Antitrypsin (100 μg/ml)	4.4 ± 0.2
Pepstatin (100 μg/ml)	4.1 ± 0.4
Leupeptin (50.0 μg/ml)	No reactivation
(12,5 μg/ml)	1.5 ± 0.3
(2.5 μg/ml)	5.2 ± 0.8
Aprotinin (1.5 μg/ml)	No reactivation
(0.6 μg/ml)	1.5 ± 0.2
(0.3 μg/ml)	6.3 ± 1.2

[a] Protease inhibitors were added to the reactivation medium at the final concentration indicated, before spermatozoa and ATP

[b] Duration: from the time the motility was initiated to the time movement stopped, mean ± SEM for three to nine preparations.

TABLE 2. Effects of Serine Protease Substrates on Motility of Demembranated Reactivated Rabbit Spermatozoa

Substrate	Motility
None (control)	+++
Benzoyl-phe-val-arg-p-nitroanilide (80 μM)	0
Carbobenzoxy-val-gly-arg-p-nitroanilide (300 μM)	0
N-benzoyl-tyr-p-nitroanilide (2,000 μM)	+++
Hydrolyzed benzoyl-phe-val-arg-p-nitroanilide (160 μM)	+++

Motility was evaluated on a 0 (no motility) to ++++ (maximum motility) scale basis.

The data suggest that a specific protease might be involved in the motility of mammalian spermatozoa. This may not be the case for sea urchin as demembranated reactivated spermatozoa from this species were not affected by concentration of aprotinin 50-fold higher than the effective dose for rabbit spermatozoa (unpublished results).

REFERENCES

1. SUMMERS, K. E. & I. R. GIBBONS. 1973. J. Cell Biol. **58:** 618–629.
2. GIBBONS, B. H. & I. R. GIBBONS. 1973. J. Cell Sci. **13:** 337–357.
3. YANO, Y. & T. MIKI-NOUMURA. 1981. J. Cell Sci. **48:** 223–239.
4. DE LAMIRANDE, E., C. W. BARDIN & C. GAGNON. 1983. Biol. Reprod. **28:** 788–796.
5. DE LAMIRANDE, E. & C. GAGNON. 1983. J. Submicrosc. Cytol. **15:** 83–87.

Sperm Motility in a
Non-mammalian Vertebrate:

The Lizard *Lacerta vivipara* Acquisition of Sperm Motility and Its Maintenance during Storage

A. DEPEIGES

Biologie Cellulaire et Génétique
Université de Clermont-Ferrand II
BP 45 63170 Aubiere, France

J. L. DACHEUX

Institut National de Recherches Agronomiques
Station de Physiologie de la Reproduction
37380 Nouzilly, France

INTRODUCTION

In mammals it is well established that spermatozoa acquire the ability to fertilize during their transit from the caput to the cauda epididymis.[1-4] Very little is known about sperm maturation and storage in lower vertebrates. However, if we consider earlier studies, it has been shown that in teleost fishes, cyclostomes, and frogs, spermatozoa emerging from the testis are motile and fertile.[2] The first important evolution appears to have taken place in an elasmobranch (the skate) and in some species of birds and reptiles. It seems evident that a better knowledge of sperm maturation and storage in these subtherian animals would be of great interest.

The lizard *Lacerta vivipara* is a seasonal breeder, copulating only during spring. We have previously shown that its epididymis produces a large amount of secretory granules made up of a central core (Ø 6 μm) and a peripheral vacuole from March to June (the reproductive period). This secretory activity is androgen dependent.[5] The peripheral vacuole contains a major protein, protein "L" (18,000 M.W.)[6] that binds to the head of spermatozoa.[38]

Our purpose was to investigate the importance of the epididymis on the acquisition of the optimal motility and on storage of viable sperm in the viviparous lizard.

MATERIAL AND METHODS

The lizard epididymis was divided in three segments [proximal, median, and distal (zone of storage)] by anatomical and histological criterions. Spermatozoa were

[a] This research was supported by a grant from the Institut national de la santé et de la recherche médicale contract no. 834009 and the Ministère de l'Education Nationale (Aide à la Recherche en Biologie 1982).

released by mincing the testis or the epididymal tubules with scissors in Tyrode solution with 5% yolk. In each case an aliquot was retained and 6 mM caffeine was added to the medium. One to thirty minutes later, a 10 μl drop was removed following further mixing, transferred to a warm slide, and observed with a dark medium contrast phase microscope.

Motility was estimated by two methods. Motile and immotile cells were counted by means of a hemocytometer and motility was expressed by percentages of all sperm or several (15 to 30) photomicrographs with four-second exposures were performed in each experimental condition and the moving spermatozoa were identified by their tracks on the film. The length of a track recorded over a known interval was used as a direct measure of the swimming speed of each single sperm.

This study have been carried out at different times during the reproductive period during the breeding period: B.P. (in April), B.P. + 15 days, and B.P. + 30 days.

RESULTS AND DISCUSSION

During the breeding Period

It has been shown that the spermatozoa that are immotile in the testis develop the ability to swim as they pass along the epididymis: 30% of motile sperm in the proximal segment, 50% in the median segment, and 85% in the distal segment were found during this period. As recorded by means of histograms, sperm velocity was about 2 to 6 μm/sec in the distal sperm. The addition of a phosphodiesterase inhibitor (caffeine) without effect on testicular sperm can induce some forward motility in the caput and median sperm and increase the velocity of sperm in the three segments. This suggests that sperm motility in this species, as in mammals, is cyclic AMP–dependent (originally reported by Frenkel et al. in the guinea pig[2]) and that the intrasperm levels of cyclic AMP may increase during the epididymal transit.

After the Breeding Period

During the month following the B.P. the sperm motility decreases significantly in percentage of all sperm and in velocity. In the distal segment, the percentage of motile sperm was 85% during the B.P., 75% on B.P. + 15 days, and 30% during B.P. + 30 days. Caffeine has less effect on sperm after than during the B.P.

In other reptiles studied there is no relationship between testicular androgens, the epididymis, and sperm viability.[3] In *Lacerta vivipara,* the sperm motility in the distal segment is maximal (85%) while plasma androgens reach the highest levels in the year (400 ng/ml testosterone) in April[10] and decrease progressively during the following month. By early June motile sperm represent only 30% of all sperm as plasma testosterone levels decline to 20 ng/ml. These data suggest an androgen dependency of sperm maturation and sperm viability during the storage.

In the lower vertebrates, there is generally a coincidence of internal fertilization and the appearance of some post-testicular maturation. This property seems peculiarly well developed in the sparrow (passerine bird) and, as shown in this work, in the viviparous lizard. Furthermore, the viviparous lizard, with its highly androgen-dependent epididymal secretory activity and sperm maturation and storage, shows a further increase in complexity of epididymal function in comparison with the other lower vertebrates studied. Placed in a comparative setting this animal is an interesting model for studying the establishment of testicular androgen involvement in the maturation and maintenance of viability of mature spermatozoa and especially for studying the role of a specific androgen-dependent epididymal protein (protein "L")[6-8] in these phenomena.

REFERENCES

1. BEDFORD, J. M. 1975. Handb. Physiol. **5:** 303–317.
2. BEDFORD, J. M. 1979. *In* The Spermatozoon. D. W. Fawcett & J. M. Bedford, Eds.: 7–21. Baltimore, MD.
3. HOSKINS, D. D. & E. R. CASILLAS. 1975. Handb. Physiol. **4:** 453–460.
4. ORGEBIN-CRIST, M. C., B. J. DANZO & J. DAVIS. 1975. Handb. Physiol. **5:** 319–338.
5. GIGON-DEPEIGES, A. & J. P. DUFAURE. 1977. Secretory activity of lizard epididymis and its control by testosterone. Gen. Comp. Endocrinol. **33:** 473–479.
6. DEPEIGES, A. & J. P. DUFAURE. 1981. Major proteins secreted by the epididymis of *Lacerta vivipara*. Identification by electrophoresis of soluble proteins. Biochim. Biophys. Acta **667:** 260–266.
7. DEPEIGES, A., G. BETAIL & J. P. DUFAURE. 1981. Caractérisation immunochimique d'une protéine majeure sécrétée par l'épididyme de lézard. C.R. Acad. Sci. **292:** 211–216.
8. DEPEIGES, A. & J. P. DUFAURE. 1983. Binding to spermatozoa of a major soluble protein secreted by the epididymis of the lizard Lacerta vivipara. Gamete Res. **4:** 401–406.
9. FRANKEL, G., R. N. PETERSON & M. FREUND. 1973. The role of adenine nucleotides and the effect of caffeine and dibutyryl cyclic AMP on the metabolism of Guinea pig spermatozoa. Proc. Soc. Exp. Biol. Med. **144:** 420–425.
10. COURTY, Y. & J. P. DUFAURE. 1980. Levels of testosterone, dihydrotestosterone, and androstenedione in the plasma and testis of a lizard (Lacerta vivipara Jacquin) during the annual cycle. Gen. Comp. Endocrinol. **42:** 325–333.

Phospholipid Methylation during
Chemotaxis of Starfish Spermatozoa

J. TEZON,[a] R. MILLER,[b] and C. W. BARDIN[a]

[a] The Population Council
New York, New York 10021

[b] Department of Biology
Temple University
Philadelphia, Pennsylvania 19122

Sperm chemotaxis has been demonstrated in a major class of echinoderms, the Asteroidea.[1] The affected spermatozoa swim up a gradient of the chemoattractant. The substances responsible for the attraction are produced by the ovaries and are of low molecular weight (3,000–5,000), sensitive to proteases, stable to heat and acid, and highly polar. They are specific at least to the family or, in some cases, the genus level. This response enhances efficient and appropriate sperm-egg interaction in the open sea where fertilization normally takes place in these animals.

Since phospholipid methylation (PLM) is believed to play a significant role in macrophage chemoattraction,[2] a series of studies was performed to investigate whether this reaction is also linked to sperm chemotaxis. Purified ovarian extracts were bioassayed for attractant activity by microinjections into one side of a suspension of motile sperm.[3] Titer for chemoattractant activity was defined as the highest number of serial half-dilutions required for complete loss of activity. Endogenous PLM was measured using motile sperm cells incubated with [^{3}H]methylmethionine. After addition of attractant the reaction was stopped and [^{3}H]phospholipids were extracted and measured as described previously.[4]

The chemoattractant produced a very rapid fall in the concentration of methylated phospholipids with only 20% of the basal activity remaining after 2 sec. This effect was dose-dependent and a 40% decrease in methylated phospholipids was produced by the amount of chemoattractant needed for positive response in the bioassay (FIGURE 1). Association of PLM with sperm chemotaxis was reinforced by experiments in which attractants from species with little cross-reactivity in the bioassay were checked for their effect on methylation using both types of sperm. Species specificity of the chemoattractants was demonstrated by the differential sensitivity of spermatozoa in both the chemotactic and the PLM assays (FIGURE 1). This figure also shows that significant reduction in [^{3}H]phospholipids always occurs before any biological effect is observed.

When the transmethylase inhibitor, homocysteine, was added to the preincubation media PLM was significantly decreased (ID_{50} 50 μM) but no change in sperm motility was observed with this inhibitor under non-stimulated conditions. However, in the presence of homocysteine there was a dose-dependent increase in the sensitivity of the sperm cells to the attractant. The concentration of inhibitor (homocysteine, 200 μM) that produced maximal inhibition of basal methylation decreased the amount of ovarian peptide required to produce a positive attractant response to 1% of that without homocysteine (FIGURE 2).

Analysis of the phospholipid fractions extracted under basal and stimulated conditions was performed using thin layer chromatography. The addition of chemoattractants resulted in a reduction in the amount of [^{3}H]phosphatidyl monomethyl ethanolamine and an increase in highly methylated phospholipids, such as

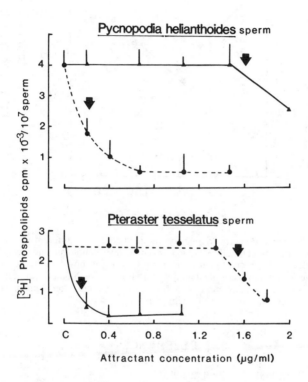

FIGURE 1. Sperm from different species of starfish challenged with homologous and heterologous attractants. The effect on methylated phopholipids is shown in the ordinates. Sperm suspensions were also bioassayed for chemoattraction and the minimal concentrations capable of showing a positive response are shown by the arrows. Attractant from *Pycnopodia* ovaries, (●---●); Attractant from *Pteraster* ovaries (▲---▲).

[^{3}H]phosphatidyl choline. Homocysteine induced accumulation of phosphatidyl monomethyl ethanolamine (FIGURE 2) so that the proportion of the different metabolites during inhibition resembled that seen in non-stimulated cells.

A reduction in PLM is linked to sperm chemotaxis. Methylation of phospholipids seems to desensitize sperm cells to the attractant and in this way might play an active role in the orientation mechanism of the spermatozoa as it swims through the gradient formed by the egg.

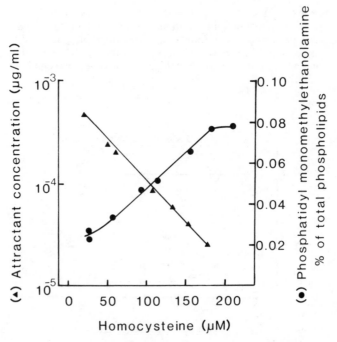

FIGURE 2. *Pycnopodia* sperm suspension preincubated with different concentrations of homocysteine for 30 min and aliquots bioassayed against homologous attractant. The minimal concentrations of attractant giving positive response are shown on the left (▲). Aliquots from the same incubation were incubated with [³H]methylmethionine and individual phospholipids separated by thin layer chromatography. The accumulation of phosphatidyl monomethyl ethanolamine is shown on the right (●).

REFERENCES

1. MILLER, R. L. 1981. Am. Zool. **21:** 985.
2. PIKE, M. C., N. M. KREDICH & R. SNYDERMAN. 1979. Proc. Natl. Acad. Sci. USA **76:** 2922–2926.
3. MILLER, R. L. 1979. Marine Bio. **53:** 115–124.
4. HIRATA, F., O. H. VIVEROS, E. DILBERTO, JR. & J. AXELROD. 1978. Proc. Natl. Acad. Sci. USA **75:** 1718–1721.

Glucose Metabolism in Rat Germ Cells: Mechanism of Action of Gossypol[a]

SVEIN MAGNE TVERMYR,[b] ANNEKE FRØYSA,
NICOLET H. P. M. JUTTE, and VIDAR HANSSON

Institutes of Medical Biochemistry and Pathology
University of Oslo
Oslo 3, Norway

It has been known for a long time that testicular germ cells (primary spermatocytes and spermatids) show an unusual dependence on glucose as a source of energy.[1] However, when primary spermatocytes or spermatids (isolated from 32-day-old rats) are incubated in a complete tissue culture medium (MEM) containing 5.5 mM of glucose, the ATP levels drop very rapidly and the cells die. Isolated primary spermatocytes and spermatids incubated in the presence of lactate or pyruvate, however, survive for up to 24 hours, indicating that there may be a yet undefined block in the glycolytic pathway. For that reason we have measured the glycolytic enzymes in five different types of cells (liver cells, primary spermatocytes, round spermatids, spermatozoa, and Sertoli cells).

TABLE 1 shows the activities of the nine glycolytic enzymes in these cells (mean values $\pm$ S.D., $N = 4$). In contrast to the other cells, primary spermatocytes and round spermatids contain very low aldolase activities; 3–4 times lower than in Sertoli cells and approximately half that observed in liver cells. Spermatozoa showed about 6–7 times higher aldolase activity than germ cells. These observations suggest that the glycolytic capacity in germ cells is limited at the level of aldolase. In support of this, exogenous addition of aldolase to cytosol from round spermatids stimulated lactate formation from fructose-1,6-diphosphate by more than 100%.

Gossypol, a polyphenolic compound from the cotton seed, is known to cause immobilization of spermatozoa and kill the more mature testicular germ cells *in vivo*. It is not known why this compound selectively affects sperm motility and germ cell viability. At relatively low concentrations (10^{-8} M–10^{-6} M), gossypol acts as an uncoupler of oxidative phosphorylation, causing a concentration-dependent increase in oxygen consumption by isolated mitochondria. At higher concentrations (10^{-6} M–10^{-4} M), it causes a concentration-dependent decrease in ATP levels both in Sertoli cells and isolated germ cells. At gossypol concentrations (10^{-6} M–10^{-4} M) that reduced cellular ATP levels, the effects of FSH on the lactate secretion from Sertoli cells were abolished. At these higher gossypol concentrations no direct effect on glycolytic enzymes in germ cells or Sertoli cells was observed, but it has been reported that several Krebs cycle enzymes as well as the germ cell–specific LDH-X are inhibited. Interestingly, the maximal uncoupling effect of gossypol on testis mitochondria was achieved at a concentration of

[a] Supported by the Rockefeller Foundation, Norwegian Research Council for Science and the Humanities (NAVF), and the Norwegian Society for Fighting Cancer (NFTKB).
[b] Correspondence to: Svein Magne Tvermyr, Institute of Medical Biochemistry, University of Oslo, P.B. 1112, Blindern, Oslo 3, Norway.

TABLE 1. Glycolytic Pathway

Enzymes (nmol/mg protein × min)	Liver	Primary Spermatocytes	Round Spermatids	Spermatozoa	Sertoli Cells
Hexokinase	15.1 ± 1.6	31.9 ± 7.1	48.2 ± 8.5	38.1 ± 4.9	30.6 ± 10.2
Glucosephosphate isomerase	730.4 ± 22.7	441.6 ± 2.6	838.7 ± 45.7	2435.0 ± 285.8	644.7 ± 65.1
Phosphofructokinase	24.4 ± 4.3	19.4 ± 5.6	41.0 ± 14.6	13.4 ± 8.5	33.0 ± 11.6
Aldolase	69.5 ± 6.4	29.4 ± 1.3	42.1 ± 1.4	223.7 ± 38.3	116.4 ± 12.8
Glyceraldehyde-3-phosphate dehydrogenase	985.9 ± 135.8	246.4 ± 24.0	234.3 ± 30.3	94.5 ± 13.4	648.4
Phosphoglycerate kinase	1147.8 ± 101.3	244.5 ± 1.1	261.2 ± 2.1	2580.6 ± 217.7	502.2 ± 39.0
Phosphoglyceromutase	369.5 ± 69.6	261.3 ± 17.2	285.2 ± 64.4	1604.7 ± 393.2	607.9 ± 127.8
Enolase	188.1 ± 18.9	58.9 ± 10.3	63.4 ± 12.3	293.9 ± 11.5	141.7 ± 157
Pyruvate kinase	176.9 ± 18.7	252.2 ± 68.2	248.0 ± 1.7	86.8 ± 2.7	399.0 ± 78.4

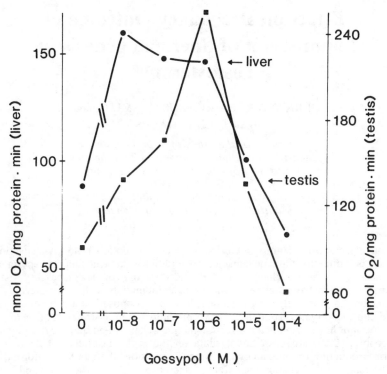

FIGURE 1. The effect of gossypol on O_2 consumption in testis and liver mitochondria.

10^{-8} M, whereas the maximal uncoupling effect on liver mitochondria was obtained at 10^{-6} M. This may explain the cell-specific effect of gossypol on germ cells and spermatozoa (FIGURE 1).

It is likely that the uncoupling effect of gossypol is central in explaining the antifertility effect of this drug. It has been reported[2] that heat as such is an uncoupling stimulus for germ cell mitochondria. Since low concentrations of gossypol cause uncoupling of germ cell mitochondria, and uncoupling produces heat, this may constitute a self-amplifying mechanism that may explain why germ cells but not somatic cells are affected by gossypol.

REFERENCES

1. FREE, M. J. 1970. *In* The Testis. A. D. Johnson, W. R. Gomes & N. L. Vandermark, Eds. **2:** 125–192. Academic Press. New York.
2. NAKAMURA, M., I. YASUMASU, S. OKINAGE & K. ARAI. 1982. Dev. Growth Differ. **24:** (3): 265–272.

Effect on Pregnancy Outcome of Suppression of Spermatogenesis by Testosterone[a]

BERNARD ROBAIRE,[b] SUSAN SMITH, and
BARBARA F. HALES

Centre for the Study of Reproduction
Department of Pharmacology and Therapeutics
Department of Obstetrics and Gynecology
McGill University
Royal Victoria Hospital
Montreal, Quebec H3G 1Y6, Canada

We have previously demonstrated that testosterone administration, via sustained release polydimethylsiloxane capsules, to adult male rats will suppress spermatogenesis.[1] There is no change in serum testosterone or sex accessory tissue weights.[1] Testosterone, either alone or in combination with other steroids or luteinizing hormone releasing hormone, has been proposed as a component of a male contraceptive.[2-4] Though we have previously demonstrated that testosterone does not have a significant effect on mating behavior and that the treatment is reversible,[5] there are no available data on the potential effects of decreasing sperm production on pregnancy outcome. In addition, there is little information on the relationship between the extent of decrease in sperm production and fertilizing potential. The objectives of the present study were to determine whether testosterone treatment, resulting in decreased spermatogenic activity by interfering with the hypothalamo-pituitary-testicular axis, can provide a situation where there is a reduced but measurable fertility and whether the resulting progeny have any apparent abnormalities.

The experimental design was to implant adult male rats subcutaneously with blank (4.0 cm) or testosterone-filled polydimethylsiloxane capsules of varying lengths (0.5, 1.0, 2.0, 3.0, 4.0, and 8.0 cm, $N = 6$). Animals were weighed at weekly intervals. Ninety days after the initiation of the treatment each male was exposed overnight to two females in proestrus. This fertility test was repeated two weeks later with two additional females. Thus, for each male treatment group, there were at least twenty-four females; in the treatment group receiving implants measuring 4.0 cm there were twenty-six females. The presence and number of seminal plugs and the presence of spermatozoa in vaginal smears was assessed within twelve hours of mating. Twenty days later the females were killed, and the ovaries and uteri removed. Numbers of corpora lutea, implantation sites, resorptions, and live normal and abnormal fetuses were counted. Fetuses were sexed, weighed, and then fixed in either Bouin's solution or ethanol for analysis by Wilson's razor blade sections[6] and skeletal staining.[7]

[a] Supported by a Reproductive Hazards in the Workplace grant from the National Foundation March of Dimes and by the Medical Research Council of Canada.

[b] Address correspondence to: Dr. Bernard Robaire, Department of Pharmacology & Therapeutics, McGill University, 3655 Drummond Street, Montreal, Quebec H3G 1Y6.

The effects of testosterone treatment on the males were similar to those previously reported. The initial animal weights ranged from 303–343 g per group and increased consistently during the three month treatment, with final body weights ranging from 502–588 g. The weights of the sex accessory tissues were increased significantly only with the 8.0 cm implants. Paired testicular weights decreased significantly in the animal groups receiving the 3.0, 4.0, and 8.0 cm implants. The largest decrease was seen in the group receiving the 4.0 cm testosterone implants (control, 3.17 ± 0.07 g versus 4.0 cm testosterone, 1.48 ± 0.02 g). The largest reduction in testicular sperm content, down to 15% of control, was also seen in this group.

Caput-corpus and caudal epididymal weights and sperm counts were significantly reduced in the groups receiving 3.0, 4.0, and 8.0 cm testosterone implants. Sperm counts in the epididymal caput-corpus region in these treatment groups were 12.6, 3.0, and 29.9% of control, respectively. Those in the caudal region of the epididymis in these groups were 19.8, 4.0, and 50.8% of control, respectively.

TABLE 1. The Effect of Testosterone Implants in the Male on Mating

Treatment Group (size of testosterone implant)	No. of plugs per male	Sperm-positive Females/No. Bred		Pregnant Females/ Sperm-positive Females	
		No.	%	No.	%
Control	5.30 ± 0.47^a	23/24	95.8	19/23	82.6
0.5 cm	5.50 ± 0.43	18/24	75.0	18/18	100
1.0 cm	3.80 ± 0.90^b	19/24	79.2	16/19	84.2
2.0 cm	5.90 ± 0.38	22/24	91.7	20/22	90.9
3.0 cm	5.00 ± 0.45	20/24	83.3	2/20	10.0^b
4.0 cm	5.18 ± 0.70	13/26	50.0	1/13	7.7^b
8.0 cm	6.00 ± 0.71	20/24	83.3	16/20	80.0

^{a} Mean $\pm$ S.E.M. ($N=12$).
^{b} $p \leq 0.05$, ANOVA or Chi square with Yate's correction for discontinuity.

Testosterone treatment had little effect on mating behavior as assessed by the number of seminal plugs (TABLE 1). The number of females with spermatozoa in the vagina after breeding was diminished only in animals mated with males treated with the 4.0 cm testosterone implants while the number of pregnant females per sperm-positive females was markedly reduced in the females mated to males with both the 3.0 cm and 4.0 cm testosterone implants. Of the fifty females exposed to males bearing 3.0 or 4.0 cm testosterone implants only three litters were obtained. It is interesting to note that caudal epididymal sperm counts in these two groups were 19.8 and 4.0% of control, respectively. Despite the low number of caudal epididymal sperm in these two groups, the percentages of sperm-positive females were 83.3% and 50.0% of the number exposed to males, respectively. Surprisingly, of the females that were sperm positive in these two groups, only 10.0 and 7.7%, respectively, were pregnant.

Since the females were not treated one would not have expected a change in the number of corpora lutea per pregnant female. This was indeed the case. The number of implantations per pregnant female ranged between 9.8 and 12.5 for the control, 0.5, 1.0, 2.0, and 8.0 cm testosterone treatment groups. For the three litters obtained with males from the 3.0 and 4.0 cm testosterone treatment groups,

TABLE 2. Effect of Paternal Testosterone Implants on Pregnancy Outcome

| Testosterone Implant | Dead or Resorbed Fetuses | | Abnormal Fetuses | |
| | Implantations | | Live Fetuses | |
	No.	%	No.	%
Control	9/164	5.49	1/221	0.45
0.5 cm	18/191	9.42	1/173	0.58
1.0 cm	4/157	2.55	2/140	0.71
2.0 cm	12/228	5.26	2/203	0.98
3.0 cm	1/9	11.11	0/9	0
4.0 cm	1/11	9.09	0/10	0
8.0 cm	4/200	2.00	1/189	0.53

the numbers of implantations were in the expected range for two (8 and 11) but in one instance there was only one implantation.

With the exception mentioned above, all of the litters had an indistinguishable number of fetuses of similar weights. The incidence of post-implantation loss (dead or resorbed fetuses) and malformations was not different in any of the treatment groups (TABLE 2). There were no significant differences in the numbers of male or female pups/litter or in the mean weights of male pups. The 2.0 cm testosterone implant did appear to decrease the mean weights of female pups/litter (control 3.47 ± 0.06 g versus 2.0 cm testosterone, 3.30 ± 0.06 g).

A number of conclusions may be drawn from these results. First, a decrease in caudal epididymal sperm content to less than 5% of control can still result in pregnancy. Second, the percentage of females that are sperm positive does not correlate directly with the percent of females pregnant. Third, a decrease in spermatogenic activity does not cause an increase in teratogenicity in the resultant progeny. These results are encouraging for those developing contraceptive formulations containing testosterone.

REFERENCES

1. ROBAIRE, B., L. L. EWING, D. C. IRBY & C. DESJARDINS. 1979. Biol. Reprod. **21:** 455–463.
2. EWING, L. L. & B. ROBAIRE. 1978. Ann. Rev. Pharmacol. Toxicol. **18:** 167–187.
3. DE KRETSER, D. M. 1976. Proc. R. Soc. London Ser. B **195:** 161–174.
4. LINDE, R., G. C. DOELLE, N. ALEXANDER, F. KIRCHNER, W. VALE, J. RIVIER & D. RABIN. 1981. N. Engl. J. Med. **305:** 663–666.
5. EWING, L. L., R. A. GORSKI, R. J. SBORDONE, J. V. TYLER, C. DESJARDINS & B. ROBAIRE. 1979. Biol. Reprod. **21:** 765–772.
6. WILSON, J. G. 1965. *In* Teratology: Principles and Techniques. J.G. Wilson & J. Warkany, Eds: 262–277. University of Chicago Press. Chicago, IL.
7. INOUYE, M. 1976. S. Congr. Anom. **16:** 171–173.

Initiation, Restoration, and Maintenance of Spermatogenesis in Non-human Primates by Testosterone

G. R. MARSHALL and E. NIESCHLAG

Max Planck Clinical Research Unit for Reproductive Medicine
University Women's Hospital of Münster
D-4400 Münster, F.R. Germany

The prevailing concept of the role of testosterone in the regulation of spermatogenesis, generally obtained from experimental results in rats, is that androgens can qualitatively maintain and restore spermatogenesis,[1,2] but not initiate the complete process.[3,4] Androgens appear to be necessary for meiosis in both mature and immature rats and can only partially stimulate spermiogenesis in immature rats. Little experimental data from primates including humans exist. We, therefore, investigated the role of testosterone in the regulation of spermatogenesis in three hypogonadotropic states in non-human primates.

IMMATURE MONKEYS

Four immature *M. fascicularis* monkeys were treated with testosterone that elevated serum androgen levels tenfold higher than those of normal adults. Testicular volumes increased sixfold over those of four other untreated immature monkeys. Motile sperm were found in some ejaculates and histological examination revealed spermatogenesis only in the treated monkeys' testes.[5]

STALK-SECTIONED MONKEYS

After allowing the testes to regress following sectioning of the pituitary stalk, four adult rhesus monkeys received twelve weekly i.m. injections of 250 mg testosterone enanthate. These resulted in peak serum testosterone values approximately 25-fold higher than presurgical levels and nadir values around tenfold higher by the seventh day. Testicular volumes that had regressed to about 25% of presurgical values increased under treatment to around 60% of presurgical volumes. Motile sperm were found in the ejaculates.[6]

HYPOPHYSECTOMIZED MONKEYS

Two adult male *M. fascicularis* monkeys were hypophysectomized and at the time of surgery, twenty 5-cm long testosterone-filled Silastic[R] capsules were implanted subcutaneously, elevating serum testosterone levels to around 160 nmol/l or tenfold higher then pre-hypophysectomy levels. After seven weeks of treatment, testicular volumes, which had decreased to 30% of presurgical values in untreated stalk-sectioned animals, were reduced only very slightly in size. Sperm counts and motility remained unchanged. Histologically, spermatogenesis occurred in every seminiferous tubule profile and appeared normal.

From the results of these three studies, we conclude that testosterone alone can not only restore and maintain spermatogenesis in hypogonadotropic adult monkeys but also initiate complete spermatogenesis in immature primates.

REFERENCES

1. BUHL, A. E., J. C. CONNETTE, K. T. KIRTON & Y.-D. YUAN. 1982. Hypophysectomized male rats treated with polydimethylsiloxane capsules containing testosterone: effect on spermatogenesis, fertility, and reproduction tract concentrations of androgen. Biol. Reprod. **27:** 183–188.
2. BOCCABELLA, A. V. 1963. Reinitiation and restoration of spermatogenesis with testosterone propionate and other hormones after a long-term post-hypophysectomy regression period. Endocrinology **72:** 787–798.
3. CHOWDHURY, A. K. & E. STEINBERGER. 1975. Effect of 5 α-reduced androgens on sex accessory organs, initiation and maintenance of spermatogenesis in the rat. Biol. Reprod. **12:** 609–617.
4. CHEMES, H. E., M. DYM & H. G. M. RAJ. 1979. The role of gonadotropins and testosterone on initiation of spermatogenesis in the immature rat. Biol. Reprod. **21:** 241–249.
5. MARSHALL, G. R., E. J. WICKINGS & E. NIESCHLAG. 1983. Testosterone (T) alone can initiate spermatogenesis in a non-human primate. Acta Endocrinol. **103** (Suppl.): 250.
6. MARSHALL, R. R., E. J. WICKINGS, D. K. LÜDECKE & E. NIESCHLAG. 1983. Stimulation of spermatogenesis in stalk-sectioned rhesus monkeys by testosterone alone. J. Clin. Endocrinol. Metab. **57:** 152–159.

FSH and Catecholamine Regulation of Sertoli Cell Adenylyl Cyclase: Requirements for Desensitization in a Cell-free System[a]

HÅVARD ATTRAMADAL,[b] TORE JAHNSEN, and
VIDAR HANSSON

Institutes of Pathology and Medical Biochemistry
University of Oslo
Oslo 1, Norway

Incubation of membrane particles from cultured immature Sertoli cells with either FSH or isoproterenol resulted in a time- and concentration-dependent loss of subsequent adenylyl cyclase (AC) response to the homologous hormone. Half-maximal refractoriness was achieved within 20–30 min of incubation. FIGURE 1 shows hormone-specific desensitization of the FSH-responsive AC in a cell-free system. Basal AC activity increased linearly throughout the 90-min incubation. In the presence of FSH, a considerably higher initial rate of cAMP formation was seen; however, the stimulated activity decreased gradually and approached that of basal AC activity. Addition of more FSH after 45 min of incubation did not further stimulate AC activity in previously FSH-treated membranes, indicating that the loss of FSH-responsive AC activity was not due to breakdown or inactivation of hormone during incubation. However, addition of isoproterenol to FSH-treated membranes at 45 min, dramatically stimulated AC activity and the non-stimulated membrane preparation (basal) responded normally to both FSH and isoproterenol. This shows that the loss of response was not due to reduced viability of the membranes. The concentration of FSH required to obtain half-maximal loss of AC response (400 ng/ml) was similar to the apparent K_m for FSH-stimulated AC activity (300 ng/ml).

Homologous desensitization was dependent on the presence of ATP. Increasing concentrations of ATP caused, in the presence of FSH (5 μg/ml), a concentration-dependent loss of response to homologous hormone (FIGURE 2). Half-maximal desensitization was achieved at an ATP concentration of 0.2 mM. Increasing concentrations of Mg^{2+} also caused, in the presence of hormone, homologous desensitization. The concentration of Mg^{2+} that caused half-maximal effect was approximately 5 mM in excess of ATP and EDTA. However, higher concentrations of free Mg^{2+}, in the absence of hormone, caused desensitization of both FSH- and isoproterenol-sensitive AC with half-maximal effect at approximately 30 mM. Homologous desensitization was obtained in the presence of GTP. However, when GTP was substituted with the non-hydrolyzable analog GMPP(NH)P the hormonal activation remained constant throughout 90 min of incubation.

[a] Supported by the Rockefeller Foundation, Norwegian Research Council for Science and the Humanities (NAVF), and the Norwegian Society for Fighting Cancer (NFTKB).

[b] Address correspondence to: Håvard Attramadal, Institute of Pathology, Rikshospitalet, Oslo 1, Norway.

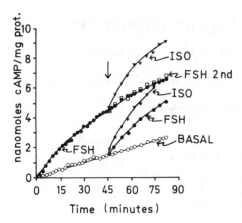

FIGURE 1. Homologous desensitization of FSH-responsive AC in a cell-free system. Membrane particles (0.02 mg/ml of protein) were incubated at 32.5°C in the absence (open circles) or presence (closed circles) of NIH-oFSH-S14 (5 µg/ml) in an AC assay.[2] At successive time intervals 50 µl aliquots were withdrawn and assayed for AC activity. After 45 min (arrow) a new dose of either oFSH-S14 (5 µg/ml) or D,L-isoproterenol (5 µg/ml) was added both to the basal and to the tube containing FSH. Note: There is a hormone-specific loss of FSH response whereas the response to isoproterenol is maintained.

The requirements of ATP and Mg^{2+} for desensitization are compatible with the hypothesis that homologous desensitization is due to a phosphorylation reaction. Furthermore, resensitization of desensitized follicular AC by exogenous phosphoprotein phosphatase[1] supports this notion. Homologous desensitization of the Sertoli cell AC is not mediated via cAMP. Homologous desensitization is associated with normal function of the N-component. AC is activated normally by Mg^{2+}, fluoride, GTP, and GMPP(NH)P. Furthermore, the typical elimination of

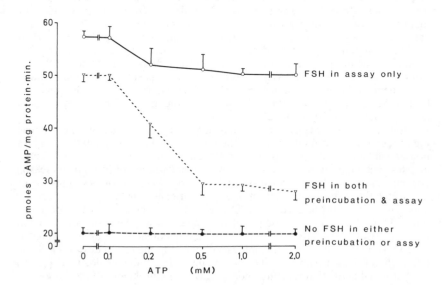

FIGURE 2. Effect of ATP on FSH-induced desensitization in a cell-free system. Membrane particles were preincubated for 45 min at 32.5°C with varying concentrations of ATP (0–2.0 mM) in the absence and presence of oFSH-S14 (5 µg/ml) followed by washing, centrifugation, and assay of AC activity.[2] Note: ATP in the presence of FSH caused a concentration-dependent decrease in FSH response (K_m = 0.2 mM).

lag time by Mg^{2+} takes place normally in densensitized membranes, whereas elimination of lag time by hormone does not occur.[2] This indicates that the lesion in homologous desensitization is associated with the hormone receptor itself. Desensitization of isoproterenol-responsive AC in turkey erythrocytes is associated with physical changes in the β-adrenergic receptor[3] strengthening the hypothesis that homologous desensitization is due to a receptor phosphorylation.

Our studies show that homologous desensitization requires an excess of free Mg^{2+}, and that hormone may accelerate desensitization of the AC by increasing its sensitivity to the actions of Mg^{2+}. It is possible that this effect of hormone on the binding affinity of Mg^{2+} to the N-component is related to the mechanism by which hormone activates the AC.

REFERENCES

1. HUNZICKER-DUNN, M., D. DERDA, R. A. JUNGMANN & L. BIRNBAUMER. 1979. Endocrinology **104:** 1785–1793.
2. IYENGAR, R., P. W. MINTZ, T. L. SWARTZ & L. BIRNBAUMER. 1980. J. Biol. Chem. **255:** 11875–1192.
3. STADEL, J. M., P. NAMBI, T. N. LAVIN, S. L. HEALD, M. G. CARON & R. J. LEFKOWITZ. 1982. J. Biol. Chem. **257:** 9242–9245.

Serum Follicle Stimulating Hormone, Androgen Binding Protein, and Regeneration of the Seminiferous Epithelium after Local Testicular Irradiation

J. I. DELIC and J. H. HENDRY

Department of Radiobiology
Paterson Laboratories
Christie Hospital
Manchester M20 9BX, U.K.

I. D. MORRIS

Department of Pharmacology
University of Manchester
Manchester M13 9PT, U.K.

S. M. SHALET

Department of Endocrinology
Christie Hospital
Manchester M20 9BX, U.K.

INTRODUCTION

The seminiferous epithelium is a rapidly proliferating tissue that is readily impaired by cytotoxic insults. Consequently, radiation and anti-tumor drugs have been widely used to investigate the relationship between the semiferous epithelium and the gonadotrophins. From these and other experiments a dual hormonal control of the testis has been postulated. The Leydig cell and androgen secretion are primarily controlled by LH. The seminiferous epithelium and the secretion of a yet unidentified hormone, inhibin, appears to be controlled by FSH. Inhibin is believed to originate from the Sertoli cell.[1] However, the evidence for the existence of inhibin is largely circumstantial as laboratory assays for inhibin are not widely available, are difficult to use, and rely upon indirect bioactivity measurements.[2] The Sertoli cell also secretes androgen binding protein (ABP) into the blood. It has been suggested that serum ABP will reflect Sertoli cell activity.[3] Inhibin is a Sertoli cell protein; changes in serum inhibin may be monitored by changes in ABP. Recently ABP has been purified and a radioimmunoassay made available so that large numbers of measurements are easily made. As part of a study that extensively documents the effects of testicular radiation, we have attempted to correlate Sertoli cell activity (measured by levels of ABP) with serum gonadotrophin concentrations.

METHODS

The testes of conscious adult male rats (11–12 weeks) were exposed to a single acute irradiation of 300(peak)kilovoltage X rays (doses of 1,2,3,4,5,10,15, or 20 Gray). The rats were then housed under standard animal house conditions together with age-matched, sham-irradiated controls and bilateral castrates and killed at 8 or 24 weeks after treatment. Serum gonadotrophins and ABP were measured with radioimmunoassay kits kindly provided by National Institute of Arthritis, Diabetes and Diseases of the Kidney. Estimations of the regeneration of the seminiferous tubules were made by light microscopy.

RESULTS

Eight weeks after treatment, testicular weights showed a dose-dependent decrease up to 5 Gy, and this decrease was maintained at higher doses. However, by 24 weeks testicular weight was recovering at doses below 5 Gy and this was associated with regeneration of the seminiferous epithelium. Recovery was not seen at higher doses and no regeneration was evident. Concentrations of serum FSH, which is associated with spermatogenesis and Sertoli cell function, were increased at 2 Gy and above, 8 weeks after treatment, a maximum being reached at 4 Gy. Castrate values at this time, were not achieved. By 24 weeks, FSH levels were still elevated at 4 Gy and above, but at lower doses levels were within the normal range. These changes with time at the lower doses may be associated with the regeneration of the seminiferous epithelium. After 8 weeks, decreased concentrations of ABP were detected after 5 Gy and reached a plateau between 5 and 10 Gy, slightly higher than in castrates. Twenty four weeks after irradiation ABP was also decreased, the plateau was reached between 4 and 5 Gy, ABP concentrations at 15 and 20 Gy were not significantly different from castrates. Serum FSH in these rats also plateaued between 4 and 5 Gy.

DISCUSSION

FSH concentrations were elevated at doses of > 2 Gy and > 3 Gy at 8 and 24 weeks, respectively. In general, ABP was low in the serum of these rats. However, at those doses of radiation where the rates of change in FSH concentrations were maximal, ABP did not change in concert. A similar lack of correlation was noted for seminiferous tubule regeneration and testicular weight. It has become apparent that the interstitial and tubular compartments of the testis cannot be considered in isolation. We have shown elsewhere[4] that in irradiated rats after 8 weeks androgen secretion was altered as the ventral prostate, seminal vesicle weights, and serum testosterone concentrations were decreased. Twenty four weeks after irradiation serum testosterone is within the normal range, yet FSH remained elevated associated with, at the high doses, castrate levels of ABP. The Leydig cell population and LH receptors are also reduced after 8 and 24 weeks.

These data unequivocally demonstrate that serum FSH and LH can be controlled independently in the male rat, these changes are associated with changes in Sertoli cell secretion monitored by serum ABP concentrations. However, as radiation also changes Leydig cell function, the existence of the tubular messenger, inhibin, and its role in the control of gonadotrophin secretion remain to be established.

REFERENCES

1. LE GAC F. & D. M. DE KRETZER. 1982. Molec. Cell. Endocrinol. **28:** 487–498.
2. SCOTT, R. S., H. G. BURGER, H. QUIGG, M. DOBOS, D. M. ROBERTSON & D. M. DE KRETZER. 1982. Molec. Cell. Endocrinol. **27:** 307–316.
3. MATHER, J. P., G. L. GUNSALUS, N. A. MUSTO, C. Y. CHENG, M. PARVINEN, W. WRIGHT, V. PEREZ-INFANTE, A. MARGIORIS, A. RIOTTA, R. BECKER, D. T. KRIEGER & C. W. BARDIN, 1983. J. Steroid Biochem. **19:** 41–51.
4. DELIC, J. I., J. H. HENDRY, I. D. MORRIS & S. M. SHALET. July 1983. C2-03 7th International Congress of Radiation Research. Amsterdam.

Spermatogenic Cells in the Germinal Epithelium Utilize α-Ketoisocaproate and Lactate, Produced by Sertoli Cells from Leucine and Glucose

J. ANTON GROOTEGOED,[a] RUUD JANSEN, and
HENK J. VAN DER MOLEN

Department of Biochemistry
(Division of Chemical Endocrinology)
Medical Faculty
Erasmus University
Rotterdam, The Netherlands

INTRODUCTION

There is convincing evidence that several steps in spermatogenesis are dependent on complex structural interactions between Sertoli cells and the developing germ cells. Some important biochemical aspects of the Sertoli cell–germ cell interaction, however, could involve a simple mechanism, such as the intracellular exchange of diffusable ubiquitous compounds.

Isolated rat spermatocytes and spermatids cannot fully support their energy requirements from glucose, but depend on exogenous pyruvate and/or lactate as an energy substrate. Sertoli cells *in vitro* release pyruvate and lactate, and the rate of glycolysis and the release of these substrates is stimulated by FSH and insulin. These observations led us to propose that one aspect of the interaction between Sertoli cells and germ cells might be the exchange of energy-yielding substrates.[1,2,4] With respect to the situation in the germinal epithelium, however, it is not certain whether Sertoli cells actually are involved in the supply of energy substrates, or which substrates are used by the germ cells *in situ*. Lactate and pyruvate may diffuse into the spermatogenic microenvironment from the circulation, and the contribution of Sertoli cells in the supply of lactate and pyruvate may not be significant.

The present results indicate that spermatogenic cells *in situ*, in contact with Sertoli cells, use lactate as an energy substrate. The contribution of Sertoli cells to the supply of lactate in the spermatogenic microenvironment is important, because a high concentration of lactate appears to be essential to support ATP synthesis by spermatocytes and spermatids. Sertoli cells were found to produce also α-ketoisocaproate (KIC) from leucine, and the germ cells reduced KIC to α-hydroxyisocaproate (HOIC) concomitant with the utilization of lactate. Thus, at least two ubiquitous compounds, lactate and KIC, are released by Sertoli cells and can be used by spermatogenic cells.

[a] Address correspondence to: J. A. Grootegoed, Department of Biochemistry II, Medical Faculty, Erasmus University Rotterdam, P.O. Box 1738, 3000 DR Rotterdam, The Netherlands.

RESULTS AND DISCUSSION

Utilization of Pyruvate and Lactate by Isolated Germ Cells

The ATP content of pachytene spermatocytes and round spermatids, isolated from rat testes, decreased during incubation in the presence of glucose, but was maintained at a high level when pyruvate or lactate was present in the incubation medium (approx. 4 nmol ATP/10^6 spermatids or 16 nmol ATP/10^6 spermatocytes). It has been reported that pyruvate cannot support ATP synthesis in rat spermatids at 37°C, although isolated spermatids may lose mitochondrial respiratory control at 37°C.[7] Under the present incubation conditions, however, the spermatocytes and spermatids had exactly the same ATP content at 32, 37, or 40°C.

The ATP content of isolated spermatids was maintained at 0.25 mM pyruvate or at 3 mM L-lactate (Eagle's Minimum Essential Medium, 5.6 mM glucose, 0.4% bovine serum albumin, 32°C). The rate of pyruvate oxidation (conversion of [U-^{14}C]pyruvate to $^{14}CO_2$; 8–9 nmol/10^6 spermatids/hr at 2 mM pyruvate) was at least two times higher than the rate of lactate oxidation (conversion of L-[U-^{14}C]lactate to $^{14}CO_2$; 3–4 nmol/10^6 spermatids/hr at 3–6 mM L-lactate). The latter result was explained by the observation that pyruvate was reduced to lactate at a high rate. Thus, NADH produced from NAD$^+$ by mitochondrial oxidation of exogenous pyruvate was reoxidized for the greater part not via the electron transport chain, but via the conversion of exogenous pyruvate to lactate. Preliminary observations indicate that the NADH/NAD$^+$ system was highly oxidized in spermatocytes and spermatids during incubation in the presence of pyruvate.

In conclusion, pyruvate appears to be an effective energy substrate at much lower concentrations than lactate, but the overall rate of pyruvate utilization (oxidation in the mitochondria plus reduction to lactate) is very high.

Germ Cells in Contact with Sertoli Cells Utilize Lactate and KIC

Indications that spermatocytes and spermatids in contact with Sertoli cells convert exogenous lactate pyruvate are derived from the following observations.

Sertoli cells, isolated from sterile rats (prenatally irradiated), metabolize the branched-chain amino acids (leucine, isoleucine, and valine) at a higher rate than other amino acids.[5] Sertoli cells, but not the germ cells, contain a high activity of branched-chain amino acid amino-transferase[5] and convert leucine to KIC (KIC was estimated using a spectrophotometric assay or using gas-liquid chromatography). For the greater part, KIC was decarboxylated at the branched-chain α-keto acid dehydrogenase complex (conversion of [1-^{14}C]leucine to $^{14}CO_2$) but in addition KIC was released from the cells.

Spermatocytes and spermatids can be kept in vitro in contact with Sertoli cells, in tubule fragments isolated by collagenase treatment from testes of 4-week-old intact rats, and incubated in the presence of glucose.[3] Apparently, the endogenous production of lactate and/or pyruvate from glucose was sufficient to maintain the germ cells. In addition, it was found that the tubule fragments produced HOIC, rather than KIC, from leucine. It can be concluded that in these tubule fragments KIC released by Sertoli cells was reduced to HOIC by the germ cells.

Isolated spermatocytes and spermatids reduced KIC to HOIC during an incubation in the presence of exogenous lactate and 0.25 mM KIC, but not when pyruvate was used as an energy substrate. The low NADH/NAD$^+$ ratio, in the presence of pyruvate, may restrict the reduction of KIC. Reduction of KIC was catalyzed most likely by the lactate dehydrogenase isozyme LDH-C_4 from male germ cells, because LDH-C_4 from rats catalyzes the reduction of branched-chain α-keto acids (from branched-chain amino acids) with NADH as coenzyme.[8]

In conclusion, the reduction of KIC to HOIC by the germ cells that are in contact with Sertoli cells in the tubule fragments, indicates that the germ cells use lactate exogenous as an energy-yielding substrate.

Is the Reduction of KIC to HOIC of Physiological Importance?

It is not certain that the reduction of KIC to HOIC by the germ cells is of physiological importance. This conversion may reflect the coincidence that the germ cells contain an LDH isozyme with a broad substrate specificity, that Sertoli cells release KIC, and that the $NADH/NAD^+$ ratio of the germ cells that use lactate is sufficiently high to cause reduction of KIC.

Perhaps KIC plays a role in the energy metabolism of the spermatogenic cells with respect to the reoxidation of cytosolic NADH. Concomitant with the conversion of lactate or glucose to pyruvate, NAD^+ is reduced to NADH in the cytosol. The rate of reoxidation of cytosolic NADH via a shuttle system for transporting reducing equivalents from cytosolic NADH into the mitochondrial matrix (such as the malate-aspartate shuttle system) may be rate-limiting in the germ cells.

It was observed that the rate of lactate oxidation (conversion of L-[U-^{14}C]lactate to $^{14}CO_2$, at 6 mM L-lactate) by spermatids was increased by 20–25% after addition of 0.25 mM KIC. In addition, it was found that the rate of conversion of [6-^{14}C]glucose to $^{14}CO_2$ by isolated spermatocytes and spermatids, at different concentrations of glucose, was increased by 40–80% in the presence of 0.25 mM KIC. This result may be explained by an increased rate of mitochondrial oxidation of endogenous pyruvate, when reoxidation of NADH in the cytosol is carried out at the reduction of KIC to HOIC, rather than at the reduction of pyruvate to lactate. The rate of glucose oxidation by the isolated germ cells incubated in the presence of both glucose and KIC, however, still was too low to maintain the ATP content.

We have concluded that spermatocytes and spermatids in tubule fragments, incubated in the presence of leucine and glucose, reduce KIC (produced by Sertoli cells) to HOIC and use lactate (produced by Sertoli cells) as an energy substrate. A high concentration of lactate (3–6 mM) seems to be required to maintain the ATP content of the germ cells. The concentration of lactate in rat blood is approximately 1 mM, and net production of lactate by Sertoli cells may be essential to raise the concentration of lactate in the spermatogenic microenvironment *in vivo* so that the energy requirements of the developing germ cells can be met.

REFERENCES

1. JUTTE, N. H. P. M., J. A. GROOTEGOED, F. F. G. ROMMERTS & H. J. VAN DER MOLEN. 1981. J. Reprod. Fert. **62:** 399–405.
2. GROOTEGOED, J. A., N. H. P. M. JUTTE, R. JANSEN, F. A. HEUSDENS, F. F. G. ROMMERTS & H. J. VAN DER MOLEN. 1982. *In* Research on Steroids. Volume X: 169–183. Excerpta Medica. Amsterdam.
3. JUTTE, N. H. P. M., R. JANSEN, J. A. GROOTEGOED, F. F. G. ROMMERTS, O. P. F. CLAUSEN & H. J. VAN DER MOLEN. 1982. J. Reprod. Fert. **65:** 431–438.

4. JUTTE, N. H. P. M., R. JANSEN, J. A. GROOTEGOED, F. F. G. ROMMERTS & H. J. VAN DER MOLEN. 1983. J. Reprod. Fert. **68:** 219–226.
5. GROOTEGOED, J. A., N. H. P. M. JUTTE, R. JANSEN & H. J. VAN DER MOLEN. 1983. *In* Hormones and Cell Regulation. **7:** 299–316. Elsevier Biomedical Press. Amsterdam.
6. MITA, M. & P. F. HALL. 1982. Biol. Reprod. **26:** 445–455.
7. NAKAMURA, M., I. YASUMASU, S. OKINAGA & K. ARAI. 1982. Develop. Growth Differ. **24:** 265–272.
8. CORONEL, C. E., C. BURGOS, N. M. GEREZ DE BURGOS, L. E. ROVAI & A. BLANCO. 1983. J. Exp. Zool. **225:** 379–385.

Rat Sertoli Cells and Epididymal Epithelium Secrete A Protein Found in Mature Sperm

S. R. SYLVESTER and M. D. GRISWOLD

Biochemistry/Biophysics Program
Washington State University
Pullman, Washington 99164-4660

Cultured rat Sertoli cells secrete many proteins into media. We have purified and characterized one of the major proteins, a dimeric acidic glycoprotein (DAG-protein). This sulfated and heavily glycosylated protein is composed of disulfide-linked monomers of 29,000 and 41,000 MW, that exhibit isoelectric points of 3.7 and 4.8, respectively. Rabbit antiserum prepared against DAG-protein immuno-precipitates a variable amount of a sulfated glycoprotein of 70,000 MW (band 4) that is electrophoretically distinct from the unreduced DAG-protein heterodimer. It is not clear if band 4 is a non-covalently bound subunit of the native structure of DAG-protein or that our antisera cross-reacts with it.

The rabbit antiserum was also used to localize DAG-protein in paraffin sections of rat testis, epididymis, and vas deferens, and in smears of washed spermatozoa by indirect immunofluorescence. Smears of spermatozoa or thin sections of the organs were incubated sequentially with antiserum, biotinylated goat anti-rabbit gamma globulin, and fluorescein isothiocyanate and conjugated avidin. Control sections were incubated with normal rabbit serum rather than DAG-protein antiserum.

In sections of the testis, fluorescence was observed in the Sertoli cell cyto-plasms between germinal cells. The heads and tails of late spermatids and the membranes of residual bodies fluoresced brightly. In the epididymis, the epithe-lium of the initial segment was uniformly but lightly stained. The membranes and stereocilia of principal cells in the caput region of the epididymis fluoresced brightly. In the corpus and cauda epididymis, the stereocilia were not as bright but halo cells were well stained. Clear cells were devoid of staining. Only the luminal ciliated surfaces of the vas deferens were stained. The heads and tails of sperm were stained throughout the sections of the organs. Indirect immunofluorescence of smears of sperm revealed staining of the acrosomal region, neck, and tail. The midpiece of the tail was stained but not nearly as brightly as the endpiece. Control sections were very weakly stained and showed no specific areas of intense staining.

The staining observed in the epithelium of the epididymis could be the result of absorption of sperm proteins. However, immunoprecipitates of epididymis organ culture media revealed the secretion of a modified form of DAG-protein. The epididymal protein was composed of monomers of lower molecular weight and of more basic isoelectric point than the Sertoli cell culture counterparts and was produced mainly by the caput epididymis.

We believe that DAG-protein is similar, if not identical, to a protein secreted by epididymis organ cultures (protein F) described by Brooks.[1] The 29,000 MW monomer of DAG-protein is similar in some respects to the acidic epididymal glycoprotein (AEG) described by Lea *et al.*[2] Unlike DAG-protein, AEG has not been shown to be associated with other glycoproteins and the immunohisto-chemistry of AEG does not concur with out findings.

The results of this study suggest that Sertoli cells and epididymal cells secrete a protein that remains a part of the developing and mature sperm.

REFERENCES

1. BROOKS, D. E. 1983. Gamete Res. **4:** 367–376.
2. LEA, O. A., P. PETRUSZ & F. S. FRENCH. 1978. Int. J. Androl. (Suppl. 2): 592–606.

Glucagon-stimulated Cyclic AMP Formation in Rat Sertoli Cells: Inhibitory Effects of Adenosine[a]

LARS EIKVAR,[b] FINN O. LEVY, HÅVARD
ATTRAMADAL, NICOLET H.P.M. JUTTE, E. MARTIN
RITZÉN, ROBERT HORN, and VIDAR HANSSON

Institutes of Medical Biochemistry and Pathology
University of Oslo
Oslo, Norway

Pediatric Research Unit
Karolinska Hospital
Stockholm, Sweden

Adenylyl cyclase activity and cyclic AMP formation in cultured immature rat Sertoli cells are stimulated by FSH and isoproterenol. Cyclic AMP subsequently stimulates glucose uptake and lactate secretion as well as aromatization. Glucagon is a primary regulator of glucose metabolism. For that reason we investigated possible effects of glucagon on cultured immature rat Sertoli cells. Cyclic AMP systems in several tissues are influenced by adenosine.[1] Possible effects of this nucleotide in our system were also studied.

Sertoli cells isolated from 19-day-old Sprague-Dawley rats were cultured for five days in Eagles MEM in the presence of 10% fetal calf serum (FCS). Unless stated otherwise, the cells were preincubated for 24 hr without FCS. At day 5 the experiments were started by adding hormones (NIH-FSH-S14, glucagon and isoproterenol) and/or methyl-isobutyl-xanthine (MIX). After 18 hr of stimulation, the media were removed and immediately heated at 80°C for 3 minutes. The samples were subsequently stored at $-70°C$. The cells were dissolved in 1 M NaOH before protein measurements. Lactate was estimated enzymatically, cyclic AMP by a competitive protein binding assay, and estradiol by radioimmunoassay. Adenylyl cyclase activity in membrane particles was analyzed using $[\alpha\text{-}^{32}P]ATP$ as radioactive substrate and isolating $[\alpha\text{-}^{32}P]cAMP$ by double chromatography on Dowex-50 and alumina.

Addition of glucagon to cultured Sertoli cells isolated from immature (10–19 days old) rats caused a time- and concentration-dependent stimulation of cyclic AMP formation, lactate secretion, and estradiol formation. The magnitude and kinetics of these responses were comparable to the effects observed with FSH. Glucagon also caused a concentration-dependent activation of adenylyl cyclase activity in Sertoli cell membrane particles (K_m 300 ng/ml) (FIGURE 1).

Intracellular concentration of cyclic AMP was maximal already 30 minutes after the addition of glucagon (0.5 μg/ml), after which it gradually decreased

[a] Supported by the Rockefeller Foundation, Norwegian Research Council for Science and the Humanities (NAVF), and the Norwegian Society for Fighting Cancer (FTKB).

[b] Address correspondence to: Lars Eikvar, Institute of Medical Biochemistry, P.b. 1112 Blindern, Oslo 3, Norway.

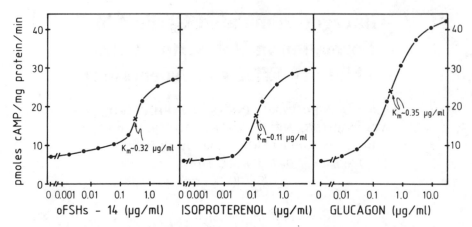

FIGURE 1. Dose-response curves for the activation of the Sertoli cell adenylyl cyclase by oFSH, isoproterenol, and glucagon. Adenylyl cyclase activity was measured in membrane particles prepared from isolated rat Sertoli cells after four days in culture, and incubated at 32.5°C for 12 min with oFSH, isoproterenol, and glucagon. All values represent the mean of duplicate measurements.

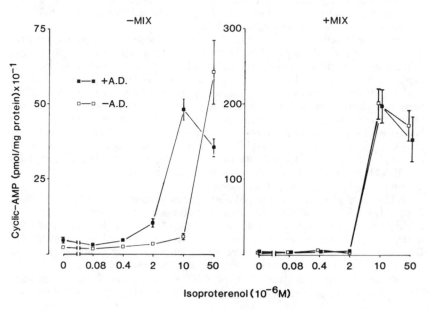

FIGURE 2. Effects of adenosine deaminase (2 μg/ml) and MIX (0.2 mM) on isoproterenol-stimulated cAMP production to media from cultured Sertoli cells. All values represent the mean ± SEM of six incubations.

towards basal. Cyclic AMP concentrations in the medium increased much more slowly and reached a plateau after approximately 6 hr. After 6 hr the level of lactate in the medium was increased twofold compared to basal level, and a fivefold increase was observed after 24 hr. The concentration of glucagon required for half-maximal stimulation (ED_{50}) of cyclic AMP formation was about 0.5 μg/ml, whereas ED_{50} for lactate secretion and estradiol formation was found to be ten to hundred times lower. This indicates that only a small proportion of the glucagon receptors needs to be occupied in order to achieve a maximal metabolic response.

Removal of adenosine by the addition of adenosine deaminase (2 μg/ml) to the incubation medium, caused a shift to the left of the dose-response curves for cyclic AMP formation (FIGURE 2) and lactate secretion compared to the controls, whereas the maximal levels were similar in both conditions. This indicates that the Sertoli cell contains adenosine receptors and that adenosine has an inhibitory effect on the hormonal effects. The effects of adenosine deaminase were observed with both glucagon, FSH, and isoproterenol.

MIX is known to stimulate cyclic AMP formation by inhibition of phosphodiesterase activity; it is also an inhibitor of adenosine binding to its receptors on the cell membrane. In our studies MIX dramatically stimulated cyclic AMP formation and lactate secretion after addition of glucagon, FSH, and isoproterenol, but eliminated the effects of adenosine deaminase (FIGURE 2).

It remains to be demonstrated whether glucagon or adenosine represent regulators of Sertoli cell function in vivo.

REFERENCE

1. WOLFF, J., C. LONDOS & D. M. F. COOPER. 1981. Adv. Cyclic Nucleotide Res. **14:** 199–214.

Metabolism of Palmitate in Cultured Sertoli Cells and Interaction with Glucose Metabolism[a]

NICOLET H.P.M. JUTTE[b] and VIDAR HANSSON

Institutes of Medical Biochemistry and Pathology
University of Oslo
Oslo, Norway

Sertoli cells have a large capacity to convert glucose to pyruvate and lactate, and the latter two substrates are essential for the viability of pachytene spermatocytes and round spermatids *in vitro*. The yield of ATP from the glycolytic pathway is limited and therefore it is likely that Sertoli cells themselves require additional energy substrates besides carbohydrates. Furthermore, the fact that Sertoli cells can survive 24 hours of incubation in a medium without glucose also suggests that the cells can use alternative energy substrates. Considering the fact that Sertoli cells often contain numerous lipid droplets, the presence of which is correlated with the endocrine status of the animals, we have investigated lipid metabolism in Sertoli cells.

Sertoli cells, isolated from 19–20-day-old rats, were used on the fifth day after plating in flasks (25 cm^2). The cells (1–2 mg protein) were, unless stated otherwise, incubated for five hours in 1–2.3 ml Krebs-Henseleit buffer in the presence of [1-^{14}C]palmitate (0.522 mM, 0.5 mCi/mmol, 0.8% BSA). The radioactivity in CO_2, perchloroacetic acid (PCA)-soluble material, and lipids was determined and expressed as nmol palmitate metabolized. Where indicated, cells and medium were separated before PCA was added. β-OH-butyrate and lactate, secreted into the medium, were estimated enzymically. Data are presented as means ± S.E.M.

As shown in FIGURE 1, increasing concentrations of palmitate caused increasing production of $^{14}CO_2$, ^{14}C-labeled acid-soluble compounds, and β-OH-butyrate by Sertoli cells. Maximum oxidation was obtained at a palmitate concentration of 0.35 mM. In the presence of a saturating concentration of palmitate, the amount of radioactivity in CO_2 and in the acid-soluble fraction of the medium (ketone bodies) increased linearly with time for at least six hours. The amount of acid-soluble radioactivity in the cells (intermediates) had reached a plateau already after three hours.

Of the total amount of [1-^{14}C] palmitate oxidized (110 ± 46 nmol/flask; $N = 5$), 65 ± 2% was recovered as CO_2 and 34 ± 2% as acid-soluble compounds. Approximately one third of the acid-soluble radioactivity was found within the cells and the rest was secreted into the medium. By enzymatic measurements it was confirmed that the Sertoli cells secreted β-OH-butyrate (28 ± 8 nmol/flask; $N = 4$). Under these conditions only a small amount of palmitate (0.9 ± 0.3 nmol/flask; $N = 3$) was esterfied into triacylglycerols (FIGURE 2). Addition of glucose (5.5 mM)

[a] Supported by the Rockefeller Foundation, Norwegian Research Council for Science and the Humanities (NAVF), and the Norwegian Society for Fighting Cancer (NFTKB).
[b] Address correspondence to: Dr. Nicolet Jutte, Institute of Medical Biochemistry, University of Oslo, P.O.Box 1112, Blindern, Oslo 3, Norway.

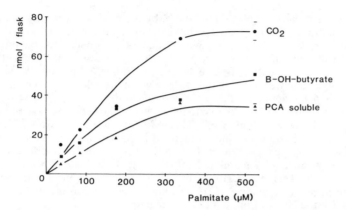

FIGURE 1. Effect of the concentration of substrate on palmitate oxidation by Sertoli cells.

to the culture medium together with [1-^{14}C]palmitate caused a small and variable decrease of $17 \pm 9\%$ ($N = 5$) in CO_2 production but a dramatic (approximately tenfold) increase in radioactivity incorporated into triacylglycerols (FIGURE 2). This increase in esterification is probably a result of an increase in available glycerophosphate.

Enzymatic measurements showed that Sertoli cells secreted β-OH-butyrate both in the absence and presence of glucose (28 ± 8 and 35 ± 7 nmol/flask respectively; $N = 4$) when palmitate was present. In the absence of exogenous

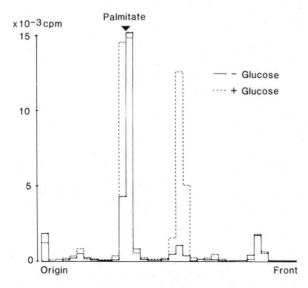

FIGURE 2. Thin-layer chromatography (silica gel) of lipids, extracted from Sertoli cells with chloroform/methanol (2:1), using diethylether:hexane:acetic acid (20:80:1) as developing fluid.

palmitate the production of β-OH-butyrate by the cells was very low both in the absence and presence of glucose. This indicates that the production of ketone bodies from endogenous lipids is negligible under these conditions. Lactate secretion by Sertoli cells incubated in the presence of glucose was hardly influenced by the presence of palmitate (2.04 ± 0.44 and 2.89 ± 0.99 μmol/flask, respectively; $N = 3$). No lactate was found in the medium when the cells were incubated in the presence of palmitate but in the absence of glucose).

Glucagon and cAMP are known to inhibit acetyl CoA-carboxylase resulting in reduced synthesis of malonyl CoA. This reduction in malonyl CoA relieves the block of fatty acid transport into mitochondria causing an increase in fatty acid oxidation and ketogenesis. Under the conditions described, FSH (0.22 μg FSH-S13/ml) or glucagon (0.43 μg/ml) did not stimulate the formation of ketone bodies by Sertoli cells. This may partly be due to the palmitate concentration used. A high concentration of palmitoyl CoA also inhibits acetyl CoA-carboxylase, which may abolish the effect of hormones on ketogenesis.

Thus, Sertoli cells have a high capacity to metabolize lipids and oxidation of lipids may represent the primary source of energy for this cell. Furthermore, lipid oxidation by Sertoli cells may also be important for germ cells; ketone bodies secreted by Sertoli cells may be additional substrates for pachytene spermatocytes and round spermatids. Glucose dramatically stimulated palmitate esterification by Sertoli cells but hardly affected palmitate oxidation. It will be of interest to see whether effects of hormones on lipid metabolism in Sertoli cells may influence the survival of germ cells.

Alteration of the Normal Age-related Decline in Sertoli Cell Responsiveness to FSH in the H^{re} Rat[a]

JERROLD J. HEINDEL

Department of Biology
University of Mississippi
University, Mississippi

ALBERT S. BERKOWITZ

Department of Obstetrics, Gynecology and
Reproductive Science
University of Texas Medical School
Houston, Texas

ANDREZEJ BARTKE

Department of Obstetrics and Gynecology
The University of Texas Health Science Center
San Antonio, Texas

We have been interested in the possible physiological significance of the age-related prematurational decline in ability of Sertoli cells to respond to FSH with an increased intracellular accumulation of cAMP.

In both the Long Evans rat and the golden hamster the decline in Sertoli cell response to FSH is related to the onset of testicular maturation.[1,2] Maximal Sertoli cell response to FSH occurred between 16–18 days of age in both species. Responsiveness then declined to adult levels by 34–36 days of age in both species.

During pineal-induced testicular regression and recrudescence in the hamster, Sertoli cell response to FSH returns to immature levels as spermatogenesis is inhibited, and again declines to adult levels during reinitiation of spermatogenesis.[3]

We have now examined rats with the autosomal H^{re} gene,[4] which results in failure of the seminiferous epithelium, in order to correlate testis weight with the *in vitro* Sertoli cell responsiveness to FSH.

At 18 days of age, testis weights were similar in H^{re} rats and control littermates. Testis weight in the H^{re} rats then changed from the controls in two distinct phases (FIGURE 1). During the first phase (20–50 days) testis weight of the H^{re} rats lagged behind the controls by 10–12 days. A testis weight of 400 mg was achieved at 30 days of age in the controls compared to 42 days of age in the H^{re} rat. In the second phase, the testis weight of the H^{re} plateaued at 650 mg at 50–60 days of age and then declined to the stable adult level of 400 mg per testis.

Sertoli cells were prepared from H^{re} rats and their control littermates at various ages from 18–120 days according to the procedure described previously.[1] After four days in culture the Sertoli cells were challenged with FSH in the presence of 1 mM isobutyl methyl xanthine for 30 min. The cAMP was extracted

[a] Supported in part by National Institutes of Health grants HD-18186 and 5 P 50 HD08338.

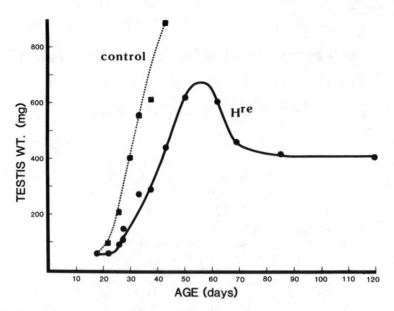

FIGURE 1. A comparison of the age-related changes in the testis weights of H^re rats and their control litter mates. Each point is the average of 2–8 values.

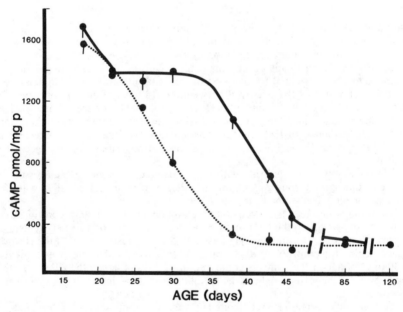

FIGURE 2. A comparison of the age-related decline in response to maximal doses of FSH in Sertoli cells from H^re and control rats. There is a shift of approximately 14 days in the age-related decline in response of Sertoli cells from H^re rats compared to control littermates. However, the response of Sertoli cells from the H^re rats is the same as that of control rats with the same testis weight. Each point is the average of quadruplicate values from an experiment repeated 2–4 times ± SEM.

from the cells with alcohol, aliquoted, and dried. cAMP was quantitated by radioimmunoassay and calculated as cAMP pmol/mg protein. Sertoli cells from 18-day-old control and H^{re} rats responded to FSH with the same maximal cAMP response (1686 ± 92 versus 1581 ± 76 pmol/mg protein, respectively) with no shift in the FSH dose-response curve. The Sertoli cells from both the control and the H^{re} rats showed an age-related loss in response to FSH, but this response was delayed by 12–15 days in the H^{re} rats (FIGURE 2). A fifty percent decline in Sertoli cell response to FSH occurred at the same testis weight (400 mg) in the H^{re} and control; however, this weight was attained at 30 days of age in the controls and at 42 days in the H^{re} rats. The response of Sertoli cells from adult control rats (testis weight 1800 mg) and adult H^{re} rats (testis weight 400 mg) were similar at about 300 pmol/mg protein. These results suggest two possible defects in the H^{re} rat. There is an initial shift in the time of the onset of spermatogenesis, which is followed by an inhibition of spermatogenesis that results in infertility. The fact that the initial shift in the onset of spermatogenesis correlates with a change in the ability of FSH to stimulate cAMP accumulation in Sertoli cells provides further evidence for a physiologically important role for this altered Sertoli cell response in the control of the onset of spermatogenesis. The stimulus for this altered Sertoli cell function or its role in the resulting infertility is not clear.

REFERENCES

1. STEINBERGER, A., M. HINTZ & J. J. HEINDEL. 1978. Biol. Reprod. **19:** 566–572.
2. HEINDEL, J. J., A. S. BERKOWITZ, R. PHILO & J. P. PRESLOCK. 1981. Am. J. Andrology **2:** 217–221.
3. BERKOWITZ, A. S. & J. J. HEINDEL. 1982. Am. Soc. Andrology Annual Meeting. Hilton Head, NC.
4. MUSTO, N. A., R. J. SANTEN, C. HUCKINS & C. W. BARDIN. 1978. Biol. Reprod. **19:** 797–806.

Effect of Purified and Cell-produced Extracellular Matrix Components on Sertoli Cell Function[a]

J. P. MATHER, S. D. WOLPE, G. L. GUNSALUS,
C. W. BARDIN, and D. M. PHILLIPS

The Population Council
New York, New York 10021

Basal lamina have been implicated in the regulation of epithelial cell function in a number of tissues. In the testis, the Sertoli cell is in direct contact with the basal lamina of the seminiferous tubule. The removal of pertiubular myoid cells from segments of seminiferous tubule alters the secretion of both androgen binding protein (ABP) and transferrin (TF) by Sertoli cells. The most marked effect being a four- to fivefold decrease in ABP secretion.[1] We have used purified components of basal lamina; including type I and IV collagen (coll), laminin (lam), fibronectin (fbn), and extracellular matrix (ECM) produced by an established testicular cell line, TR-M, to explore the effects of these components on Sertoli cell function *in vitro*.

The TR-M cell line[2] has many characteristics of peritubular myoid cells. It forms contact-inhibited monolayers, does not secrete plasminogen activator, and forms aggregates on co-culture with Sertoli cells. The TR-M cells secrete an extensive extracellular matrix *in vitro*. Antibodies raised to fibronectin and laminin show strong binding to ECM. Antisera raised against ECM bind to purified laminin and fibronectin. Cross-linked collagen and an amorphous elastin-like material have been identified in the matrix with electron microscopy. Using these approaches, collagen, fibronectin, laminin, and elastin have been tentatively identified as components of the matrix (Mather, Wolpe, and Phillips, submitted for publication).

To explore the role of the ECM on Sertoli cell function, TR-M monolayers were maintained at confluency for three weeks to allow deposition of matrix. Cells were removed from the ECM by treatment with 0.01 N NH_4OH and the ECM washed extensively with medium. Controls were cultured on tissue culture plastic or plastic coated with collagen, laminin, fibronectin, serum, or serum-spreading factor[3] (SSF, gift of Dr. David Barnes, University of Pittsburgh). Primary cultures enriched for Sertoli cells were prepared from 20-day-old rats as previously described[4] and plated on the various substrates in serum-free medium containing insulin (10 μg/ml), human transferrin (5 μg/ml), and EGF (2.5 ng/ml) (3F); 3F + FSH (200 ng/ml) or 3F + retinoic acid (RA, 50 ng/ml). Secreted rABP and TF were assayed in the medium by specific RIA. Cross-reactivity of hTF with the anti-rTF antibody was <0.1%. Conversion of [^{3}H]adenine to [^{3}H]cAMP was measured as previously described[5] during a 20 min incubation without hormone (NS) or with NIH oFSH.S14 (1 μg/ml), isoproterenol (10^{-6} M), or forskolin (10 μM).

[a] This work was supported by National Institutes of Health P50 grant #HD-13541.

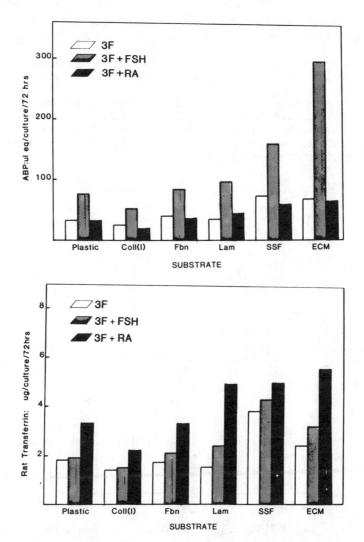

FIGURE 1. Effect of substrate and hormones on rABP and rTF secretion from Sertoli cell–enriched cultures from 20-day-old rats. Medium was changed on day 3 and collected on day 6 of culture. Abbreviations as described in the text.

The results shown in FIGURE 1A show that Sertoli cells cultured on ECM have an increased ABP secretion in all hormone supplements. However, the most marked effect is seen on FSH-stimulated ABP secretion where there is a four- to fivefold increase over control. In contrast, collagen, fibronectin, and laminin substrates do not significantly affect ABP secretion. SSF increases basal secretion but the FSH-stimulated secretion is equivalent to that seen in cells cultured on plastic (2.2-fold).

In contrast, TF secretion was influenced to a much smaller extent than ABP secretion by substrate (FIGURE 1B). SSF precoat had the most stimulatory effect on TF secretion with 3F while RA-stimulated secretion was increased approximately 50% over control in cells cultured on laminin, SSF, and ECM. Collagen (type IV) and serum pre-coat gave the same results as collagen (type I) (data not shown).

It is notable that FSH is an important stimulator of ABP secretion whereas RA has no effect. In contrast, FSH does not stimulate TF secretion while RA stimulates two- to threefold.

The increased response to FSH of ABP secretion shown by cells plated on matrix led us to explore the response of adenyl cyclase to FSH in these cultures. Basal (NS) cyclase levels were not affected by substrate, however the hormone-stimulated conversion of [3H]adenine for cells plated on ECM was less than that of cells on plastic or fibronectin (FIGURE 2).

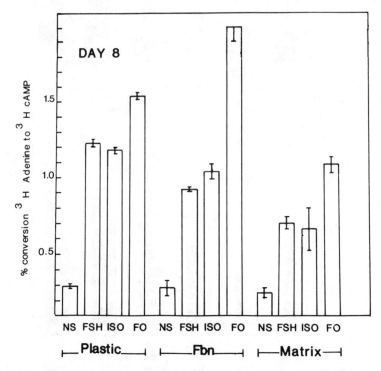

FIGURE 2. Effect of substance on the stimulation of the conversion of [3H]adenine to [3H]cAMP by various hormones. Cultures were prepared from 20-day-old rats and cultured in 3F-supplemented medium with one medium change on day 4. Assay conditions are described in the text.

In conclusion, ECM can modulate Sertoli cell function *in vitro*. The effect of the TR-M cell–produced ECM cannot be mimicked by the purified components of the ECM tested, suggesting that either two or more of these components are required or, other components of ECM, as yet unidentified, are important to the response. The major effect of ECM is to increase the FSH stimulation of ABP production. The decrease in FSH-stimulated conversion of [3H]adenine to

[^{3}H]cAMP in cells cultured on ECM suggests that the effect on rABP occurs at a point after cAMP production. rTF and rABP are independently regulated with TF secretion stimulated by RA (but not FSH) and relatively independent of substrate, while ABP secretion is stimulated by FSH (but not RA) and is strongly affected by substrate (ECM).

ACKNOWLEDGMENT

We wish to thank Ms. A. L. Byer for technical assistance.

REFERENCES

1. MATHER, J. P., G. L. GUNSALUS, N. A. MUSTO, C. Y. CHENG, M. PARVINEN, W. WRIGHT, A. MARGIORIS, A. LIOTTA, V. PEREZ-INFANTE, R. BECKER, D. T. KRIEGER & C. W. BARDIN. 1983. The hormonal and cellular control of Sertoli cell secretion. J. Ster. Biochem. **19:** 41–51.
2. MATHER, J. P., L.-Z. ZHUANG, V. PEREZ-INFANTE & D. M. PHILLIPS. 1985. Culture of testicular cells in hormone supplemented serum-free medium. Ann. N.Y. Acad. Sci. **383:** 44.
3. BARNES, D., J. VAN DER BOSCH, H. MASUI, K. MIYAZAKI & G. SATO. 1981. The culture of human tumor cells in serum-free medium. Meth. Enzymol. **79:** 68–390.
4. MATHER, J. P. & D. M. PHILLIPS. 1984. Primary culture of testicular somatic cells. *In* Methods in Molecular and Cell Biology. D. Barnes, D. Sirbasque & G. Sato, Eds.: 29–45. Alan R. Liss, Inc. New York.
5. SALOMON, Y. 1979. Adenylate cyclase assay. Adv. Cycl. Nucl. Res. **10:** 35–55.

Sertoli Cell Adenylyl Cyclase Is Stimulated by a Factor Associated with Germ Cells

MICHAEL J. WELSH, MARK E. IRELAND, and
GLENN J. TREISMAN[a]

Department of Anatomy and Cell Biology
[a] Department of Pharmacology
University of Michigan School of Medicine
Ann Arbor, Michigan 48109

It is not yet apparent how Sertoli cell functions are regulated to coordinate and support differentiation of the adjacent germ cells (GC) in the seminiferous tubules of the testis. Studies have shown that FSH binding and response by cells of the seminiferous tubule,[1,2] as well as activities of specific enzymes,[3] can be correlated with the stage of spermatogenesis existing within isolated tubule segments. Because the hormonal milieu of the testis is essentially constant, these observations support the hypothesis of a mechanism within the seminiferous tubule for localized regulation of morphological and biochemical events.[3] GC may directly affect Sertoli cell function by essentially the same series of biochemical events as the FSH response mechanism.[1,3] To examine the possibility of direct GC effects on Sertoli function, we have studied the effects of GC and GC fractions of adenylyl cyclase (AC) activity in membrane preparations from highly enriched populations of rat Sertoli cells. We observe stimulation of AC by GC and GC fractions.

Basal AC activity of membranes from Sertoli cells cultured for three days in hormone and serum-free medium was found to be low, ranging from 2 to 14 pmoles cAMP/min/mg protein. When the Sertoli membranes were treated with FSH or isoproterenol in the presence of 1 μM GTP, conditions that elicit maximal AC responses, AC was stimulated to average rates of 104 and 76 pmoles cAMP/min/mg, respectively (FIGURE 1a). If freshly prepared GC (50–150 μg protein/assay) instead of hormone were added to Sertoli membranes, AC activity was measured to average 62 pmoles cAMP/min/mg Sertoli protein. When GC alone were assayed, they were found to exhibit no AC activity under the conditions employed. GC were also separated into membrane and cytosol fractions. Both fractions were able to stimulate AC activity of Sertoli membranes to levels significantly higher than basal (FIGURE 1b). The results did not offer any clear evidence concerning the subcellular localization of the GC factor that was activating Sertoli AC.

The possibility of the activation being due to calmodulin was considered. Because calmodulin has been shown to be heat stable with a half-life of 7 min at 100°C,[4] the effect of heat on the GC fractions' ability to activate Sertoli AC was examined (FIGURE 1c). Treatment at 60°C did not diminish the capacity of GC preparations to activate AC. However, 100°C for 1 min abolished completely the ability of GC preparations to activate AC. The results indicate that the stimulatory activity associated with the GC possesses limited heat stability and cannot be attributed to the heat-stable activator calmodulin.

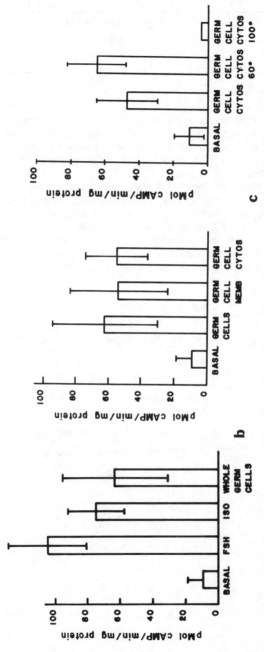

FIGURE 1. (a) Stimulation of Sertoli AC by hormones or whole GC. With all treatments AC activities were significantly higher than basal. (b) Stimulation of Sertoli AC by whole GC or GC fractions. Germ cells, 30,000 × *g* pellet or supernatant fractions stimulated Sertoli AC significantly. (c) Heat stability of GC stimulation of Sertoli AC. Unheated and 60°C-treated GC cytosol fractions significantly stimulated Sertoli AC.

TABLE 1. Response of TRST Adenylyl Cyclase to Various Treatments

Treatment	FSH (5 μg/assay)	Isoproterenol (10 μM)	Whole Germ Cells
Average stimulation (above basal)	Twofold	Fivefold	Threefold

The specific germ cell developmental stage that possesses the most potent ability to stimulate Sertoli AC is not yet evident. The GC preparations used for the experiments contained spermatocytes and virtually all stages of spermatids. The GC stimulator of AC is not limited to AC from Sertoli cells, however. GC and GC fractions have been found to be able to stimulate AC in membrane fractions of the Sertoli-derived cell line TRST (TABLE 1).

Taken together, our results indicate that a factor associated with GC is able to stimulate Sertoli cell AC. The factor is heat labile and does not require calcium for activation. Therefore, the observed stimulatory activity cannot be attributed to calmodulin. The GC factor may be similar in nature to the heat-labile cytoplasmic factors that have recently been reported to be present in lung,[5] or may be similar to the AC-stimulating factor associated with a particulate fraction from bovine epididymal sperm,[6] as reported while this work was in progress.

REFERENCES

1. GORDELADZE, J. O., M. PARVINEN, O. P. F. CLAUSEN & V. HANSSON. 1982. Arch. Androl. **8:** 43–51.
2. RITZEN, E. M., C. BOITANI, M. PARVINEN, F. C. FRENCH & M. FELDMAN. 1982. Molec. Cell. Endocrinol. **25:** 25–33.
3. PARIVINEN, M. 1982. Endocr. Rev. **3:** 404–417.
4. BEALE, E. G., A. J. DEDMAN & A. R. MEANS. 1977. Endocrinology **101:** 1621–1634.
5. NIJJAR, M. S., A. W. Y. AU & K. C. CHAUDHARY. 1981. Biochim. Biophys. Acta **677:** 153–159.
6. JOHNSON, R. A., J. A. AWAD, K. H. JAKOBS & G. SHULTZ. 1983. FEBS Lett. **152:** 11–16.

Low Molecular Weight Factors in Bovine Serum which Inhibit FSH Binding to Calf Testis Receptors[a]

THOMAS T. ANDERSEN, PATRICK M. SLUSS, and
LEO E. REICHERT, JR.

Department of Biochemistry
Albany Medical College
Albany, New York

We[1-5] and others[6] have reported the presence in serum and other biological fluids of low molecular weight factors (FSH-BI) that inhibit the binding of FSH to receptor *in vitro*. These factors are of interest because of their possible physiologic relevance as local regulators of FSH action, as possible pharmacologic agents that may interfere with FSH effects *in vivo,* as a tool in understanding mechanisms of the hormone-receptor interaction, and because it is essential to account for their effects when interpreting results based on binding of FSH to receptor (as in FSH radioligand receptor assays or analysis of hormone binding by Scatchard analysis or related techniques).

Bovine serum appears to have at least two "classes" of binding inhibitors, separable by diafiltration through membranes of selected pore size, and with apparent molecular weights (MW) of <500, and 500 to 5000, respectively. Monovalent ions, which are normal constituents of serum with MW less than 500, have been shown to have FSH-BI activity[7] and presumably represent the bulk of one "class" of low MW binding inhibitors. Such ions inhibit FSH binding by reducing the affinity of ^{125}I-labeled hFSH-calf testis receptor interactions, but do not significantly alter the number of receptors.[7,8] In *in vitro* situations it is likely that the inhibitory effect of most of these ions is due to alterations in physicochemical interactions between solutes, water, and macromolecules since the degree of binding inhibition could be related to the B coefficient of viscosity of the various monovalent ions.[8] However, the monovalent cation Na^+ appeared to have a unique interaction with calf testis receptor or with FSH since it was a more potent binding inhibitor than expected on the basis of its B coefficient. This, together with its presence in physiological fluids, suggests that Na^+ may be a regulator of FSH binding *in vivo* as well as *in vitro*.

The second class of inhibitors (500 to 5000 MW) can be resolved into three fractions with FSH-BI activity by gel filtration on a Sephadex G-10 column equilibrated with water. These fractions have been designated as G10-1 (V_e/V_o ratio = 1.1), G10-2 (V_e/V_o = 1.4), and G10-3 (V_e/V_o = 1.6). It is probable that the G10-3 fraction contains residual salt that is responsible for much of its FSH-BI activity. The G10-1 and G10-2 fractions each contain at least two components that react with dansyl chloride and therefore presumably contain a primary amino group. Thin layer chromatography of dansylated derivatives of G10-1 and G10-2 was

[a] Supported by National Institutes of Health grant HD-16716 (T.T.A.) and a grant from the Andrew W. Mellon Foundation (L.E.R.).

TLC (SILICA-G) OF DANSYLATED (DNS) DERIVATIVES

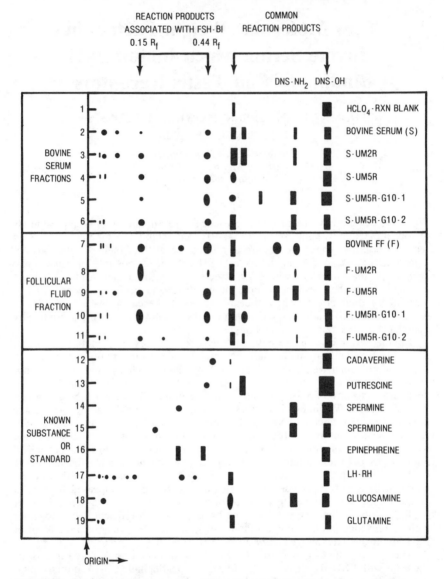

FIGURE 1. Thin-layer chromatography (Silica-G) of dansylated derivatives. 300 μl aliquots of serum or follicular fluid (150 μl gave about 50% FSH-BI) were acidified with an equal volume of 0.4 N perchloric acid and incubated for 24 hr at 4°C. Samples were then centrifuged and components in 200 μl of the supernate were derivatized with dansyl chloride in the presence of excess Na_2CO_3. After 24 hr at 24°C, these samples were extracted with 0.5 ml benzene. Ten to 20 μl of benzene extracts were applied to the preadsorbant layer of 250 μm Silica G prechanneled plates. Plates were developed in cyclohexane: ethylacetate (3:2, vol/vol) for approximately 1 hr in a saturated atmosphere TLC tank. After drying, the plates were fixed with triethanolamine:propanol (1:4, vol/vol) and viewed under ultraviolet light. This figure represents a composite of five individual plates. R_f values are based on DNS-OH

performed on Silica G multichannel plates (FIGURE 1). Correlation of the chromatograms with inhibitory potency demonstrated that two components ($R_f = 0.15$ and $R_f = 0.44$) are uniquely present in all fractions that have FSH-BI activity. It is noteworthy that follicular fluid also contains factors with similar R_fs (FIGURE 1) and that co-purify with FSH-BI activity during molecular sieving. Additionally, low MW FSH-BI activity in both serum and follicular fluid distributes in a similar fashion during membrane filtration and gel filtration chromatography. Thus the properties of follicular fluid FSH-BIs appear to be qualitatively similar to those found in serum.

Our data suggest that FSH-BI activity due to the <500 MW component of bovine serum may be caused in part by salt effects on hormone binding to receptor, an observation that should serve as a general caution. The FSH-BI activity of the fractions of MW between 500 and 5,000 cannot be attributed totally to salt effects. Amine-containing (dansyl-positive) components, such as peptides or polyamines, which are known to be present in serum and follicular fluid, may be involved in the local regulation of FSH-receptor interactions.

REFERENCES

1. DARGA, N. C. & L. E. REICHERT, JR. 1978. Some properties of the interaction of follicle stimulating hormone with bovine granulosa cells and its inhibition by follicular fluid. Biol. Reprod. **19:** 235–241.
2. DARGA, N. C. & L. E. REICHERT, JR. 1979. Evidence for the presence of a low molecular weight follitropin binding inhibitor in bovine follicular fluid. Adv. Exp. Med. Biol. **112:** 383–388.
3. FLETCHER, P. W., J. A. DIAS, M. A. SANZO & L. E. REICHERT, JR. 1982. Inhibition of FSH action on granulosa cells by low molecular weight components of follicular fluid. Molec. Cell. Endocrinol. **25:** 303–315.
4. REICHERT, L. E. JR., M. A. SANZO, P. W. FLETCHER, J. A. DIAS & C. Y. LEE. 1982. Properties of follicle stimulating hormone binding inhibitors found in physiological fluids. *In* Intraovarian Control Mechanisms. C. Channing & B. Segal, Eds.: 135–143. Plenum Publ. Corp. New York.
5. SLUSS, P. M., P. W. FLETCHER & L. E. REICHERT, JR. 1984. Inhibition of ^{125}I-human follicle stimulating hormone binding to receptor by a low molecular weight fraction of bovine follicular fluid: Inhibitor concentration is related to biochemical parameters of follicular development. Biol. Reprod. **29:** 1105–1113.
6. HILLENSJO, T., S. CHARI, L. NILSSON, L. HAMBERGER, E. DAUME & G. STURM. 1983. Inhibition of progesterone secretion in cultured human granulosa cells by a low molecular weight fraction of human follicular fluid. J. Clin. Endocrinol. Metab. **56:** 835–838.
7. ANDERSEN, T. T. & L. E. REICHERT, JR. 1982. Follitropin binding to receptors in testis: Modulation by monovalent salts and divalent cations. J. Biol. Chem. **257:** 11551–11557.
8. ANDERSEN, T. T. & L. E. REICHERT, JR. 1984. Correlation of B coefficient of viscosity for monovalent salts with effects on binding of human follitropin to receptors. Molec. Cell. Endocrinol. **35:** 41–46.

($R_f = 1.0$) that usually migrated 60 to 65 mm from the origin in this system. Standard compounds were dissolved in 0.2 N perchloric acid, which was used as a reaction blank. Note that dansylated substances having $R_f = 0.15$ and 0.44 are the only sample specific substances observed in all FSH-BI containing serum and follicular fluid samples.

Evidence for a Soluble Fetal Urogenital Sinus–derived Growth Factor(s)

TIMOTHY C. THOMPSON and LELAND W. K. CHUNG

Pharmacology/School of Pharmacy
University of Colorado
Boulder, Colorado 80309

The inductive capacity of fetal urogenital sinus mesenchyme (UGM) has been established previously.[1,2] Recently, our laboratory described a new rodent model for prostatic hyperplasia whereby a marked prostatic overgrowth (10- to 20-fold) can be induced *in situ* by direct implantation of either intact fetal urogenital sinus (UGS) or UGM into the adult prostate glands.[3,4]

In an effort to elucidate the underlying mechanism for the induction of prostatic overgrowth by fetal urogenital sinus tissues, a tissue culture system was developed whereby the UGS was co-cultured with non-confluent primary culture cells derived from adult rat ventral prostatic stroma (Wistar strain, three to five months). To test for the possible existence of a soluble fetal urogenital sinus–derived growth factor(s), attempts were made to prevent cell-cell contact during the culturing procedures. Modified procedures resulted in the proliferation of two cell populations (i.e., adult ventral prostatic stroma and fetal UGS-derived embryonic cells) interacting only through the exchange of certain soluble and diffusible factor(s).

In brief, experiments were performed as follows. Ventral prostates were excised aseptically from the adult male rats. Ventral prostatic stromal cells were isolated from minced tissues by mild collagenase digestion.[5] They were plated in 35 mm plastic dishes at 6.5×10^5 cells/dish. Twelve hours later, UGSs removed from 18-day-old Nb rat embryos[1] were co-cultured in small glass dishes (one UGS/dish) which had been placed within the larger plastic 35 mm dishes containing the previously seeded adult stroma. Cells were then grown under standard conditions of 95% air, 5% CO_2 in F12K media containing 20% fetal calf serum, 5 μg/ml transferrin, 5 μg/ml bovine insulin, 0.1 μg/ml dihydrotestosterone, 1 mg/ml bovine serum albumin, and penicillin (50 units)-streptomycin (50 μg) per ml. Medium was changed every 48 hours and growth was assessed immediately afterwards by histological and biochemical methods as discussed below.

FIGURE 1 provides morphological evidence of increased proliferation of adult stroma (comparison with control stroma, FIGURE 1a) co-cultured with the intact fetal UGS and its derived cells. Areas selected for their representative histomorphology were obtained by staining the culture dishes with Giemsa dye seven days after the control and UGS-induced growth. In addition to increased cell number observed under fetal UGS-induced growth, the induced stromal cells were also larger and appeared more "stretched," a condition that has been previously observed to indicate a more tenacious, trypsin-resistant attachment to the substrata.[6] We have also observed increased size of cell nuclei and number of nucleoli in the UGS co-cultured adult stromal cells. These results suggest polyploidy in the induced cells. FIGURE 1 demonstrates the outgrowth of both embryonic epithelia (c) as well as embryonic mesenchyme (d) from the UGS in culture.

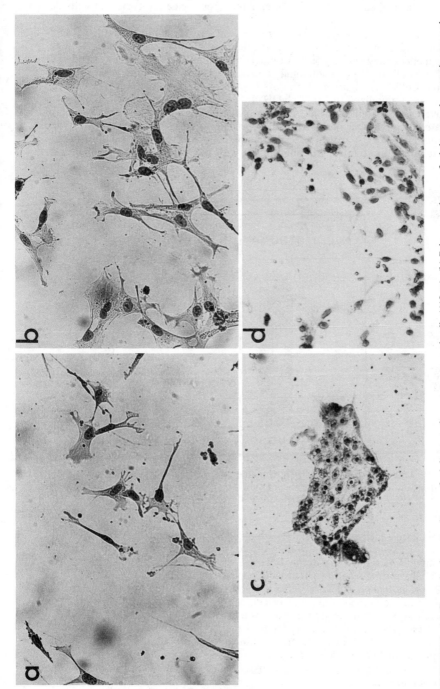

FIGURE 1. (a) Control primary cultures of adult ventral prostate stromal cells (412 ×). (b) Primary cultures of adult ventral prostatic stromal cells co-cultured with fetal urogenital sinus (UGS) and its derived cells (412 ×). (c) Fetal urogenital sinus epithelial cells derived from fetal UGS (412 ×). (d) Outgrowth of fetal urogenital sinus mesenchymal cells from fetal UGS (412 ×). The vacant area in the center represents the site where UGS had previously attached. Figure reduction, 80%.

The smaller cell sizes and less differentiated appearance are typical of cells derived from embryonic tissues.

FIGURE 2 demonstrates total incorporation of [³H]thymidine into the acid-
insoluble fractions of the adult stromal cells harvested seven days after seeding.
Upon media change on day 5, 5 μCi of [³H]thymidine (2.0 Ci/mmol) was added to
duplicate culture dishes containing control and UGS co-cultured adult prostatic
stroma. Cells were harvested on day 7, washed twice with phosphate-buffered
saline, and solubilized in 1.0 N NaOH. Intact UGS and UGS-derived cells were
removed and treated likewise. Aliquots of the NaOH-solubilized cells were precipitated on glass fiber filters with 2.0 N perchloric acid (PCA) and washed twice
with both 0.4 N PCA as well as 95% ethanol. Filters were then dried and counted
in a scintillation counter. In confirmation with the morphological studies, total

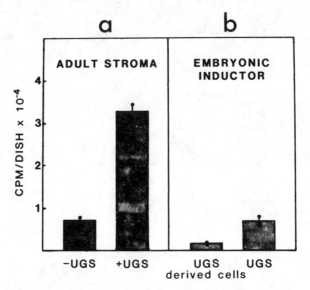

FIGURE 2. (a) Incorporation of [³H]thymidine into the acid-insoluble fraction of adult
ventral prostatic stromal cells. (b) Incorporation of [³H]thymidine into the acid-insoluble
fraction of UGS and UGS-derived cell populations.

[³H]thymidine incorporation into acid-insoluble materials (DNA) was fourfold
higher in UGS-induced samples than the controls. The embryonic growth inductors, intact UGS and UGS-derived cells, also were proliferative as indicated by
their ability to incorporate [³H]thymidine into cellular DNA (FIGURE 2b). The
mitogenic action of UGS and UGS-derived cells on the adult prostatic stroma
occurred in the complete absence of cell-cell contact between the inductors and
the adult stroma, suggesting the existence of certain soluble and diffusible fetal
growth factor(s). In more recent experiments we have observed only a 20–30%
stimulation of [³H]thymidine incorporation into prostatic stromal DNA by co-
culturing with fetal UGS over shorter culturing and incorporation periods. It
appears that the reduced mitogenic activity observed may result from the altered
culture conditions.

Evidence is presented herein for a soluble and diffusible UGS-derived growth factor(s). A culture system that provides physical separation, yet allows "media communication" between responding adult prostatic stroma and embryonic inductor cells was developed in order to ascertain the presence of fetal UGS-derived growth factor(s). Our study is consistent with the recent demonstration that hyperplastic dog (Story *et al.,* unpublished results) and human prostatic tissues contained soluble growth factor(s) that exert mitogenic actions on cultured human fibroblasts.[7] Further elucidation of the chemical nature of this growth-promoting substance(s) may provide further insight in the regulation of prostatic growth and regeneration in prostatic hyperplasia.[3,4,7]

REFERENCES

1. CUNHA, G. R. 1972. Anat. Rec. **172:** 179–196.
2. LASNITZKI, I. & T. MIZUNO. 1979. J. Endocrinol. **82:** 171–178.
3. CHUNG, L. W. K., J. MATSUURA, A. K. ROCCO, T. C. THOMPSON, G. J. MILLER & M. N. RUNNER. 1984. *In* New Approaches for Benign Prostatic Hyperplasia. A. Buhl, D. Carter & F. Kimball (Eds.): 291–306. Alan. R. Liss, Inc. New York.
4. CHUNG, L. W. K., J. MATSUURA, A. K. ROCCO, T. C. THOMPSON, G. J. MILLER & M. N. RUNNER. 1984. Ann. N.Y. Acad. Sci. (This volume.)
5. YANG, J., R. GUZMAN, J. RICHARD & S. NANDI. 1980. *In Vitro* **16:** 502–506.
6. FISHER, H. W., T. T. PUCK & G. SATO. 1958. Proc. Natl. Acad. Sci. USA **44:** 4–10.
7. LAWSON, R. K., M. T. STORY & S. C. JACOBS. 1981. *In* The Prostatic Cell: Structure and Function, Part A. G. Murphy, A. Sandberg & J. Karr, Eds.: 325–336. Alan R. Liss, Inc. New York.

Maturational and Androgen-dependent
Aspects of Sertoli Cell Function[a]

B. M. SANBORN,[b,c,d] J. R. WAGLE,[b,d] and

A. STEINBERGER[b,d]

[b] Departments of Reproductive Medicine and Biology
[c] Biochemistry and Molecular Biology and
[d] Obstetrics, Gynecology and Reproductive Sciences
University of Texas Medical School at Houston
Houston, Texas 77025

The Sertoli cell (SC) is a potential androgen target cell in the seminiferous tubule. In support of this premise, the Sertoli cell has been shown to contain macromolecules with the properties of cytosol androgen receptors, to accumulate androgen into the cell nucleus in a time- and temperature-dependent, saturable manner, to possess chromatin acceptor sites for androgen-receptor complexes, and to respond to androgen stimulation with an increase in RNA polymerase II activity and poly A^+ RNA production.[1]

Cytoplasmic receptor concentrations in hormone-sensitive target tissues often reflect the capacity of those systems to respond to hormones.[2] Cytoplasmic receptor concentrations can be regulated by hormones.[2] In order to investigate the possible control of cytoplasmic androgen receptor levels by androgens, rats were hypophysectomized at 21 days and subsequently injected with oil or testosterone propionate (0.5 mg/day). Cytoplasmic androgen receptor concentrations in cultured Sertoli cells from these animals were reduced to 40 and 20% of levels in cells from age-matched controls by 15 and 21 days after surgery, respectively ($p < 0.05$). Testosterone propionate treatment prevented this decline (120 and 108% of control, respectively).

When Sertoli cells in culture were exposed to ^{3}H-R1881(methyltrienolone), cytoplasmic androgen receptor concentrations rapidly declined to a minimum in < 20 min, while nuclear concentrations of bound label increased.[3] However, upon continued exposure to ^{3}H-R1881 (5 nM, 34°C) cytoplasmic androgen receptor concentrations gradually returned to levels comparable to those in unexposed cells. Nuclear-bound label reached a maximum by 2 hr and only declined by 30% over 16 hr. Longer exposure of Sertoli cells to R1881 or testosterone (3 days) did not increase cytoplasmic androgen receptor concentrations further. These data suggest that androgens can influence the concentration of cytoplasmic androgen receptor as well as affecting its distribution within the Sertoli cell.

The Sertoli cell undergoes a number of morphological and biochemical changes over the period between 15 and 35 days of age in the rat. Among the biochemical changes are increases in the protein/DNA and RNA/DNA ratios and changes in soluble ribonucleotide pool sizes and composition.[4] As an extension of the study of biochemical features of Sertoli cell maturation, an investigation of Sertoli cell protein synthesis and the effects of R1881 treatment (10 nM, 18 hr) in cells from 15, 25, and 35 days was undertaken. ^{35}S-Met (20 μCi/ml, 18 hr) was

[a] Supported by National Institutes of Health grants NIH-P50-HDO8338 and NIH-R01-17795.

incorporated into secretory and soluble cellular proteins in comparable amounts per mg protein but in increasing amounts per mg DNA as a function of age. Examination of newly synthesized protein patterns by two-dimensional PAGE (pH 3–10, 5–20% acrylamide) revealed specific changes. Soluble cellular proteins designated Scl and Sc2 were observed only in cells treated with R1881. Appearance of Scl was noted only in cells from 25-day-old and 35-day-old animals. Secretory protein patterns from 15- and 25-day-old animals were similar, but five additional spots were present in the medium from Sertoli cells from 35-day-old animals. No significant effects of R1881 treatment on these patterns were noted.

These data suggest that hormonal regulation of androgen receptor concentrations may be important in modulating some aspects of Sertoli cell function. Furthermore, the maturational changes taking place in the Sertoli cell during the interval when the first meiotic divisions occur in seminiferous tubules may reflect important changes in Sertoli cell function that could influence germ cell maturation.

REFERENCES

1. Sanborn, B. M., J. R. Wagle, A. S. Steinberger & D. J. Lamb. 1983. The Sertoli cell as an androgen target. *In* Recent Advances in Male Reproduction: Molecular Basis and Clinical Implications. R. D'Agata, M. Lipsett, P. Polosa & H. van der Molen, Eds.: 69. Serono Symposium. Raven Press. New York.
2. Clark, J. H. & E. J. Peck, Jr. 1979. Female Sex Steroids: Receptors and Function. Springer Verlag. New York.
3. Sanborn, B. M., A. Steinberger & A. Lee. 1981. Subcellular distribution of androgen binding sites in cultured Sertoli cells before and after exposure to androgens. J. Steroid Biochem. **14:** 133.
4. Lamb, D. J., M. J. Kessler, D. S. Shewach, A. Steinberger & B. M. Sanborn. 1982. Characterization of Sertoli cell RNA synthetic activities in vitro at selected times during sexual maturation. Biol. Reprod. **27:** 374.

Detection of Estrogen Receptors in Cultured Sertoli Cells

A. M. NAKHLA, O. A. JÄNNE, J. P. MATHER, and
C. W. BARDIN[a]

The Population Council
The Rockefeller University
New York, New York 10021

Although Sertoli cells respond to estrogens,[1,2] the presence of receptors for this class of steroid has not been reported in these cells. We therefore examined several Sertoli cell lines and demonstrated that they contain a specific estradiol binding protein in cytosol that has the characteristics of an estrogen receptor.

Sertoli cells for primary cultures were isolated from 20-day-old Sprague-Dawley rats by collagenase treatment. The TM_4 (Sertoli cell, immature mice), TR-ST (Sertoli cell, adult rats), TR-1 (rat endothelial cells), and TR-M (rat myoid cells) cell lines were employed.[2] They were maintained in either F12/DME medium containing 7.5% serum or in serum-free medium containing insulin, transferrin, and epidermal growth factor, and used at confluency (4–5 days of culture). Cytosol and nuclear receptor assays were performed with the exchange methods (10 nM [³H]estradiol and 15 nM [³H]methyltrienolone as ligands for estrogen and androgen, respectively).[3]

Low capacity (50 fmoles/mg cytosol protein), high affinity ($K_D = 1.1$ nM) binding sites of estradiol were present in the cytosol of TR-ST cells (FIGURE 1). A similar estradiol-binding component (85 fmoles/mg cytosol protein; $K_D = 0.9$ nM) was also found in TM_4 cells. Steroid binding was estrogen specific, since only estradiol and diethylstilbesterol competed for estradiol binding sites in the cell lines. Specific androgen receptors were also demonstrated in these cells. The concentration of estrogen and androgen receptors in different cell lines is shown in TABLE 1. The estrogen receptor content in Sertoli cells is higher than that in Leydig cells.

Exposure of the cells to estradiol (10 nM at 37°C) caused translocation of cytosol receptors to nuclei. A maximal accumulation of nuclear estrogen receptors occurred within 30 min and thereafter declined despite a continuous presence of estradiol in the medium. This was in contrast to the androgen receptors where there was a progressive increase of nuclear receptors over a period of 24 hr during incubation with [³H]methyltrienolone. These results suggest that estrogen binding protein in the cytosol of Sertoli cell lines is an estrogen receptor rather than an extracellular steroid-binding protein, such as androgen binding protein (ABP) or testosterone-estradiol binding globulin (TeBG).

Estrogen receptors were not detectable in freshly isolated Sertoli cells. However, after 15 days in culture 42 fmoles/mg protein of estrogen binding sites were detected. The appearance of the receptors in the cytosol of the primary cultures with time in culture suggests that these cells are capable of expressing estrogen

[a] Address correspondence to: Dr. C. Wayne Bardin, Population Council, 1230 York Avenue, New York, NY 10021.

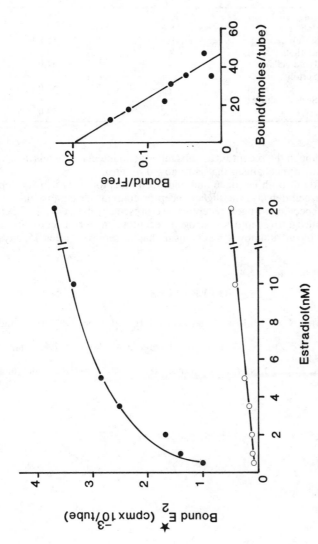

FIGURE 1. Binding of [^{3}H]estradiol to estrogen receptors in the cytosol of TR-ST Sertoli cell line. (●) Total binding and (○) nonspecific binding using 1,000-fold molar excess of estradiol. (Inset) specific binding data plotted according to the method of Scatchard.

TABLE 1. Estrogen and Androgen Receptor Concentrations in the Cytosol of Some Established Cell Lines

	Receptor Content/mg Cytosol Protein	
Cell Line	Estrogen Receptor	Androgen Receptor
TM$_3$ (Leydig cells)	12.9	58.2
TM$_4$ (Sertoli cells)	85.6	47.1
TR-ST (Sertoli cells)	49.9	55.8
TR-1 (Endothelial cells)	–	19.0
TR-M (Myoid cells)	–	44.0
Primary Sertoli cultures (3 days)	–	52.0
Primary Sertoli cultures (15 days)	41.7	79.0

receptors even though the receptors are absent or at undetectable levels *in vivo* by an, as yet, unknown mechanism that is removed *in vitro*.

The expression of both estrogen and androgen receptors was density dependent. The higher cell density, the higher receptor content per mg protein.

Conclusion: specific estrogen receptors are present in the cytosol of Sertoli cells. Unlike androgen receptors, estrogen receptors in Sertoli cells are suppressed *in vivo* by an unknown mechanism that is removed after 15 days in culture.

REFERENCES

1. NAGENDRANATH, N., T. M. JOSE, A. R. SHETH & H. S. JUNEJA. 1982. Arch. Androl. **9:** 217–222.
2. MATHER, J. P., L-Z. ZHUANG, V. PEREZ-INFANTE & D. M. PHILLIPS. 1982. Ann. N.Y. Acad. Sci. **383:** 44–68.
3. ISOMAA, V., A. E. I. PAJUNEN, C. W. BARDIN & O. A. JANNE. 1982. Endocrinology **111:** 833–843.

Properties and Compartmentalization of the Testicular Receptor for 1,25-Dihydroxyvitamin D_3^a

FINN OLAV LEVY,[b] LARS EIKVAR,
NICOLET H. P. M. JUTTE, and VIDAR HANSSON

Institutes of Medical Biochemistry and Pathology
University of Oslo
Oslo 3, Norway

$1\alpha,25$-dihydroxyvitamin D_3 ($1,25\text{-}(OH)_2D_3$), the most active form of vitamin D_3, is a major calcium homeostatic hormone. The hormone is a seco-steroid and is believed to act via a classical steroid hormone mechanism. The best characterized target organs for $1,25\text{-}(OH)_2D_3$ are the intestine, bone, parathyroid glands, and kidney, but receptors for $1,25\text{-}(OH)_2D_3$ have been shown in other organs, including the pancreas, pituitary, skin, mammary gland, placenta, uterus, ovary, avian shell gland, and, recently, also in the rat testes.[1,2] In this study we have confirmed the presence and examined the properties and compartmentalization of a testicular receptor for $1,25\text{-}(OH)_2D_3$ in the rat.

Seminiferous tubules and interstitial tissue from adult rats were prepared by wet dissection. The isolated tissues were homogenized in buffer KTEDMo (10 mM Tris/HCl, 1.5 mM EDTA, 1 mM dithiothreitol, 10 mM sodium molybdate, and 300 mM KCl, pH 7.4 at 0°C), and a 105,000 g supernatant was prepared (cytosol). Cultured Sertoli cells were obtained from 19-day-old rats by enzyme treatment (trypsin, collagenase, and DNase) and cultured for five days before scraping and sonication in KTEDMo buffer. Crude germ cells were obtained from whole testes of 32-day-old rats by enzyme treatment (collagenase and trypsin) and sonicated in KTEDMo buffer.

Free and receptor-bound steroids were separated by hydroxylapatite and sucrose gradient centrifugation. Labeled cytosol (100 μl) was added to 500 μl hydroxylapatite slurry (50% vol/vol, in 10 mM K_2HPO_4/KH_2PO_4, pH 7.5, 100 mM KCl) and incubated 15 min at 0°C with frequent vortexing. The hydroxylapatite was then washed three times with 2.0 ml buffer KTED + 0.5% Triton-X-100 by centrifugation at 3000 rpm for 5 min. Radioactivity was extracted from the final hydroxylapatite pellet with 2.0 ml ethanol and counted.

As shown in FIGURE 1, receptors for $1,25\text{-}(OH)_2D_3$ are present in KCl extracts from both seminiferous tubules and interstitial tissue. Using bovine serum albumin (4.4 S) and chymotrypsinogen (2.5 S) as standards, the steroid-receptor complex had a sedimentation coefficient of 3.2 $S_{20,w}$ in high-salt gradients (0.3 M KCl), while it aggregated in low-salt gradients (without KCl). The receptor shows high affinity for $1,25\text{-}(OH)_2D_3$ but low capacity. Using the hydroxylapatite assay

[a] Supported by the Rockefeller Foundation, Norwegian Research Council for Science and the Humanities (NAVF), and the Norwegian Society for Fighting Cancer (NFTKB).

[b] Address correspondence to: Finn Olav Levy, Institute of Medical Biochemistry, University of Oslo, P.B. 1112, Blindern, Oslo 3, Norway.

591

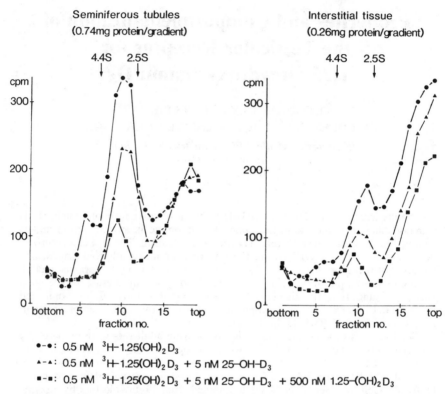

Seminiferous tubules
(0.74mg protein/gradient)

Interstitial tissue
(0.26mg protein/gradient)

•-•: 0.5 nM ^{3}H-1.25(OH)$_2$D$_3$

▲-▲: 0.5 nM ^{3}H-1.25(OH)$_2$D$_3$ + 5 nM 25-OH-D$_3$

■-■: 0.5 nM ^{3}H-1.25(OH)$_2$D$_3$ + 5 nM 25-OH-D$_3$ + 500 nM 1.25-(OH)$_2$D$_3$

FIGURE 1. Sucrose gradient analysis of [^{3}H]1,25-(OH)$_2$D$_3$ binding in seminiferous tubules and interstitial tissue. Aliquots of cytosol, preincubated with the indicated concentrations of steroids at 0°C for 3 hr, were treated with charcoal to remove free steroid. Cytosol was then layered over 5 to 20% sucrose gradients (4.2 ml) prepared in hypertonic buffer and centrifuged for 16 hr at 225,000 g_{av}. Fractions of eight drops each were collected from the bottom and counted for radioactivity.

we obtained values for K_d and N_{max} of 2.7×10^{-11} M and 8.3 fmol/mg cytosol protein, respectively, while sucrose gradient analysis yielded corresponding values of 3.8×10^{-11} M and 6.0 fmol/mg protein. The affinities reported here are in good agreement with that found for 1,25-(OH)$_2$D$_3$ receptors in other tissues, while the capacity is much lower than in the intestinal mucosa. Incubation of tubular cytosol with [^{3}H]1,25-(OH)$_2$D$_3$ alone or with [^{3}H]1,25-(OH)$_2$D$_3$ and increasing concentrations of various cold analogues of vitamin D$_3$ showed that the affinity of these analogues for the receptor decreased in the following order: 1,25-(OH)$_2$D$_3$ > 1α,24R,25-(OH)$_3$D$_3$ > 25-OH-D$_3$ > 1α-OH-D$_3$ > 24R,25-(OH)$_2$D$_3$. Other steroid hormones or synthetic analogues (E$_2$, T, Dex, Prog, R-5020) did not show any ability to compete for the receptor. This shows that the receptor is specific for 1,25-(OH)$_2$D$_3$. At 0°C, and at hormone concentrations of 0.5–1.0 nM, maximal receptor binding was achieved after three hours. At lower concentrations of hormone, the equilibration time was longer. The occupied receptors were stable for more than 24 hours at 0°C, and at this temperature the rate of dissociation of hormone-receptor complexes was very slow ($t_{1/2} > 48$ hr). At 29°C, the half-life of dissociation was about one hour.

Little or no specific binding of [^{3}H]1,25-$(OH)_2D_3$ was detected in cultured Sertoli cells or in crude germ cells. In the Sertoli cell cytosol there was a high level of a low affinity, high capacity binding moiety sedimenting significantly faster than the receptor. If neither the Sertoli cells nor the germ cells contain these receptors, the most likely candidates to contain the tubular 1,25-$(OH)_2D_3$ receptors would seem to be the peritubular cells. Which of the cells in the interstitial compartment contain these receptors also remains to be shown.

REFERENCES

1. MERKE, J., W. KREUSSER, B. BIER & E. RITZ. 1983. Eur. J. Biochem. **130:** 303–308.
2. WALTERS, M. R., D. L. CUNEO & A. P. JAMISON. 1983. J. Steroid Biochem. **19**(1): 913–920.

Gonadotropin-induced Changes in the LH Receptors in Cultured Leydig Cells: Measurement of the Immunoactive Bound Hormone

JOSÉ LINO S. BARAÑAO and MARIA L. DUFAU

Section on Molecular Endocrinology
National Institute of Child Health and Human Development
National Institutes of Health
Bethesda, Maryland 20205

Protein hormones are known to modulate the sensitivity of their target tissues by regulating the number of receptors in the cell surface. Exposure to high levels of the hormone usually produce negative autoregulation of the homologous receptors. In many systems this phenomenon is associated with a rapid internalization and degradation of the ligand. In the rat testis, however, internalization of the hormone-receptor complex after *in vivo* administration of ^{125}I-hCG is a relatively slow process.

It was previously reported that when ^{125}I-hCG is added to cultured rat Leydig cells a high percentage of the radioactivity remains on the cell surface even after three hours and that only a small proportion of the hormone is spontaneously degraded.[1] In the present study the degradation of the bound hCG was evaluated by measuring the amounts of the immunoactive bound hormone (IBH). Changes in this parameter were correlated with the onset of the desensitization of the steroidogenic responses after exposure to the gonadotropin. Adult rat Leydig cell cultures, steroid measurements, and ^{125}I-hCG binding to cultured cells were performed as previously described.[1] For the determination of the IBH, the cells were removed from the plates, resuspended in Medium 199, and the cell-bound unlabeled hormone was released by heating at 65°C for 30 min. The cells were then centrifuged at 3,000 rpm for 15 min and hCG was determined in the supernatant by radioimmunoassay. Non-specific binding was evaluated in parallel incubations using ^{125}I-hCG in the presence of an excess of unlabeled hormone and was always less than 5%.

FIGURE 1 (top) shows the levels of IBH as a function of the incubation time with unlabeled hCG. Maximal values, comparable to the amounts of ^{125}I-hCG that could be initially bound by the cells, were achieved four to eight hours after the addition of a saturating dose of hCG (20 ng/ml). The increase in the IBH was associated with the decline in the number of available sites for ^{125}I-hCG. Parallel measurements of the testosterone and pregnenolone responses showed that the cells were desensitized two to four hours after exposure to the hormone (FIGURE 1, bottom).

When Leydig cells were cultured for 24 hours with increasing doses of unlabeled hCG the levels of IBH and the decrease in the number of available binding sites for ^{125}I-hCG showed a similar ED_{50} for the gonadotropin (2.5 ng/ml) (FIGURE 2, top). Comparatively lower concentrations of hCG were required for the stimu-

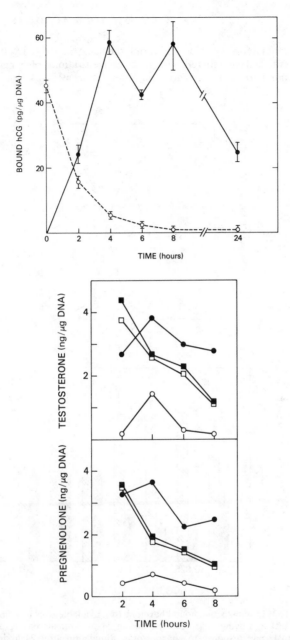

FIGURE 1. (*Top*) Immunoactive bound hormone (●) and available sites for ^{125}I-hCG (○) in cultured Leydig cells at different times after the addition of a saturating dose of hCG (20 ng/ml). (*Bottom*) Time course of the desensitization of the testosterone and pregnenolone responses to gonadotropin stimulation. Leydig cells were cultured in the presence (□, ■) or absence (○, ●) of 20 ng/ml hCG. At the times indicated media were changed and the cells further incubated with (●, ■) or without (○, □) 100 ng/ml of hCG for 3 hr. Pregnenolone production was measured in the presence of cyanoketone (10^{-6} M) and spironolactone (10^{-5} M).

lation of the testosterone production during the same period (ED$_{50}$ 0.2 ng/ml). On the other hand, cells incubated with hCG concentrations of 5 ng/ml or higher failed to respond to acute gonadotropin stimulation after 24 hours (FIGURE 2, bottom).

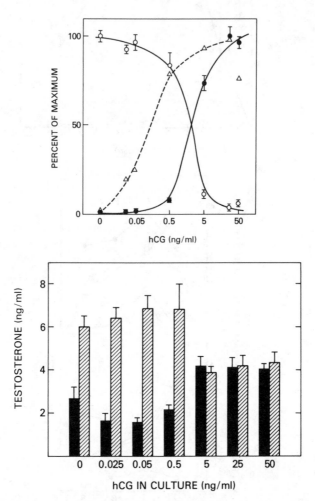

FIGURE 2. (Top) Immunoactive bound hormone (●), available sites (○), and testosterone accumulation (△) in Leydig cells cultured during 24 hr with increasing doses of hCG. (Bottom) Testosterone response to gonadotropin stimulation after 24 hr in Leydig cells cultured with different doses of hCG. (■) − hCG; (□) + hCG, 100 ng/ml.

In order to evaluate the degradation rate of the IBH, cells were incubated with a saturating dose of hCG for three hours at 37°C, washed (time 0), and then incubated at 37°C in the absence of the hormone for different periods. After 4.5 and 9 hours the amounts of IBH were 48 and 37%, respectively, of the time 0 value.

The negative correlation between the levels of IBH and the number of available binding sites would indicate that the receptor loss observed within 24 hours of exposure to high doses of hCG is mainly due to receptor occupancy. This is consistent with previous observations in rat testis membranes after the *in vivo* administration of hCG.[2] Data presented here also indicate that the receptor-bound hCG remains considerably intact for several hours suggesting that the degradation rates are slower than those described for other ligands.

The half-life for the internalization and degradation of hCG in cultured cells seems to vary according to the cell type. Thus, the half-life of approximately 4.5 hours reported here would be intermediate between the values of 50 min reported for Leydig tumor cells[3] and that of 9.6 hours determined in ovine luteal cells.[4] In addition, recent studies of cultured pig Leydig cells have also demonstrated the presence of hCG at the cell membrane level up to 48 hours after exposure to the hormone.[5]

In conclusion, extensive internalization and degradation of the bound hCG do not seem to be required for the early phase of the process of desensitization of the Leydig cell to gonadotropin stimulation.

REFERENCES

1. Baranao, J. L. S. & M. L. Dufau. 1983. J. Biol. Chem. **258:** 7322–7328
2. Hsueh, A. J. W., M. L. Dufau & K. J. Catt. 1976. Biochem. Biophys. Res. Commun. **72:** 1145–1152.
3. Ascoli, M. 1982. J. Biol. Chem. **25:** 13306–13311.
4. Ahmed, C. E., H. R. Sawyer & G. D. Niswender. 1981. Endocrinology **109:** 1380–1387.
5. Saez, J. M., M. Benahmed, J. Reventos, M. L. Bommelaer, C. Mombrial & F. Haour. 1983. J. Steroid Biochem. **19:** 375–384.

Structural Characteristics of the Leydig Cell Lactogen Receptors

JUAN S. BONIFACINO and MARIA L. DUFAU

Section on Molecular Endocrinology
Endocrinology and Reproduction Research Branch
National Institute of Child Health and Human Development
National Institutes of Health
Bethesda, Maryland 20205

Several reports have suggested that prolactin plays an important role in the modulation of Leydig cell function, probably supporting LH-stimulated androgen production.[1-3] Specific receptors that could mediate prolactin action have been demonstrated in Leydig cells using autoradiographic[4] as well as radioligand binding techniques.[5,6]

We have found that these receptors can be solubilized from Leydig cell membranes with 1% (w/vol) Triton X-100. The solubilized preparation is able to bind ^{125}I-hGH, displaying an affinity constant of 3.8×10^9 M$^-$ and a binding capacity of 167 fmol/mg of proteins. Lactogenic hormones such as hGH, oPRL, hPRL, and hPL inhibit binding of ^{125}I-hGH to the solubilized receptors whereas non-lactogenic hormones do not cause any effect up to concentrations of 0.01 mg/ml.

With the aim of studying the structural characteristics of these receptors. ^{125}I-hGH was covalently coupled to the receptor molecules with the bifunctional cross-linking reagent disuccinimidyl suberate (DSS) and the reaction products were analyzed by SDS-PAGE and autoradiography.

The procedure employed consisted of incubating ^{125}I-hGH (1.4–2.1×10^5 cpm) with a 1% (w/vol) Triton X-100 extract of membrane-rich Leydig cell particles (100–200 μg of proteins) in 200 μl of 0.1% bovine serum albumin (BSA)/Dulbecco's PBS pH 7.4 for 5 hr at 22°C. Samples were then cross-linked with 3–8 μl of freshly prepared 25 mM DSS in dimethyl sulfoxide for 15 min at 0°C. The reaction was terminated by the addition of 30 μl of 1 M Tris/HCl buffer, pH 7.4. Samples were boiled for 10 min in 60 mM Tris/HCl buffer, pH 6.8/10% (vol/vol) glycerol/2% SDS/5 mM EDTA/0.7 m β-mercaptoethanol and analyzed by SDS-PAGE on 7.5% acrylamide gels. Dried gels were subjected to autoradiography.

The patterns obtained in the absence of cross-linking reagent (lane A) or in the presence of 0.4 mM DSS (lane B) and 1 mM DSS (lane C) are shown in FIGURE 1 (left panel). Two sets of radioactive bands could be observed. The first set was composed of a band at an approximate M_r of 103,000 and of a fainter and sometimes not well resolved band at a M_r of 113,000. The second set was composed of two bands at $M_r = 59,000$ and $M_r = 53,000$. Since ^{125}I-hGH has a M_r of 22,000, therefore the labeled hormone was coupled to molecules having approximate M_rs of 91,000, 81,000, 37,000, and 31,000. All of these molecules appear to be components of the lactogen receptors, since incubation in the presence of hGH or hPRL significantly decreased the intensity of the higher M_r doublet and completely abolished the lower M_r doublet; whereas bGH, oLH, and oFSH had no effect. The same pattern of cross-linking was observed using other bifunctional reagents such as ethylene glycol bis succinimidyl succinate and bis 2-succinimido oxycarbonyloxy ethyl sulfone. No changes in the distribution of the bands were evident

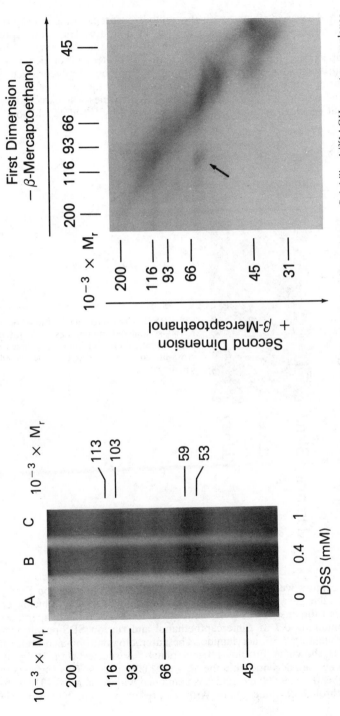

FIGURE 1. (Left panel) Cross-linking of ^{125}I-hGH to Triton X-100–solubilized Leydig cell membranes. Solubilized ^{125}I-hGH receptor complexes were reacted with DSS at the concentrations indicated. The cross-linked products were analyzed by SDS-PAGE/autoradiography. (Right panel) Effect of β-mercaptoethanol. See text for details.

when ^{125}I-hGH was incubated with the solubilized preparation in the presence of various protease inhibitors such as trypsin inhibitor, leupeptin, aprotinin, pepstatin A, TLCK, and PMSF. This indicates that the receptor components detected upon cross-linking were not originated by proteolysis of higher M_r components during incubation. However, it does not rule out the occurrence of proteolysis during preparation of the receptors or even in the intact cells.

The relationship between the different labeled species was explored by two-dimensional gel electrophoresis. Complexes formed by ^{125}I-hGH and solubilized

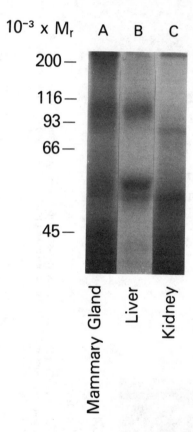

FIGURE 2. Cross-linking of ^{125}I-hGH to Triton X-100–solubilized membranes from rat mammary gland, liver, and kidney. Samples were cross-linked and analyzed as described for Leydig cells.

lactogen receptors were cross-linked with 0.5 mM DSS and run on SDS-polyacrylamide tube gels containing 7.5% acrylamide, under non-reducing conditions. The first-dimension gels were then soaked for 1 hr at room temperature in a solution containing 0.7 M β-mercaptoethanol and run on SDS-polyacrylamide slab gels containing 7.5% acrylamide. The autoradiogram obtained under these conditions is shown in FIGURE 1 (right panel). A species with $M_r = 59,000$ (arrow) can be seen deriving from the $M_r = 103,000$ species. This suggests that a fraction of the $M_r = 59,000$ molecules is contained within the $M_r = 103,000$ form, associated through disulfide bonds. With the present protocol, however, it is not possible to accurately quantitate the extent of this association since the cross-linking that occurred within subunits did not allow the covalently linked complexes to dissociate under reducing conditions. The structural relationship among these and the other two forms is not clear at the present time.

Coupling of ^{125}I-hGH to Triton X-100–solubilized membranes from ovary,[7] mammary gland, liver, and kidney resulted in patterns of cross-linking resembling that observed in Leydig cells (FIGURE 2). However, single bands and not doublets were observed in some cases. Also, the M_rs of homologous species were slightly different according to the organ that served as source of prolactin receptors.

REFERENCES

1. HAFIEZ, A. A., C. W. LLOYD & A. BARTKE. 1972. J. Endocrinol. **52:** 327–332.
2. BARTKE, A. & S. DALTERIO. 1976. Biol. Reprod. **15:** 90–93.
3. PURVIS, K., O. P. CLAUSEN, A. OLSEN, E. HAUG & V. HANSSON. 1979. Arch. Androl. **3:** 219–230.
4. COSTLOW, M. E. & W. L. McGUIRE. 1977. J. Endocrinol. **75:** 221–226.
5. ARAGONA. C. & H. G. FRIESEN. 1975. Endocrinology **97:** 677–684.
6. CHARREAU, E. H., A. ATTRAMADAL, P. A. TORJESEN, K. PURVIS, R. CALANDRA & V. HANSSON. 1977. Mol. Cell. Endocrinol. **6:** 303–307.
7. BONIFACINO, J. S. & M. L. DUFAU. 1984. J. Biol. Chem. **259:** 4542–4549.

Effect of hCG on Testicular Steroidogenesis and Gonadotropin and Prolactin Receptors in Unilaterally Cryptorchid Rats

ILPO HUHTANIEMI,[a,b] ANDERS BERGH,[c] HANNU
NIKULA,[a] and JAN-ERIK DAMBER[d]

[a] Department of Clinical Chemistry
Department of Immunology and Bacteriology
University of Helsinki
Helsinki, Finland

[c] Department of Anatomy
[d] Department of Clinical Chemistry
University of Umeå
Umeå, Sweden

The profound tubular damage in cryptorchidism, with atrophy of the germinal epithelium, is associated with clear-cut morphological and functional changes in Sertoli and Leydig cells.[1,2] It is possible that the changes observed in this condition are partly caused by altered response of the abdominal testis to tropic regulation. This concept was studied further by assessing the functional response of the scrotal and contralateral abdominal testis to hCG stimulation in unilateral cryptorchidism.

Sprague-Dawley rats were made unilaterally cryptorchid by cutting the gubernaculum testis at birth.[3] At 100 days of age the rats were injected with 600 IU/kg of hCG (Pregnyl, Organon), and the testicular levels of testosterone (T) and progesterone (P), and receptors for LH, FSH, and prolactin (Prl) were measured up to 10 d after hormone injections in the abdominal and scrotal testes. The steroids were measured by radioimmunoassay after diethylether extraction of testis homogenates. The receptors of the testicular homogenates were measured using ^{125}I-hCG, ^{125}I-hFSH, and ^{125}I-hGH as ligands.[4]

Intratesticular T was significantly ($p < 0.01$) higher in the scrotal than abdominal testes (30 ± 4.0 versus 13 ± 2.8 ng/g, S.E., $N = 16$). A reverse situation was observed with testicular P, being 1.0 ± 0.094 and 1.4 ± 0.19 ng/g in the scrotal and abdominal testes, respectively ($p < 0.05$). A biphasic T response was seen in the scrotal testis in response to hCG (FIGURE 1), with maxima at 1 hr and 3 days after injection. A similar acute peak was observed in the abdominal testis, but the secondary peak was less prominent, with no significant elevation in testicular T between 1 day and 3 days. The response of testicular P to hCG stimulation showed a maximum at 1 day in both testes (FIGURE 1), but the response was 12–20-fold higher in the abdominal testis in two experiments performed, with

[b] Address correspondence to: Dr. Ilpo Huhtaniemi, Department of Clinical Chemistry, University of Helsinki, Meilahti Hospital, SF-00290 Helsinki 29, Finland.

maximum concentrations of 900–1,200 ng/g versus 50–100 ng/g in the abdominal and scrotal testes, respectively ($p < 0.001$).

The affinities of hCG, hFSH, and hGH binding to scrotal and abdominal testes were similar (results not shown). The concentration of LH receptors was 50% higher in the abdominal than scrotal testes (3.3 ± 0.2 versus 2.1 ± 0.1 pmol/g, $N = 11$, $p < 0.001$). Conversely, the Prl receptor concentrations were about 30% lower in the abdominal than scrotal testes (190 ± 14 versus 260 ± 15 fmol/g, $N = 11$, $p < 0.001$). The FSH receptor levels were similar in both cases (180–210 fmol/g).

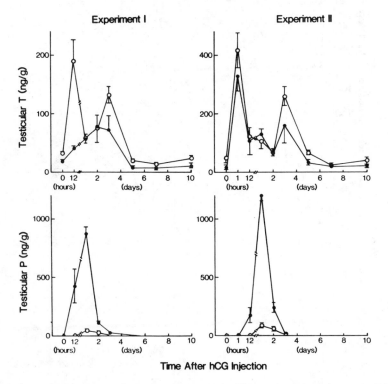

FIGURE 1. Intratesticular T (upper panels) and P (lower panels) in the scrotal (○) and abdominal (●) testes of the unilaterally cryptorchid rats after a single injection of 600 IU/kg hCG. Note that the 1-hr samples were only taken in Experiment II. The number of individual animals analyzed per time-point was 3–6 in Experiment I and 5 in Experiment II.

After hCG injection, the loss of free LH receptors was faster in the abdominal testes (FIGURE 2). Likewise, the recovery of binding was faster in the abdominal testes, being at 10 days 102 ± 5% of the starting level versus 52 ± 4% in the scrotal testes ($p < 0.01$), when the starting levels were used as reference points. Similar days in the abdominal testis only ($p < 0.05$) (FIGURE 2). Thereafter, on days 5–10, the FSH binding of the abdominal testes was 20–40% higher than in the scrotal testes ($p < 0.01$), when the starting levels were used as reference points. Similar

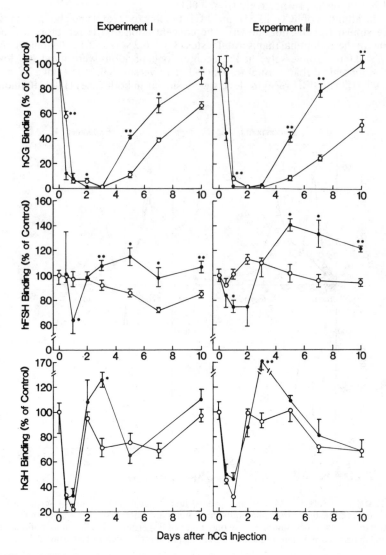

FIGURE 2. hCG-induced changes in the levels of testicular receptors for LH (upper panels), FSH (middle panels), and Prl (lower panels). The open symbols (○) show receptor levels in the scrotal testes and the closed symbols (●) in the abdominal testes. The binding in each case is expressed as percents of the 0-hr level. The asterisks indicate statistically significant differences in the percents of initial binding at the individual times between the scrotal and abdominal testes (*, $p < 0.05$; **, $p < 0.01$). The numbers of individual measurements per time point are as in FIGURE 1.

heterologous down-regulation of 50–80% of Prl receptors was found in both testes between 12–24 hr (FIGURE 2). However, the abdominal testes showed a transient elevation of 25–70% at day 3 ($p < 0.01$), which was not seen in the scrotal testes.

It is concluded from these studies that the abdominal testis displays, besides lowered basal T production, a dramatically enhanced blockade of C21 steroid side-chain cleavage in response to gonadotropin stimulation. The kinetics of testicular LH, FSH, and Prl receptors in response to hCG stimulation is faster in the abdominal testis, and these receptor levels display transient up-regulatory responses that are not observed in the scrotal testis. The results indicate clearly altered responses to tropic stimulation in Leydig and Sertoli cells of the abdominal testis, and may be indicative of direct functional changes in these cells in the elevated intra-abdominal temperature or changes in the paracrine component of testicular endocrine regulation.

REFERENCES

1. KERR, J. B., K. A. RICH & D. M. DE KRETSER. 1979. Effects of experimental cryptorchidism on the ultrastructure and function of the Sertoli cells and peritubular tissue of the rat testis. Biol. Reprod. **21:** 823–838.
2. BERGH, A. 1983. Early morphological changes in the abdominal testes in immature unilaterally cryptorchid rats. Int. J. Androl. **6:** 73–90.
3. BERGH, A., H. F. HELANDER & L. WAHLQVIST. 1978. Studies on factors governing testicular descent in the rat. —Particularly the role of gubernaculum testis. Int. J. Androl. **1:** 342–356.
4. CATT, K. J., J.-M. KETELSLEGERS & M. L. DUFAU. 1976. Receptors for gonadotropic hormones. *In* Methods in Receptor Research. M. Blecher, Ed. **1:** 175–250. Marcel Dekker. New York.

Changes in Gonadotropin and Isoproterenol Stimulated Adenylate Cyclase Activities in Rat Testicular Tissue during Cryptorchidism

T. JAHNSEN,[a] B. KARPE,[b] H. ATTRAMADAL,[a]
A. ERICHSEN,[a] E. HAUG,[c] M. RITZEN,[d] and
V. HANSSON[a,e]

[a] Institute of Pathology
Rikshospitalet
Oslo 1, Norway

[b] Department of Pediatric Surgery
St. Gøran Hospital
11281 Stockholm, Sweden

[c] Aker Hospital
Oslo, Norway

[d] Pediatric Endocrinology Unit
Karolinska Hospital
10401 Stockholm, Sweden

[e] Institute of Medical Biochemistry
University of Oslo
Blindern, Oslo 3, Norway

During unilateral cryptorchidism (3–28 days) in adult rats there was a selective decrease in the adenylate cyclase responses to gonadotropin stimulation in the abdominal testis (FIGURE 1). This was associated with a parallel decrease in specific FSH and LH binding. There was no reduction in the response of testicular adenylate cyclase to PGE_1 or fluoride stimulation, indicating that both the GTP binding protein (N-component) and the catalytic subunit of the adenylate cyclase complex were intact. The reduction in FSH-responsive adenylate cyclase activity in the abdominal testis was not due to a change in the K_m for adenylate cyclase activation, but a reduction in maximal velocities. The desensitization of the gonadotropin-responsive adenylate cyclases and the loss of gonadotropin receptors in Leydig and Sertoli cells were not due to changes in plasma gonadotropin values because LH concentrations were within normal limits and plasma FSH was only marginally elevated during unilateral cryptorchidism. No significant alterations of any of these parameters (gonadotropin receptors, adenylate cyclase activities) were seen in the scrotal testis of unilaterally cryptorchid rats when compared to values for intact controls.

In a second experiment, rats in groups of five were either sham-operated or made unilateral or bilateral cryptorchid at both 20 and 80 days of age. The animals were killed four weeks later. This experiment showed that cryptorchidism was associated with an increased responsiveness of the isoproterenol-sensitive adenylate cyclase in testicular membrane particles from abdominal testes.

In a third experiment, using 72 rats, we examined the effects of bilateral cryptorchidism and orchidopexy (cryptorchidism started at 17 days of age) on the response of the isoproterenol-sensitive adenylate cyclase (FIGURE 2). Maximal isoproterenol responses were seen three to four weeks after the rats were made

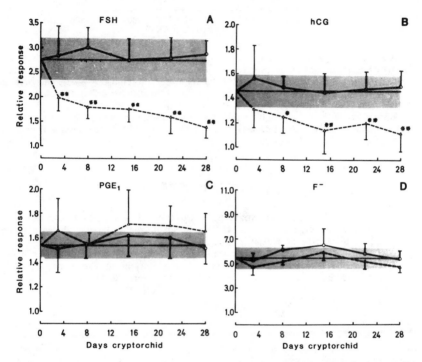

FIGURE 1. Changes (mean ± s.d. for 4 testes) in adenylate cyclase responsiveness to (A) FSH, (B) hCG, (C) PGE-1, and (D) fluoride in whole testis tissue membrane particles from abdominal (△-----△) and scrotal (○——○) testes of unilaterally cryptorchid rats. The shaded area indicates the mean ± s.d. of 10 control animals. Relative responses significantly different from control animals are indicated: * $p < 0.05$, ** $p < 0.01$ (Wilcoxon's rank test). (From Jahnsen *et al.*[1] With permission from *Journal of Reproduction and Fertility*.)

cryptorchid. Following orchidopexy there was a gradual normalization of the isoproterenol response and two to three months after orchidopexy the isoproterenol response in the rat testis had decreased to normal control values.

Thus, experimental cryptorchidism in rats is associated with a decreased responsiveness of gonadotropin-sensitive adenylate cyclase activity, and increased responsiveness of isoproterenol-sensitive adenylate cyclase activity in testicular membrane particles from abdominal testes.

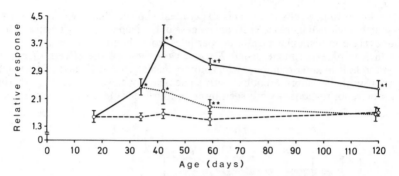

FIGURE 2. Changes (mean ± s.d., $N = 6$) in relative response (stimulated activities divided by basal activities), of isoproterenol-stimulated adenylate cyclase activity in testicular membrane particles from control (O--O), bilaterally cryptorchid (△——△), and orchidopexic rats (□---□). The abscissa shows the age of the animals when killed. *$p < 0.01$, **$p < 0.05$: values for cryptorchid and orchidopexic animals compared with control animals (Wilcoxon's rank test). † $p < 0.01$: values for orchidopexic animals compared with cryptorchid animals (Wilcoxon's rank test). (From Jahnsen et al.[2] With permission from *Journal of Reproduction and Fertility*.)

REFERENCES

1. JAHNSEN, T., J. O. GORDELADZE, E. HAUG & V. HANSSON. 1981. Changes in rat testicular adenylate cyclase activities and gonadotrophin binding during unilateral experimental cryptorchidism. J. Reprod. Fert. **63**: 381–390.
2. JAHNSEN, T., B. KARPE, H. ATTRAMADAL, M. RITZEN & V. HANSSON. 1984. Changes in isoproterenol-stimulated adenylate cyclase activity in rat testicular tissue during cryptorchidism and after orchidopexy. J. Reprod. Fert. **70**: 443–448.

Development of Adenosine Responsiveness after Isolation of Leydig Cells

F. F. G. ROMMERTS,[a] R. MOLENAAR,
J. W. HOOGERBRUGGE, and H. J. VAN DER MOLEN

Department of Biochemistry
Division of Chemical Endocrinology
Medical Faculty
Erasmus University
Rotterdam, The Netherlands

Adenosine can modify intracellular cAMP concentrations and physiological functions in several tissues and isolated cells, e.g. brain tissue, fat cells, coronary artery, and platelets.[1] Effects of adenosine on steroidogenesis have been described for Leydig and adrenal tumor cell lines.[5] Moreover, receptors for adenosine have been detected in testicular tissue.[2,4] Thus, adenosine may act *in vivo* as a (local) modulator of Leydig cell function. In this respect we have investigated the effects of adenosine and related compounds on the steroidogenic activity of isolated Leydig cells. Leydig cells were prepared from testes of 21-day-old rats according to Rommerts *et al.*[3] After attachment of the isolated cells to plastic and incubation periods of 1 and 24 hr, the basal steroidogenic activity and the effects of various additions were determined (TABLE 1). Stimulation of steroid production by LH or 22R-hydroxycholesterol in freshly prepared cells or after 24 hr incubation of the cells was not different, indicating that cells remain viable. Moreover, cellular ATP levels did not decrease during culture, but rather increased with 80%.

Addition of adenosine or N6-(1-2-phenyl-isopropyl) adenosine (PIA) had no effects after 1 hr incubation, but stimulated steroid production after 24 hr incubation to the same extent as LH (TABLE 1). Cells incubated for 24 hr with 100 ng LH/ml or 200 μM adenosine were as active as cells incubated without these additions. Specificity studies showed that ATP, NADP, NADPH, and other compounds containing both adenine and ribose were also active, whereas inosine was inactive. Leydig cells prepared enzymatically from adult rat testes or mechanically from mouse testes also became responsive to adenosine after 24 hr incubation, although the effects of adenosine were less pronounced than with cells from immature rats. Steroid production in testis tissue from immature rats was 5–25-fold stimulated by LH, but not with 100–200 μM adenosine, indicating the absence of adenosine sensitivity of Leydig cells *in situ*. The time course of the induction of adenosine sensitivity of collagenase-dispersed Leydig cells was investigated with cells isolated from immature rats. The first significant effect of adenosine on pregnenolone production could be shown three hours after isolation

[a] Address correspondence to: F. F. G. Rommerts, Department of Biochemistry II, Faculty of Medicine, Erasmus University Rotterdam, P.O. Box 1738, 3000 DR Rotterdam, The Netherlands.

of the cells and the stimulation increased almost linearly during the next few hours (FIGURE 1).

Levels of cyclic AMP were measured in cells incubated in the presence of 1-methyl-3-isobutyl xanthine (MIX). In fresh cells 100 ng LH/ml stimulated cAMP production more than tenfold, but no effects of adenosine could be shown. After 24 hr incubation, the effect of 100 ng LH/ml on cAMP production was not changed and in addition a small, but significant ($p < 0.02$) stimulation of cAMP levels by adenosine and PIA could be demonstrated (control 3.1 ± 0.6; adenosine 6.3 ± 1.1; PIA 5.9 ± 0.6). These small changes in cAMP concentrations can stimulate protein phosphorylation of the 17,000 dalton protein and steroid production (TABLE 1) to the same degree as LH (100 ng/ml).

The results of the present study demonstrate that dispersed Leydig cells develop a responsiveness to adenosine several hours after isolation. LH- and 22R-hydroxycholesterol–stimulated steroidogenesis, LH-stimulated cAMP production, and ATP levels were not decreased for at least 24 hr, indicating that cells remain intact and viable during this period. Specificity studies showed that all compounds with an adenosine moiety could stimulate cAMP and steroid production. The lack of adenosine sensitivity immediately after cell isolation may be caused by a loss of existing receptors after exposure to proteolytic enzymes used in the cell isolation procedure. It may also be a consequence of new membrane properties induced by the *in vitro* conditions. The first explanation appears unlikely, because mouse Leydig cells prepared mechanically without collagenase showed no response when exposed to adenosine immediately after isolation. Moreover, Leydig cells in intact testicular tissue from immature rats did not respond to adenosine.

Adrenal and Leydig tumor cells grown in culture also respond to adenosine,[5] whereas the results in this paper show that freshly prepared (tumor) Leydig cells cannot be stimulated by adenosine. The different results obtained with freshly or cultured normal Leydig cells and tumor Leydig cells indicate that adenosine responsiveness is most likely induced by the *in vitro* conditions. These results indicate that caution is required when effects of adenosine or related compounds

TABLE 1. Pregnenolone Production by Leydig Cells from Immature Rats[a]

Incubation Condition	Pregnenolone (ng/hr per 10^6 cells)	
	Fresh Cells	24 hr Incubation
Control	1.1 ± 0.3 (6)[b]	1.7 ± 0.3
LH (1 ng/ml)	n.e.	20 ± 7 (6)[a]
LH (100 ng/ml)	32 ± 9 (6)[b]	24 ± 5 (6)[a]
22R-Hydroxycholesterol (30 μM)	250 ± 72 (6)[b]	275 ± 91 (6)[a]
Adenosine (50 μM)	1.5 ± 0.2 (6)	23 ± 4 (6)[a]
N[6]-(L-2-phenyl-isopropyl)-adenosine (50 μM)	1.4 ± 0.3 (4)	21 ± 6 (4)[a]
LH (100 ng/ml) + adenosine (50 μM)	n.e.	28 ± 6 (6)[a]

[a] Attached to plastic dishes preincubated for 1 hr or 24 hr in culture medium without hormones.
Means ± S.D. and number of observations, n.e. = not estimated.
[b] $p < 0.01$ versus control.

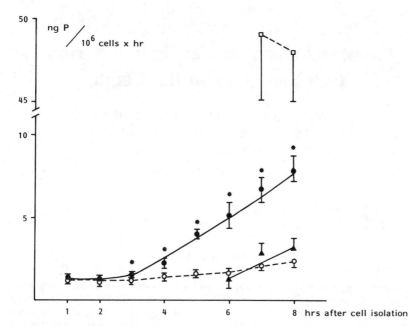

FIGURE 1. Effect of nucleosides and LH on steroidogenesis by Leydig cells isolated from testes of 21-day-old rats at various times after isolation: (O---O) controls; (▲——▲) inosine 50 μM; (●——●) adenosine 50 μM; and (□···□) LH 100 ng/ml. Points represent mean values ± S.D. of six incubations. Steroid production per hour was measured in culture medium and each aliquot portion of cells was used during three subsequent periods. * Significantly different from control values ($p < 0.01$).

on isolated Leydig cells are interpreted as physiologically important for the Leydig cells *in vitro*.

REFERENCES

1. FAIN, J. N. & C. C. MALBON. 1979. Molec. Cell. Biochem. **25:** 143–169.
2. MURPHY, K. M. M. & S. H. SNYDER. 1981. Life Sci. **28:** 917–920.
3. ROMMERTS, F. F. G., M. J. A. VAN ROEMBURG, L. M. LINDH, J. A. J. HEGGE & H. J. VAN DER MOLEN. 1982. J. Reprod. Fert. **65:** 289–297.
4. WILLIAMS, M. & E. RISKY. 1980. Proc. Natl. Acad. Sci. USA **77:** 6892–6896.
5. WOLFF, J. & G. H. COOK. 1977. J. Biol. Chem. **252:** 687–693.

Effects of Temporary or Permanent Cryptorchidism on Leydig and Sertoli Cell Functions in the Lamb

C. MONET-KUNTZ, B. BARENTON, M. BLANC,
A. LOCATELLI, J. PELLETIER, C. PERREAU and
M. T. HOCHEREAU-de-REVIERS

Institut National de la Recherche Agronomique
Reproductive Physiology
37380 Nouzilly, France

INTRODUCTION

Experimentally induced cryptorchidism results in a disruption of spermatogenesis although gonadotrophin levels increase. We wanted to know how the populations of Leydig and Sertoli cells evolve from a morphological point of view, whether the testis retains its sensitivity to gonadotrophins and androgens, whether the secretory activity of Leydig and Sertoli cells is modified by cryptorchidism, and whether the effects of cryptorchidism are reversible when testes are redescended into the scrotum.

MATERIAL AND METHODS

Ile-de-France × Romanov lambs were divided into three groups: intact (I, $N = 5$), cryptorchidized at two months of age (C, $N = 5$), and cryptorchidized at two months with testes redescended at four months (temporary cryptorchid, TC, $N = 5$). All animals were slaughtered at seven months. Lambs were rendered bilaterally cryptorchid. For TC, Teflon prostheses were left in the scrotum so that the testes could be later redescended. Histological analysis of both intertubular and tubular tissue was performed.[1] Before slaughtering, blood was sampled every 30 min for 7 hr. Plasma levels of LH,[2] FSH,[3] and testosterone[4] were measured by radioimmunoassays. LH and FSH receptors were both assayed in the same testicular membrane preparations.[5] Androgen receptors were assayed in testicular cytosols using dextran-coated charcoal.[6] Androgen-binding protein (ABP) was assayed in testicular cytosols by steady-state polyacrylamide gel electrophoresis.[7]

RESULTS

Testicular growth was much reduced by cryptorchidism since testis weight was 190 g in I and 24 g in C. It recommenced when the testes were redescended (94 g in TC). The volume of lymphatic and blood vessels was 12 cm^3 in I, 1.4 cm^3 in C, and

TABLE 1. Influence of Cryptorchidism on Leydig Cell Characteristics

	Intact (I)	Cryptorchid (C)	Temporary Cryptorchid (TC)
Total number of Leydig cells per testis ($\times 10^{-8}$)	10.1	2.1[a]	5.7[a]
Individual volume of Leydig cells (μm^3)	400	421	370
LH receptors (pmoles/testis)	8.5	2.6[a]	5
Mean plasma testosterone (ng/ml)	6.6	4.9	5.4

[a] Significantly different from intact lambs ($p < 0.05$).

5.5 cm^3 in TC. Mean plasma LH levels (3.3 ng/ml in I) were raised by cryptorchidism (8.3 ng/ml in C) and lowered to normal values when testes were redescended. Mean plasma FSH levels (5.2 ng/ml in I) were raised by cryptorchidism (29.5 ng/ml in C), and lowered to intermediate values when testes were redescended (14.8 ng/ml in TC). TABLE 1 shows that the number of Leydig cells was severely decreased by cryptorchidism due to complete cessation of their divisions. Their individual volume was not affected by cryptorchidism. Total number of LH receptors was decreased by cryptorchidism, essentially due to the decrease in the number of Leydig cells. LH receptors were partly restored when the testes were redescended. However, mean plasma testosterone levels were not modified by cryptorchidism. TABLE 2 shows that the total number of Sertoli cells was not affected by cryptorchidism, but their cross-sectional surface area was slightly decreased. Total numbers of FSH receptors and androgen receptors were greatly reduced by cryptorchidism. Both were poorly restored when testes were redescended. Testicular content of ABP was greatly reduced by cryptorchidism and poorly restored when testes were redescended. Daily production of round spermatids per testis (2.03 $\times$ 10^9 in I) was zero in C lambs. It was partly restored in TC lambs (0.59 $\times$ 10^9), but 40% of the tubules remained inactive.

TABLE 2. Influence of Cryptorchidism on Sertoli Cell Characteristics

	Intact (I)	Cryptorchid (C)	Temporary Cryptorchid (TC)
Total number of Sertoli cells per testis ($\times 10^{-8}$)	50	42	54
Mean surface area of Sertoli cells (μm^2)	56.4	44.4[a]	48.6[a]
FSH receptors (pmoles/testis)	68.7	2.5[a]	16.2[a]
Androgen receptors (pmoles/testis)	187	26.7[a]	47.9[a]
ABP (pmoles/testis)	360	41.7[a]	122[a]

[a] Significantly different from intact lambs ($p < 0.05$).

CONCLUSION

This study demonstrates that, in the lamb, the spermatogenic disruption that results from the induction of cryptorchidism is accompanied by changes in Leydig and Sertoli cell function. These changes may be related to the elevation of temperature, which is known to affect Sertoli cells,[8] as well as to the spermatogenic damage.[9]

REFERENCES

1. HOCHEREAU-DE-REVIERS, M. T., M. R. BLANC, C. CAHOREAU, M. COUROT, J. L. DACHEUX & C. PISSELET. 1979. Histological testicular parameters in bilateral cryptorchid adult rams. Ann. Biol. Anim. Biochim. Biophys. **19:** 1141–1146.
2. PELLETIER, J., G. KANN, J. DOLAIS & G. ROSSELIN. 1968. Dosage radioimmunologique de l'hormone lutéinisante plasmatique de mouton. Mise au point de la technique de dosage. C. R. Hebd. Séanc. Acad. Sci. Paris D. **266:** 2291–2294.
3. BLANC, M. R. & J. C. POIRIER. 1979. A new homologous radioimmunoassay for ovine follicle stimulating hormone: development and characterization. Ann. Biol. Anim. Biochim. Biophys. **19:** 1011–1026.
4. GARNIER, D. H., Y. COTTA & M. TERQUI. 1978. Androgen radioimmunoassay in the ram: results of direct plasma testosterone and dehydroepiandrosterone measurement and physiological evaluation. Ann. Biol. Anim. Biochim. Biophys. **18:** 265–281.
5. BARENTON, B., M. R. BLANC, A. CARATY, M. T. HOCHEREAU-DE-REVIERS, C. PERREAU & J. SAUMANDE. 1982. Effect of cryptorchidism in the ram: changes in the concentrations of testosterone and estradiol and receptors for LH and FSH in the testis, and its histology. Mol. Cell. Endocrinol. **28:** 13–25.
6. MONET-KUNTZ, C., M. TERQUI & A. LOCATELLI. 1979. Characterization of a cytoplasmic androgen receptor in the ram testis. Mol. Cell. Endocrinol. **16:** 57–70.
7. CARREAU, S., M. DROSDOWSKY & M. COUROT. 1979. Age related effects on androgen binding protein (ABP) in sheep testis and epididymis. Int. J. Androl. **2:** 49–61.
8. HAGENÄS, L., E. M. RITZEN, J. SVENSSON, V. HANSSON & K. PURVIS. 1978. Temperature dependence of Sertoli cell function. Int. J. Androl. Suppl. **2:** 449–456.
9. JEGOU, P., A. O. LAWS & D. M. DE KRETSER. 1983. The effect of cryptorchidism and subsequent orchidopexy on testicular function in adult rats. J. Reprod. Fert. **69:** 137–145.

Effects of 20-α-Hydroxy-4-pregnen-3-one Treatment on the Hypophyseal Testicular Axis in Rats

KARL E. FRIEDL, STEPHEN R. PLYMATE,
BRUCE L. FARISS, MINA J. GARRISON, and
LOUIS A. MATEJ

Department of Clinical Investigation
Madigan Army Medical Center
Tacoma, Washington 98431

In vitro biochemical studies have demonstrated that 20α-hydroxy-4-pregnen-3-one (20α-OHP) inhibits 17α-hydroxylase[1] and 20α-OHP is suggested to be a regulator of intratesticular androgen biosynthesis. The activity of 20α-hydroxysteroid dehydrogenase has been found in the rat seminiferous tubule[2,3] and this association with the germinal epithelium offers the possibility of a regulatory function of 20α-OHP in the testis-hypophyseal axis. In this study, we examined the effects of exogenously administered 20α-OHP on gonadotrophins, testosterone, and rat androgen binding protein (ABP). In order to distinguish direct effects of 20α-OHP on gonadotrophin secretion, FSH and LH were also studied in treated castrate animals.

Thirty-two Sprague-Dawley rats (250 ± 15 g) were divided into four groups and received daily 0.2 ml intramuscular injections for 21 days of either vehicle (sesame oil), 1 mg progesterone, 1 mg 20α-OHP, or 5-mg 20α-OHP (Sigma Co). Animals were sacrificed and trunk blood was collected 12 hours after the last treatment. Testosterone was measured by radioimmunoassay. Rat LH (compared to NIADDK-rLH-RP2), rat FSH (compared to NIAMD-rFSH-RP1), and rat ABP were measured by double antibody radioimmunoassay (RIA) using reagents obtained from the National Institutes of Health. Tissue levels of rat ABP and testosterone were measured after tissue homogenization in phosphate-buffered saline (with 0.5% bovine serum albumin) and centrifugation. Protein concentrations were determined by the Lowry technique. Organ weights were obtained for testes, epididymides, ligated seminal vesicles (with coagulating glands removed), seminal vesicles with contents expressed, ventral prostate, and adrenals.

Median plasma testosterone values were significantly reduced for progesterone (1.9 ng/ml) and 20α-OHP treated groups (1.7, 1.8 ng/ml) compared to controls (3.2 ng/ml) ($p < 0.05$, Mann-Whitney U-test). Progesterone treatment resulted in a significant reduction in plasma LH concentration (0.36 ng/ml). In spite of the fall in plasma testosterone concentrations, there was no change in the plasma LH levels in either of the 20α-OHP–treated groups (0.49, 0.43 ng/ml) compared to controls (0.43 ng/ml). Plasma FSH concentrations also remained unchanged with 20α-OHP treatments (253 ± 18, 246 ± 26 ng/ml) in comparison with the control group (246 ± 31 ng/ml).

Tissue concentrations of testosterone were significantly reduced for all steroid treatment groups. ABP concentration was significantly elevated in the testis and epididymis of the 5 mg 20α-OHP treated animals (TABLE 1). There were no significant differences between mean body weights or between reproductive organ weights for any of the treatment groups. Seminal vesicular contents were significantly increased in the 5 mg 20α-OHP group and decreased in the progesterone group.

A second experiment with 32 rats divided into four similar treatment groups examined the effect of 20α-OHP in castrate rats treated for 21 days beginning within one week of castration. There were no significant differences detected for plasma LH or FSH between groups. There were no differences for mean organ weights (ligated seminal vesicles, ventral prostate, and adrenals) between 20α-OHP–treated groups and controls. These castrate experiment results are consistent with the findings of other investigators.[4]

TABLE 1. Mean Testosterone, Androgen Binding Protein, and Gonadotrophin Concentrations after 21 Days of Daily Treatments (± SEM)

Intact Animals	Controls	Progesterone	20α-OHP (1 mg)	20α-OHP (5 mg)
Plasma FSH (ng/ml)	246 ± 31	223 ± 23	253 ± 18	247 ± 26
Plasma LH (ng/ml)	0.49 ± 0.05	0.37 ± 0.06[a]	0.52 ± 0.10	0.47 ± 0.10
Plasma T (ng/ml)	4.2 ± 1.2	1.9 ± 0.3[a]	2.2 ± 0.4[a]	2.5 ± 0.7[a]
Intratesticular T (ng/g testis)	56.2 ± 2.9	36.1 ± 3.6[a]	41.5 ± 3.0[a]	35.6 ± 2.7[a]
Testicular ABP (pmoles/mg Pr−)	0.34 ± 0.02	0.35 ± 0.02	0.33 ± 0.02	0.40 ± 0.01[a]
Epididymal ABP (pmoles/mg Pr−)	2.24 ± 0.15	2.76 ± 0.23[a]	2.52 ± 0.23	3.36 ± 0.38[a]
Castrate Animals	Controls	Progesterone	20α-OHP (1 mg)	20α-OHP (5 mg)
Plasma FSH (ng/ml)	1162 ± 105	1151 ± 45	1120 ± 94	1259 ± 85
Plasma LH (ng/ml)	9.63 ± 0.66	9.46 ± 0.78	11.32 ± 0.95	9.49 ± 0.81

[a] $p < 0.05$ for medians compared to controls (Mann-Whitney U test).

The testicular action of 20α-OHP was further investigated by studies on LH-stimulated testosterone production with a Leydig cell preparation from six-week-old Swiss-Webster mice. Complete inhibition of testosterone production with 10^{-4} to 10^{-8} M 20α-OHP was observed. At concentrations of less than 10^{-8} M, testosterone response to LH improved; however, even at the lowest dose of 20α-OHP, 10^{-16} M, testosterone response was still less than controls without 20α-OHP.

These findings support a regulatory role for 20α-OHP within the testis. The principal effects are an inhibition of testosterone production and an increase in ABP. The results are intriguing in view of the recent suggestion that progestins may be associated with spermiation and Sertoli cell enlargement.[5]

ACKNOWLEDGMENTS

The authors wish to thank Dr. W. J. Bremner for laboratory support and Ms. Eugenia Hough for secretarial assistance.

REFERENCES

1. FAN, D., H. OSHIMA, B. R. TROEN & P. TROEN. 1974. Studies of the human testis. IV. testicular 20α-hydroxysteroid dehydrogenase and steroid 17α-hydroxylase. Biochim. Biophys. Acta **360:** 88–99.
2. LACY, D. & A. J. PETTITT. 1970. Sites of hormone production in the mammalian testis, and their significance in the control of male infertility. Brit. Med. Bull. **26:** 87–91.
3. INANO, H. 1974. Studies on enzyme reactions related to steroid biosynthesis—III. distribution of the testicular enzymes related to androgen production between the seminiferous tubules and interstitial tissue. J. Steroid Biochem. **5:** 145–149.
4. SWERDLOFF, R. S., P. K. GROVER, H. S. JACOB & J. BAIN. 1973. Search for a substance which selectively inhibits FSH—effects of steroids and prostaglandins on serum FSH and LH levels. Steroids **21:** 703–721.
5. UEDA, H., G. YOUNG, L. W. CRIM, A. KAMBEGAWA & Y. NAGAHAMA. 1983. 17α,20β-dihydroxy-4-pregnen-3-one: plasma levels during sexual maturation and *in vitro* production by the testes of amago salmon and rainbow trout. Gen. Comp. Endocrinol. **51:** 106–112.

Characteristics of Leydig Cells and Macrophages from Developing Testicular Cells

RINKJE MOLENAAR,[a] FOCKO F. G. ROMMERTS, and
HENK J. VAN DER MOLEN

Division of Chemical Endocrinology
Department of Biochemistry
Medical Faculty
Erasmus University
Rotterdam, The Netherlands

INTRODUCTION

Leydig cells and macrophages are present in the interstitial tissue of the testis. It is well known that properties of Leydig cells change during development, but little is known about the function and development of testicular macrophages. Recently the presence of F_c receptors on Leydig cell membranes (Haour, personal communication) and specific binding of lymphocytes to Leydig cells (rosette formation)[1,4] have been described. This indicates that Leydig cells and macrophages may have common properties.

We have investigated with cytological and histochemical techniques in interstitial cell preparations from 21–23-day-old rats and 60–90-day-old rats the cellular localization of 3β-hydroxysteroid dehydrogenase (3β-HSD) activity (marker for Leydig cells), α-naphtyl esterase (α-NE) activity (marker for Leydig cells and macrophages), and the phagocytic uptake of microbeads as well as the presence of macrophage membrane antigens (markers for macrophages). In addition, changes in steroidogenic activities during development have been investigated. Details of methods used for isolation of cells, histochemistry, and measurement of steroids have been described previously.[3] Further details are given in TABLE 1.

RESULTS AND DISCUSSION

Steroidogenic activities of Leydig cells obtained from 21–23- and 60–90-day-old rats have been compared. The basal, LH-, and dbcAMP-stimulated pregnenolone production as well as the cholesterol side-chain cleavage (CSCC) activity in the presence of 22R-hydroxycholesterol was significantly higher in Leydig cells obtained from mature rats than in cells from immature rats (TABLE 1), indicating an increase in steroidogenic capacity per Leydig cell during maturation. Testosterone and pregnenolone production by Leydig cells from mature rats were similar in control cells and in cells stimulated with LH. In the presence of 22R-hydroxycholesterol, however, the testosterone production was significantly lower than the

[a] Address correspondence to: R. Molenaar, Department of Biochemistry II, Faculty of Medicine, Erasmus University Rotterdam, P.O. Box 1738, 3000 DR Rotterdam, The Netherlands.

pregnenolone production (TABLE 1). This indicates that *in vitro,* with maximal CSCC activity in the presence of an excess 22R-hydroxycholesterol, a rate-limiting step exists between pregnenolone and testosterone. In the presence of LH this step is not rate limiting. Under *in vivo* conditions, however, pregnenolone metabolism appears to be always rate limiting, because Cigorraga[2] demonstrated the presence of substantial amounts of 17α-hydroxy metabolites in testis tissue. This apparent discrepancy in capacity for pregnenolone metabolism *in vivo* and *in vitro* may be caused by the presence of a certain amount of damaged cells in isolated cell preparations.[3] If such damaged cells cannot be stimulated by LH, but are active in pregnenolone metabolism, an overestimation of the rate of pregnenolone metabolism can be expected.

The conversion of pregnenolone to testosterone (expressed as the ratio $\frac{\text{testosterone production}}{\text{pregnenolone production}} \times 100\%$) in cells from rats 21–23, 35–40, and 60–90 days old was 5.0 ± 1.7 ($N = 4$), 23.5 ± 11.4 ($N = 4$), and 71.2 ± 16.6 ($N = 4$)

TABLE 1. Steroid Production by Isolated Leydig Cells

Incubation Conditions	21–23-Day-Old Rats (ng Pregnenolone/hr/ 10^6 3β-HSD+ Cells)	60–90-Day-Old Rats (ng Steroid/hr/10^6 3β-HSD+ Cells)	
		Pregnenolone	Testosterone
Control	7 ± 2	60 ± 27^a	50 ± 26
LH (100 ng/ml)	153 ± 19	635 ± 231^a	433 ± 124
dbcAMP (0.5 mM)	143 ± 21	562 ± 201^a	n.d.
22R-Hydroxycholesterol (7.5 μg/ml)	1079 ± 358	5541 ± 2341^a	1088 ± 403^b

Means ± S.D. of four cell preparations are given.
n.d. — not detected.
[a] Significantly different from 21–23-day-old rats ($p < 0.005$).
[b] Significantly different from pregnenolone production ($p < 0.005$).

(means ± S.D.), respectively. This indicates that a greater proportion of pregnenolone is converted to testosterone in matured cells. This developmental change in steroid production is correlated with a change in the number of α-NE–positive Leydig cells (FIGURE 1). In preparations from immature rats, 40–50% Leydig cells (3β-HSD positive) and no α-NE–positive cells are present, α-NE–positive Leydig cells emerge from approximately 30 days onwards and in mature rats all 3β-HSD–positive (Leydig) cells are also α-NE positive. In addition approximately 10% of the cells are α-NE positive, but not 3β-HSD positive (FIGURE 1).

The presence of macrophage characteristics was investigated in cell preparations from 21–23- and 60–90-day-old rats by studying the presence of phagocytic cells and specific macrophage antigens. Phagocytosis was determined by incubation of the cells in the presence of fluorescent beads (ϕ 1.7 μm) and macrophage antigens were detected by labeling with monoclonal antibodies against macrophages (raised in mice).

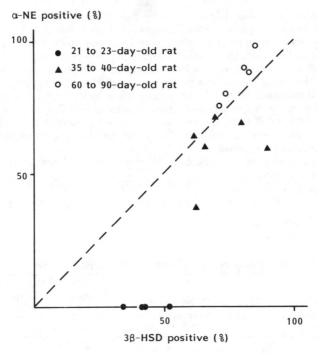

FIGURE 1. Age-dependent correlation between 3β-HSD and α-NE activity.

In cell preparations from immature rats, 50% of the 3β-HSD–positive cells were phagocytic. No binding of macrophage antibodies on these cells was observed. In cell preparations from mature rats, 3β-HSD–positive cells are not active in phagocytosis whereas less than 10% of α-NE–positive cells showed activity. Specific binding of macrophage antibodies was observed on approximately 90% of the cells. This indicates that membranes from Leydig cells contain specific macrophage antigens. Binding of rabbit immunoglobulins, but not of the F_{ab} fragment, was observed, indicating that F_c receptors are present on the Leydig cell membrane. These results are summarized in TABLE 2. Preparations of peritoneal

TABLE 2. Summary of Properties of Leydig Cells and Macrophages

Property	Immature Rats	Mature Rats	
	Leydig Cell/Macrophage?	Leydig Cell	Macrophage
3β-HSD activity	+	+	−
α-NE activity	−	+	+
Phagocytosis	+	−	+
Macrophage membrane antigen	−	+	+
F_c receptor	−	+	+
Steroid production	+	+	?

macrophages were highly active in phagocytosis but negative in 3β-HSD and α-NE activity and no binding of antibodies was observed.

The results indicate that in immature rats steroidogenic activities and phagocytic activity may reside in one cell type, whereas in mature rats these functions occur in different cell types. Furthermore, it appeared that during maturation Leydig cells acquire α-NE activity and membrane antigens that are also present on macrophages.

We have concluded from these results that functional properties of Leydig cells and macrophages change during development and similar functions may be present in both cell types. This may indicate that regulation of Leydig cell and macrophage functions involves partly similar mechanisms.

REFERENCES

1. BORN, W. & H. WEKERLE. 1981. Eur. J. Cell Biol. **25:** 76–81.
2. CIGORRAGA, S. B., S. SORRELL, J. BATOR, K. J. CATT & M. L. DUFAU. 1980. J. Clin. Invest. **65:** 699–705.
3. MOLENAAR, R., F. F. G. ROMMERTS & H. J. VAN DER MOLEN. 1983. Int. J. Androl. **6:** 261–274.
4. RIVENSON, A., T. OHMORI, M. HAMAZAKI & R. MADDEN. 1981. Cell. Molec. Biol. **27:** 49–56.

"Antigonadal" Activity of the Neurohypophysial Hormones: Direct in Vivo Regulation of Leydig Cell Function[a]

ELI Y. ADASHI and CAROL E. RESNICK

Division of Reproductive Endocrinology
Department of Obstetrics & Gynecology
University of Maryland School of Medicine
Baltimore, Maryland 21201

The neurohypophysial hormones were recently shown to exert a direct inhibitory effect on gonadotropin-stimulated androgen biosynthesis by cultured rat testicular cells.[1] The present study was undertaken to investigate this "antigonadal" activity of the neurohypophysial principles under *in vivo* conditions and to further characterize their mechanism(s) and site(s) of action. Control and FSH-maintained immature hypophysectomized male rats received either vehicle or arginine vasotocin (AVT, 25 μg/rat, s.c.) for five days. The testes of each *in vivo* treatment group were pooled, weighed, and assayed for their LH/hCG binding capacity and affinity or incubated for 3 hr in the presence of MIX (10^{-4} M), with or without hCG (500 ng/ml) or forskolin (10^{-5} M). Media were assayed for their cAMP and androgen (total testosterone immunoreactivity) content by radioimmunoassays.

Control rats receiving vehicle or AVT did not differ significantly in testicular weight, LH/hCG binding capacity (FIGURE 1) and affinity, or *in vitro* responsiveness to hCG stimulation (FIGURE 2). Relative to controls, treatment with FSH increased testicular weight (1.4-fold), LH/hCG binding capacity (1.6-fold), (FIGURE 1) as well as the hCG-stimulated accumulation of extracellular cAMP (63-fold) (FIGURE 2), and androgen (3.5-fold). However, concomitant treatment with AVT substantially decreased the FSH-maintained testicular LH/hCG binding capacity (64% inhibition) (FIGURE 1) as well as the hCG-stimulated accumulation of extracellular cAMP (98% inhibition) (FIGURE 2) and androgen (46% inhibition). Treatment with AVT also decreased forskolin-stimulated androgen biosynthesis but was without significant effect on the FSH-maintained testicular weight (FSH 128 ± 4 mg; FSH + AVT = 119 ± 3 mg) and LH/hCG binding affinity ($K_d = 1.6 ± 0.4 \times 10^{-10}$ M). These findings suggest that the direct "antigonadal" activity of the neurohypophysial hormones, previously demonstrated *in vitro*, can be fully reproduced *in vivo*. The mechanisms underlying this "antigonadal" effect may thus include a decrease in testicular LH/hCG binding capacity and inhibition of hCG-sensitive Leydig cell adenylate cyclase activity and androgen biosynthesis. The ability of AVT to suppress forskolin-stimulated Leydig cell androgen biosynthesis suggests that the "antigonadal" activity of the neurohypophysial hormones is exerted, in large part, at post LH/hCG receptor site(s).

[a] Supported in part by the Frank G. Bressler Research Fund

AVT has previously been shown to exert profound pharmacological inhibitory effects on male reproductive functions *in vivo*.[2-5] Although AVT may have exerted its inhibitory effect *in vivo* by reducing the release of pituitary gonadotropins,[6,7] the possibility of a direct antigonadal effect could not be ruled out. The present findings using hypophysectomized rats suggest that the *in vivo* "antigonadal" activity of AVT in the intact animal is due, in part, to direct inhibition of testicular function. Since the reported circulating concentrations of the neurohypophysial hormones in various adult mammals including humans are of the order

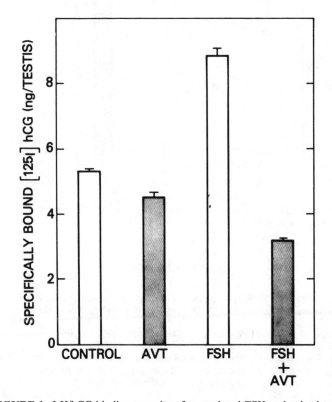

FIGURE 1. LH/hCG binding capacity of control and FSH-maintained testes.

of 10^{-12}–10^{-11} M, and since the minimal effective "antigonadal" dose *in vitro* is 10^{-10} M, it is unlikely that endogenous, blood-borne neurohypophysial principles are of physiologic relevance to testicular function. It is therefore tempting to speculate that the putative, pressor-selective testicular recognition sites subserve neurohypophysial hormones or closely related peptides that may be produced within the testis, yielding local concentrations high enough ($>10^{-10}$ M) to exert *in situ* paracrine or autocrine regulation of testicular functions.

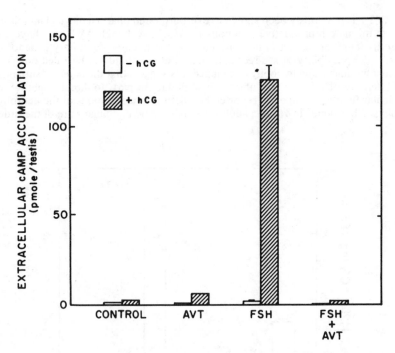

FIGURE 2. Basal and hCG-stimulated accumulation of extracellular cAMP *in vitro* by control and FSH-maintained testes. Modulation by AVT.

REFERENCES

1. ADASHI, E. Y. & A. J. W. HSUEH. 1981. Direct inhibition of testicular androgen biosynthesis revealing antigonadal activity of neurohypophysial hormones. Nature **293:** 650–652.
2. VAUGHAN, M. K., G. M. VAUGHAN & D. C. KLEIN. 1974. Arginine vasotocin: Effects on development of reproductive organs. Science **186:** 938–939.
3. VAUGHAN, M. K., R. J. REITER, T., MCKINNEY & G. M. VAUGHAN. 1974. Inhibition of growth of gonadal dependent structures by arginine vasotocin and purified bovine pineal fractions in immature mice and hamsters. Int. J. Fertil. **19:** 103–106.
4. YAMASHITA, K., M. MIENO & E. R. YAMASHITA. 1979. Suppression of the luteinizing hormone releasing effect of luteinizing hormone releasing hormone by arginine vasotocin. J. Endocrinol. **81:** 103–108.
5. YAMASHITA, K., M. MIENO & E. R. YAMASHITA. 1980. Suppression of the luteinizing hormone releasing effect of luteinizing hormone releasing hormone by arginine vasotocin in immature male dogs. J. Endocrinol. **84:** 449–452.
6. VAUGHAN, M. K., D. E. BLACK, L. Y. JOHNSON & R. J. REITER. 1979. The effect of subcutaneous injections of malatonin, arginine vasotocin and related peptides on pituitary and plasma levels of luteinizing hormone, follicle-stimulating hormone, and prolactin in castrated adult male rats. Endocrinology **104:** 212–217.
7. PAVEL, S., N. LUCA, M. CALB & R. GOLDSTEIN. 1979. Inhibition of release of luteinizing hormone in the male rat by extremely small amounts of arginine vasotocin: Further evidence for the involvement of 5-hydroxytryptamine-containing neurons in the mechanism of action of arginine vasotocin. Endocrinology **104:** 517–523.

Comparison of LH and LHRH Agonist Action on Steroidogenesis in Rat Leydig Cells

AXEL P. N. THEMMEN,[a] FOCKO F. G. ROMMERTS, and
HENK J. VAN DER MOLEN

Division of Chemical Endocrinology
Department of Biochemistry
Medical Faculty
Erasmus University
Rotterdam, The Netherlands

INTRODUCTION

Steroidogenesis in rat Leydig cells is regulated mainly by the pituitary hormone LH. The cholesterol side-chain cleavage enzyme (CSCC), which converts cholesterol into pregnenolone, is the rate-limiting step in Leydig cell steroidogenesis. Stimulation of this enzyme by LH is accompanied by increased levels of cAMP, protein kinase activation, stimulated protein phosphorylation of at least six proteins, and requires continuous protein synthesis.[2] Ca^{2+} and calmodulin may be involved also in CSCC activation.[3] Recently it has been shown that LHRH and its agonists also can stimulate steroid production in Leydig cells, but the mechanism of action is unknown. We have studied effects of LHRH agonist on cAMP levels, protein phosphorylation, Ca^{2+} involvement, and steroid production in collagenase-dispersed Leydig cells from immature (21 day old) rats. Methods used for isolation and incubation of Leydig cells as well as analytical methods have been described elsewhere.[1,4]

RESULTS AND DISCUSSION

Short-term and long-term effects of LHRH agonist (LHRHa) were investigated with a maximally stimulating dose of the LHRH agonist (Hoe-766; 50 ng/ml), according to Sharpe and Cooper.[6] This dose of LHRHa stimulated steroid production ninefold. Steroid production was stimulated 30–60-fold when a maximally stimulating dose of LH was used. This effect of LHRHa, but not that of LH, was abolished when the LHRH antagonist ORG-30093D (0.5 μg/ml) was present. The maximally LH-stimulated steroid production could not be further stimulated when LHRH was present. Steroid production in cells incubated for 48 hr without hormones could still be stimulated by LH, but not by LHRHa. No significant effect on the maximally LH-stimulated steroid production could be shown when cells were incubated for 48 hr either in the presence of LH or LHRHa. However,

---

[a] Address correspondence to: A. P. N. Themmen, Department of Biochemistry II, Medical Faculty, Erasmus University Rotterdam, P.O. Box 1738, 3000 DR Rotterdam, The Netherlands.

the LH-stimulated steroid production was decreased when cells had been cultured for 48 hr with LH together with LHRHa. This inhibitory effect of LHRHa was abolished when ORG-30093D was present during the 48 hr incubation period.

Steroid production in isolated Leydig cells can be stimulated by LH within several minutes.[5] Effects of LHRH, however, have only been observed after several hours.[6] This difference in kinetics of LH and LHRH action may reflect that the mechanism of action of these hormones is not the same. Kinetic studies with LH and LHRH were therefore carried out. Cells were incubated with or without hormones for 3 hr and steroid concentrations in the incubation media were measured every 10 min. The results in FIGURE 1 show that stimulation of

KINETICS OF LH AND LHRH-A ACTION

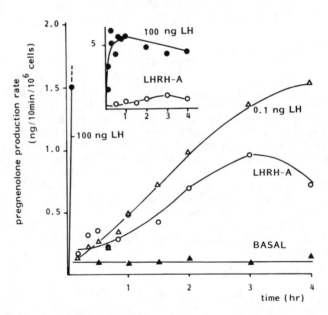

FIGURE 1. Kinetics of LH and LHRH agonist action on pregnenolone production by isolated Leydig cells. Pregnenolone production per 10 min was calculated from the concentrations of pregnenolone in culture media from cells incubated during different periods. Mean results of triplicate determinations are shown.

steroid production by 100 ng/ml LH starts a few minutes after addition of LH and that full stimulation was obtained within approximately 30 min. The first significant effects of LHRHa could be detected after approximately 20 min, whereas for the maximum effect 3 hr were required. The results also show that more than 3 hr are required to reach a steady-state stimulation of steroid production with 0.1 ng LH/ml. Stimulatory effects of low concentrations of LH may therefore be underestimated when relatively short incubation periods are used. As a consequence, the dose-response relationship of LH action on steroid production becomes dependent on the duration of the incubation period. The results also indicate that the mechanism of action of high and low concentrations of LH may be different and that the mechanism of action of LHRH and the low dose of LH appear similar in this respect. Moreover, comparisons between the effects of LH and LHRH analogues must at least include experiments with concentrations of LH and LHRHa that stimulate steroid production to the same degree.

It is generally accepted that LH stimulates steroid production via cAMP as second messenger and that phosphoproteins are somehow involved in the ultimate regulation of the CSCC activity. The effect of LHRHa on cellular cAMP levels in Leydig cells sometimes incubated in the presence of 1-methyl-3-isobutyl-xanthine (MIX) was therefore compared with that of LH. In the presence of 100 ngLH/ml cAMP levels were approximately sixfold increased (basal: 6.4 ± 2.1; 100 ng/ml LH: 37.4 ± 9.1 pmol cAMP/10^6 cells), but no significant effects could be shown when 0.2 ng LH/ml or 50 ng/ml LHRHa were used. Pregnenolone production stimulated by 0.2 ng LH/ml, however, was further stimulated by addition of MIX (0.2 ng/ml LH: 5.9 ± 1.6; with MIX: 27.6 ± 4.0 ng pregnenolone/hr $\times$ 10^6 cells; cAMP: 0.2 ng/ml LH: 7.7/9.8; with MIX: 7.1 ± 1.8 pmol cAMP/10^6 cells), which indicates an involvement of cAMP action with this dose of LH. LHRHa action was not affected by MIX, which argues against an important role of cAMP. The results show also that small and almost undetectable changes in cAMP can cause complete stimulation of steroid production. Measurements of cAMP are thus inadequate for discerning the mechanisms of action of hormone concentrations, which do not overstimulate the cell. In order to compare with more sensitive techniques the effects of LH and LHRH, we have measured endogenous protein phosphorylation in intact cells as a parameter for intracellular cAMP action on protein kinase activity. The patterns of ^{32}P-labeled phosphoproteins after separation of cellular proteins on SDS gels showed that the intensity of the 17,000 and 33,000 dalton phosphoproteins was increased after incubations of cells with 100 ng LH/ml, confirming earlier observations.[2] The highest increase was observed for the phosphorylation of the 17,000 dalton protein. The effect of 0.2 ng LH/ml on protein phosphorylation was much less, although effects of LH could still be detected for both proteins. It appears that the resolution of the one-dimensional separation system is a major limitation for the detection of the other LH-dependent phosphoproteins. When LHRHa was employed to stimulate steroid production, no changes in protein phosphorylation could be shown. Apparently, LHRH acts differently from LH (not via cAMP?) and it could be possible that the LH-dependent phosphoproteins are not a prerequisite for stimulation of CSCC activity. Calcium appears to be involved in regulation of steroid production in Leydig cells.[3] Increasing concentrations of the calcium ionophore A23187 caused a progressive inhibition of the effect of high concentrations of LH on steroid production. However, the production of pregnenolone in the presence of 25-hydroxycholesterol, which is independent of LH action, was also inhibited by the ionophore. This indicates that 1–10 μM ionophore acts aspecifically, which makes it difficult to draw definite conclusions about the mechanisms of hormone stimulation. On the other hand, no effects of any ionophore concentration on the action of LHRHa or low concentrations of LH could be demonstrated. These results may suggest that these LH or LHRHa actions are not affected by increased intracellular calcium levels. For expression of LH and LHRHa action extracellular calcium is required. Low concentrations of extracellular calcium reduce the maximal steroidogenic response triggered by LH or LHRHa and the effects of LH and LHRHa at the various calcium concentrations are inhibited in a similar fashion. In this respect LH and LHRHa action have the same requirements for calcium.

The different effects of low and high concentrations of LH on protein phosphorylation and kinetics of steroid production as well as the different effects of A23187 on high and low dose LH-stimulated steroid production, may indicate that, depending on the concentration, LH action on Leydig cells may require other mediators in addition to cAMP. LHRH action may depend more on other mediators than on cAMP and the role of calcium should be investigated further as a possible alternative mediator in Leydig cells.

REFERENCES

1. BAKKER, G. H., J. W. HOOGERBRUGGE, F. F. G. ROMMERTS & H. J. VAN DER MOLEN. 1981. Biochem. J. **198:** 339–346.
2. BAKKER, G. H., J. W. HOOGERBRUGGE, F. F. G. ROMMERTS & H. J. VAN DER MOLEN. 1982. Biochem. J. **204:** 809–815.
3. HALL, P. F., S. OSAWA & J. MROTEK. 1981. Endocrinology **109:** 1677–1682.
4. MOLENAAR, R., F. F. G. ROMMERTS & H. J. VAN DER MOLEN. 1983. Int. J. Androl. **6:** 261–274.
5. ROMMERTS, F. F. G., M. J. A. VAN ROEMBURG, L. M. LINDH, J. A. J. HEGGE & H. J. VAN DER MOLEN. 1982. J. Reprod. Fertil. **65:** 289–297.
6. SHARPE, R. M. & I. COOPER. 1982. Mol. Cell. Endocr. **27:** 199–211.

Acute Stimulation of Rat Leydig Cell Steroidogenesis by Gonadotropin-releasing Hormone: Investigation of the Mechanism of Action[a]

WILLIAM H. MOGER

Departments of Physiology & Biophysics
and of Obstetrics & Gynecology
Dalhousie University
Halifax, Nova Scotia B3H 4H7, Canada

Whether a gonadotropin-releasing-hormone analog (GnRHa) acutely stimulates Leydig cell steroidogenesis via receptor-mediated adenylate cyclase activation has been studied by comparing the effect of forskolin (which augments such activation in a variety of tissues[1]) on LH and GnRHa concentration-response curves. In addition, three steroidogenesis inhibitors that block LH-induced androgen formation at steps beyond cAMP formation have been investigated for their ability to inhibit GnRHa-induced steroidogenesis.

Collagenase-dispersed interstitial cells from adult Sprague-Dawley rats were prepared and incubated as described by Sharpe and Cooper.[2] Forskolin (Calbiochem-Behring), LH (NIH-LH-B9), des Gly[10],D-Ala[6] N-ethylamidine GnRH (GnRHa, Sigma), cobalt chloride (BDH), cycloheximide (Sigma), and/or Nα-p-tosyl-lysylchloromethylketone (TLCK, Sigma) were added at the start of the incubation.

In the presence or absence of 0.1 μM forskolin, increasing concentrations of LH stimulated androgen output from 3.25 $\pm$ 0.16 ng/10^6 cells/4 hr to a maximum of 13.1 $\pm$ 0.92 ng/10^6 cells/4 hr. However, forskolin caused a left-shift in the LH concentration-response curve (FIGURE 1, upper panel) reducing the concentration of LH required for half-maximum stimulation (EC$_{50}$) from 0.82 ng/ml to 0.16 ng/ml and the EC$_{100}$ from 3 ng/ml to 1 ng/ml.

As shown in FIGURE 1 (lower panel) forskolin (0.1 μM) had very little effect on the GnRHa concentration-response curve. Forskolin alone increased basal androgen production from 5.36 $\pm$ 0.31 ng/10^6 cells/4 hr to 7.22 $\pm$ 0.33 ng/10^6 cells/4 hr and the response to maximum GnRHa stimulation was also increased from 16.3 $\pm$ 0.9 to 22.3 $\pm$ 1.0 ng/10^6 cells/4 hr. However, forskolin had no effect on the GnRHa EC$_{100}$ (1 nM) and caused only a small, though significant, reduction in the GnRHa EC$_{50}$ from 0.24 nM to 0.15 nM. Similar results were obtained with 0.3 μM forskolin, except that forskolin did not significantly alter the GnRHa EC$_{50}$ (data not shown).

As forskolin potentiates agonists that are generally believed to activate steroidogenesis via cAMP formation,[3,4] the lack of a consistent and substantial reduction in the EC$_{50}$ for GnRHa-activated steroidogenesis in the presence of

[a] Supported by Grant MT-5401 from the Medical Research Council (Canada).

629

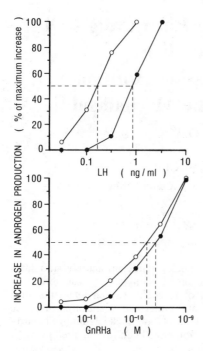

FIGURE 1. GnRHa (lower panel) and LH (upper panel) concentration-response curves in the absence (closed symbol) or presence (open symbol) of 0.1 μM forskolin. Each point is the mean of five replicates. The SEM (not shown) are less than 10% of the mean. Dashed lines lead to the EC_{50}.

forskolin is evidence that GnRHa does not stimulate androgen production via cAMP formation. However, three steroidogenesis inhibitors that inhibit LH-induced androgen secretion at sites between cAMP formation and cholesterol side-chain cleavage[5-7] also inhibit GnRHa-evoked steroidogenesis (TABLE 1).

A hypothesis to account for these results is that GnRHa-receptor interaction causes the activation of a non-cAMP-dependent protein kinase (possibly a calcium- and phospholipid-dependent kinase). If the GnRHa-activated kinase phosphorylates the same, or some of the same, proteins phosphorylated by the cAMP-dependent protein kinase activated by LH-receptor interaction, the pathway to increased steroidogenesis would be common from this point.

TABLE 1. Effect of Steroidogenesis Inhibitors on LH- and GnRHa-induced Androgen Production

	Agonist		
Inhibitor	None	LH (30 ng/ml)	GnRHa (10 nM)
None	2.1 ± 0.2[a]	22.8 ± 1.1	9.4 ± 0.3
CoCl$_2$ (1mM)	1.4 ± 0.2	2.7 ± 0.1	1.6 ± 0.1
None	5.6 ± 0.2	89.1 ± 4.0	24.8 ± 5.7
Cycloheximide (3 μM)	4.1 ± 0.4	17.5 ± 1.7	5.3 ± 0.5
None	4.9 ± 0.1	57.9 ± 1.6	17.5 ± 0.5
TLCK (1 mM)	2.9 ± 0.1	2.5 ± 0.3	3.4 ± 0.1

[a] Androgen production (ng/10⁶ cells/4 hr), mean ± SEM of five replicates.

REFERENCES

1. SEAMON, K. B. & J. W. DALY. 1983. Trends Pharmacol. Sci. **4:** 120–123.
2. SHARPE, R. M. & I. COOPER. 1982. Mol. Cell. Endocrinol. **26:** 141–150.
3. MORIWAKI, K., Y. ITOH, S. IIDA & K. ICHIHARA. 1982. Life Sci. **30:** 2235–2240.
4. MOGER, W. H. & O. O. ANAKWE. 1984. Biol. Reprod. (In press.)
5. MOGER, W. H. 1983. Biol. Reprod. **28:** 528–535.
6. COOKE, B. A., L. M. LINDH & H. J. VAN DER MOLEN. 1979. Biochem. J. **184:** 33–38.
7. MOGER, W. H. In preparation.

Testicular Tyrosine-specific Protein Kinase Activity: High Levels in Purified Leydig Cells

MICHAEL H. MELNER,[a,b] DAVID PUETT,[a,b]
DAVID L. GARBERS,[c,d,e] and LARRY DANGOTT[c,d]

*aDepartments of Biochemistry,[c] Pharmacology, [e]Physiology and
the [d]Howard Hughes Medical Institute Laboratory
Vanderbilt University School of Medicine
Nashville, Tennessee 37232*

The tyrosine protein kinases are a group of enzymes that phosphorylate the tyrosine side chains of proteins.[1,2] These kinase activities have been found associated with retrovirus-transforming proteins, e.g. pp60[src] of Rous sarcoma virus,[3] and a number of mitogenic growth factor receptors, e.g. for epidermal growth factor,[2,4] insulin,[5-7] platelet-derived growth factor,[8-9] and insulin-like growth factor 1.[7] These findings indicate that a relationship may exist between tyrosine protein kinase activity and the regulation of cell growth, but the exact role of the enzymes is not known.

Recently it was reported in a study using a synthetic peptide as substrate, that a substantial amount of tyrosine protein kinase activity occurs in rat testes and other tissues.[8] Herein, the peptide, NH_2-GLU-ASP-ALA-GLU-TYR-ALA-ALA-ARG-ARG-ARG-GLY-COOH, was used as substrate to measure tyrosine-specific protein kinase activity in different cellular fractions of the rat testis including two purified populations of Leydig cells.

Leydig cells, germinal cells, and red blood cells were isolated on discontinuous Metrizamide density gradients by the method of O'Shaughnessy *et al.*[9] Individual tubules were collected after brief collagenase treatment. Cells were homogenized in 10 mM HEPES, 150 mM NaCl, 1 mM MgCl, pH 7.2, and subcellular fractions prepared by centrifugation. Following a $1,000 \times g$ pellet, 90% of the tyrosine kinase activity was localized in the $30,000 \times g$ pellet, which was used for all assays described. Peptide substrates were synthesized[10] and phosphorylation was performed as described earlier.[8]

Tyrosine-specific protein kinase activity in Leydig cells was consistently 6–20-fold higher than in any other cell type purified from rat testes (FIGURE 1). The activity in particulate fractions from population I Leydig cells was ~50% higher than that observed in fractions from population II Leydig cells.

The effect of amino acid deletions or insertions in the peptide substrates on specific activity was measured in the particulate fractions from the Leydig cell populations and is presented in TABLE 1. As expected, replacement of a single tyrosine with phenylalanine (E_{10}-F-G_1) eliminates phosphorylation of the peptide. A comparison of activities using $E_{11}G_1$ and $E_{10}G_1$ suggests that an additional arginine residue doubles the apparent specific activity of the enzyme.

[b] Present address: The Reproductive Sciences and Endocrinology Laboratories, Department of Biochemistry, University of Miami School of Medicine, P.O. Box 016129, Miami, Florida 33101.

TABLE 1. Tyrosine Protein Kinase Activity in Rat Leydig Cell Particulate Fractions Using Different Synthetic Peptide Substrates

Peptide Designation	Amino Acid Sequence	Specific Activity (% of maximum)	
		Leydig I	Leydig II
A8-G1	ALA-GLU-*TYR*-ALA-ALA-ARG-ARG-GLY	42	23
E10-G1	GLU-ASP-ALA-GLU-*TYR*-ALA-ALA-ARG-ARG-GLY	56	48
E10-F-G1	GLU-ASP-ALA-GLU-*PHE*-ALA-ALA-ARG-ARG-GLY	0	0
E11-G1	GLU-ASP-ALA-GLU-*TYR*-ALA-ALA-ARG-ARG-ARG-GLY	100	100
L13-G1	LEU-ILE-GLU-GLU-ASP-ALA-GLU-*TYR*-ALA-ALA-ARG-ARG-ARG-GLY	44	17

All assays performed at a peptide concentration of 1 mM with 60 μM [γ-^{32}P]ATP, 50 mM MgCl$_2$, 10 μM vanadate, and 0.02% NP-40. The amount of protein assayed was 2.0 μg for population I and II Leydig cell particulate fractions, respectively. The amino terminal residue is shown to the far left in each peptide.

These studies have demonstrated the presence of high tyrosine protein kinase activity (56–165 pmol/mg/min) in purified Leydig cells from rat testis relative to other testicular cells. The finding that population I Leydig cells exhibit nearly twice the tyrosine protein kinase activity of population II cells is of interest in light of the suggestion by Chase and Payne that population II Leydig cells may be derived from population I cells during sexual maturation.[11]

Although tyrosine protein kinase activity has been implicated in the processes of cell transformation and growth,[2,12] its function remains unclear. Further studies on Leydig cells and other normal cells may help elucidate the physiological role of these kinases.

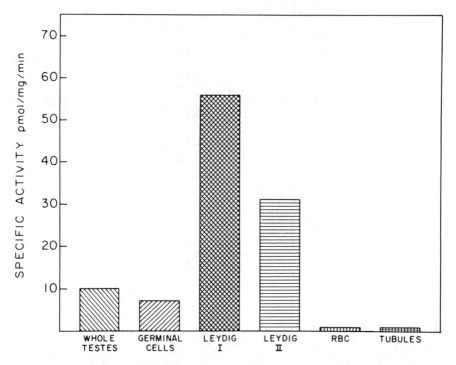

FIGURE 1. Tyrosine protein kinase activity in particulate fractions from purified cells in normal rat testes. All assays were performed at 30°C for 10 min with 60 μM [γ-^{32}P]ATP, 50 mM MgCl$_2$, 10 μM *ortho*vanadate, 1 mM E$_{11}$G$_1$ peptide, and 0.02% NP-40.

REFERENCES

1. ERICKSON, R. L., M. S. COLLETT, E. ERICKSON, A. F. PURCHIO & J. S. BRUGGE. 1980. Cold Spring Harbor Symp. Quant. Biol. **44:** 907–917.
2. USHIRO, H. & S. COHEN. 1980. J. Biol. Chem. **255:** 8363–8365.
3. HUNTER, T. & B. M. SEFTON. 1980. Proc. Natl. Acad. Sci. USA **77:** 1311–1315.
4. COHEN, S., R. A. FAVA & S. T. SAWYER. 1982. Proc. Natl. Acad. Sci. USA **79:** 6237–6241.

5. KASUGA, M., Y. ZICK, D. L. BLITHE, M. CRETAZZ & C. R. KAHN. 1982. Nature **298:** 667–669.
6. KASUGA, M., Y. FUJITA-YAMAGUCHI, D. L. BLITHE & C. R. KAHN. 1983. Proc. Natl. Acad. Sci. USA **80:** 2137–2141.
7. SHIA, M. A. & P. F. PILCH. 1983. Biochemistry **22:** 717–721.
8. SWARUP, G., J. D. DASGUPTA & D. L. GARBERS. 1983. J. Biol. Chem. **258:** 10341–10347.
9. O'SHAUGHNESSY, P. J., K. L. WONG & A. H. PAYNE. 1981. Endocrinology **109:** 1061–1066.
10. GARBERS, D. L., H. D. WATKINS, J. R. HANSBROUGH, A. SMITH & K. S. MISONO. 1982. J. Biol. Chem. **257:** 2734–2737.
11. CHASE, D. J. & A. H. PAYNE. 1983. Endocrinology **112:** 29–34.
12. HUNTER, T. & J. A. COOPER. 1981. Cell **24:** 741–752.

Ultrastructural, Morphometric, and Functional Characterization of Interstitial Cells from Mouse Testes Fractionated on Percoll Density Gradients

J. B. KERR, D. M. ROBERTSON, and D. M. de KRETSER

Department of Anatomy
Monash University
Clayton 3168, Victoria, Australia.

Previous studies on isolated rat[1-4] and mouse[4-5] Leydig cells present in enriched fractions of interstitial cells obtained by density gradient centrifugation have demonstrated two or more bands of interstitial cells that differ in buoyant density and exhibit peaks of specific binding of ^{125}I-hCG. The presence of hCG binding has been interpreted to represent different populations of Leydig cells. The cells of greater density show significantly greater testosterone (T) production *in vitro* in response to luteinizing hormone (LH)/hCG stimulation.[1-4,6-8] An alternative interpretation is that differences in steroidogenesis are more likely an artifact resulting from damage to the Leydig cells during tissue dissociation and cell isolation in the density gradients. The latter suggestion has been supported by recent reports[6,9-11] indicating that different dissociation methods applied to rat or mouse testes (mechanical and/or collagenase dispersion) may result in significant variations in Leydig cell yield, viability, and receptor and steroidogenic properties. The ability of isolated interstitial cell suspensions to respond to *in vitro* LH/hCG stimulation used in these studies relies upon expressing the production of T in relation to the estimated number of Leydig cells present in suspension. Accurate identification of a Leydig cell within mixtures of interstitial and germ cells is therefore of importance in deriving conclusions from these experiments. Leydig cell morphology is a most reliable guide for identification of these cells. Yet in most studies the histochemical demonstration of 3β-hydroxysteroid dehydrogenase, phenyl esterase, the presence of LH/hCG receptors, or the observation of yellow haloes seen with phase-contrast microscopy have each been considered as acceptable markers for identification of isolated Leydig cells. In this study adult mouse testes were dissociated by mechanical or collagenase dispersion and comparison of the ultrastructure, hCG receptor properties, and hCG-stimulated T production of interstitial cells was obtained following separation in Percoll density gradients. Gradients were fractionated according to specific gravity and all cell types were quantitated using morphometric techniques. Three peaks of ^{125}I-hCG binding of density 1.0667 g/cm^3 (fractions 2–3), 1.045 g/cm^3 (fractions 6–7), and 1.0365–1.0215 g/cm (fraction 9) were noted following collagenase but not mechanical dispersion, the second peak being absent from the latter. Morphometry (light microscopy) was applied to fractions of the first and second binding peaks, the third not being studied further as it contained germ cells and membrane debris. In both methods

636

of preparation, morphologically intact Leydig cells represented 60–80% and 7–10% of the cells in respective fractions 2–3 and 6–7 associated with the first and second peaks of hCG binding. Similar numbers of hCG receptors were found on mechanically dispersed Leydig cells but hCG-stimulated T production per Leydig cell was significantly greater for denser Leydig cells containing few lipid inclusions, in contrast to the lipid-rich lighter Leydig cells. T production by dense and light collagenase-dispersed Leydig cells was not significantly different. The second hCG binding peak in collagenase-dispersed cell fractions was associated with 40–60% interstitial mesenchymal cells, whose ultrastructure and limited ^{125}I-hCG binding capacity suggested that they may represent Leydig cell precursors preferentially released from the testes by collagenase treatment. It is concluded that the identification and quantitation of different cell types in isolated testicular cell fractions are of central importance in the interpretation of receptor and secretory capacities of enriched preparations of Leydig cells.

REFERENCES

1. JANSZEN, F. H. A., B. A. COOKE, M. J. A. VAN DRIEL & H. J. VAN DER MOLEN. 1976. J. Endocr. **70:** 345–359.
2. PAYNE, A. H., J. R. DOWNING & K. L. WONG. 1980. Endocrinology 106: 1424–1429.
3. BROWNING, J. Y., R. D'AGATA & H. E. GROTJAN. 1981. Endocrinology 109: 667–669.
4. COOKE, B. A., R. MAGEE-BROWN, M. GOLDING & C. J. DIX. 1981. Int. J. Androl. 4: 355–366.
5. SCHUMACHER, M., G. SCHAFER, A. F. HOLSTEIN & H. HILZ. 1978. F.E.B.S. Lett. **91:** 333–338.
6. DEHEJIA, A., K. NOZU, K. J. CATT & M. L. DUFAU. 1982. J. Biol. Chem. **257:** 13781–13786.
7. PAYNE, A. H., D. J. CHASE & P. J. O'SHAUGHNESSY. 1982. *In* Cellular Regulation of Secretion and Release. P.M. Conn, Ed.:355–408. Academic Press. New York.
8. PAYNE, A. H., P. J. O'SHAUGHNESSY, D. J. CHASE, G. E. K. DIXON & A. K. CHRISTENSEN. 1982. Ann. N.Y. Acad. Sci. 383: 174–200.
9. SHARPE, R. M. & I. COOPER. 1982. J. Reprod. Fertil. **65:** 475–481.
10. ALDRED, L. F. & B. A. COOKE. 1982. Int. J. Androl. **5:** 191–195.
11. MOLENAAR, R., F. F. G. ROMMERTS & H. J. VAN DER MOLEN. 1983. Int. J. Androl. **6:** 261–274.

A Model System to Study the Morphogenic and Steroidogenic Effects of Various Gonadotropins on the Leydig Cell of the Boar

M. MESURE-MORAT and J. P. DUFAURE

Laboratory of Cell Biology
University of Clermont-Ferrand II
B.P. 45
63170 Aubière, France

INTRODUCTION—MATERIALS AND METHODS

The boar testis was chosen because it contains a great number of large polyhedric Leydig cells providing a good opportunity to perform morphometric analysis. Our model system consists of small pieces of testis from adult animals hypophysectomized since 1 to 3 months of age, which were maintained in static organ cultures with medium 199, 10% calf serum, and 250 I.U./ml of penicillin (Trowell's method,[1] modified by Lasnitzski,[2] adapted to pig testis material[3]). This medium was supplemented or not with hormones (hCG, LH, or FSH) or other components (related antihormones, cAMP, and dibutyryl cAMP). Results were analyzed both by microscopic examination and measures at histological and cytological levels,[4] and by measurements (radioimmunoassays[5]) of the steroids released into the medium for 24 hours (testosterone, dihydrotestosterone, androstenedione, and dehydroepiandrosterone sulfate).

We have previously shown that hypophysectomy[4,6] was followed by a dramatic reduction in the size of the Leydig cells, of their nucleus, and of their organelles (particularly those involved in steroidogenesis), but by only a slight decrease in their number, although testosterone was not more detectable in the plasma.[7] *In vivo*, these modifications were reversed by injection of hCG.[6,8] From 2 days to 10 days of culture with 10 I.U./ml of hCG, the size of the cells and of their nucleus increased, cytoplasmic structures associated to steroidogenesis developed, and the four steroids were released into the medium. The full activity was reached after 10 days of culture (testosterone: 80 ng/ml of medium/24 hr corresponding to 13.2 ng/mg of tissue/24 hr); then activity decreased regularly and irreversibly (except for one case).[9]

The system was further used to study the dose-response effects of hCG, of various hypophyseal gonadotropins (porcine, ovine, bovine, and human LH and FSH),[a] given alone or combined with their related antihormone, and of the intracellular mediator cAMP.

---

[a] Ovine LH NIH-LH-S20, × 1.19 NIH-LH-S1 units/mg, <5% NIH-FSH-S1. Bovine LH NIH-LH-B19, × 1.06 NIH-LH-S1 units/mg, <5% NIH-FSH-S1. Human LH LER-960, very slight FSH contamination. Ovine FSH NIH-FSH-S12, × 1.25 NIH-FSH-S1 units/mg, <1% NIH-LH-S1. Bovine FSH NIH-FSH-B1, × 0.49 NIH-FSH-S1 units/mg, <1% NIH-LH-S1. Porcine FSH NIH-FSH-P2, × 0.69 NIH-FSH-S1 units/mg, <1% NIH-LH-S1. Human FSH NIH-FSH-HS-1, = 3.7% LH.

RESULTS AND DISCUSSION

Dose-response Effects of hCG

The best reactivation was obtained with a concentration of 10 I.U./ml (testosterone production: 80 ng/ml of medium/24 hr) (FIGURE 1). We have estimated at 0.06 pg/cell/24 hr the release of testosterone into the medium. For Christensen and Peacock[10] the normal rat Leydig cell produces 0.22 pg of testosterone/cell/24 hr. When we increased (100 I.U./ml) or reduced (1, 0.1, 0.01, 0.001 I.U./ml) the concentration, the steroids production decreased by half at the 0.01 I.U./ml concentration and to control level for the lowest concentration.

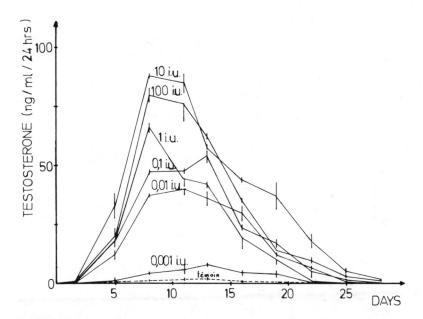

FIGURE 1. Dose-response curves of the testosterone released in the medium in function of time, in organ culture of testicular tissue from a three month hypophysectomized boar: comparative effects of several hCG concentrations (100, 10, 1, 0.1, 0.01, 0.001 I.U./ml). Each point is the mean of three measurements performed on nine pooled culture dish (vertical bars: SEM). The results are expressed in ng/ml of medium/24 hr.

Effects of Various Hypophyseal Gonadotropins

Among the hypophyseal gonadotropins, human LH appeared to be the most potent when investigated at the lowest concentration (28 ng/ml of medium). Concentrations of 280 or 2,800 ng/ml were necessary to reach the optimal secretion of steroids with the ovine, bovine, and porcine LH.[a] In any case, time-response graphs were identical to those obtained with hCG. Similar effects have been observed on different mammals with LHs of mammalian[11,12] and non-mammalian[13] origin. These effects reported in the pig were abolished by anti-LH (human and porcine) at 1:15,000 as final dilution in the medium, when it was added at the start of a culture with LH, and after 10 days of culture with LH alone (at the time when cells were perfectly stimulated).

The various FSHs induced the same effects that LH did at a hundred-fold higher concentration. But the FSHs used were never pure; they were contaminated by about 1% LH. The production of an LH effect to explain the stimulation

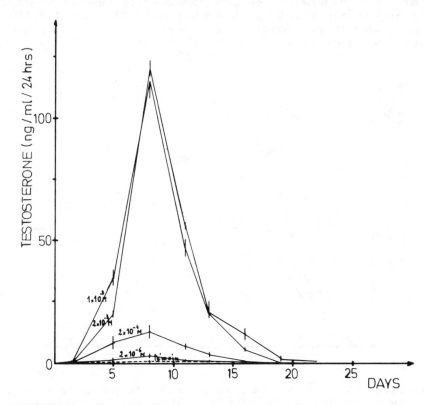

FIGURE 2. Dose response curves of the testosterone released in the medium in function of time, in organ culture of testicular tissue from a three month hypophysectomized boar: comparative effects of several dibutyryl cAMP concentrations (2×10^{-3} M; 1×10^{-3} M; 2×10^{-4} M; 2×10^{-6} M). Each point is the mean of three measurements performed on nine pooled culture dish (vertical bars: SEM). The results are expressed in ng/ml of medium/24 hr.

observed with FSH was confirmed by a suppression of this effect obtained by decreasing the amounts of FSH and by using combined appropriate anti-LH (final concentration 1:15,000).

Effects of cAMP and Dibutyryl cAMP

The explants in culture with 2×10^{-3} M and 1×10^{-3} M cAMP dibutyrate were perfectly restored at histological level and produced a higher amount of testosterone (125 ng/ml of medium/24 hr) than with hCG (FIGURE 2). This stimulation was faster but less durable. With lower dbcAMP concentrations, the response decreased: for 2×10^{-4} M, the testosterone level was 9 ng/ml 24 hr, for 2×10^{-6} M it remained at the control level. With cAMP, we never obtained either trophic effect or steroidogenic activity.

In conclusion, this system of organ culture allows the study of long-term effects of hormones in conditions respecting the relationships between the different cells of the testis and the extracellular matrix. It provides results that could be compared with some benefit to those obtained with other systems, such as cell cultures using isolated and reassociated cells.

REFERENCES

1. TROWELL, O. A. 1959. The culture of mature organs in a synthetic medium. Exp. Cell Res. **16:** 118.
2. LASNITZKI, I. 1964. The effect of hydrocortisone on the ventral and anterior prostate gland of the rat grown in culture. J. Endocr. **30:** 225–233.
3. MORAT, M., M. CHEVALIER & J. P. DUFAURE. 1971. Culture "in vitro" de fragments de testicules de porc: étude morphologique et histoenzymologique. C. R. Soc. Biol. **165:** 1894–1898.
4. MORAT, M. 1977. Action morphogène des hormones gonadotropes sur les cellules de Leydig du testicule de verrat. I. Effet de l'hypophysectomie. Arch. Anat. Micr. Morph. Exp. **66:** 119–142.
5. MORAT, M. & Y. COURTY. 1979. Dosage simultané, par radioimmunologie, de l'androstènedione, de la testostérone et de la dihydrotestostérone. Application à l'étude du fonctionnement des cellules de Leydig. C. R. Soc. Biol. **6:** 1070–1077.
6. DUFAURE, J. P., F. DU MESNIL DU BUISSON, M. MORAT, M. CHEVALIER & A. LOCATELLI. 1974. Effets de l'hypophysectomie et de l'administration. d'hormone gonadotrope (hCG) sur les cellules de Leydig du testicule de verrat. C. R. Ac. Sc. Paris **279:** 1907–1910.
7. MORAT, M., A. LOCATELLI, M. TERQUI, M. CHEVALIER, M. CHAMBON & J. P. DUFAURE. 1980. Effets de l'hypophysectomie, puis de l'administration de la gonadotropine hCG sur le taux de testostérone plasmatique et sur la structure de l'épididyme et des glandes accessoires chez le verrat (*Sus scrofa* L.). Reprod. Nutr. Develop. **20:** 61–76.
8. MORAT, M. 1977. L'action morphogène des hormones gonadotropes sur les cellules de Leydig du testicule de verrat. II. Effets de l'administration de gonadotropine chorionique après hypophysectomie. Action "in vivo" et en culture organotypique. Arch. Anat. Micr. Morph. Exp. **66:** 181–205.
9. MORAT, M. & J. P. DUFAURE. 1979. Production d'androstènedione, de testostérone et de dihydrotestostérone par le tissu testiculaire de verrat hypophysectomisé, sous l'action de hCG, en cultures organotypiques de longue durée. C. R. Soc. Biol. **6:** 1078–1082.
10. CHRISTENSEN, A. K. & K. C. PEACOCK. 1980. Increase in Leydig cell number in testis of adult rats treated chronically with an excess of human chorionic gonadotropin. Biol. Reprod. **22:** 383–392.
11. DUFAU, M., C. R. MENDELSON & K. J. CATT. 1974. A highly sensitive "in vitro" bioassay for luteinizing hormone and chorionic gonadotropin: testosterone production by dispersed Leydig cells. J. Clin. Endocr. Metab. **39:** 610–613.
12. DUFAU, M. L., R. POCK, A. NEUBAUER & K. J. CATT. 1976. "In vitro" bioassay of LH in human serum: the rat interstitial cell testosterone (RICT) assay. J. Clin. Endocr. Metab. **42:** 958–969.
13. FARMER, S. W., A. SUYAMA & H. PAPKOFF. 1977. Effect of diverse mammalian and non mammalian gonadotropins on isolated rat Leydig cells. Gen. Comp. Endocrinol. **32:** 488–494.

Direct Stimulation of Phospholipid Labeling and Steroidogenesis by Gonadotropin Releasing Hormone in Purified Rat Leydig Cells

TU LIN[a] and JOHN L. ORCHARD

Medical Service
Wm. Jennings Bryan Dorn Veterans Hospital
and Department of Medicine
University of South Carolina School of Medicine
Columbia, South Carolina 29201

In short-term incubations, gonadotropin-releasing hormone (GnRH) and its analogs (GnRHa) have a direct stimulating effect on Leydig cell steroidogenesis.[1,2] This stimulating effect is abolished in the absence of calcium in the incubation medium and is blocked by the addition of the calcium-channel blocking agent, nifedipine. Furthermore, GnRH has no significant effect on cyclic AMP–dependent protein kinase. These results suggest that the major stimulating effect of GnRH is calcium dependent.[2]

It is suggested that phospholipids may regulate cell processes by controlling the flux of calcium across cellular membrane.[3] It is hypothesized that ligand-receptor interaction may stimulate phosphatidylinositol degradation, which in turn increases the influx of extracellular calcium and biological responses.[3] Since GnRH-stimulated steroidogenesis is calcium dependent, the present studies were conducted to evaluate the effect of GnRH on phospholipid turnover, which may be important in mediating its biological effects.

Interstitial cells were obtained from adult Sprague-Dawley rats, 60–90 days of age, following collagenase treatment of decapsulated testes. Purified Leydig cells were then obtained by metrizamide density centrifugation. More than 85% of cells were stained positively for 3β-hydroxysteroid dehydrogenase enzyme. Purified Leydig cells (10^6 cells/0.5 ml) were incubated for 60 min at 34°C, 95% O_2/5% CO_2 in medium 199, 0.1% bovine serum albumin, 0.1 mM 1-methyl-3-isobutyl xanthine with 40 μCi[^{32}P]P$_i$ per tube. GnRH analog (des-Gly^{10}(D-Ala^6)GnRH N-ethyl-amide), with or without GnRH antagonist (DpGlu^1-D-Phe^2, D-Tyr^{3,6}-GnRH), and nifedipine were then added. Incubations were terminated at specific time period by adding 8 ml of chloroform/methanol/HCl (2/1/0.25%, vol/vol/vol) followed by 1.5 ml of 0.1 N HCl. Phospholipids were then purified by Supelco thin layer chromatography plates. The phospholipids were identified by comparison with authentic standards following autoradiography.[4] Spots were scraped and counted in a liquid scintillation spectrometer. Data were analyzed by Student's t test.

GnRHa in concentrations of 10^{-9} to 10^{-7} M caused dose-dependent increments of testosterone formation. Concomitant with increased testosterone formation, [^{32}P]P$_i$ incorporation into phosphatidylinositol (PI) and phosphatidic acid

---

[a] Address correspondence to: Tu Lin, M.D., Medical Service, WJB Dorn Veterans' Hospital, Columbia, SC 29201.

(PA) increased markedly. Labeling of PI increased $258 \pm 13\%$ (mean $\pm$ SE), whereas labeling of PA increased to $292 \pm 16\%$ of respective controls in response to 10^{-7} M of GnRHa (FIGURE 1). Time course of GnRHa-stimulated phospholipid labeling was next investigated. Increased $[^{32}P]P_i$ incorporation into PI and PA was detected as early as 2 min after the addition of GnRHa. GnRH antagonist (10 $\mu g/$ ml) completely abolished GnRHa-stimulated testosterone formation and $[^{32}P]P_i$ incorporation into PA and PI. Finally, the effect of nifedipine on phospholipid turnover was studied. The addition of nifedipine (1 μg and 10 $\mu g/$ ml) inhibited GnRH-stimulated testosterone formation, but had no significant effect on GnRH-induced phospholipid turnover.

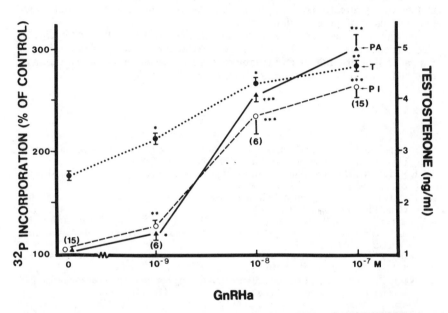

FIGURE 1. The effects of GnRHa on testosterone formation and phospholipid labeling. Purified Leydig cells (10^6 cells/0.5 ml) were incubated with 40 μCi$[^{32}P]P_i$ for 60 min. Various concentrations of GnRHa (10^{-9}–10^{-7} M) were then added and incubations were carried out for an additional 60 min. Phospholipids were extracted and purified on thin layer chromatography plates. Results are the mean $\pm$ SE. Numbers in the parentheses are the number of determinations. $*p < 0.05$, $**p < 0.01$, $***p < 0.001$ as compared with respective controls. (PA) phosphatidic acid, (PI) phosphatidylinositol, (T) testosterone.

Evidence has been accumulating that the effect of GnRH is not mediated by cyclic AMP or cyclic GMP, but is calcium dependent. In the pituitary cells, GnRH stimulates phosphatidylinositol turnover and the release of arachidonic acid. Inhibition of the release of arachidonic acid from phospholipids blocks GnRH-stimulated LH release.[5] In cultured ovarian granulosa cells, Naor and Yavin[6] reported that GnRH stimulates phospholipid labeling. Similar to that of granulosa cells, we now report that GnRH significantly increased PA and PI labeling of testicular Leydig cells. GnRH antagonist completely blocked GnRH-stimulated testosterone formation and phospholipid labeling. This suggests that the effect of GnRH on testosterone formation and phospholipid labeling is specific and receptor mediated.

It is still unclear how the changes in phospholipid metabolism lead to the opening of calcium channels and subsequent biological responses. One hypothesis is that the altered phospholipid of the cell membrane results in an alteration of membrane fluidity with subsequent opening of calcium channels. Another possibility is that newly synthesized phosphatidate may act as a calcium ionophore. In our purified Leydig cell system, addition of nifedipine inhibited GnRH-stimulated steroidogenesis but had no significant effect on phospholipid labeling. This strongly suggests that GnRH-induced phospholipid labeling is calcium independent. This also supports the hypothesis by Michell[3] that phosphatidylinositol metabolism is directly triggered by receptor activation and is the cause, rather than the result of increased influx of calcium.

We have provided evidence that the stimulatory effect of GnRH on Leydig cell steroidogenesis is calcium dependent and correlates with phospholipid turnover. Similar to that of pituitary and granulosa cells, increased phospholipid turnover may be involved in the cellular action of GnRH in Leydig cells.

REFERENCES

1. SHARPE, R. M. & I. COOPER. 1982. Stimulatory effect of LHRH and its agonist on Leydig cell steroidogenesis in vitro. Mol. Cell. Endocrinol. 26: 141–150.
2. LIN, T. 1983. Direct stimulating effects of gonadotropin releasing hormone on Leydig cell steroidogenesis. J. Andrology 4: 55.
3. MICHELL, R. H. 1975. Inositol phospholipids and cell surface receptor function. Biochim. Biophys. Acta 415: 81–147.
4. ORCHARD, J. L., J. S. DAVIS, R. E. LARSON & R. V. FARESE. 1984. Effects of carbachol and cholecystokinin on polyphosphoinositide metabolism in the rat pancreas in vitro. Biochem. J. 271: 281–287.
5. NAOR, Z. & K. J. CATT. 1981. Mechanism of action of gonadotropin-releasing hormone. J. Biol. Chem. 256: 2226–2229.
6. NAOR, Z. & E. YAVIN. 1982. Gonadotropin-releasing hormone stimulates phospholipid labeling in cultured granulosa cells. Endocrinology 111: 1615–1619.

Changes in Testosterone Hydroxylase Activity in Rat Testis following Administration of 2,3,7,8-Tetrachlorodibenzo-p-dioxin

J. C. MITTLER,[a] N. H. ERTEL,[a] R. X. PENG[B]

C. S. YANG,[b] and T. KIERNAN[a]

[a] Medical Service
Veterans Administration Medical Center
East Orange, New Jersey 07019
Departments of [b] Biochemistry and [a]Medicine
University of Medicine and Dentistry of New Jersey
New Jersey Medical School
Newark, New Jersey 07103

Microsomal cytochrome P-450-dependent monooxygenase systems, each consisting of NADPH-cytochrome P-450 reductase and different forms of cytochrome P-450, are a heterogeneous group of enzymes, most extensively studied as drug-inducible enzymes in liver.[1] Similar enzymes are also found in other tissues such as testis[2] and the lung[3] and are known to catalyze the oxygenation of a variety of endogenous and exogenous substrates. In the liver and lung, the major functions of the monooxygenase systems are related to detoxification and catabolism. In the testes, some of these systems, such as the 7α-hydroxylase, may participate in local regulatory mechanisms since 7α-hydroxylated androgens inhibit several steroid-metabolizing enzymes.[2]

The 6β-, 7α-, and 16α-hydroxylases active on androgens are found in both liver and testis. Many compounds have been shown to alter the monooxygenase activities by inducing different cytochrome P-450 isozymes. In the liver, treatment with 2,3,7,8-tetrachlorodibenzo-p-dioxin (TCDD) increases the androgen 7α-hydroxylase markedly.[4] The effects of TCDD on testicular androgen hydroxylation have not previously been studied, although Goldstein and Linko[5] showed that TCDD increases certain cytochromes in liver and testis. In this work, we studied the effect of TCDD treatment on the hydroxylation of testosterone by testicular microsomes.

Male Sprague-Dawley rats, body weight 90 g were given a single intraperitoneal injection of 5.0, 1.0, 0.2, or 0 μg/kg TCDD in 0.1 ml olive oil. Testes were collected 90 hours later.

Six testes from each group were decapsulated and treated with collagenase (Worthington, Freehold, NJ, 1.6 mg/ml) in medium 199 with agitation until seminiferous tubules were cleanly separated from interstitial tissue. Interstitial cells were collected by centrifugation. Seminiferous tubules were collected on cheesecloth and washed thoroughly. Selected whole testes and fractions were fixed in Bouin's solution and prepared for histological examination using PAS-hematoxylin stain.

Enzyme activities were measured as described by Sunde *et al.*[2] in low speed supernatants of testis homogenates. Identities of tritiated steroids were confirmed

TABLE 1. Testosterone Hydroxylase Activities in Low Speed Supernatants of Whole Testis, Interstitial Tissue, and Seminiferous Tubules of Control and TCDD-treated Rats

Treatment	Whole Testis (pg/mg protein/hour, mean ± standard error of the mean, 3 testes/group)			Interstitial Fraction (pg/mg protein/hour)			Seminiferous Tubules (pg/mg protein/hour)		
	16α-Hydroxytestosterone	6β-Hydroxytestosterone	7α-Hydroxytestosterone	16α-	6β-	7α-	16α-	6β-	7α-
				Hydroxytestosterone			Hydroxytestosterone		
Vehicle only (control)	0.96 ± 0.22	0.79 ± 0.01	0.14 ± 0.02	0.60	0.10	0.09	0.00 ± 0	ND	ND
0.2 µg/kg body wt	1.67 ± 0.19[a]	1.14 ± 0.11[b]	0.21 ± 0.003	1.50	0.40	0.18	0.12	ND	ND
1.0 µg/kg body wt	1.66 ± 0.31[a]	1.01 ± 0.11	0.12 ± 0.06	0.76	0.35	0.12	0.14 [c]	ND	ND
5.0 µg/kg body wt	1.29 ± 0.32	0.76 ± 0.15	0.19 ± 0.05	0.82	0.43	0.12	0.07	ND	ND

ND = Not detectable.

[a] Two groups combined vs. control: $p < 0.05$.

[b] $p < 0.05$ vs. control.

[c] 6 controls vs. 3 treatment groups: $p < 0.001$.

by multiple chromatographies and recrystallization. These values are not corrected for recovery. We estimate losses from further metabolism as 10% of the 6β-hydroxytestosterone, 7% of the 7α-hydroxytestosterone, and 5% of the 16α-hydroxytestosterone. Means ± SEM are presented. Student's *t*-test was used to determine significance of differences between means.

Whereas the two lower doses of TCDD (0.2 and 1.0 μg/kg) did not produce any discernible effect on morphology, high dose TCDD (5.0 μg/kg) was associated with shrunken, hyperchromatic nuclei in the two layers of the seminiferous tubules closest to the basement membrane. Since only one time interval was studied, i.e. 90 hours, we cannot speculate on the possible reversibility of the observed lesion in the testis.

Biochemical data are shown in TABLE 1. In the three control rats, 16α-hydroxytestosterone production by whole testes was 0.96 ± 0.22 pg/mg protein/hour. After TCDD treatment, the values were 1.67 ± 0.19 for the low dose (0.2 μg/kg body weight) and 1.66 ± 0.31 for the medium dose (1.0 μg/kg) testes. When these two TCDD-treated groups are combined, there is significant increase in the 16α-hydroxylase activity (170% of control, $p < 0.05$). Further analysis with pooled fractions of testes indicated that all of the 16α-hydroxylase activity was in the interstitial fraction of control animals; there was none in the seminiferous tubules. The seminiferous tubule fractions from treated animals, however, had induced 16α-hydroxylase activity: 0.12 pg/mg/hour in the low dose group, 0.14 in the medium dose group, and 0.07 in the high dose group. There was significant stimulation when the latter three means are compared with the six control testes, which were devoid of 16α-hydroxylase activity ($p < 0.001$). 16α-hydroxytestosterone is a precursor to estriol, which is a significant estrogen in pregnancy and biologically active in some assay systems. For this reason, we considered 16α-hydroxytestosterone important for study, but more work will be necessary to determine the significance of the stimulation observed in both interstitial and tubular fractions.

6β-hydroxylase activity was confined to the interstitial fraction and was stimulated by the low dose of TCDD (144% of control, $p < 0.05$). The decreased values for 16α-, 6β-, and 7α-hydroxylase activities in animals treated with the highest dose of TCDD (5 μg/kg) compared to the two lower doses, suggest inhibition of all three hydroxylases, perhaps due to tissue damage or to a direct effect of residual TCDD on the enzyme system.

7α-hydroxylase activity in these immature testes was confined to the interstitial tissue and was not affected by TCDD treatment.

No differences in 5α-reductase activity among groups were observed. Also, no differences in unmetabolized testosterone were noted. Therefore, it is unlikely that depletion of substrate influenced these results.

The present results suggest that the 16α-, 6β-, and 7α-hydroxylases active on testosterone may be differentially affected in the testis by a microsomal inducing agent.

REFERENCES

1. COON, M. J., D. R. KOOP, A. V. PERSSON & E. T. MORGAN. 1980. *In* Biochemistry, Biophysics and Regulation of Cytochrome P-450. J. Gustaffsson, A. Carlstedt-Duke, A. Mode, J. Rafter, Eds.: 7–16. Elsevier/North Holland Biomedical Press. Amsterdam.
2. SUNDE, A., K. TVETER & K. B. EIK-NES. 1980. Acta Endocrinol. (Kbh). **93:** 243–249.

3. SLAUGHTER, S. R., C. R. WOLF, C. J. SERABJIT-SINGH, J. P. MACINISZYN & R. M. PHILPOT. 1980. *In* Biochemistry, Biophysics and Regulation of Cytochrome P-450. J. Gustaffsson, A. Carlstedt-Duke, A. Mode & J. Rafter, Eds.: 41–48. Elsevier/North Holland Biomedical Press. Amsterdam.
4. SHIVERICK, K. 1980. *In* Program, 62nd Annual Meeting, The Endocrine Society. 255. Washington, D.C.
5. GOLDSTEIN, J. A. & P. LINKO. 1983. Fed. Proc. **42:** 806.

Microsomal Cytochrome P-450 Enzyme Damage in Cultured Leydig Cells: Relation to Steroidogenic Desensitization[a]

PATRICK G. QUINN[b] and ANITA H. PAYNE

*Departments of Biological Chemistry and Obstetrics
and Gynecology
Reproductive Endocrinology Program
The University of Michigan
Ann Arbor, Michigan 48109*

It is well established that treatment of animals with a single high dose of LH or hCG results in steroidogenic desensitization of Leydig cells.[1,2] Desensitized Leydig cells exhibit a decreased capacity to produce testosterone in response to subsequent stimulation with gonadotropins or cAMP analogues, and have decreased activities of the microsomal P-450 enzymes, 17α-hydroxylase, and C_{17-20} lyase. The present study provides evidence that the decreases in microsomal P-450 activities are caused by oxygen-derived, free-radical damage of the enzymes, and, furthermore, that the decrease in microsomal P-450 activities are not the primary cause of the decrease in testosterone-producing capacity observed in desensitized Leydig cells.

Primary cultures of purified, adult mouse Leydig cells were maintained in serum-free medium at 32°C, in a humidified atmosphere of 19% O_2 (95% air/5% CO_2) or 1% O_2, in the presence and absence of the antioxidant dimethyl sulfoxide. The culture medium was changed daily and the activities of microsomal enzymes were determined by quantifying the conversion of ^3H-substrate to ^3H-products during a 1 hr incubation at 37°C, in an atmosphere of 19% O_2. The maximal capacity to produce testosterone was determined by incubating replicate cultures with 1 mM 8-Br-cAMP for a 3 hr period and measuring testosterone in the medium by radioimmunoassay.

1 mM 8-Br-cAMP was added to half of the Leydig cells, during the initial 24 hr of culture only, to induce steroidogenic desensitization. The other half served as controls. Testosterone production by desensitized Leydig cells was 15-fold and threefold greater than that of controls on days one and two of culture, respectively. The addition of dimethyl sulfoxide to the culture medium and/or reduction of the oxygen tension had no effect on testosterone production by control or desensitized Leydig cells.

The data presented in TABLE 1 demonstrate that, when control Leydig cell cultures are incubated in 19% O_2, the microsomal P-450 activities, 17 α-hydroxylase and C_{17-20} lyase, are stable during the first 24 hr but decrease markedly by 48

[a] This study was supported by National Institutes of Health Grant HD-08538. Patrick G. Quinn is supported in part by National Institutes of Health Training Grant HD-07048.

[b] Address correspondence to: Patrick G. Quinn, Steroid Research Unit, L 1221 Women's Hospital, The University of Michigan, Ann Arbor, MI 48109.

TABLE 1. Microsomal Enzyme Activities and Maximal Testosterone Production of Cultured Leydig Cells

Treatment	nmol products · h⁻¹ · 10⁵ Leydig cells⁻¹			
	17α-Hydroxylase Activity	C_{17-20} Lyase Activity	Δ^{5}-3β-Hydroxysteroid Dehydrogenase Activity	Maximal Testosterone Production
I. 19% O_2				
Day 0	2.062 ± 0.200[a]	3.750 ± 0.950	2.310 ± 0.206	0.147 ± 0.008
Day 1 control	1.753 ± 0.284	3.650 ± 0.248	N.D.[b]	0.160 ± 0.006
Day 1 desensitized	0.971 ± 0.054	2.272 ± 0.157	N.D.	0.079 ± 0.003
Day 2 control	0.473 ± 0.043	1.234 ± 0.161	2.333 ± 0.139	0.150 ± 0.021
Day 2 desensitized	0.163 ± 0.027	0.327 ± 0.147	2.269 ± 0.020	0.037 ± 0.008
II. 19% O_2 + Dimethyl sulfoxide				
Day 0	2.033 ± 0.137	3.481 ± 0.109	2.259 ± 0.103	0.176 ± 0.035
Day 1 control	1.945 ± 0.056	3.601 ± 0.083	N.D.	0.185 ± 0.005
Day 1 desensitized	1.184 ± 0.185	2.557 ± 0.241	N.D.	0.079 ± 0.006
Day 2 control	1.041 ± 0.217	2.171 ± 0.137	2.205 ± 0.014	0.193 ± 0.005
Day 2 desensitized	0.348 ± 0.105	0.967 ± 0.112	1.987 ± 0.030	0.039 ± 0.001
III. 1% O_2				
Day 0	2.139 ± 0.226	3.221 ± 0.323	2.342 ± 0.160	0.161 ± 0.010
Day 1 control	2.452 ± 0.342	4.170 ± 0.560	N.D.	0.237 ± 0.011
Day 1 desensitized	2.287 ± 0.470	3.838 ± 0.811	N.D.	0.107 ± 0.021
Day 2 control	1.560 ± 0.085	3.418 ± 0.370	2.145 ± 0.047	0.239 ± 0.014
Day 2 desensitized	1.436 ± 0.054	2.952 ± 0.483	1.954 ± 0.090	0.085 ± 0.012
IV. 1% O_2 + Dimethyl sulfoxide				
Day 0	3.050 ± 0.110	4.132 ± 0.198	2.866 ± 0.475	0.175 ± 0.023
Day 1 control	3.198 ± 0.777	5.522 ± 0.288	N.D.	0.229 ± 0.009
Day 1 desensitized	2.691 ± 0.623	5.047 ± 0.278	N.D.	0.106 ± 0.020
Day 2 control	2.851 ± 0.641	5.317 ± 0.739	2.131 ± 0.455	0.289 ± 0.007
Day 2 desensitized	2.085 ± 0.371	4.075 ± 0.644	1.721 ± 0.202	0.083 ± 0.008

[a] $\bar{X} \pm$ S.D. [b] Not determined.

hr. This decline in P-450 activities was partially prevented by addition of the antioxidant dimethyl sulfoxide to the medium or by reduction of the oxygen tension. The combined effects of these treatments were synergistic in preserving the P-450 activities of control Leydig cells. In contrast, the P-450 activities of desensitized Leydig cells maintained at 19% O_2 were reduced to 50 and 33% of control values at 24 and 48 hr, respectively. However, when Leydig cells were cultured in an atmosphere of 1% O_2, the cAMP-induced decrease in the P-450 activities was essentially prevented. The activity of Δ^5-3β-hydroxysteroid dehydrogenase-isomerase, a microsomal enzyme that is not P-450–dependent, was stable in both control and desensitized Leydig cells during the 48 hr culture period, indicating that the decrease in microsomal P-450 activities was specific and not due to damage of the cells and/or the smooth endoplasmic reticulum. These data are consistent with the hypothesis that oxygen-mediated damage is responsible for the time-dependent decrease in 17α-hydroxylase and C_{17-20} lyase activities of control Leydig cells, and is the mechanism by which these activities are further decreased in desensitized Leydig cells. The large and rapid reduction of hydroxylase and lyase activities of desensitized Leydig cells at 19% O_2 is consistent with the model described by Hornsby for inactivation of the adrenal P-450 enzyme, 11β-hydroxylase, by the product, cortisol.[3] In this model, interaction of products (pseudosubstrates) with the enzyme leads to release of damaging free radicals from the P-450·pseudosubstrate complex, due to the inability of the steroid product to be hydroxylated. In this regard, it should be noted that during the desensitization process, Leydig cells are exposed to high concentrations ($\sim 2 \mu M$) of the product, testosterone. Recent results, which indicate that a 24 hr incubation of Leydig cells with high (2 μM) but not low (0.2 μM) concentrations of testosterone causes the same extent of decrease in P-450 activities as incubation with cAMP, and that this decrease is prevented by reduction of the oxygen tension, support the hypothesis that decreases in microsomal P-450 activities of desensitized Leydig cells are caused by steroid pseudosubstrate-induced, oxygen-derived, free-radical damage of these P-450 enzymes.

The capacity of control Leydig cells to produce testosterone in response to cAMP was not diminished at any time or under any culture conditions tested, even though P-450 activities of cultures maintained at 19% O_2 had decreased by 75% after 48 hr. In contrast, the capacity of desensitized Leydig cells had decreased by 50% at 24 hr under all culture conditions, in spite of the fact that Leydig cells maintained at 1% O_2 did not exhibit decreased P-450 activity at this time. Thus, the decrease in maximal capacity for testosterone production of desensitized Leydig cells cannot be attributed to the decrease in 17α-hydroxylase and C_{17-20} lyase activities and must be caused by other factors, such as a decrease in cholesterol side-chain cleavage activity[4] or depletion of cholesterol stores.[5,6]

REFERENCES

1. CIGORRAGA, S. B., M. L. DUFAU & K. J. CATT. 1978. J. Biol. Chem. **253:** 4297–4304.
2. O'SHAUGHNESSY, P. J. & A. H. PAYNE. 1982. J. Biol. Chem. **257:** 11503–11509.
3. HORNSBY, P. J. 1980. J. Biol. Chem. **255:** 4020–4027.
4. LUKETICH, J. D., M. H. MELNER, F. P. GUENGERICH & D. PUETT. 1983. Biochem. Biophys. Res. Commun. **111:** 424–429.
5. QUINN, P. G., L. J. DOMBRAUSKY, Y-D. I. CHEN & A. H. PAYNE. 1981. Endocrinology **109:** 1790–1792.
6. FREEMAN, D. A. & M. ASCOLI. 1982. Proc. Natl. Acad. Sci. USA **79:** 7796–7800.

Use of Inherited Differences among Strains of Inbred Mice to Study Genetic Determinants of Steroid Biosynthesis[a]

JOHN R. D. STALVEY[b] and ANITA H. PAYNE

Reproductive Endocrinology Program
Departments of Obstetrics and Gynecology and
Biological Chemistry
The University of Michigan
Ann Arbor, Michigan 48109

Testosterone biosynthesis by Leydig cells is the result of extensive sequential enzymatic modification of the parent molecule, cholesterol. Genetic differences that exist between and within species can result in alterations of structure and/or activity of the enzymes responsible for metabolism of cholesterol to testosterone. Thus, the genetic differences in laboratory animals can be used to study the influence of variation in structure and/or activity of the enzymes on the production of testosterone. We have recently adopted this approach, using purified Leydig cells from genetically defined inbred mice, to study the relationships between maximal testosterone production and the activities of steroidogenic enzymes of the smooth endoplasmic reticulum (SER) that catalyze the synthesis of testosterone from pregnenolone.

Various strains of inbred mice were screened for differences in maximal testosterone production. Through this screening process it became apparent that Leydig cells from C57BL/10J (BL/10) and C57BL/6J (BL/6) mice produced twice as much testosterone in response to maximal hCG or dibutyryl-cAMP stimulation as did Leydig cells from DBA/2J (DBA) or C3H/HeJ (C3H) mice.[1] Furthermore, there was no correlation between maximal testosterone production per Leydig cell and the number of LH receptors per Leydig cell.[1] These observations indicated that these four strains would be useful to study steps distal to the formation of cAMP that might influence differences in testosterone production.

Leydig cells were purified from testes of BL/10, BL/6, DBA, and C3H mice. Decapsulated testes were completely dissociated by treatment with collagenase and Leydig cells were purified by centrifugation in a continuous 12–27% gradient of Metrizamide.[1] Maximal testosterone production was assessed by incubating cells for 2 hr at 34°C with a saturating concentration of hCG. Testosterone was measured in cells plus medium by radioimmunoassay. Activities of 3β-hydroxysteroid dehydrogenase-isomerase (3βHSD), 17α-hydroxylase, C_{17-20} lyase, and 17-ketosteroid reductase were determined by incubating homogenized Leydig cells for 5 min at 37°C with saturating concentrations of the appropriate cofactor and the appropriate ^{3}H-labeled substrate and measuring the amount of ^{3}H-labeled product formed.

[a] Supported by National Institute of Child Health and Human Development grants HD-08358 and HD-17916, and a National Research Service Award HD-06392 to J.R.D.S.

[b] Address correspondence to: John R. D. Stalvey, Steroid Research Unit, L 1221 Women's Hospital, The University of Michigan, Ann Arbor, MI 48109.

TABLE 1. Maximal Testosterone Production in Response to hCG Stimulation and the Activity of the Smooth Endoplasmic Reticular Steroidogenic Enzyme, 3β-Hydroxysteroid dehydrogenase-isomerase, in Leydig Cells from Four Strains of Inbred Mice

Strain	Testosterone Production (ng/10^6 Leydig cells/2 hr)	3β-Hydroxysteroid dehydrogenase-isomerase Activity (pmol/min/10^6 Leydig cells)
C57BL/10J (3)	1168 ± 126[a]	1683 ± 209[x]
C57BL/6J (6)	1255 ± 97[a]	1142 ± 111[y]
DBA/2J (6)	640 ± 76[b]	758 ± 41[z]
C3H/HeJ (3)	655 ± 59[b]	697 ± 69[z]

For statistical analysis, data were subjected to analysis of variance and Duncan's new multiple range test ($\alpha = 0.05$).

Groups sharing the same superscript ([a–b] or [x–z]) are not significantly different.

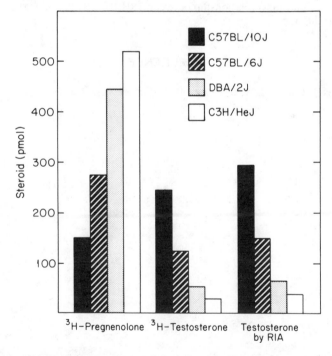

FIGURE 1. Testosterone production by intact Leydig cells incubated with pregnenolone. Equivalent numbers of whole Leydig cells were incubated for 2 hr at 34°C with 1 μM [^{3}H]pregnenolone or 1 μM nonradioactive pregnenolone. The group of bars to the left represent unmetabolized [^{3}H]pregnenolone. The group of bars in the middle and to the right represent the amount of testosterone produced as measured by determining the amount of [^{3}H]testosterone formed from [^{3}H]pregnenolone or the amount of nonradioactive testosterone formed from nonradioactive pregnenolone. The latter value was measured by radioimmunoassay.

Leydig cells from BL/10 and BL/6 mice produced twice as much testosterone as did Leydig cells from DBA and C3H mice (TABLE 1). Of the SER enzymes, only 3βHSD activity differed significantly among Leydig cells from the four strains (TABLE 1), and there was a significant interstrain correlation ($r = 0.82$) between maximal testosterone production and 3βHSD activity. When intact Leydig cells from the four strains were incubated for 2 hr with equal concentrations of pregnenolone, Leydig cells from BL/10 and BL/6 mice, the strains that exhibited high hCG-stimulated testosterone production, metabolized considerably more of the added pregnenolone to testosterone than did Leydig cells from DBA and C3H mice, the strains that exhibited low hCG-stimulated testosterone production (FIGURE 1).

The inverse relationship between unmetabolized pregnenolone and the amount of testosterone produced, in addition to the interstrain correlation between hCG-stimulated testerone and 3βHSD activity, indicates that 3βHSD activity is important in maximal testosterone production. Also, these results suggest that genetic analysis of the steroidogenic enzymes can be used to study the regulation of testosterone biosynthesis. Further studies using standard genetic crosses as well as recombinant inbred lines should allow us to establish whether or not there is a causal relationship between 3βHSD activity and maximal testosterone production.

REFERENCE

1. STALVEY, J. R. D. & A. H. PAYNE. 1983. Endocrinology 112:1696–1701.

A Transplantable Rat Leydig Cell Tumor: Binding Properties, Hormonal Responsiveness, and Tumor Growth[a]

AAGE ERICHSEN,[b] TORE JAHNSEN, HÅVARD
ATTRAMADAL, DRUDE ANDERSEN, and
VIDAR HANSSON

Institutes of Pathology and Medical Biochemistry
University of Oslo
Oslo, Norway

In the present study we have examined the properties and binding capacities of the LH and prolactin receptors and the adenylyl cyclase (AC) response to various hormones in a transplantable rat Leydig cell tumor. We also examined the rate of tumor growth and to what extent this may be influenced by the endocrine status of the host animal (intact, castrated, and hypophysectomized rats). The study was undertaken to examine to what extent the tumor Leydig cells differ from normal adult Leydig cells; judged by the quality and the number of receptors as well as the response of the AC to various hormones.

The tumors originally arose spontaneously in male Fisher rats.[1] They were implanted subcutaneously on the back of adult male intact, castrated, or hypophysectomized Sprague-Dawley rats, and harvested six weeks (intact and castrated rats) or 18 weeks (hypophysectomized rats) after tumor implantation. Details concerning isolation of membrane particles, iodination of LH, and the binding assay have been presented elsewhere.[2] The AC activity was determined in membrane particles employing $[\alpha\text{-}^{32}P]ATP$ and the $[^{32}P]cAMP$ formed was isolated by Dowex and alumina chromatography.[3]

Tumor Leydig cells were shown to contain membrane receptors for LH and prolactin with qualitative properties (specificity, stability, and affinity) identical to those in normal Leydig cells. The apparent K_d and the number of LH and prolactin receptors in the tumor Leydig cells, testis and prostate are shown in TABLE 1. As shown in the table, the number of LH receptors in tumor Leydig cells was greatly reduced compared to normal Leydig cells (1–2%), whereas the number of prolactin receptors was closer to normal. Using the same hormone preparations, the ration of LH/prolactin receptors in the adult testis is approximately 20–25. In the tumor Leydig cell this ratio is close to one. Tumors grown in hypophysectomized rats showed lower levels of LH and prolactin receptors (TABLE 1). The properties of the LH and prolactin receptors appear to be normal; they are severely (LH) or moderately (prolactin) reduced in number compared to normal adult Leydig cells. Furthermore, it appears that the receptors for LH and prolactin in the tumor Leydig cells are stimulated by gonadotropins. The properties of

[a] This work was supported by the Norwegian Society for Fighting Cancer (NFTKB) and the Norwegian Research Council for Science and Humanities (NAVF).

[b] Address correspondence to: Aage Erichsen, Institute of Pathology, Rikshospitalet, Oslo, Norway.

TABLE 1. Affinity and Capacity of LH and Prolactin Receptors in Adult Rat Testis (LH) and Ventral Prostate (prolactin) and in Tumor Leydig Cells Grown in Intact, Castrated, and Hypophysectomized Rats

		Prolactin Receptors				LH Receptors			
		Intact Rats	Castrated Rats	Hypophysectomized Rats	Prostate	Intact Rats	Castrated Rats	Hypophysectomized Rats	Testes
K_d (10^{-10} M)	Range	3.2–8.1	2.6–7.4	0.94–9.1	1.4–2	0.77–1.4	0.78–1.9	0.24–1.9	0.67–1.6
	Mean ± S.D.	4.5 ± 1.7	4.2 ± 2.2	4.54 ± 3.4	3.25 ± 1.7	1.04 ± 0.23	1.22 ± 0.48	1.28 ± 0.91	1.04 ± 0.44
Binding sites	Range	14.4–30.7	17.7–29.4	3.3–6.3	22.1–61.5	7.1–11.2	6.7–11.36	0.35–5.42	18.4–57.0
(fmol/mg prot.)	Mean ± S.D.	25.1 ± 6.0	23.18 ± 5.8	5.0 ± 1.4	44.8 ± 18.8	8.74 ± 1.5	8.7 ± 2.13	3.03 ± 2.55	36.6 ± 19.2
Number of experiments		7	4	4	5	5	4	3	4

the receptor AC system (ATP, GTP, and Mg^{2+} dependence) in tumor Leydig cells appear to be similar to those of AC system in other somatic cells. In contrast, the hormonal activation of the tumor Leydig cell AC is quite different from that of normal Leydig cells in that the response to hCG is decreased and the responses to prostaglandin E_1 and isoproterenol are increased (FIGURE 1). In addition, both tumor Leydig cells and normal rat Leydig cell AC can be activated by glucagon in physiological concentrations (FIGURE 1). Growth of the Leydig cell tumors is clearly dependent of the endocrine status of the host animal; tumor Leydig cells grown in castrated rats revealed the fastest growth whereas those implanted into hypophysectomized rats showed the slowest growth. In contrast, the endocrine status of the host animal, did not appear to influence the response pattern of the

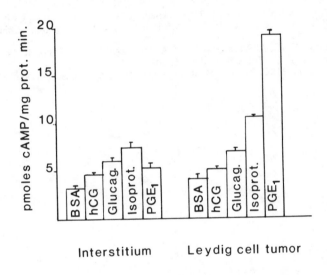

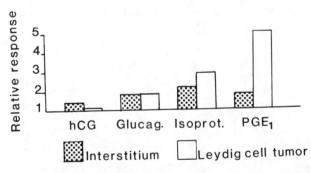

FIGURE 1. Activation of tumor Leydig cell AC by hCG (5 I.U.), isoproterenol (5 µg/ml), glucagon (5 µg/ml), and prostaglandin E_1 (5 µg/ml). Membrane particles were incubated at 35°C for 12 min in the presence of ATP (1.0 mM), GTP (0.04 mM), and Mg^{2+} (0.4 mM, in excess of ATP and EDTA). The upper panel shows absolute activities whereas the lower panel shows the relative responses (stimulated activities divided on basal activities). The bars show mean values ± SD.

tumor Leydig cell AC, and the tumor Leydig cells have not during multiple transplantations changed their characteristics with regard to receptor content, receptor specificity, or hormonal responsiveness of the AC.

Thus, although the tumor Leydig cells contain LH receptors and produce testosterone, these results show that the functional properties of the tumor Leydig cells in many regards are different from that of normal Leydig cells. This should be taken into account when using the tumor Leydig cells in studies on Leydig cell function and regulation.

REFERENCES

1. COOKE, B. A., L. M. LINDH, F. H. A. JANSZEN, M. J. A. VAN DRIEL, C. P. BAKKER, M. P. I. VAN DER PLANK & H. J. VAN DER MOLEN. 1979. Biochim. Biophys. Acta 583: 320–331.
2. CHARREAU, E. H., A. ATTRAMADAL, P. A. TORJESEN, R. CALANDRA, K. PURVIS & V. HANSSON. 1977. Mol. Cel. Endocr. 6: 303–307.
3. SALOMON, Y., M. C. LONDOS & M. RODBELL. 1974. Anal. Biochem. 58: 541–548.

Expression of Pro-opiomelanocortin-like Gene in the Testis and Leydig Cell Lines

C.-L. C. CHEN, J. P. MATHER, P. L. MORRIS, and
C. W. BARDIN

The Population Council
The Rockefeller University
New York, New York 10021

Adrenocorticotropin (ACTH) and β-endorphin, which are derived from a common precursor, pro-opiomelanocortin (POMC), have been shown to be present in a variety of tissues other than the pituitary.[1] The *de novo* synthesis of POMC peptides has also been demonstrated in the pituitary, hypothalamus, and human placenta. In addition, the messenger RNA coding for POMC protein has been identified in the pituitary, hypothalamus, and other regions of the rat brain (amygdala and cortex).[2]

Recently, immunoreactive β-endorphin has been detected in human semen[3] and rat testicular extract.[1,4] Immunocytochemical studies revealed that β-endorphin and α-MSH–like materials were localized in the cytoplasm of Leydig cells and in the epithelium of the epididymis, seminal vesicle, and vas deferens. No immunoreactive staining was found in the Sertoli, myoid, endothelial, or germ cells.[5] In order to determine whether POMC peptides are synthesized in the reproductive tissue, in this report, we have studied the existence of POMC mRNA in the testis, epididymis, and the Leydig cell lines.

Messenger RNAs were extracted from various rat tissues and Leydig cell lines. POMC-like mRNAs were determined by Northern blot analysis using rat POMC cDNA (pI13) as a hybridization probe. The POMC cDNA (pI13) was isolated from rat neurointermediate pituitary mRNA and identified to contain sequences coding from the middle portion of the NH_2-terminal glycopeptide to the poly(A) tail.[6] Using pI13 as a probe, POMC-like mRNAs were detected in the pituitary, testis, and epididymis (FIGURE 1). The POMC-like mRNAs were also present in the established normal mouse Leydig cell line, TM_3, (FIGURE 1) and tumor originating from Leydig cells (I10A). The hybridizable species of POMC-like mRNA in the testis, epididymis, and mouse Leydig cells have the same mRNA size. However, they were approximately 150 bases shorter than those in the pituitary (FIGURE 1) or in the hypothalamus (data not shown). Herbert and his colleagues have also found similar results in some regions of the brain. POMC-like mRNAs from amygdala and cerebral cortex of the brain were shorter than that from pituitary or hypothalamus.[2] In fact, we have found that POMC-like mRNAs in the testis, epididymis, or mouse Leydig cells were the same size as those detected in the amygdala.

The concentrations of POMC mRNA in the testis and epididymis have also been determined by dot blot analysis (FIGURE 2). Equal amount of poly(A) RNA from testis, epididymis, hypothalamus, and liver was spotted on nitrocellulose filter and the concentration of POMC mRNA in each tissue was determined by hybridization to POMC cDNA (pI13) probe. The POMC mRNA is almost as concentrated in the testis as in the hypothalamus. The POMC mRNA level in the neurointermediate pituitary is 10–20 times higher than in the anterior pituitary. In turn, the POMC mRNAs in the anterior pituitary are approximately 20–30 times as concentrated as in the hypothalamus or testis.

One of the possible explanations for the variation in the size of POMC mRNA is the existence of the tissue specific heterogeneous length of poly(A) tails. Poly(A) tails are known to vary in size within a specific mRNA class. The smaller size of POMC-like mRNA in the testis may be due to the shorter length of poly(A) tail. In addition, the POMC mRNAs may be transcribed from multiple non-allelic POMC genes in different tissues. The POMC mRNAs in the testis, epididymis, or amygdala are expressed from one POMC gene and the POMC mRNAs in the pituitary or hypothalamus are derived from the other gene. The number of POMC

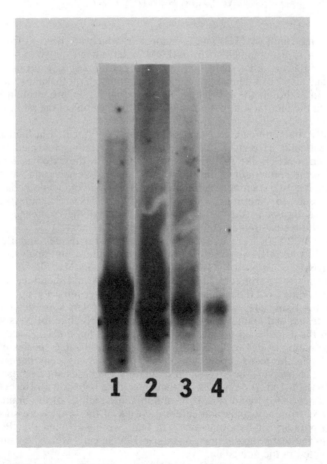

FIGURE 1. POMC-like mRNAs in various tissues and Leydig cell lines. The poly A-containing RNAs were subjected to Northern blot analysis: (1) neurointermediate pituitary, 43 ng; (2) testis, 30 μg; (3) mouse normal Leydig cell line, TM$_3$, 25 μg; and (4) epididymis, 18 μg. The POMC-like mRNAs were identified using rat POMC cDNA (pI13) as a hybridization probe.

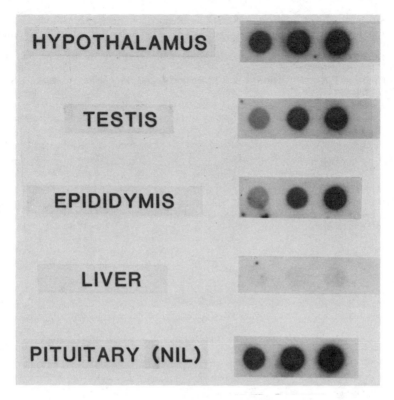

FIGURE 2. Comparison of POMC-like mRNA concentration by dot blot analysis. Poly A-containing RNAs were spotted on a nitrocellulose filter and POMC-like mRNAs were detected as described above. 1, 2, and 4 µg of poly A RNA isolated from hypothalamus, testis, epididymis, or liver were spotted. The amount of neurointermediate pituitary mRNA used here is 4.3, 8.6, and 17.2 ng.

genes present in the rat is less clear. So far, only one POMC gene has been identified in the rat system. However, two POMC-like genes have been found in the mouse. Another alternative explanation is that the POMC mRNAs may be transcribed from the same gene, however, the processing of the nuclear precursor RNA to its mature mRNA is tissue specific. The best example of this is the calcitonin gene system, in which selective splicing of gene transcripts results in the production of two distinct mRNAs in the thyroid and hypothalamus. The possible mechanisms involved in the presence of heterogeneous POMC-like mRNAs are currently under investigation in our laboratory.

REFERENCES

1. MARGIORIS, A. N., A. S. LIOTTA, H. VAUDRY, C. W. BARDIN & D. T. KRIEGER. 1983. Endocrinology **113:** 663–671.
2. CIVELLI, O., N. BIRNBERG & E. HERBERT. 1982. J. Biol. Chem. **257:** 6783–6787.

3. SHARP, B. & A. E. PEKARY. 1981. J. Clin. Endocrinol. Metab. **52:** 586–588.
4. TSONG, S. D., D. PHILLIPS, N. HALMI, A. S. LIOTTA, A. N. MARGIORIS, C. W. BARDIN
   & D. T. KRIEGER. 1982. Endocrinology **110:** 2204–2206.
5. TSONG, S. D., D. M. PHILLIPS, N. HALMI, D. T. KRIEGER & C. W. BARDIN. 1982. Biol.
   Reprod. **27:** 775–764.
6. CHEN, C.-L. C., F. T. DIONNE & J. L. ROBERTS. 1983. Proc. Natl. Acad. Sci. USA **80:**
   2211–2215.

Regulation of 3β-Hydroxysteroid Dehydrogenase Activity by Human Chorionic Gonadotropin, Androgens, and Antiandrogens in Cultured Testicular Cells[a]

C. M. R. GALARRETA, L. F. FANJUL, E. Y. ADASHI, and
A. J. W. HSUEH

Department of Reproductive Medicine
University of California, San Diego
La Jolla, California 92093

Using a primary culture of rat testicular cells, we previously reported that a synthetic androgen (R1881) decreases, whereas a synthetic antiandrogen (cyproterone acetate) increases, the gonadotropin-stimulated accumulation of testosterone through an androgen receptor–mediated process.[1] The present study attempts to further characterize the cellular mechanisms whereby androgens regulate their own production by investigating their effects on the activity of the key steroidogenic enzyme, Δ^5-3β-hydroxysteroid dehydrogenase (3β-HSD).

Basal 3β-HSD activity of cultured testicular cells was inhibited following treatment with testosterone, dihydrotestosterone, and R1881, but not R5020, a highly specific and metabolically stable progestin. The testosterone-mediated inhibition of basal 3β-HSD activity was blocked by cyproterone acetate. Treatment of testicular cells with human chorionic gonadotropin (hCG) results in progressive and time-dependent increases in testosterone accumulation associated with a biphasic alteration of 3β-HSD activity. Specifically, initial stimulation (52%) of 3β-HSD activity observed between 3 and 12 hours of culture when medium testosterone was low, gave way to significant inhibition of 3β-HSD activity on days 2 and 3 of culture when medium testosterone was elevated. Concomitant treatment of hCG-primed cells for three days with R1881 (10^{-6} M) further decreased, whereas treatment with cyproterone acetate (CA; 10^{-6} M) increased testosterone accumulation and 3β-HSD activity (FIGURE 1A and B). Significantly, the ability of R1881 to inhibit hCG-stimulated testosterone accumulation and 3β-HSD activity was completely reversed by concomitant treatment with cyproterone acetate. In contrast, treatment with hCG in the absence of endogenous androgens (effected by 10^{-5} M spironolactone),[2] increased 3β-HSD activity in a time- and dose-related

[a] Supported in part by National Institutes of Health Research Grant HD-15667 and Program Project Grant HD-12303. A.J.W.H. is the recipient of Research Career Development Award HD-00375. C.M.R.G. and L.F.F. were visiting scientists supported by the Spanish American Joint Committee for Scientific and Technological Cooperation.

manner (FIGURE 2). Furthermore, the ability of hCG to stimulate 3β-HSD activity of spironolactone-treated cells was unaffected by cyproterone acetate (CA; 10^{-6} M) but was decreased by R1881 (10^{-6} M). This inhibitory effect of R1881, however, was reversed by cyproterone acetate.

The present studies confirm and extend previous *in vivo*[3-5] and *in vitro*[6,7] observations wherein androgens have been shown to regulate their own production through an intratesticular, ultra short-loop negative feedback mechanism. The mechanism by which androgens block 3β-HSD activity was also studied. When added *in vitro* to the enzyme assay, no effect of the steroid on 3β-HSD activity could be observed. Thus, possible interference of androgens with the active site of the enzyme is ruled out. Furthermore, incubation with testosterone or hCG decreases the apparent V_{max} without affecting the apparent K_m of the enzyme. Likewise, hCG stimulates the apparent V_{max}, but not the K_m, of the enzyme in spironolactone-treated cells. Thus, the effect of androgens on 3β-HSD activity is not due to a modification of the affinity of the enzyme to its substrate. Instead, androgens may interfere with the synthesis of the enzyme. Since cycloheximide treatment partially inhibits the androgen suppression of 3β-HSD activity without affecting basal enzyme activity (data not shown), one can postulate that androgens may induce the formation of an inhibitory factor(s) that inhibits 3β-HSD activity.

Conclusions: (1) Androgens inhibit basal and hCG-stimulated 3β-HSD activity through an androgen receptor–mediated process. (2) hCG stimulates 3β-HSD activity under androgen-free conditions. (3) Androgen-mediated inhibition of 3β-HSD activity may account, in part, for the intratesticular ultra short-loop negative feedback mechanism whereby androgens regulate their own production.

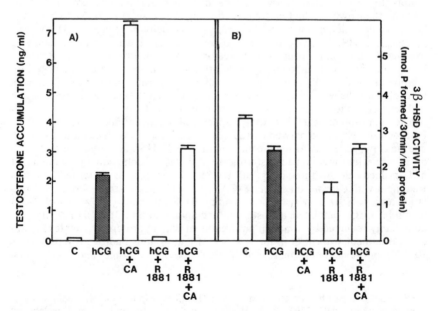

FIGURE 1. hCG-stimulated testosterone accumulation and 3β-HSD activity: Modulation by cyproterone acetate and R1881.

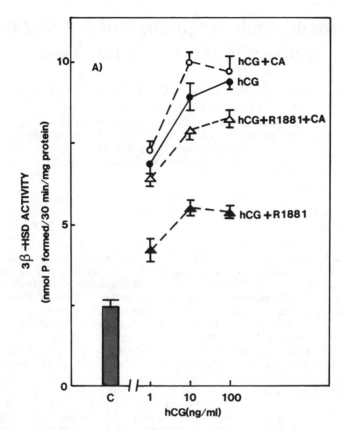

FIGURE 2. hCG-stimulated 3β-HSD activity: Modulation by cyproterone acetate and R1881 under spironolactone-treated androgen-free conditions.

REFERENCES

1. ADASHI, E. Y. & A. J. W. HSUEH. 1981. Autoregulation of androgen production in a primary culture of rat testicular cells. Nature **293:** 737–738.
2. MENARD, R. H., T. M. GUENTHNER, H. KON & J. R. GILLETTE. 1979. Studies on the destruction of adrenal and testicular cytochrome P-450 by spironolactone. J. Biol. Chem. **254:** 1726–1733.
3. CHEN, Y-D., M. J. SHAW & A. H. PAYNE. 1977. Steroids and FSH action on LH receptors and LH sensitive testicular responsiveness during sexual maturation of the rat. Mol. Cell. Endocrinol. **8:** 291–299.
4. PURVIS, K., O. P. F. CLAUSEN & V. HANSSON. 1979. Androgen effects on rat Leydig cells. Biol. Reprod. **20:** 304–309.
5. PURVIS, K. & V. HANSSON. 1978. Hormonal regulation of Leydig cell function Mol. Cell. Endocrinol. **12:** 123–138.
6. EWING, L. L., C. E. CHUBB & B. ROBAIRE. 1976. Macromolecules, steroid binding and testosterone secretion by rabbit testis. Nature **264:** 84–86.
7. DARNEY, JR., K. J. & L. EWING. 1981. Autoregulation of testosterone secretion in perfused rat testes. Endocrinology **109:** 993–995.

Gonadotropic Regulation of Aromatase Activity in the Adult Rat Testis

C. H. TSAI-MORRIS, D. R. AQUILANO, and M. L. DUFAU

Molecular Endocrinology Section
Endocrinology and Reproduction Research Branch
National Institute of Child Health and Human Development
National Institutes of Health
Bethesda, Maryland 20205

The steroidogenic lesion responsible for impaired conversion of progesterone to androgen in gonadotropin-treated Leydig cells has been attributed to an inhibitory effect of estrogen on 17α-hydroxylase and 17,20-desmolase activity. The mediation of estrogen in the desensitizing process was further supported by the nuclear translocation of estrogen receptors,[1] the estrogen-dependent activation of RNA polymerase,[2] and the synthesis of an estrogen-dependent protein[3] in the Leydig cell after treatment with hCG. In LH/hCG-treated rats, an acute elevation of intratesticular estrogen precedes the appearance of the steroidogenic lesion by 3–6 hr.[1,3] However, the nature of the increase in testicular estrogen after a desensitizing dose of hCG has not yet been defined. A detailed study on aromatase activity and levels of testosterone and estradiol was made in purified adult rat Leydig cell (prepared by centrifugal elutriation) during gonadotropin-induced *in vitro* and *in vivo* desensitization. Aromatase activity was measured by a tritiated water release method using saturating concentrations of 1β-^{3}H-testosterone (1.5 μCi/1.0 μM) as a substrate.[4,5] Estradiol was separated from testosterone by toluene-NaOH partition and measured by radioimmunoassay (RIA) with sensitivity of 0.5 pg using ^{125}I-estradiol-17β-tyrosine methyl ester as a tracer.

After *in vitro* stimulation by hCG, aromatase activity of the Leydig cell increased by 30% ($p < 0.05$) within 30 min and rapidly returned to the control level for up to 16 hr of culture (FIGURE 1, upper panel). Net testosterone accumulation in the incubation medium increased at 30 min, and reached a plateau by 4 hr. A small but significant increase in estradiol levels was observed at 30 min ($p < 0.05$), maintained constant until 2 hr, and then followed by a sharp rise parallel to that of testosterone (FIGURE 1, lower panel). This biphasic pattern suggested that the initial increase in estrogen production was induced by activation of the aromatase, whereas the second rise in the levels of estradiol was more related to an increased availability of the substrate. For *in vivo* stimulation, animals were injected with a single subcutaneous dose of 5 μg hCG and killed at various times. Aromatase activity was stimulated (10–20%) ($p < 0.05$) 1 hr after hCG injection with no change in the K_m for testosterone (1.7 μM) (FIGURE 2, lower panel). The basal levels of testosterone in Leydig cells isolated from these animals increased gradually from 1 hr to reach a maximum at 6 hr, and then returned to the control value (FIGURE 2, middle panel). The maximum testosterone response *in vitro* was observed at 40–60 min (20-fold increase) after *in vivo* hCG treatment. However, testosterone responses started to decrease at 3 hr while the stimulated levels of pregnenolone remained as in control up to 6 hr indicating the presence of a steroidogenic lesion caused by a partial blockade of the microsomal enzymes 17α-hydroxylase and 17,20-desmolase. Testosterone and estradiol levels in testicular homogenates showed small but significant increases within 40 or 60 min ($p < 0.05$) respectively, after hCG treatment. Testicular testosterone content reached a peak

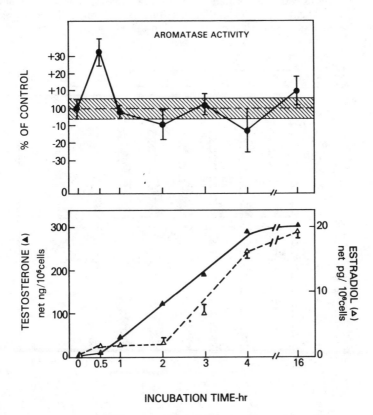

FIGURE 1. *In vitro* temporal effect of hCG (100 ng) on the activity of aromatase in the Leydig cell expressed as percentage of its respective control at each time (*upper panel*); and the net (stimulated minus basal) levels of testosterone and estradiol in the incubation medium (*lower panel*).

at 1 hr (768 ± 80 ng/testis) and preceded the peak level of estradiol (92 ± 4 pg/testis) by 2 hr. This pattern resembled that observed *in vitro*, and suggests that the early aromatase activation induced a minute and presumably compartmentalized increase in estradiol that in turn caused the early events leading to the estradiol-mediated desensitization.

Aromatase activity was also studied in testis from immature rats (5 and 15 days old), and was found to be localized in both Leydig and Sertoli cells. The capacity to aromatize androgens increased in Leydig cells but decreased in Sertoli cells during testicular development (FIGURE 3). The highest aromatase activity was found in the adult rat Leydig cell indicating the importance of estradiol as an endogenous modulator of the androgen synthesis.

In conclusion, we propose that the estradiol-mediated desensitization of the Leydig cell steroidogenesis observed after the administration of hCG is initiated by an early activation of the aromatase, and is subsequently magnified by a significant rise in estradiol formation due to an increased substrate availability. The low aromatizing capacity of the immature rat Leydig cell could partially explain the lack of desensitization observed in these animals.[6]

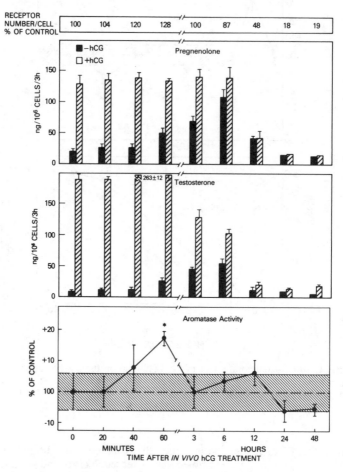

FIGURE 2. LH/hCG binding sites (*upper panel*); pregnenolone and testosterone production (*middle panel*); and aromatase activity expressed as percentage of control at time 0 (*lower panel*) in purified Leydig cells isolated from adult rat testes after *in vivo* subcutaneous hCG (5 μg) injection. Cells were incubated for 3 hr in the presence or absence of 100 ng hCG. Each value represents the mean ± S.E. of three determinations.

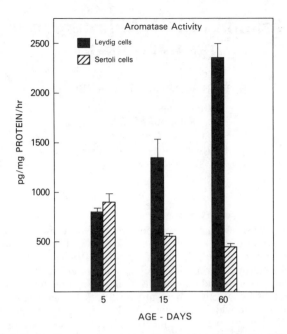

FIGURE 3. Cellular localization of aromatase activity during testicular maturation. Aromatase activity was measured in purified Leydig and Sertoli cells from 5-, 15-, 60-day-old rats. Each value represents the mean ± S.E. of three determinations.

REFERENCES

1. Nozu, K., M. L. Dufau & K. J. Catt. 1981. Estradiol receptor-mediated regulation of steroidogenesis in gonadotropin-desensitized Leydig cells. J. Biol. Chem. **256:** 1915–1922.
2. Aquilano, D. R. & M. L. Dufau. 1983. Changes in ribonucleic acid polymerase activities in gonadotropin-treated Leydig cells: An estradiol-mediated process. Endocrinology **113:** 94–103.
3. Nozu, K., A. Dehejia, K. J. Catt & M. L. Dufau. 1981. Gonadotropin-induced receptor regulation and steroidogenic lesions in cultured Leydig cells: Induction of specific protein synthesis by chorionic gonadotropin and estradiol. J. Biol. Chem. **256:** 12875–12882.
4. Thompson, E. A. & P. K. Siiteri. 1973. Studies on the aromatization of C-19 androgens. Ann. N.Y. Acad. Sci. **212:** 378–391.
5. Gore-Langton, R., H. McKeracher & J. Dorrington. 1980. An alternative method for the study of follicle-stimulating hormone effects on aromatase activity in Sertoli cell cultures. Endocrinology **107:** 464–471.
6. Huhtaniemi, I. T., K. Nozu, D. W. Warren, M. L. Dufau & K. J. Catt. 1982. Acquisition of regulatory mechanisms for gonadotropin receptors and steroidogenesis in the maturing rat testis. Endocrinology **111:** 1711–1720.

Localization of [³H]Aldosterone in the Rat Epididymis[a]

B. T. HINTON and D. A. KEEFER[b]

Department of Anatomy
School of Medicine
University of Virginia
Charlottesville, Virginia 22908

Several studies have shown that there is considerable movement of ions and water across the epithelium of the mammalian epididymis and that this movement appears to be under the control of certain androgens. In view of the well known functions of aldosterone in renal electrolyte and water balance, we wanted to determine whether this steroid may play a similar role in the epididymis. Our first goal was to determine whether there are receptors for aldosterone within the epididymis and if so, in which cell types. Adult male rats were adrenalectomized for four days and then given either saline, or 50 μg of aldosterone, testosterone, or desoxycorticosterone. Each animal received either saline or the steroid 1 hr before the administration of 0.59 μg [³H]aldosterone (sp. act. 77.0 Ci/mM). One hour later, each animal was sacrificed, epididymides excised, cut into three regions (caput, corpus, and cauda) and frozen quickly in Freon (−150°C). The epididymal regions were then sectioned (4 μm) at −30°C and freeze-dried overnight. Individual sections were mounted onto dessicated emulsion-coated slides and exposed for 400 days at −20°C. The sections were photographically processed and stained. For each animal silver grains were counted over nuclei of 40 cells for each cell type using a Zeiss microscope at 1250×. Labeled cells were determined by the Poisson distribution. The clear cell contained silver grains; occasional labeling was noted in endothelial and stromal cells but other epididymal cell types (basal, principal, etc.) were not labeled. At the concentrations used, aldosterone, desoxycorticosterone, and testosterone reduced the labeling by approximately 65%, 40%, and 0%, respectively. In view of the known absorptive role of the clear cell in the epididymis, we suspect that aldosterone plays a role in absorption of ions into its interior or it may have a local intracellular role in concentrating macromolecules after they have been absorbed from the epididymal lumen. In preliminary experiments, we have found that the absorption of luminally perfused horseradish peroxidase by the clear cell is under the control of aldosterone. Further experiments are underway to define the exact role of aldosterone in this epididymal cell type.

[a]Supported by grants: Research career development award (DAK) HD00243 from the National Institutes of Health, grant AM 22125 from the Diabetes Research Training Center and grant 5S07RR05431-22 from the Biomedical Research Support Award (BTH), University of Virginia.

[b] Present address: Department of Biology, Loyola College, Baltimore, MD 21210.

670

Induction of Testicular Development in the Fetal Mouse Ovary[a]

TERUKO TAKETO and SAMUEL S. KOIDE

Center for Biochemical Research
The Population Council
New York, New York 10021

HORACIO MERCHANT-LARIOS

Instituto de Investigaciones Biomedicas
Universidad Nacional de Mexico
Mexico D. F.

An experimental approach to elucidate the mechanism controlling gonadal differentiation is to study the condition(s) in which gonadal sex is reversed. It has been reported that fetal rat ovaries develop testicular structures after transplantation into various sites of adult rats.[1-3] However, the tubular structures in ovarian grafts were not considered to be testicular by some investigators.[4] In the present study, we succeeded in inducing frequent ovotestes development from fetal mouse ovaries following transplantation. Electron microscopic examination confirmed that testicular structures of ovotestes were comparable to those of normal neonatal testes.

Between the 11th and 16th day of gestation (d.g.), fetal mouse gonads were transplanted into a site beneath the kidney capsules of adult mice. An inbred mouse strain (SLJ/J) and an outbred mouse strain (NCS Swiss from the Rockefeller University) were used. The day when copulation plugs were found was defined as 0 d.g. Between the 12th and the 16th d.g., gonadal sex was determined under a dissecting microscope for the presence or absence of testis cords; one of each pair of gonads was transplanted into an adult male mouse, and the other into an adult female mouse. The sex of gonadal primordia on the 11th d.g. could be determined after culturing one side of gonads for seven days[5]; contralateral gonads were transplanted into male or female adult mice. All transplants were examined with light and electron microscopy after 4 to 30 days.

Fetal ovaries isolated on the 12th d.g. developed testicular structures in addition to follicular structures (ovotestes, FIGURE 1, center) by the 14th day after transplantation into male mice of the same strain. Ovotestes developed in 20 of 25 ovarian grafts in the NCS strain and 6 of 13 ovarian grafts in the SJS/J strain. In contrast, fetal ovaries that had been transplanted into female mice developed only ovarian structures (FIGURE 1, right) (12 grafts in NCS and 14 grafts in SJL/J). Fetal testes developed only testicular structures (FIGURE 1, left) in hosts of either sex.

[a] Partly supported by Rockefeller Foundation Grant GA PS 8310 and National Institute of Child Health and Human Development Grant RO-HD-13184.

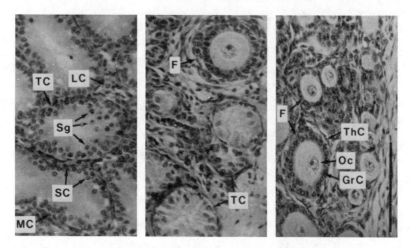

FIGURE 1. Fetal testis (*left*) or ovaries (*center and right*) on the 14th day after transplantation. Bar indicates 0.1 mm. Hematoxylin and Eosin staining. (*Left*) A fetal testis transplanted into an adult female mouse. Testis cords (TC) containing Sertoli cells (SC), germ cells undergoing spermatogenesis (Sg) are surrounded by myoid cells (MC). Leydig cells (LC) are occasionally seen in the interstitial region. (*Center*) A fetal ovary transplanted into an adult male mouse. Note a follicle (F) enclosing an oocyte (top) and testis cords containing Sertoli cells but no germ cells (bottom). (*Right*) A fetal ovary transplanted into an adult female mouse. Follicular structures at various developmental stages are seen around each oocyte (Oc). Granulosa cells (GrC) and theca cells (ThC) line the inside and outside borders, respectively, of the basement membrane of follicles. Steroidogenic cells are absent from the interstitial region.

Fetal ovaries developed testicular structures only when transplanted during early stages of development; the crucial time for the NCS strain was between the 13th and 14th d.g. and that for the SJL/J strain was between the 12th and 13th d.g. Castration of male hosts (4 weeks before receiving grafts) slightly decreased the frequency of ovotestis development in NCS (7 of 10), but did not change the frequency in SJL/J (4 of 8).

Electron microscopic examination revealed that the testicular portion of ovotestes contained all types of testicular somatic cells, i.e., Sertoli cells, myoid cells, and Leydig cells (FIGURE 2). Gap junction complexes typical of Sertoli cells, called "intersertoli contact specializations,"[6] were present in the testicular part, while these structures were not observed between granulosa cells in the ovarian part. Myoid cells contained microfilaments occupying the cytoplasm,[7] but theca cells surrounding follicles did not. Steroidogenic cells containing many lipid droplets and mitochondria with tubular cristae were seen in the interstitial region of testicular structures but not in the same region of ovarian structures. Although all types of testicular somatic cells were present in ovotestes, no spermatogenic cells were observed inside the testis cords.

Our results show that transplanted gonadal somatic cells differentiate as testicular cells in male mice regardless of the genetic sex of the gonads, suggesting that a male factor induces testicular differentiation, and the production of this factor is not limited to the testis.

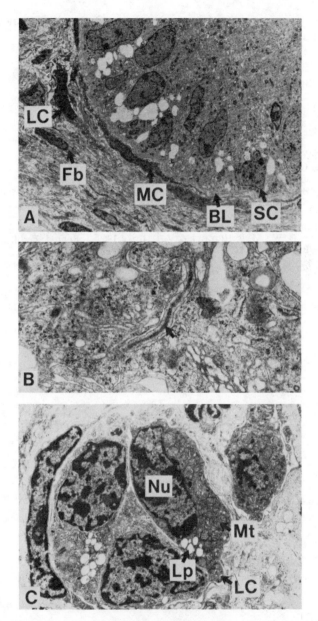

FIGURE 2. Electron micrographs of the testicular structure of ovotestes. (A) A part of testis cords developed in an ovarian graft. Sertoli cells occupy the inside of the basal lamina (BL). Myoid cells with abundant microfilaments surround the outside of the basal lamina. Leydig cells and fibroblasts (Fb) are seen in the interstitial region ($\times 1,600$). (B) A part of an intersertoli contact specialization (*arrow*) that is characterized by the presence of an intercellular space (about 7–9 nm) and a flat cisternum of endoplasmic reticulum running parallel to juxtaposed Sertoli cell plasma membranes with some ribosomes on the cytoplasmic side. Note the accumulation of a layer of electron-dense filamentous material between the plasma membrane and the associated cisterna of the endoplasmic reticulum. ($\times 15,000$). (C) Four Leydig cells with abundant lipid droplets (Lp) and large mitochondria (Mt) with tubular cristae. Nu, nuclei. ($\times 4,200$).

ACKNOWLEDGMENT

We thank Braulio Centeno for technical assistance.

REFERENCES

1. BUYSE, A. 1935. J. Expl. Zool. **70:** 1–41.
2. MOORE, C. R. & D. PRICE. 1942. J. Expl. Zool. **20:** 229–265.
3. TORREY, T. W. 1950. J. Expl. Zool. **115:** 37–38.
4. OZDZENSKI, W., T. ROGULSKA, M. BATAKIER, M. BRZOZOWSKA, A. BEMBISZEWSKA & A. V. STEPINSKA. 1976. Arch. d'Anat. Microscop. **65:** 285–294.
5. TAKETO, T. & S. S. KOIDE. 1981. Develop. Biol. **84:** 61–66.
6. FLICKINGER, J. C. 1967. Z. Zellforsch. **78:** 92–113.
7. FAWCETT, D. W., M. P. HEIDGER & V. L. LEAK 1969. J. Reprod. Fertil. **19:** 109–119.

Ontogenic Changes in the Ability of Estradiol to Suppress Androgen Secretion in the Rat

DAVID K. POMERANTZ

Medical Research Council
Group in Reproductive Biology
Departments of Physiology and Obstetrics and Gynecology
University of Western Ontario
London, Ontario, Canada N6A 5Cl

An intratesticular site of action has been demonstrated for the ability of estradiol to suppress testosterone secretion.[1-5] The physiologic importance of these observations remains unclear. It is known that the secretion of estradiol and testosterone, as well as testicular content of estrogen receptors, changes during testicular development.[6-12] Such studies suggested an intratesticular role for estradiol in some of the endocrine changes that occur during development. The present experiments compared testes from 12-day-old and adult rats for the ability of *in vivo* estradiol treatment to decrease *in vitro* testosterone secretion in response to LH (1 ng LH-24/ml) and dibutyryl cAMP (1.0 mM).

In vitro responsiveness was estimated by radioimmunoassay (RIA) measurement of androgen secretion after five days of treatment with estradiol as well as daily LH (100 ng/g BW) to maintain Leydig cell stimulation. This intact animal model was chosen because hypophysectomy of the infant rats was not possible and the experimental design sought to minimize the differences between experimental groups, except for their age. In adult tissues responsiveness to LH and cAMP was decreased to 20% of normal by 500 ng estradiol/g BW. Other doses of estradiol produced a dose-related suppression of androgen secretion. Using 10 or 100 ng LH/ml did not overcome the suppression. Similar results were obtained from infant's tissue except that the inhibitory effect of estradiol disappeared when a higher (10 ng/ml) dose of LH was used. In 12-day-old animals estradiol treatment had no inhibitory effect on the response to *in vitro* dibutyryl cAMP. *In vivo* treatment with estradiol alone decreased responsiveness at both ages. *In vivo* treatment with LH alone decreased *in vitro* responsiveness of the adult testes, but increased responsiveness to LH in the infant tissue.

The data suggest that in the adult, estrogen pretreatment decreases the ability of the Leydig cell to form testosterone and that one site for the lesion is distal to cAMP generation. This confirms earlier results from other laboratories.[2-5] The Leydig cell of the infant may also be sensitive to estradiol, but the mechanism of action is different. Because the estradiol-induced suppression of androgen secretion could be overcome by sufficient dibutyryl cAMP or LH, the Leydig cell of the infant rat may respond to estradiol by activation of phosphodiesterase and/or by decreased synthesis of cAMP in response to submaximal stimulation with LH.

REFERENCES

1. MOGER, W. H. 1976. Biol. Reprod. **14:** 115–117.
2. VAN BEURDEN, W. M. O., B. ROODNAT, F. H. DE JONG, E. MULDER & H. J. VAN DER MOLEN. 1976. Steroids **28:** 847–866.
3. CHEN, Y. D. I., M. SHAW & A. PAYNE. 1977. Mol. Cell. Endocrinol. **8:** 291–299.
4. HSUEH, A. J. W., M. L. DUFAU & K. J. CATT. 1978. Endocrinology **103:** 1096–1102.
5. KALLA, N. R., B. C. NISULA, R. MENARD & D. L. LORIAUX. 1980. Endocrinology **106:** 35–39.
6. ABNEY, T. O. & M. H. MELNER. 1979. Steroids **34:** 413–427.
7. ARMSTRONG, D. T. & J. H. DORRINGTON. 1977. Estrogen biosynthesis in the ovaries and testes. *In* Regulatory Mechanisms Affecting Gonadal Hormone Action. J. A. Thomas & R. L. Singhal, Eds.: 217–258. University Park Press. Baltimore, MD.
8. DE BOER, W., E. MULDER & H. J. VAN DER MOLEN. 1976. J. Endocrinol. **70:** 397–407.
9. HUHTANIEMI, I. T., K. NOZU, D. W. WARREN, M. L. DUFAU & K. J. CATT. 1982. Endocrinology **111:** 1711–1720.
10. POMERANTZ, D. K. 1980. Biol. Reprod. **23:** 948–954.
11. ROMMERTS, F. F. G., F. H. DE JONG, A. O. BRINKMANN & H. J. VAN DER MOLEN. 1982. J. Reprod. Fertil. **65:** 281–288.
12. VALLADARES, L. E. & A. H. PAYNE. 1981. Biol. Reprod. **25:** 752–758.

Adrenocorticotropin Stimulates Testosterone Production by Fetal Rat Testes

DWIGHT W. WARREN, CHERYL A. SCHMITT, and
STEPHEN J. FRANZINO

Department of Physiology and Biophysics
School of Medicine
University of Southern California
Los Angeles, California 90033

Chronic stress applied to pregnant rats will affect the male fetuses resulting in increased feminine and decreased masculine adult sexual behavior.[1-4] Serum testosterone in affected male rat fetuses reaches maximal levels at day 17.5 of gestation, one day earlier than controls, then decreases to a level significantly below controls later in fetal and postnatal life.[5] It is speculated that the increase in testosterone prematurely sets the hypothalamus to respond to lower testosterone levels.[5] The mechanism that induces the early peak and subsequent lowered serum testosterone in these fetuses is not known. The usual response to stress in the adult animal is increased secretion of adrenocorticotropin (ACTH). However, luteinizing hormone (LH) and gonadal steroids decrease after chronic stress.[6-9] Thus, secretion of ACTH by the fetal or maternal pituitary gland rather than LH would be the most likely response to stress. It has been shown that the fetal testis can use steroid substrates for testosterone production.[10,11] ACTH could increase fetal adrenal secretion of potential steroid substrates that would then be available to the fetal testis. The maternal adrenal gland could also provide steroid substrates for use by the fetal testis. This study is designed to determine if maternal and/or fetal adrenal steroids might contribute to fetal testosterone production.

METHODS

Rat fetuses, 20.5 days of gestation, and mothers were injected with 0.125 and 1.25 USP units of ACTH (Cortrosyn, Organon, West Orange, NJ), respectively. The doses of ACTH exceeded those needed to elicit maximal corticosterone secretion. Fetuses were sacrificed at varying times up to 4 hours, and testes and trunk blood collected for determination of testosterone by radioimmunoassay (RIA). In order to determine the mechanism by which ACTH stimulates the fetal testes to produce testosterone, fetal testes were incubated in Medium 199 alone or containing 100 IU human chorionic gonadotropin (hCG) (Pregnyl, Organon) or 0.25 USP units ACTH. Additionally, fetal testes and adrenals were incubated together in the presence of ACTH and fetal adrenals were incubated with ACTH. Testosterone was measured by RIA.

677

RESULTS AND DISCUSSION

The results of measurement of intratesticular testosterone (IT) after ACTH injection are shown in FIGURE 1. Fetal serum testosterone levels paralleled testis values. The peak IT concentration occurred one-half hour after ACTH injection and remained elevated at one hour but returned to control levels by two hours. Maternal ACTH injection was without effect. Thus, fetal ACTH is capable of increasing fetal IT production while maternal ACTH is not. If the fetus is able to respond to maternal stress with an increase in ACTH secreted by the fetal pituitary gland, this might be the mechanism that causes the premature increase in fetal plasma testosterone that is observed in male fetal rats of chronically stressed mothers.

Testosterone produced by fetal testes and/or adrenal glands during incubation is shown in FIGURE 2. ACTH had no direct effect on fetal testes and ACTH-stimulated fetal adrenal glands did not produce measurable amounts of testosterone. However, ACTH did stimulate testosterone production when testes and adrenal glands were combined but not to the extent that hCG was able to stimulate testosterone production by fetal testes. Thus, the implication for the increase in *in vivo* testosterone in response to ACTH stimulation is that this rise is due to an indirect action of ACTH mediated via the fetal adrenal gland.

Stimulation of the fetal adrenal gland would increase secretion of steroids such as progesterone and dehydroepiandrosterone as well as corticosterone. These

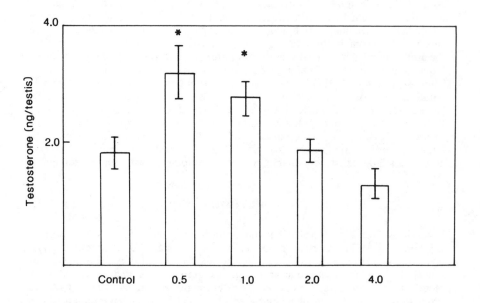

FIGURE 1. Intratesticular testosterone concentration after injection of rat fetuses with ACTH. A significant elevation above control levels is seen at 0.5 and 1 hour after treatment. * = significantly different than control at $p < 0.05$. Bar is mean ± SEM.

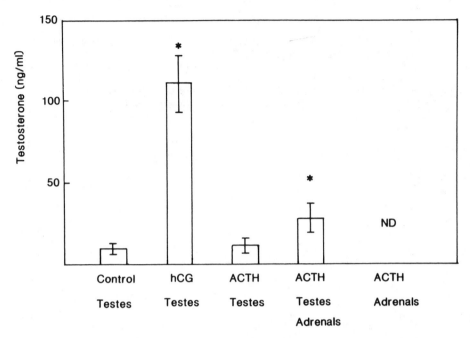

FIGURE 2. Testosterone concentration in media after 4 hours of incubation. Fetal testes treated with ACTH in the presence fetal adrenal glands and fetal testes treated with hCG were the only groups producing significantly elevated levels of testosterone. ND = non-detectable. * = significantly different than controls at $p < 0.05$. Bar is mean ± SEM.

steroids could then serve as precursors for testosterone synthesis by the fetal testis.[10,11] A less likely explanation is that ACTH stimulates the fetal adrenal gland to produce a substance that might act like LH to increase testosterone production. Further studies are being conducted to determine the nature of the adrenal contribution to testosterone production by the fetal testis.

This study demonstrates that the fetal adrenal gland may play an important role in the regulation of testosterone production by the fetal testis and may help to understand the mechanism of chronic maternal stress on fetal testosterone production. Also, it is clear from this work that any study of *in vivo* androgen production by fetal testes must take into account the possible role of fetal stress and the fetal adrenal gland.

REFERENCES

1. WARD, I. L. 1972. Science **175:** 82–84.
2. MASTERPASQUA, F., R. H. CHAPMAN & R. K. LORE. 1976. Dev. Psychobiol. **9:** 403–411.
3. WHITNEY, J. B. & L. R. HERRENKOHL. 1977. Physiol Behav. **19:** 167–169.
4. MEISEL, R. L., G. P. DOHANICH & I. L. WARD. 1979. Physiol. Behav. **22:** 527–530.
5. WARD, I. L. & J. WEISZ. 1980. Science **207:** 328–329.

6. MATSUMOTO, K., K. TAKEYASU, S. MIZUTANI, Y. HAMANAKA & T. UOZUMI. 1970 Acta Endocrinol. **65:** 11–17.
7. KREUZ, L. E., R. M. ROSE & J. R. JENNINGS. 1972. Arch. Gen Psychiat. **26:** 479–482.
8. REPCEKOVA, D. & L. MIKULAJ. 1977. Hormone Res. **8:** 51–57.
9. GRAY, G. D., E. R. SMITH, D. A. DAMASSA, J. R. L. EHRENKRANZ & J. M. DAVIDSON. 1978. Neuroendocrinol. **25:** 247–256.
10. NOUMURA, T., J. WEISZ & C. W. LLOYD. 1966. Endocrinology **78:** 245–253.
11. SANYAL, M. K. & C. A. VILLEE. 1977. Biol. Reprod. **16:** 174–181.

Cyclic Regulation of Rat Leydig Cell Testosterone Production by Seminiferous Tubules

MARTTI PARVINEN

Institute of Biomedicine
Department of Anatomy
University of Turku
SF-20520 Turku 52, Finland

HANNU NIKULA and ILPO HUHTANIEMI

Department of Clinical Chemistry, Immunology, and
Bacteriology
University of Helsinki
SF-00290 Helsinki 29, Finland

Testosterone is generally considered the main hormone regulating spermatogenesis through an action on Sertoli cells. Recent observations suggest that local cell-to-cell interactions are important modifiers of hormone responses in the testis. Sertoli cells obviously communicate with Leydig cells through a GnRH-like factor,[1] or through other types of factors.[2] The cyclic function of the Sertoli cells throughout the cycle of the seminiferous epithelium implies a local interaction between the Sertoli and germ cells. Both biochemical and morphological observations suggest that in the rat stages VII and VIII of the cycle are preferentially dependent on androgen stimulation.[3] Adjacent Leydig cells may be involved in this, as has been suggested by morphometric observations.[4] To obtain direct evidence, we isolated adult rat Leydig cells and seminiferous tubules and incubated them together. The stage-dependent influence of seminiferous tubules on hCG-stimulated testosterone production was measured.

Leydig cells were isolated by collagenase dispersion,[5] yielding 25–30% purity as judged by 3β-hydroxysteroid dehydrogenase staining, or by subsequent purification by Percoll gradient (75–85% purity).[6] The seminiferous tubules were isolated using transillumination-assisted microdissection procedure.[3] The concentration of the Leydig cells was adjusted to 500,000/ml. The incubation with seminiferous tubules of various lengths (0.1–16 cm) was performed in 0.35 ml of Medium 199 supplemented with 0.1% BSA at 34°C in a water bath in an atmosphere containing 95% O_2 and 5% CO_2. After preincubation of 2 hr, a maximally stimulating dose of hCG (Pregnyl®, Organon, 500 ng/ml) was added to half of the samples, and the incubation was continued for an additional 2 hr. Thereafter, the media were separated by centrifugation and analyzed for testosterone by radioimmunoassay.

hCG alone (no tubules) stimulated testosterone production of crude and purified Leydig cells 5–10 fold. Co-incubation of crude Leydig cell preparations with seminiferous tubules (stages VII–VIII, IX–XII, XIII–I, and II–VI, 1–16 cm) had an inhibitory effect on hCG-stimulated testosterone production that was slightly more prominent at stages VII and VIII than at other stages. No stimulatory effects were observed. Similar inhibitory effects were found when epididymal, liver, kidney, or muscle tissues were co-incubated with crude Leydig cell preparations.

No consistent effect was observed on basal testosterone production of Percoll-purified Leydig cells, but significant (up to 140%) potentiation of hCG-stimulated secretion was found with as small an amount as 0.5 cm of seminiferous tubules from stages VII–VIII. Maximal stimulation was induced by 0.5–2 cm of tubules, but 16 cm was inhibitory. No stimulation was found with epididymal, liver, kidney, or muscle tissues or with boiled seminiferous tubules.

Seminiferous tubules at stages VII and VIII have significantly greater potentiating effect on hCG-stimulated testosterone production of Percoll-purified Leydig

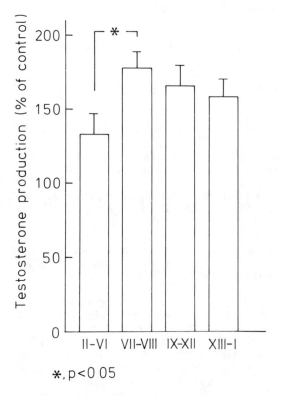

FIGURE 1. Seminiferous tubules at stages VII and VIII have significantly greater potentiating effect on hCG-stimulated testosterone production of Percoll-purified Leydig cells than stages II–VI (summary of seven experiments). Other stages have intermediate values without significant differences.

cells than stages II–VI (FIGURE 1). Stages IX–I have intermediate values without significant differences. The stimulatory effect of stages VII–VIII was additive to that of a potent GnRH agonist (Buserelin®, Hoechst, 10^{-6} M, and it could not be blocked in the presence of a GnRH antagonist. This suggests that the stimulatory effect found is distinct from the action of the putative testicular GnRH-like factor.

Although the chemical nature of the regulation remains obscure, two observations may be helpful in designing appropriate experiments in the future: (1) The stimulatory effect of seminiferous tubules on Leydig cell testosterone production can only be demonstrated in Percoll-purified Leydig cells. (2) Stages VII and VIII of the cycle in the seminiferous epithelium stimulate testosterone production most. This is in agreement with the concept of preferential androgen dependency of these stages.

REFERENCES

1. SHARPE, R. M., H. M. FRASER, I. COOPER & F. F. G. ROMMERTS. 1981. Sertoli-Leydig cell communication via an LHRH-like factor. Nature **290:** 785–787.
2. GROTJAN, H. E. JR. & J. J. HEINDEL. 1982. Effect of spent media from Sertoli cell cultures on in vitro testosterone production by rat testis interstitial cells. Ann. N.Y. Acad. Sci. **383:** 456–457.
3. PARVINEN, M. 1982. Regulation of seminiferous epithelium. Endocr. Rev. **3:** 404–417.
4. BERGH, A. 1983. Paracrine regulation of Leydig cells by the seminiferous tubules. Int. J. Androl. **6:** 57–65.
5. CATT, K. J. & M. L. DUFAU. 1973. Interactions of LH and hCG with testicular gonadotropin receptors. Adv. Exp. Med. Biol. **36:** 379–418.
6. SCHUMACHER, M., G. SCHÄFER, A. F. HOLSTEIN & H. HILZ. 1978. Rapid isolation of mouse Leydig cells by centrifugation in Percoll density gradients with complete retention of morphological and biochemical integrity. FEBS Lett. **91:** 333–337.

Synergistic Effects of Sertoli Cell and FSH on Leydig Cell Function: *In Vitro* Study

M. BENAHMED, J. REVENTOS, E. TABONE,[a] and
J. M. SAEZ

INSERM U.162
Hôpital Debrousse
29 rue Soeur Bouvier
69322 Lyon Cedex 1, France

[a]*Centre Léon Bérard*
Centre de Morphologie Cellulaire et Tissulaire

Leydig cells are the androgen-producing cells situated in the interstitial tissue of the testes. Although luteinizing hormone (LH) is the primary trophic hormone controlling Leydig cell function, a great number of studies suggest that follicle stimulating hormone (FSH) also exerts stimulatory effects on Leydig cell function. FSH pretreatment increases LH-stimulated testosterone secretion by Leydig cell both *in vivo*[1] and *in vitro*[2] and the number of testicular LH receptors.[3] However, binding of FSH to the Leydig cells has never been demonstrated[4] although it has been shown that FSH binds to Sertoli cells.[5] In addition, the stimulatory influence of FSH on Leydig cells does not seem to be the result of the small amounts of LH contaminating the FSH preparations.[6] These data suggest that the observed effects of FSH on Leydig cell function could be mediated by Sertoli cells.

In order to determine the role of Sertoli cells in the action of FSH on Leydig cells, the two cell types were cultured either separately or together for three days, in the presence or absence of FSH. Leydig cell activity was then evaluated using three parameters: the number of hCG binding sites, acute hCG-stimulated testosterone secretion, and ultrastructural morphology of Leydig cell.

Leydig cells and Sertoli cells were prepared using collagenase (Leydig cells)[7] and trypsin (Sertoli cells)[8] treatments. The cells were then purified on a discontinuous Percoll gradient.[9] The purities of Leydig and Sertoli cell preparations were confirmed by the fact that purified Leydig cells bind ^{125}I-hCG but not ^{125}I-FSH and respond to hCG stimulation while Sertoli cells bind ^{125}I-FSH but not ^{125}I-hCG and do not secrete measurable amounts of testosterone after hCG stimulation. The two cell types were cultured in a defined serum-free medium (Ham's F12 medium and Dulbecco Modified Eagle's medium, 1:1), supplemented with insulin (5 μg/ml), transferrin (5 μg/ml), vitamin E (10 μg/ml), and low density lipoprotein (20 μg/ml).[7]

RESULTS AND DISCUSSION

Effect of in Vitro *FSH Pretreatment on the Activity of Leydig Cells Cultured Alone or with Sertoli Cells*

In these experiments, Leydig and Sertoli cells were cultured separately or together, in the presence or absence of 50 ng/ml of porcine FSH (pFSH) (TABLE 1). FSH pretreatment did not modify the function of Leydig cells cultured alone. However, the activity of these cells, co-cultured with Sertoli cells, was increased by FSH pretreatment as measured by a significant increase in the number of hCG binding sites ($p < 0.01$) and in hCG-stimulated testosterone secretion ($p < 0.01$). These results indicate that the stimulatory effect of FSH is not exerted directly on Leydig cells but mediated by Sertoli cells.

TABLE 1. Effects of pFSH on Leydig Cell Functions Cultured Alone or With Sertoli Cells

	Leydig		Sertoli		Leydig + Sertoli	
	Control	FSH	Control	FSH	Control	FSH
^{125}I-hCG binding (cpm $\times$ $10^{-3}/10^6$ cells)	52 ± 2	54 ± 3	0.2	—	62 ± 3	95 ± 6
^{125}I-FSH binding (cpm $\times$ $10^{-3}/10^6$ cells)	0.1	—	25 ± 2	—	26 ± 2	—
hCG stimulated testosterone secretion (ng/10^6 cells/4 hr)	54 ± 5	56 ± 5	<1	<1	60 ± 5	98 ± 8

Purified Leydig and Sertoli cells were cultured separately or together (Leydig/Sertoli cells ratios = 1/4) for 3 days in the presence or absence (control) of 50 ng/ml pFSH. On the last day, the specific binding of ^{125}I-hCG, of ^{125}I-FSH, and hCG-stimulated testosterone secretion were measured. Each value represents the mean ± SEM of triplicate incubations for ^{125}I-hCG and ^{125}I-FSH binding and the mean ± SEM of triplicate determinations of three separate cultures for testosterone secretion.

Effect of Co-culture with Increasing Number of Sertoli Cells on Leydig Cell Function

A constant number of Leydig cells were co-cultured with increasing number of Sertoli cells, in the absence or presence of 50 ng/ml pFSH. As shown in TABLE 2, co-culture of Leydig and Sertoli cells, in the absence of pFSH did not modify the binding of hCG, but increased the acute steroidogenic response to hCG. These effects were dependent on the number of Sertoli cells. pFSH pretreatment of the co-culture increased the hCG binding site numbers as well as hCG-stimulated testosterone secretion in a manner dependent on the number of Sertoli cells.

Our results clearly indicate the mediating role of Sertoli cells in the stimulatory action of FSH on Leydig cells. These data also suggest a positive influence of Sertoli cells on Leydig cell activity. Moreover, these functional modifications of Leydig cells co-cultured with Sertoli cells were also accompanied by marked ultrastructural modifications. As compared to *in vivo* aspect, purified Leydig cells cultured alone presented some regression of smooth endoplasmic reticulum and mitochondria. These alterations were not modified by FSH treatment. However, Leydig cells co-cultured with Sertoli cells presented some development of these organelles and FSH treatment induced further development of these organelles.

Since no contact occurs *in vivo* between the two cell types, it is likely that the interaction between Leydig and Sertoli cells is mediated by diffusible factor(s). Two factors, estradiol and LHRH-like factor, have been reported to be secreted by Sertoli cells. However, in our model, neither estradiol[10] nor LHRH[11] has any effect on porcine Leydig cell steroidogenesis. The secretion by Sertoli cells of factor(s) that increase steroidogenic activity of Leydig cells has been suggested by the use of spent media from Sertoli cells. Indeed, both basal and LH-stimulated testosterone secretion were increased by spent media from Sertoli cells. However such stimulatory effect does not seem to be specific since it has been observed with spent media from other cell lines.[12]

In summary, our results show that the stimulatory effect of FSH on Leydig cell activity is mediated by Sertoli cells but the factor(s) mediating the FSH action remain unknown.

TABLE 2. Effects of Co-culture of Leydig Cells with Sertoli Cells at Different Ratios and Under pFSH Treatment on Leydig Cells Function

Cell Type Ratio	^{125}I-hCG Bound (% of Leydig Cells Alone)		hCG-stimulated Testosterone Secretion (ng/4 h/10^6 cells)	
	Control	FSH	Control	FSH
Leydig	100 ± 3	100 ± 3	13.5 ± 2.2	11 ± 1.3
Leydig + Sertoli 1/4	97.3 ± 3	129.1 ± 4	.22 ± 0.8	59.5 ± 4.2
Leydig + Sertoli 1/8	93 ± 2	144 ± 5	34.5 ± 2	77.5 ± 7.1
Leydig + Sertoli 1/12	108 ± 4	152.2 ± 6	51.8 ± 9.7	97.5 ± 13.5

Purified Leydig cells (2×10^5 cells) were cultured alone or co-cultured with increasing numbers of purified pig Sertoli cells (Leydig/Sertoli cells ratios = 1/4 to 1/12) without (control) or with pFSH (50 ng/ml) for three days. At the end of the culture, some dishes were used to measure ^{125}I-hCG binding while the others were incubated with hCG (10^{-9} M) for three additional hours to measure testosterone secretion. Each value represents the mean ± SEM of triplicate incubations for ^{125}I-hCG binding and the mean ± SEM of triplicate determinations of three dishes for testosterone secretion.

REFERENCES

1. ODELL, W. O. & R. S. SWERDLOFF. 1975. J. Steroid Biochem. **6:** 853–857.
2. VAN BEURDEN, W. M. O., B. ROODNAT, F. H. DE JONG, E. MULDER & H. VAN DER MOLEN. 1976. Steroids **28:** 847–866.
3. CHEN, Y. D. I., A. H. PAYNE & R. P. KELCH. 1976. Proc. Soc. Exp. Biol. Med. **153:** 473–475.
4. MEANS, A. R. & J. VAITUKAITIS. 1972. Endocrinology **90:** 39–46.
5. ORTH, J. & A. K. CHRISTENSEN. 1977. Endocrinology **101:** 262–278.
6. MOGER, W. H. & P. R. MURPHY. 1982. Biol. Reprod. **26:** 422–426.
7. MATHER, J. P., J. M. SAEZ & F. HAOUR. 1981. Steroids **38:** 35–44.

8. VERHOEVEN, G., P. DIERICK & P. DE MOOR. 1979. Mol. Cell. Endocrinol. **13:** 241–253.
9. LEFEVRE, A., J. M. SAEZ & C. FINAZ. 1983. Horm. Res. **17:** 114–120.
10. BENAHMED, M., M. BERNIER, J. DUCHARME & J. M. SAEZ. 1982. Mol. Cell. Endocrinol. **28:** 705–716.
11. SAEZ, J. M., M. BENAHMED, J. REVENTOS, M. C. BOMMELAER, C. MOMBRIAL & F. HAOUR. 1983. J. Steroid Biochem. **19:** 375–384.
12. GROTJAN, H. E. JR. & J. J. HEINDEL. 1982. Ann. N. Y. Acad. Sci. **383:** 456.

The Nongerminal Cell Lines of the Testis Contain Five Acid Phosphatases

T. VANHA-PERTTULA, J. P. MATHER, and
C. WAYNE BARDIN[a]

The Population Council
New York, New York 10021

Four acid phosphatases (E I–IV) have been identified in the testes of many mammalian species.[1-4] Marked changes take place in acid phosphatases (AcP) activities in various experimental conditions.[5-7] Particularly E IV, a divalent metal-activated AcP, has been found to correlate to active spermatogenesis. Due to its solubility the exact cellular location has not, however, been demonstrated. The availability of differentiated nongerminal cell lines originating from Sertoli (TR-ST, TM₄), Leydig (TM₃), myoid (TR-M), and endothelial (TR-1) cells[8] provided the possibility to analyze their AcP patterns and eventual contribution to the testicular AcP composition.

The cells were cultured in serum-free (with insulin, transferrin, and epidermal growth factor) or serum-supplemented F12/DME medium,[8] harvested after confluency, homogenized in 0.025 M imidazole-HCl buffer, pH 7.4, and fractionated by chromatofocusing with a gradient of pH 7.4–4.0 followed by a salt gradient (0–0.3 M). Enzyme activities were assayed with *p*-nitrophenyl phosphate (p-NPP), α-naphthyl phosphate (α-NP), and β-naphthyl phosphate (β-NP) as substrates. The pI, pH-optimum, and some modifier characteristics of pooled activities were recorded.

Cells grown in serum-free and serum-supplemented medium gave identical enzyme patterns with some relative changes in the size of the enzyme peaks. All cell lines showed an AcP with pI 7.3 that hydrolyzed all three substrates with relative preference for α-NP and β-NP (FIGURE 1). The enzyme was highly sensitive to fluoride (F) and tartrate (tar) and had an optimum at pH 3.5–4.0. This enzyme was regarded as identical to E II, a lysosomal AcP. Two activity peaks with pI 6.3 and 5.8 were also found in all cell lines with p-NPP and β-NP but not with α-NP. They had optimal activity at pH 4.5. Both peaks were resistant to F/tar but highly sensitive to heavy metals (Cu, Hg, Mo, V). These activities, which showed a relative augmentation in serum-free medium, appear to correspond to the soluble E III.

A F/tar-sensitive AcP hydrolyzing all three substrates optimally at pH 3.5–4.0 was eluted with pI 5.0 in all cell lines but was most prominent in TR-1 and TR-M. It was tentatively identified as E-I, classified also as a lysosomal AcP. A separate activity visualized with p-NPP only in the Sertoli cell lines (TR-ST, TM₄) was eluted with pI 4.5–4.0. It showed an optimum activity at pH 5.0 and was activated by Co, Mg, Mn, Ni, and Zn with moderate resistance to F/tar. These properties are identical to those described for E IV in the testicular tissue. A new F/tar-resistant AcP was identified that hydrolyzed all three substrates was eluted from the chromatofocusing column with NaCl and was slightly activated by Co at an optimum of pH 4.5. This AcP was found only in TR-1 and TR-M cells.

---

[a] To whom correspondence should be addressed.

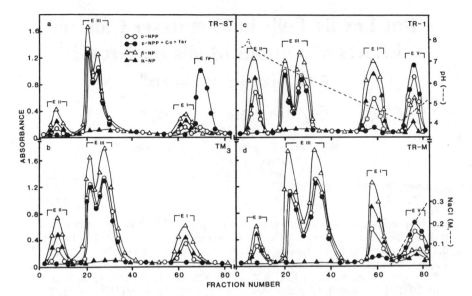

FIGURE 1. Separation of acid phosphatases of the TR-ST (a), TM₃ (b), TR-1 (c), and TR-M (d) cell lines by chromatofocusing with a pH-gradient of 7.4–4.0 followed by a linear NaCl-gradient (0–0.3 M). AcP activity in the fractions (3 ml) was determined with *p*-nitrophenyl phosphate (p-NPP) without and with Co (1 mM) and tartrate (tar, 1 mM) in the incubation medium as well as with α-naphthyl phosphate (α-NP) and β-naphthyl phosphate (β-NP). The separated AcP peaks are called E I–E V according to previously adopted criteria.[1]

It is concluded that all nongerminal testicular cell lines have variable levels of lysosomal AcP (E I, E II) with wide substrate spectrum and high sensitivity to fluoride and tartrate. All cell lines also contained the F/tar-resistant and heavy metal-sensitive E III with restricted substrate specificity. Only cells of Sertoli cell origin contained E IV, which is characterized by its activation with various divalent metal ions. An additional F/tar-resistant AcP with some activation by Co was present only in myoid and endothelial cells. This activity (called E V) has not previously been demonstrated in the testicular homogenates. The variable enzyme pattern in the five nongerminal cells indicates the maintenance of their differentiated state and the probable location of multiple enzymes in the testis.

REFERENCES

1. VANHA-PERTTULA, T. 1971. Biochim. Biophys. Acta **227**: 390–401.
2. GUHA, K., R. RYTOLUOTO-KARKKAINEN & T. VANHA-PERTTULA. 1979. Med. Biol. **57**: 52–57.
3. GUHA, K. & T. VANHA-PERTTULA. 1980. Int. J. Androl. **3**: 256–266.
4. GUHA, K. & T. VANHA-PERTTULA. 1980. Arch. Androl. **4**: 331–339.
5. VANHA-PERTTULA, T. & V. NIKKANEN. 1973. Acta Endocr. (Kbh.) **72**: 376–390.
6. GUHA, K. & T. VANHA-PERTTULA. 1980. Andrologia **12**: 252–260.
7. GUHA, K. & T. VANHA-PERTTULA. 1983. Arch. Androl. **10**: 7–16.
8. MATHER, J. P., L.-Z. ZHUANG, V. PEREZ-INFANTE & D. M. PHILLIPS. 1982. Ann. N. Y. Acad. Sci. **383**: 44–68.

Rat Leydig Cells in Monolayer Culture: Effects of Various Media on Growth and Steroidogenesis[a]

C. D'ARVILLE and B. A. COOKE

Department of Biochemistry
Royal Free Hospital School of Medicine
University of London
London NW3, U.K.

Percoll-purified rat Leydig cells[1] (Fraction III, $p = 1.072$ g/ml) were cultured for 0–3 days in either 0.7 cm (1×10^4 cells/0.1 ml medium) or 1.6 cm (0.5×10^5 cells/0.5 ml medium) wells containing the following media. (a) Dulbecco's modified Eagle's medium (DMEM) containing $NaHCO_3$ (3.7 g/l), BSA (0.1%) and kanamycin (0.1 mg/ml), incubated at 32°C in 10% CO_2:90% air. (b) Ham's-F12 medium 1:1 with DMEM containing 4.5 g glucose/l together with $NaHCO_3$ (4.88 g/l), HEPES (15 mM), kanamycin (0.1 mg/ml), and a cocktail composed of transferrin (5 μg/ml), insulin (5 μg/ml), and EGF (10 ng/ml). (c) DMEM (medium a) 1 : 1 with spent medium (charcoal treated 4°C 10 min; filter sterilized) removed from purified rat Leydig tumor cells maintained in culture. (d) medium as in (b) but containing 5% FCS in place of cocktail. Cells maintained in media (b)–(d) were incubated at 32°C in 5%:95% air.

Cells were stimulated for 2 hr with sheep lutropin (NIH, S20 1.9 of NIH-Sl/mg) (100 ng/ml final concentration) and the media assayed for testosterone production by RIA.[2] Parallel cultures were incubated for 3 hr at 37°C with [6-³H]thymidine (2 μCi/ml), trypsinized, and counted in a hemocytometer.

Media (a) and (b) maintained a comparable cellular steroidogenic potential up to day 3 when the response in (a) was between 17–20% that on days 1 and 2, whereas in medium (b) the reduction was 50%. Most of the cells were rounded on day 0 with a small proportion elongating by day 1, whilst the majority had elongated by day 2. A number of the cells displayed broad cytoplasmic extensions.

On days 0 and 1, cells in media (c) and (d) responded similarly to those above but were significantly inhibited by day 2 (39% of day 1 in (c) and 2% of day 1 in (d)). Stimulated values were similar for medium (c) whether or not the spent medium was charcoal treated, but basal levels were markedly reduced after treatment. In the presence of spent medium (c) a number of the cells were seen to elongate as soon as four hours after initial plating in contrast to those in FCS supplemented medium, where elongation was first observed on day 1. However by day 2 cells maintained in both media had formed complex lattices, the cells displaying long broad cytoplasmic extensions. A greater proportion of rounded cells remained in medium (d).

Preliminary results indicated that when compared to values obtained for medium (a) thymidine uptake was potentiated in cells maintained in medium containing growth factors, as well as serum-supplemented media. [6-³H]Thymidine up-

[a] Supported by the Wellcome Trust Fund.

take appeared greatest in cells maintained in medium (c). However, cell number increased only in media containing FCS and spent medium.

In conclusion, therefore, rat Leydig cells retain their steroidogenic responsiveness in serum-free media for up to 48 hr after which, response is improved if growth factors are present. Preliminary data suggest that the addition of growth factors insulin, transferrin, and EGF, increase mitogenesis but not cell proliferation. In contrast, the proliferation, elongation, and DNA synthesis of cells in Band III is potentiated in serum-containing media. This is particularly marked for cells maintained in spent medium. Therefore rat tumor cells maintained in monolayer culture may secrete into their culture media an additional factor other than those present in FCS, which promotes certain cellular functions.

REFERENCES

1. SCHUMACHER, M., G. SCHAFER, A. F. HOLSTEIN & H. HILZ. 1978. FEBS Lett. **91:** 333.
2. VERJANS, H. L., B. A. COOKE, F. M. DE JONG, C. M. M. DE JONG & H. J. VAN DER MOLEN. 1973. J. Steroid Biochem. **4:** 665.

Index of Contributors

Subject Index